Electroencephalography: Advanced Techniques

Electroencephalography: Advanced Techniques

Edited by Garrick Davenport

hayle
medical

New York

Hayle Medical,
750 Third Avenue, 9ᵗʰ Floor,
New York, NY 10017, USA

Visit us on the World Wide Web at:
www.haylemedical.com

ISBN: 978-1-63241-685-8

Trademark Notice: Registered trademark of products or corporate names are used only for explanation and identification without intent to infringe.

Cataloging-in-Publication Data

Electroencephalography : advanced techniques / edited by Garrick Davenport.
     p. cm.
Includes bibliographical references and index.
ISBN 978-1-63241-685-8
1. Electroencephalography. 2. Brain--Diseases--Diagnosis. I. Davenport, Garrick.
RC386.6.E43 E54 2019
616.804 754 7--dc23

Contents

Preface

Electroencephalography or EEG is an electrophysiological monitoring technique that records the electrical activity of the brain. A clinical EEG lasts between 20-30 minutes. It is used for making differential diagnoses of several conditions related to epileptic seizures and spells, organic encephalopathy or delirium and catatonia, etc. It is also used to assess the depth of anesthesia, monitor non-convulsive seizures, localize the source of epileptic brain activity, etc. It is used in various studies of neuroscience, cognitive psychology, cognitive science, neurolinguistics and psychophysiology. Research is being conducted across the world to make EEG devices smaller, easier to use and portable. The benefits of applying machine learning techniques like neural networks to classify mental states and mental emotional states are also being researched. This book is compiled in such a manner, that it will discuss the clinical applications of electroencephalography. It elucidates the concepts and innovative models around prospective developments with respect to this field. As this technology is emerging at a rapid pace, the elaborate content of this book will help the readers understand the modern concepts of this subject.

The researches compiled throughout the book are authentic and of high quality, combining several disciplines and from very diverse regions from around the world. Drawing on the contributions of many researchers from diverse countries, the book's objective is to provide the readers with the latest achievements in the area of research. This book will surely be a source of knowledge to all interested and researching the field.

In the end, I would like to express my deep sense of gratitude to all the authors for meeting the set deadlines in completing and submitting their research chapters. I would also like to thank the publisher for the support offered to us throughout the course of the book. Finally, I extend my sincere thanks to my family for being a constant source of inspiration and encouragement.

Editor

Internal Consistency of Event-Related Potentials Associated with Cognitive Control: N2/P3 and ERN/Pe

Wim J. R. Rietdijk[1]*, **Ingmar H. A. Franken**[2], **A. Roy Thurik**[1,3,4]

1 Department of Applied Economics, Erasmus School of Economics, Erasmus University Rotterdam, Rotterdam, The Netherlands, **2** Institute of Psychology, Erasmus University Rotterdam, Rotterdam, The Netherlands, **3** Panteia, Zoetermeer, The Netherlands, **4** GSCM-Montpellier Business School, Montpellier, France

Abstract

Recent studies in psychophysiology show an increased attention for examining the reliability of Event-Related Potentials (ERPs), which are measures of cognitive control (e.g., Go/No-Go tasks). An important index of reliability is the internal consistency (e.g., Cronbach's alpha) of a measure. In this study, we examine the internal consistency of the N2 and P3 in a Go/No-Go task. Furthermore, we attempt to replicate the previously found internal consistency of the Error-Related Negativity (ERN) and Positive-Error (Pe) in an Eriksen Flanker task. Healthy participants performed a Go/No-Go task and an Eriksen Flanker task, whereby the amplitudes of the correct No-Go N2/P3, and error trials for ERN/Pe were the variables of interest. This study provides evidence that the N2 and P3 in a Go/No-Go task are internally consistent after 20 and 14 trials are included in the average, respectively. Moreover, the ERN and Pe become internally consistent after approximately 8 trials are included in the average. In addition guidelines and suggestions for future research are discussed.

Editor: Bart Rypma, University of Texas at Dallas, United States of America

Funding: Funding (4×100 euro) was obtained from the host university of the corresponding author (Erasmus University) to pay the winning participant. The funder had no role in study design, data collection and analysis, decision to publish, or preparation of the manuscript.

Competing Interests: The authors have no conflicts of interest regarding the authorship or publication of this article. The affiliation of Roy Thurik with Panteia does not influence the adherence of the study to the PLOS ONE policies on sharing data and materials and did not influence the design or execution of the study. Panteia is involved in policy research and management advice, which is unrelated to the subject of the present study.

* Email: rietdijk@ese.eur.nl

Introduction

Event-related potentials (ERPs) of cognitive control are increasingly used in clinical studies to examine the relevance in several forms of psychopathology [1], such as addiction [2] and obsessive-compulsive disorder [3]. Although ERPs have certain advantages over self-reporting (e.g., they are more objective) and behavioral measures (e.g., they provide more information on the neural level), relatively little attention has been paid to their psychometric properties, especially their reliability [4]. Reliability is a key psychometric criterion of physiological tasks [5,6], and it is a necessary prerequisite to demonstrate their validity (i.e., the degree to which an ERP represents the intended underlying construct) [5,6,7,8].

Reliability is frequently examined in terms of internal consistency (e.g., Cronbach's alpha) [7,8]. The internal consistency of an ERP is defined as the similarity of the ERP across trials in a single task [8]. ERPs are usually derived by averaging (many) trials, and if the trial-to-trial waveforms are unreliable, the participant's average will also be unreliable (i.e., less internally consistent) [7,8,9]. Olvet and Hajcak [1] and Cohen and Polich [9] were among the first to examine the internal consistency of several cognitive control task ERPs, such as the ERN, Pe, and P300. Among others, Riesel et al. [4] stated that there is ample room for more studies examining the reliability (especially, the internal consistency) of ERPs in cognitive control tasks (e.g., [1,4,8,9,10,11]), such as the N2 and P3 in a Go/No-Go task. This study addresses the internal consistency of four frequently used ERP measures in two cognitive control tasks: the N2/P3

components measured during a Go/No-Go task, and the ERN/Pe components measured during an Eriksen Flanker task.

In a Go/No-Go task, two major ERP components are enhanced for No-Go trials compared with Go trials, suggesting that they reflect brain activity related to inhibitory control. The first component is the N2, which is a negative wave emerging approximately 200–300 ms after stimulus onset. The N2 reflects the first stage of inhibition, and/or it is related to conflict monitoring [12,13,14]. The other ERP component is the P3, which is a positive wave emerging approximately 300–500 ms after stimulus onset. Several studies suggest that the P3 reflects a later stage of the inhibition process that is closely related to actual inhibition of the motor response in the premotor cortex [13]. Previous studies have reported differences in the electrophysiological correlates of inhibitory control (i.e., the N2 and P3) that are driven by variations of the specific characteristics of the Go/No-Go task set up (e.g., single, multiple and semantic Go/No-Go stimuli) [15]. Therefore, it is important to understand these variations and study the consequences for the internal consistency of the electrophysiological measures of inhibitory control (i.e., the N2 and P3) [15]. In a previous study, Clayson and Larson [14] examined the internal consistency of the N2 in an Eriksen Flanker task and found an internally consistent N2 after 30 trials. Furthermore, Cohen and Polich [9] found the P3 to be internally consistent after 21 trials, measured in an oddball task. To our knowledge, ours is the first study to examine the internal consistency of both the N2 and P3 in a Go/No-Go task.

Previous research also identified two major ERPs that are enhanced for incorrect behavioral response trials (i.e., an error) compared with correct behavioral response trials, the Error-Related Negativity (ERN) and Positive error related wave (Pe) [16,17]. The ERN is an automatic response-locked negative deflection, emerging between 0–150 ms after the onset of an incorrect behavioral response [18,19]. The second positive deflection is the Pe, which peaks around 200–400 ms after the onset of an erroneous behavioral response. Although there is discussion about the exact meaning of the Pe [20], most studies indicate that the Pe is related to error recognition [20,21,22,23]. Olvet and Hajcak [1] and Pontifex et al. [11] found an internally consistent ERN and Pe after 6 and 8 trials were included to the participant's average, respectively.

In cognitive control tasks, the participants usually perform about 500 trials of a speeded reaction time task in relatively rapid succession. Errors and correct No-Go trials (i.e., successful inhibition of a participant's motor response) tend to be rare, resulting in a relatively low number of trials in the ERP averages. In fact, the number of trials for these conditions and participants varies greatly [1,9,10]. It has been suggested that only 6 and 8 trials are required for ERN and Pe, respectively [1]. However, guidance on the actual number of trials required to obtain an internally consistent ERP component for the N2 and P3 is largely lacking [1,14]. As a result, the current study is set up to test the internal consistency of the N2 and P3 in a Go/No-Go task. Moreover, to ensure the quality of our inferences about the internal consistency of the N2 and P3, we attempt to replicate the results of previous studies that address the internal consistency of the ERN/Pe in the same sample [1,11,22,23].

Method

Participants and Procedure

118 healthy right handed participants (M_{age} = 21.7 years, SD_{age} = 2.8, 61 males) participated in the electroencephalographic (EEG) task. Data from 10 participants were not analyzable due to computer errors during recording of the data. Only participants with at least 30 correct No-Go trials (N = 95, 87%) were included in the EEG analysis. Additionally, only participants with at least 14 errors in the Eriksen Flanker (N = 70, 65%) were included. These sample selection criteria, and sample inclusion rates are similar to that of Olvet and Hajcak [1], Pontifex et al. [11], and Meyer et al. [22,23]. Using an online questionnaire, participants were screened for previous brain surgeries, pregnancy, or history of psychiatric disorders (no participants had to be excluded due to these criteria). Participants were asked not to drink coffee or smoke for 1.5 hours before the experiment. The study was conducted in accordance with the Declaration of Helsinki, and written consent was obtained from each participant prior to participation. The study was approved by the Ethics Committee of the Erasmus Medical Center, Erasmus University Rotterdam.

Tasks

Participants performed a Go/No-Go task [24]. A letter (A, I, E, O, or U) was presented for 200 ms. Each stimulus was followed by a black screen for a randomly varying duration (1020 ms–1220 ms) [24,25]. Participants were instructed to respond to the letters in the Go trials by pressing a button with the index finger as fast as possible, and in the No-Go trials, participants were instructed to withhold their response (i.e., when the letter was similar to the previous letter). The task had 500 trials, 125 of which were No-Go trials (25%) [25].

Participants also performed an Eriksen Flanker task (200 congruent trials: SSSSS, HHHHH; and, 200 incongruent trials: SSHSS, HHSHH) [26,27]. Participants were instructed to

respond to the central letter. On a response box, they had to press H with their right index finger when the central letter was an H and S with their left index finger if the central letter was an S. Each trial started with a fixation cue (^) for 150 ms. Letter strings were presented for 52 ms, followed by a blank screen for 648 ms. The participants had 700 ms from stimulus onset to respond. At the end of the respond period, a feedback symbol appeared indicating whether the response was correct (ooo), incorrect (xxx), or too late (!). An interval of 100 ms was used [27].

ERP Measurement & Statistical Analysis

EEG was recorded using a Biosemi Active-Two amplifier system (Amsterdam, the Netherlands) at 32 scalp sites (positioned following the 10–20 International System and two additional electrodes: FCz and CPz) with active Ag/AgCl electrodes mounted in an elastic cap. Six additional electrodes were attached to the left and right mastoids, the two outer canthi of both eyes (HEOG), and the infraorbital and supraorbital region of the right eye (VEOG). All signals were digitalized with a sample rate of 512 Hz and 24-bit A/D conversion, with a band pass of 0–134 Hz. The data were off-line referenced to compute mastoids. Off-line, EEG and EOG activities were filtered with a band pass of 0.15–30 Hz (phase shift free Butterworth filters; 24 dB/octave slope). During offline processing, no more than four bad channels per participant were removed from the EEG signal, and new values per channel were calculated using topographic interpolation [24]. Data were segmented in epochs of 1000 ms (−200–800 ms after stimulus presentation) and 700 ms (−100–600 ms after the response) for inhibitory control and error processing, respectively [24,25,27]. The average of 200 ms before stimulus onset in the Go/No-Go task and 100 ms before the response in the Eriksen Flanker period served as a baseline which was subtracted from all subsequent time points [25,27]. Segments with incorrect responses (i.e., false alarm for No-Go trials, incorrect Go response, or false alarms for Eriksen Flanker trials) were all excluded from the EEG analysis [24,25]. After ocular correction [28], epochs, including an EEG signal exceeding ±100 μV, were excluded from the average [23]. All epochs were also visually inspected for other artifacts. Average ERP waves were calculated after baseline correction for artifact-free trials at each scalp site in each condition.

Go/No-Go inhibitory control studies have predominantly examined and observed inhibition-related N2 and P3 effects at Fz, Cz, Pz (e.g., [29,30,31,32]). Therefore, in the current study we examine the internal consistency of the N2 and P3 at Fz, Cz, and Pz. The N2 is defined as the average value in the 175–250 ms time interval after stimulus onset [24,25]. The P3 is defined as the average value in the 300–500 ms time interval after stimulus onset [25]. In the Eriksen Flanker task, the ERN is defined are the as the average value of FCz in the 25–75 ms time segment after response onset. The Pe is defined as the average value of Pz in the 200–400 ms time segment after response onset [24,25]. Note that later on in the study, the grand average waveform figures represent the difference waveforms (No-Go – Go and error – correct) of the electrodes important in the Go/No-Go (Fz, Cz, Pz) and Eriksen Flanker (FCz and Pz) task, respectively. The grand average difference waveforms are more informative for observing the temporality of the ERP measures, compared to the average waveforms of the Go and No-Go correct and Eriksen Flanker error and correct trials separately. However, in our analysis we took the amplitudes for correct No-Go N2 and P3 and ERN and Pe error trials as the variables of interest, similar to [1,11,22,23]. The separate figures for Go/No-Go and error/correct trials are available upon request from the corresponding author.

The current study employed a methodology similar to that described by Olvet and Hajcak [1], Pontifex et al. [11], and Meyer et al. [22,23]. For the ERPs of inhibitory control and error processing, we measured the average of N2/P3 and ERN/Pe trials, respectively. Random pairs of trials were included in the average (i.e., 2, 4, 6, 8, 10, …, and the participants' average, across all trials), and paired t-tests were used to determine statistically significant differences. Signal-to-Noise ratios (SNRs) were estimated using a process available in Brain Vision Analyzer Version 2.0 software (www.brainproducts.com). First, noise is estimated by summing the squares of the difference between each data point and the average EEG value; this sum is then divided by the number of data points minus one. Second, average total power is estimated by taking the average of the squared values of each data point. Average power of the signal then equals the average total power minus the average noise power [1]. SNRs of the trial pair averages were assessed using paired t-tests. Additionally, we assessed internal consistency measuring the correlation between these smaller trial averages and the N2/P3 and ERN/Pe participants' average (i.e., all trials), and Cronbach's alpha when an increasing number of trials were included in the average [1,11,22,23], both available in SPSS 19.0. The thresholds in the current study are similar to previous studies, where internal consistency is indicated when correlations reached 0.8 and Cronbach's alpha reached 0.6 [1,11,22,23].

Results

Inhibitory Control

The purpose of this study is to examine internal consistency of the N2 and P3 in a Go/No-Go task. On average, the participants had 73.87 (SD = 19.87; 60% No-Go correct) correct No-Go trials (i.e., participants successfully inhibited their motor response while performing the task). Figure 1 presents the grand average difference waveforms for Go/No-Go task for the midline electrodes Fz, Cz, and Pz. Moreover, Figure 2 presents for all three midline electrodes the average (Figure 2A) and Pearson's correlations (Figure 2B), and the Cronbach's alpha (Figure 2C) all as a function of an increasing number of trials. Paired t-tests were performed using the N2 area measures, for all three midline electrodes (Fz, Cz, and Pz). Significant differences were only observed for electrodes Fz (30 vs. participants' average, $p<0.05$), and Pz (18 vs. 20 trials, and 30 vs. participants' average, $p<0.05$), while all other pairs comparing increasing numbers of trial averages (2 vs. 4 trials, 4 vs. 6 trials, 6 vs. 8 trials, 8 vs. 10 trials, 10 vs. 12 trials, …, 28 vs. 30 trials, and 30 trials vs. participants' average (i.e., all trials) were insignificant (all $ps>0.05$); this suggests that the N2 average is still relatively instable after 30 trials.

When comparing increasing trial numbers for the P3 significant differences at the three electrodes (Fz, Cz, Pz) were found for Fz (6 vs. 8 trials, $p=0.02$; 8 vs. 10 trials, $p=0.04$; 14 vs. 16 trials, $p=0.04$), while all other pairs comparing increasing numbers of trial average were insignificant (all $ps>0.05$). Significant differences between increasing trials averages were found for Cz (6 vs. 8 trials, $p=.018$; 8 vs. 10 trials, $p=.043$; 14 vs. 16 trials, $p=.045$; 30 vs. grand average, $p=.013$), while all other pairs comparing increasing number of trial averages were insignificant (all $ps>0.05$). Significant differences between increasing trials averages were found for Pz (6 vs. 8 trials, $p=.019$; 26 vs. 28 trials, $p=.039$; 30 vs. grand average, $p=.02$), while all other pairs comparing increasing number of trial averages were insignificant (all $ps>0.05$). This suggests that the P3 is still relatively instable after 30 trials. Estimates of the SNR for N2 and P3 at Fz, Cz and Pz were also examined. SNR scores for the Fz electrode, starting with at

least 6 errors, ranged from 0.43 to 0.14. Paired t-tests show that there were significant differences for 6 vs 8 trials, 8 vs. 10 trials, 10 vs. 12 trials, 22 vs. 24 trials, 24 vs. 26 trials, 28 vs. 30 trials and 30 vs. participants' average ($p<0.05$). SNR scores for the Cz electrode, starting with at least 6 errors, ranged from 0.67 to 0.28. Paired t-tests show that there were significant differences for 6 vs. 8 trials, 8 vs. 10 trials, 10 vs.12 trials, 16 vs. 18 trials, 22 vs. 24 trials, 24 vs. 26 trials, 30 vs. participants' average ($p<0.05$). SNR scores for the Pz electrode, starting with at least 6 errors, ranged from 0.61 to 0.30. Paired t-tests show that there were significant differences for 6 vs. 8 trials, 8 vs. 10 trials, 24 vs. 26 trials and 30 vs. participants' average ($p<0.05$). Taken together, one can conclude that the signal-to-noise ratio remains relatively unstable even when including as many as 30 trials.

Additionally, we explored the relationship between each trial average and the N2/P3 participants' averages using Pearson's correlation coefficient for Fz, Cz and Pz (Figure 2B). All pairs were highly significant ($p<0.001$), suggesting that individual trial averages share a degree of similarity with the participants' average when including only a couple of ERP trials. However, high correlations ($rs>0.8$; i.e., higher internal consistency) were reached after including 18 and 14 trials to the N2 and P3 averages, respectively. These data indicate that the ERP measures become similar to the participants' average (i.e., across all trials) after including 18 trials for both the N2 and P3.

Next, we determined the Cronbach's alpha for the N2 and P3 as progressively more trials were considered (Figure 2C). They both show an increasing trend. However, in order to obtain an adequate Cronbach's alpha ($\alpha>0.6$) for the N2, at least 20 trials should be included in the participants' average. For the P3, an adequate Cronbach's alpha ($\alpha>0.6$) was obtained after 14 trails were included in the average. It is important to note that the Cronbach's alpha for the N2 remains low compared to that for the P3. Taken together, these data demonstrate that in order to obtain an internally consistent estimate for the N2 and P3, 20 and 14 trials are required taking into account both the Pearson's correlations and Cronbach's alpha analyses, respectively.

Error processing

To support the quality of our results regarding the internal consistency of the N2 and P3 in a Go/No-Go task, we attempted to replicate previous findings regarding the internal consistency of the ERN and Pe initially performed by Olvet and Hajcak [1]. On average, the participants made 26.31 errors (SD = 17.06) while performing the Eriksen Flanker task. The grand average difference waveforms for the Eriksen Flanker task for the electrodes FCz and Pz are presented in Figure 3. Moreover, Figure 4 presents for all three midline electrodes the average (Figure 4A), Pearson's correlation (Figure 4B), and the Cronbach's alpha (Figure 4C) as a function of an increasing number of trials. Paired t-tests were performed on the ERN area measures, and significant differences were observed only when comparing increasing numbers of trial averages for 4 vs. 6 trials ($p=0.03$), and 6 vs. 8 trials ($p=0.03$), while all other pairs were statistically insignificant (2 vs. 4 trials, 8 vs. 10 trials, 10 vs. 12 trials, 12 vs. 14 trials, and 14 vs. participants' average [i.e., all trials]; all $ps>0.05$); meaning that the average became stable after 8 trials were added to the participants' average. For the Pe, no significant differences were found ($p>0.05$); meanings that the Pe was relatively stable after 4 trials were included in the participants' average.

We also estimated the SNR for the ERN and Pe. SNR scores for the ERN starting with at least 6 errors ranged from 0.43 to 0.29, which is comparable to the magnitude reported in previous studies [1,11]. For the ERN, only significant difference between SNR of

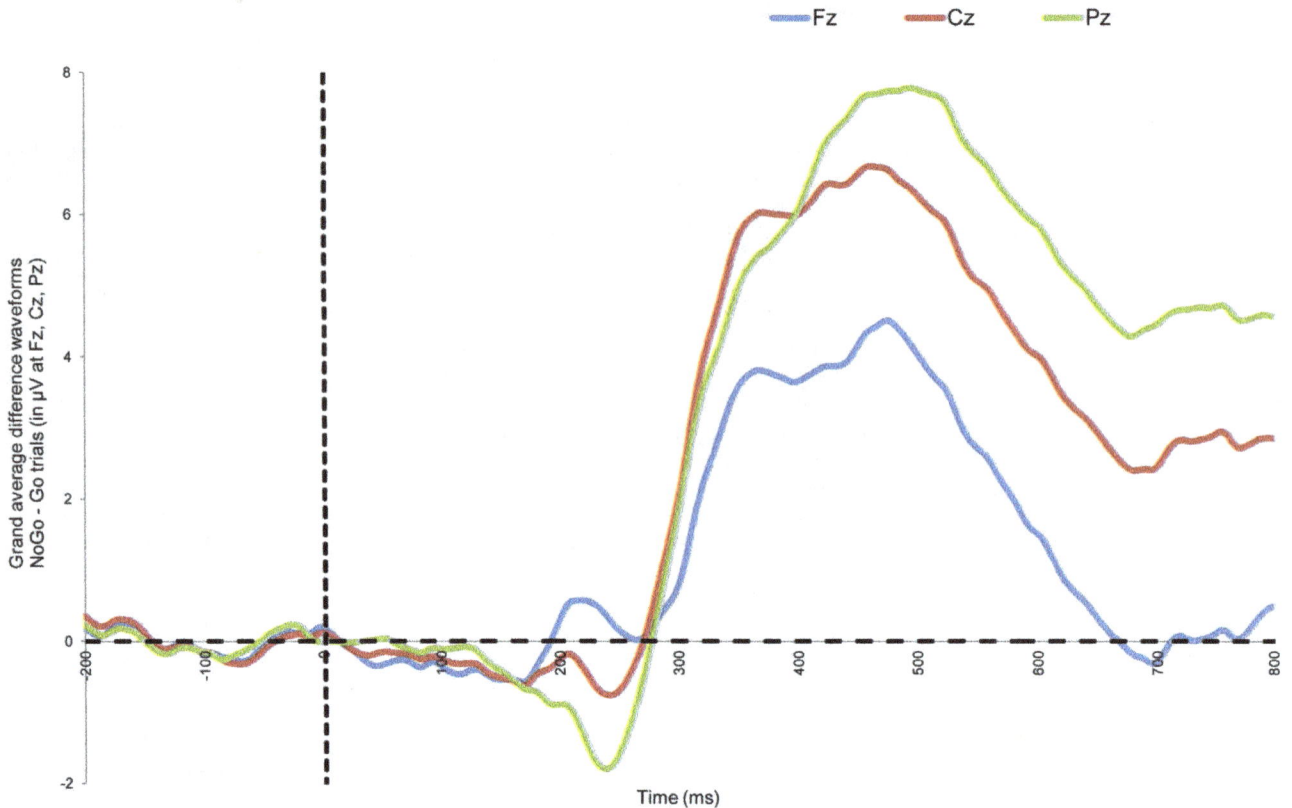

Figure 1. Grand average difference waveform: No-Go – Go trials. Figure 1 presents the grand average difference waveforms (i.e., average of all trials, across all participants) of the No-Go minus Go trials for electrodes Fz, Cz, and Pz. Note: we use the grand average difference waveforms for this figure as this is more informative compared to separate waveforms of No-Go correct trials and Go correct trials. However, in further analysis we took the amplitude for correct No-Go trials N2 and P3 at the midline electrodes Fz, Cz and Pz as the variables of interest.

trials averages 6 vs. 8 trials, 8 vs. 10 trials, and 10 vs. 12 trials, 12 vs. 14 trials ($p<0.05$), while for 14 trials vs. participants' average ($p>0.05$) was insignificant different. This means that after 14 trials the ERN signal-to-noise ratio became stable. As for the Pe SNR significant differences were observed for 12 vs. 14 trials and 14 trials vs. participants' average ($p<0.05$). This means that signal-to-noise for the Pe remained relatively unstable after 14 trials were included in the participants' average.

Additionally, we explored the relationship between each trial average and the ERN/Pe grand average using Pearson's correlation coefficient (Figure 4B). All pairs were highly significant (all ps<0.001), suggesting that individual trial averages share a degree of similarity with the participants' average when including only several ERP trials. However, the ERN and Pe trial averages showed high Pearson's correlations (i.e., higher internal consistency) after approximately 8 trials (rs>0.8) were included in the participants' average.

We also calculated the Cronbach's alpha for the ERN and Pe as progressively more trials were considered (Figure 4C). The Cronbach's alpha for the ERN and Pe were adequate ($\alpha>0.6$) after 8 trials were included in the participants' average. Thus, the ERN and Pe were both internally consistent around 8 trials were included in the participants' average, respectively.

Discussion

The present study examined the minimum number of trials required to obtain an internally consistent measure for ERPs in cognitive control tasks, the N2 and P3 in a Go/No-Go task and

the ERN and Pe in an Eriksen Flanker task. The N2 in the Go/No-Go task displayed a less favorable internal consistency pattern compared to the Eriksen Flanker task ERPs. In the Go/No-Go task, the N2 showed high Pearson's correlation coefficients after 14 trials were included in the participants' average. However, adequate Cronbach's alpha was obtained only after approximately 20 trials. This suggests that approximately 20 trials are required to obtain an internally consistent estimate for the No-Go N2. As for the P3 in the Go/No-Go task, high Pearson's correlation coefficients were reached after 14 trials were included in the participants' average, and an adequate Cronbach's alpha was already obtained after including 8 trials. Thus, 14 trials are required to obtain an internally consistent estimate for the P3. Cohen and Polich [9] found an internally consistent P3 in an oddball task after 21 trials were included in the participants' average.

In addition, we replicate in the same sample the study by Olvet and Hajcak [1], Pontifex et al. [11], and Meyer et al. [22,23]. In the current study, we found that approximately 8 trials are required to obtain an internally consistent estimate for the ERN and Pe. These recommendations are similar to previous studies [1,11,22,23].

In the current design of the Go/No-Go task, participants are required to withhold a response when a letter (A, E, I, O, or U) was repeated. This adds two components to the Go/No-Go task: a working memory component and a response conflict component (i.e., in which a participant must withhold a response to a stimulus to which the participant just responded). Maguire et al. [15,31]

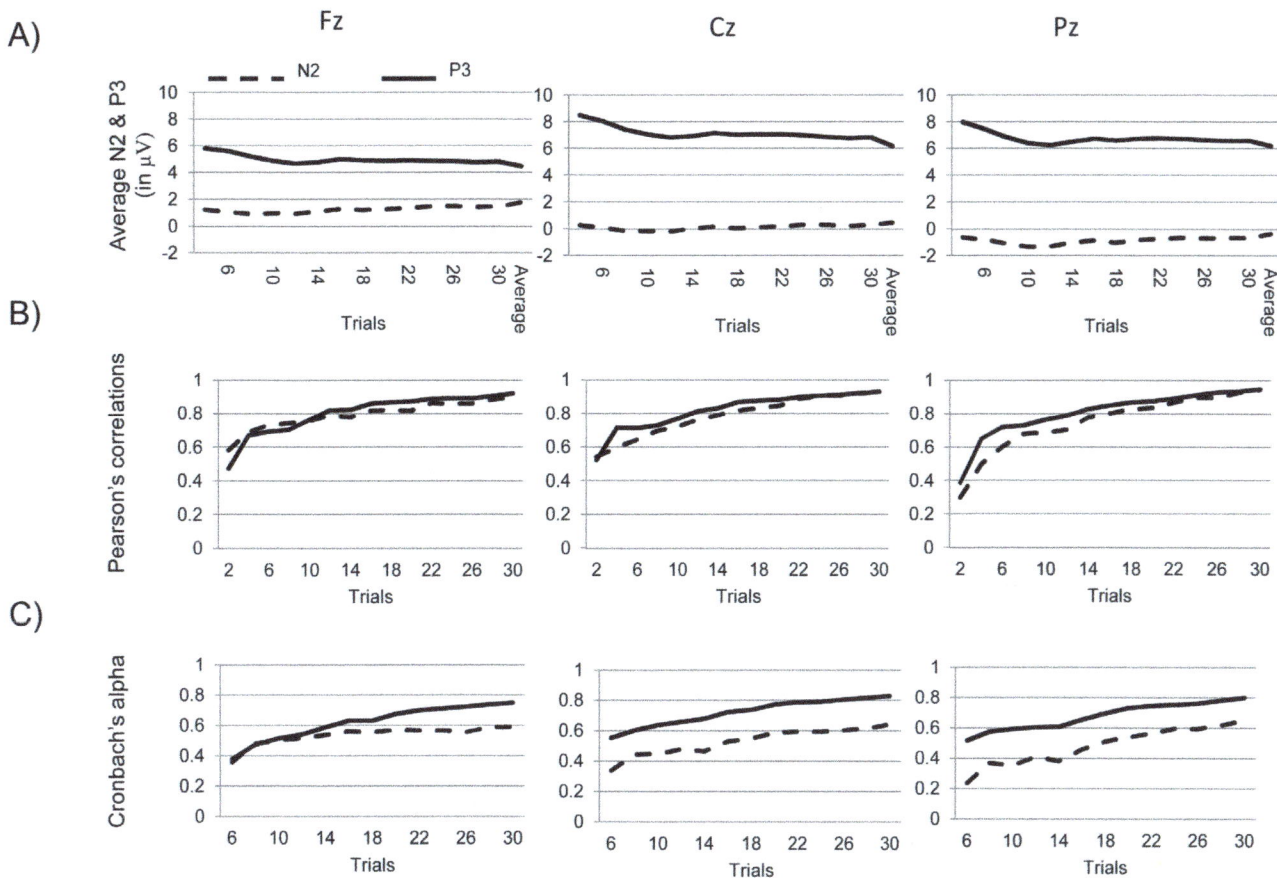

Figure 2. Correct No-Go N2 and P3– Internal consistency analysis. Figure 2 presents (A) the average N2 and P3, (B) Pearson's correlations, and (C) Cronbach's alpha as progressively more trials are included in the participants' average, all for the three midline electrodes Fz (left), Cz (middle), and Pz (right). The average presented in this figure refers to the grand average (all trials and all participants).

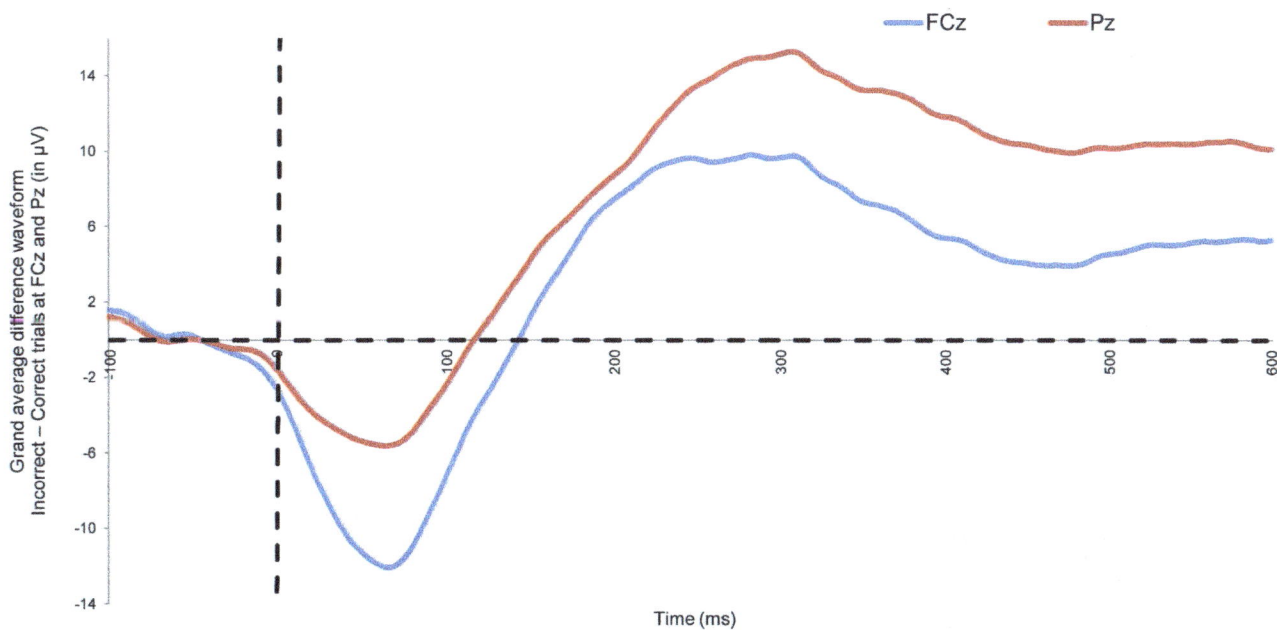

Figure 3. Grand average difference waveform: error - correct trials. Figure 3 presents the grand average difference waveforms (i.e., average of all trials, across all participants) of the error minus correct trials in the Eriksen Flanker task. Note: we use the grand average difference waveforms for this figure as this is more informative compared to separate waveforms of error and correct trials. However, in further analysis we took the amplitude for ERN (at FCz) and Pe (at Pz) error trials as the variables of interest.

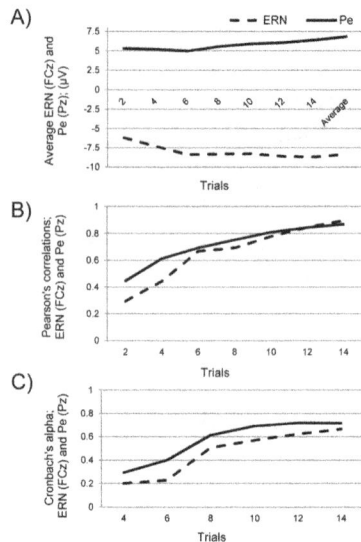

Figure 4. Error trials – Internal consistency analysis. Figure 4 presents the (A) average ERN and Pe, (B) Pearson's correlations, and (C) Cronbach's alpha as progressively more trials are included in the participants' average, for the ERN (at FCz) and Pe (at Pz). The average presented in this figure refers to the grand average (all trials and all participants).

found that both the N2 and P3 amplitudes decrease with task difficulty (e.g., adding working memory components); which implies that the amplitudes of the N2 and P3 in the current study may be affected by task complexity, and this could potentially influence the internal consistency of the N2 and P3. Therefore, for

future research it is important to examine the internal consistency of the N2 and P3 in three ways: (a) in a Go/No-Go task with lower complexity levels of the No-Go stimuli (e.g., a single Go and No-Go stimuli), see [15,31]; (b) other cognitive control tasks eliciting the N2 (e.g., stop-signal task); and/or (c) a context-specific N2 and P3, e.g., [25].

Based on the present findings, we recommend including at least 20 and 14 trials when measuring the N2 and P3 in a Go/No-Go task, respectively. Further, we recommend that at least 8 trails are required to measure the ERN and Pe in an Eriksen Flanker task.

The current study was set up to examine the internal consistency of brain activity related to error processing and inhibitory control. In line with previous findings, we have similar advice for the N2/P3 and ERN/Pe [1,8,9,11,14,22,23]. However, replication is needed to uncover the internal consistency of especially the N2 for similar as well as different behavioral tasks to confirm our conclusions and generalize the findings to other tasks (e.g., stop-signal task). Lastly, we employed a number of commonly employed statistical approaches to determine the internal consistency of the N2, P3, ERN and Pe. Future research may further examine this issue using more sophisticated statistical methods (e.g., simulation based methods).

Acknowledgments

The Erasmus Behavioral Lab and Jill Naaijen are gratefully acknowledged for their support in data collection and data management.

Author Contributions

Conceived and designed the experiments: WR IF ART. Performed the experiments: WR. Analyzed the data: WR IF. Contributed reagents/materials/analysis tools: WR IF. Wrote the paper: WR IF ART.

References

1. Olvet DM, Hajcak G (2009) The stability of error-related brain activity with increasing trials. Psychophysiology 46: 957–961.
2. Luijten M, Machielsen MW, Veltman DJ, Hester R, de Haan L, et al. (2013) Systematic review of ERP and fMRI studies investigating inhibitory control and error processing in people with substance dependence and behavioural addictions. J psych neurosci 38(1): 130052–130052.
3. Gehring WJ, Himle J, Nisenson LG (2000) Action-monitoring deficits in obsessive compulsive disorder. Psychol Sci 11: 1–6.
4. Riesel A, Weinberg A, Endrass T, Meyer A, Hajcak G (2013) The ERN is the ERN is the ERN? Convergent validity of error-related brain activity across different tasks. Biol Psychol 93: 377–385.
5. Anastasi A, Urbina S (1997) Psychological testing (7th ed.). Upper Saddle River, NJ: Prentice Hall.
6. Cook DA, Beckman TJ (2006) Current concepts in validity and reliability for psychometric instruments: Theory and application. Am J Med 119(2).
7. Cronbach LJ, Meehl PE (1955) Construct validity in psychological tests. Psychol Bull 52: 281–302.
8. Wostmann NM, Aichert DS, Costa A, Rubia K, Moller HJ, et al. (2013) Reliability and plasticity of response inhibition and interference control. Brain and Cognition 81(1): 82–94.
9. Cohen PH, Polich J (1997) On the number of trials needed for P300. Int J Psychophys 25: 249–255.
10. Kiang M, Patriciu I, Roy C, Christensen BK, Zipursky RB (2013) Test-re-test reliability and stability of N400 effects in a word-pair semantic priming paradigm. Clin Neurophysiol 4: 667–674.
11. Pontifex MB, Scudder MR, Brown ML, O'Leary KC, Wu CT, et al. (2010) On the number of trials necessary for stabilization of error-related brain activity across the life span. Psychophysiology 47(4): 767–773.
12. Falkenstein M, Hoormann J, Hohnsbein J (1999) ERP components in Go/No-Go tasks and their relation to inhibition. Acta Psychol 101: 267–291.
13. Garavan H, Ross TJ, Stein EA (1999) Right hemispheric dominance of inhibitory control: an event-related functional MRI study. Proc Natl Acad Sci USA 96: 8301–8306.
14. Clayson PE, Larson MJ (2013) Psychometric Properties of conflict monitoring and conflict adaption indices: Response time and Conflict N2 event-related potential. Psychophysiology 50: 1209–1219.
15. Maguire MJ, White J, Brier MR (2011) How semantic categorization influences inhibitory processing in middle-childhood: An Event Related Potentials study. Brain and cognition 76(1): 77–86.
16. Gehring WJ, Goss B, Coles MGH, Meyer DE, Donchin E (1993) A neural system for error detection and compensation. Psychol Sci 4: 385–390.
17. Falkenstein M, Hohnsbein J, Hoormann J, Blanke L (1991) Effects of cross modal divided attention on late ERP components. II. Error processing in choice reaction tasks. Electroen Clin Neuro 78(6): 447–455.
18. Hajcak G (2012) What we've learned from our mistakes: Insights from error-related brain activity. Current Directions in Psychol Sci 21: 101–106.
19. Bernstein PS, Scheffers MK, Coles MG (1995) "Where did I go wrong?" A psychophysiological analysis of error detection. J Exp Psychol Hum Percept Perform 21: 1312–1322.55.
20. Overbeek TJM, Nieuwenhuis S, Ridderinkhof KR (2005) Dissociable components of Error Processing. J Psychophysiol 19: 319–329.
21. Falkenstein M, Hoormann J, Christ S, Hohnsbein J (2000) ERP components on reaction errors and their functional significance: a tutorial. Biol Psychol 51: 87–107.
22. Meyer A, Riesel A, Proudfit GH (2013) Reliability of the ERN across multiple tasks as a function of increasing trials. Psychophysiology 50(12): 1220–1225.
23. Meyer A, Bress JN, Proudfit GH (2014) Psychometric properties of the error-related negativity in children and adolescents. Psychophysiology in press.
24. Littel M, van den Berg I, Luijten M, Van Rooij AJ, Keemink LM, et al. (2012) Error-processing and response inhibition in excessive computer game players: an ERP study. Addict Biol 17: 934–947.
25. Luijten M, Littel M, Franken IHA (2011) Deficits in inhibitory control insmokers during a Go/No-Go task: an investigation using event-related brain potentials. PloS ONE 6(4): e18898.
26. Franken IHA, Kroon LY, Hendriks VM (2000). Influence of individual differences in craving and obsessive cocaine thoughts on attentional processes in cocaine abuse patients. Addictive Behaviors 25(1): 99–102.
27. Marhe R, Van de Wetering BJM, Franken IHA (2013) Error-Related Brain Activity Predicts Cocaine Use after Treatment at 3-Month Follow-up. Biol Psychiat 73(8): 782–788.
28. Gratton G, Coles MG, Donchin E (1983) A new method for off-line removal of ocular artifact. Electroenceph Clin Neurophysiol 55: 468–484.

29. Donkers FC, van Boxtel GJ (2004) The N2 in go/no-go tasks reflects conflict monitoring not response inhibition. Brain and cognition 56(2): 165–176.

30. Bokura H, Yamaguchi S, Kobayashi S (2001) Electrophysiological correlates for response inhibition in a Go/NoGo task. Clinical Neurophysiology, 112(12): 2224–2232.

31. Maguire MJ, Brier MR, Moore PS, Ferree TC, Ray D, et al. (2009) The influence of perceptual and semantic categorization on inhibitory processing as measured by the N2–P3 response. Brain and cognition 71(3): 196–203.

32. Falkenstein M, Hoormann J, Hohnsbein J (1999) ERP components in Go/Nogo tasks and their relation to inhibition. Acta Psychologica, 101: 267–291.

2

Mice Lacking the Circadian Modulators SHARP1 and SHARP2 Display Altered Sleep and Mixed State Endophenotypes of Psychiatric Disorders

Paul C. Baier[1,2,9], Magdalena M. Brzózka[3,9], Ali Shahmoradi[4], Lisa Reinecke[4], Christina Kroos[4], Sven P. Wichert[3], Henrik Oster[5,6], Michael C. Wehr[3], Reshma Taneja[7], Johannes Hirrlinger[4,8], Moritz J. Rossner[3,4]*

1 Department of Neurology, University of Kiel, Kiel, Germany, 2 Department of Clinical Neurophysiology, University of Göttingen, Göttingen, Germany, 3 Department of Psychiatry, Ludwig-Maximilian-University, Munich, Germany, 4 Research Group Gene Expression, Max Planck Institute of Experimental Medicine, Göttingen, Germany, 5 Circadian Rhythms Group, Max Planck Institute of Biophysical Chemistry, Göttingen, Germany, 6 Medical Department I, University of Lübeck, Lübeck, Germany, 7 Department of Physiology, National University of Singapore, Singapore, Singapore, 8 Carl-Ludwig Institute of Physiology, University of Leipzig, Leipzig, Germany

Abstract

Increasing evidence suggests that clock genes may be implicated in a spectrum of psychiatric diseases, including sleep and mood related disorders as well as schizophrenia. The bHLH transcription factors SHARP1/DEC2/BHLHE41 and SHARP2/DEC1/BHLHE40 are modulators of the circadian system and SHARP1/DEC2/BHLHE40 has been shown to regulate homeostatic sleep drive in humans. In this study, we characterized Sharp1 and Sharp2 double mutant mice (S1/2$^{-/-}$) using online EEG recordings in living animals, behavioral assays and global gene expression profiling. EEG recordings revealed attenuated sleep/wake amplitudes and alterations of theta oscillations. Increased sleep in the dark phase is paralleled by reduced voluntary activity and cortical gene expression signatures reveal associations with psychiatric diseases. S1/2$^{-/-}$ mice display alterations in novelty induced activity, anxiety and curiosity. Moreover, mutant mice exhibit impaired working memory and deficits in prepulse inhibition resembling symptoms of psychiatric diseases. Network modeling indicates a connection between neural plasticity and clock genes, particularly for SHARP1 and PER1. Our findings support the hypothesis that abnormal sleep and certain (endo)phenotypes of psychiatric diseases may be caused by common mechanisms involving components of the molecular clock including SHARP1 and SHARP2.

Editor: Valérie Mongrain, Hôpital du Sacré-Coeur de Montréal, Canada

Received May 16, 2014; **Accepted** September 11, 2014; **Published** October 23, 2014

Funding: H. Oster is a Lichtenberg Fellow of the Volkswagen Foundation. This work was supported by the Deutsche Forschungsgemeinschaft (CMPB and grant Klinische Forschergruppe (KFO: RO 4076/1-1) 241). The funders had no role in study design, data collection and analysis, decision to publish, or preparation of the manuscript.

Competing Interests: The authors have declared that no competing interests exist.

* Email: Moritz.Rossner@med.uni-muenchen.de

⑨ These authors contributed equally to this work.

Introduction

The circadian system has been implicated in the control of alertness and clock genes have been associated with sleep and mood disorders, such as familial advance sleep phase syndrome (FASPS), depression, mania or bipolar disease (BD) [1–8], and therapeutic approaches modulating the circadian system ('chronotherapy') may be promising to improve treatment of psychiatric diseases [9,10]. Sleep-wake behavior represents the most obvious behavioral output of the circadian system and nearly all psychiatric diseases including autism and schizophrenia (SZ) are characterized by irregular sleep-wake profiles [8,11,12]. In addition to the circadian control, homeostatic processes regulate vigilance states by increasing sleep drive and endurance [13–15].

Sleep serves a variety of vital functions. Prolonged wakefulness results in compensatory or rebound sleep, and disruption of normal sleep-wake cycles may contribute to psychiatric symptoms

and inflammatory as well neurodegenerative processes [16,17]; however, sleep deprivation has been shown to have short term beneficial effects in depressive patients [18,19]. Reduced or disturbed sleep likely contributes to cognitive impairments and mood-related symptoms in psychiatric patients [8,20]. Recent data support the notion that sleep is not only a distinct behavioral state but is rather characterized by defined cellular processes, as shown by monitoring sleep or wake associated cortical gene expression at a global scale [21,22], and by progress in attributing sleep associated brain oscillations, i.e. in the theta or delta range, to functions in higher order neuronal plasticity [20,23].

Sleep-wake behavior is altered in clock gene mutant mice, although the discrimination between circadian and homeostatic processes in mutants with a disturbed clock is difficult [24–28]. The mechanisms that link clock gene function with sleep-wake control and psychiatric diseases are just beginning to be explored [8]. For example, mice expressing a truncated version of the

CLOCK protein ($Clock^{\Delta 19}$) are characterized by hyperactivity, reduced sleep, lowered anxiety and depression-like behavior as well as impaired neuronal synchronizations [29,30]. Moreover, mice lacking NPAS2, the functionally redundant paralog of CLOCK [31] which is, in contrast to CLOCK, prominently expressed in the forebrain [32], are also hyperactive, display reduced sleep and show altered sleep associated oscillations [25,28].

SHARP1 (DEC2, BHLHE41) and SHARP2 (DEC1, BHLHE40) are negative regulators of CLOCK and NPAS2 and act as adaptation factors of the molecular clock [33–35]. Both genes are involved in the entrainment of the circadian system to altered external cues, yet the corresponding single and double null mutants are characterized by a slight period shift but do not display a disrupted circadian rhythm which indicates mainly functional core clock mechanisms [35,36]. Period analysis, resetting to advanced and delayed light-dark (LD) cycles as well as nocturnal light pulses revealed gene dosage dependent functional redundancy between both genes [35] and genetic interactions with *Per1* and *Per2* [36,37]. Moreover, SHARP1/DEC2 is involved in the regulation of sleep homeostasis in mice and humans [38]. A single point mutation in the C-terminal domain (P385R) found in a human family of 'short' sleepers reduces the transcriptional repressive activity of SHARP1. In a corresponding humanized mouse model, the duration of sleep is reduced and more fragmented compared to control animals, and the latter phenotype is strongly enhanced on a *Sharp1* null background [38]. With respect to sleep architecture, only a moderate increase of non-rapid eye movement (NREM) sleep during the early dark phase has been observed in *Sharp1* null mutants [38]. Therefore, the P385R mutant SHARP1 protein was considered to act in a dominant-negative fashion.

Given the mild sleep architecture phenotype in *Sharp1* null mutants and the functional redundancy of SHARP1 and -2 in the entrainment to external cues [35] it is possible that SHARP2 could at least partially compensate for the loss of SHARP1. Consequently, we analyzed sleep-wake behavior in *Sharp1* and *-2* double null mutant ($S1/2^{-/-}$) mice. Our analysis revealed altered sleep architecture in $S1/2^{-/-}$ mice with markedly attenuated light-to-dark amplitude of the different vigilance states. Moreover, daytime dependent changes in cortical gene expression and behavioral analyses revealed associations of SHARP1/2 function with endophenotypes of psychiatric diseases beyond the homeostatic control of sleep.

Results

Attenuated Sleep-Wake Amplitudes in $S1/2^{-/-}$ mice

Given the relatively mild sleep phenotype of *Sharp1* single mutants [38] and the functional redundancy of SHARP1 and -2 [35], we focussed on the analysis of *Sharp1* and *-2* double mutant mice ($S1/2^{-/-}$). We performed EEG and EMG recordings on male mice to monitor for sleep-wake patterns over consecutive 24 h light-dark (LD) cycles. We determined the relative amounts of NREM (or slow-wave), REM (or paradoxical) sleep and wakefulness over 12 h light (L) and 12 h dark (D) periods and for the entire 24 h LD period. Total wakefulness, REM and NREM during 24 h of undisturbed sleep were similar in wild-type (WT) and $S1/2^{-/-}$ animals (Figure 1A). However, there was a clear difference in the distribution of sleep and wakefulness during L and D. WT animals showed a substantial difference in the amount of wakefulness, NREM- and REM-sleep between L and D, whereas the sleep/wake amplitude was attenuated in $S1/2^{-/-}$ animals (Figure 1B,C). Sleep-wake behavior was quantified as

relative L-D differences, which were significantly reduced in $S1/2^{-/-}$ animals for all three vigilance states ($p < 0.01$ for wake, $p < 0.05$ for REM and NREM sleep) (Figure 1B). The relative difference in the amount of wakefulness during the light and dark episodes is exemplified for individual WT and $S1/2^{-/-}$ mice (Figure 1C). We plotted the cumulated EEG data in 2 h bins to increase temporal resolution (Figure 1D-F). NREM sleep was most prominently altered in the two hours preceding lights-off (zeitgeber time (ZT) 10-12; reduced NREM) and in the middle of the dark phase (ZT19-21; increased NREM; $p < 0.05$; post-hoc test after 2-way ANOVA with significant genotype×time interaction $p < 0.05$) (Figure 1E). REM sleep was reduced at ZT4-8 ($p < 0.05$: post-hoc test after 2-way ANOVA with significant genotype $p < 0.01$ and time $p < 0.0001$ effects without significant genotype×time interaction) (Figure 1F).

We sleep deprived $S1/2^{-/-}$ and control mice by gentle handling (ZT0-6 = L1, 97±1% efficient for both genotypes) to analyze homeostatic sleep drive (Figure S1A–C). The amount of NREM sleep after sleep deprivation (SD) revealed no significant differences in L2 (ZT7-12), at the beginning of D2 (ZT17) NREM sleep was increased in $S1/2^{-/-}$ compared to WT mice ($p < 0.05$) (Figure S1B). The relative amount of REM sleep, however, was significantly reduced in $S1/2^{-/-}$ mice ($p < 0.05$) compared to WT mice 2–4 h after the SD episode (ZT8-10) (Figure S1C). The analysis of slow-wave activity (SWA) or NREM delta power after SD revealed similar levels of rebound sleep in WT and $S1/2^{-/-}$ mice compared to baseline values (Figure S2A). Nonetheless, we observed consistent but not significantly elevated SWA in $S1/2^{-/-}$ mice at almost all time points independent of SD (Figure S2A). We also analyzed the REM sleep dominating synchronized oscillations in the 5–9 Hz range (theta) (Figure S2B-D). Theta peak frequency (TPF) was significantly higher at ZT7-12 in sleep deprived $S1/2^{-/-}$ animals (TPF $S1/2^{-/-}$: 7.60±0.12 Hz) compared to undisturbed (TPF WT 7.17±0.12 Hz; $p < 0.05$) and sleep deprived WT mice (TPF WT: 7.22±0.03 Hz; $p < 0.01$) (Figure S2B). Without SD, no spectral theta differences were observed in $S1/2^{-/-}$ versus WT mice at ZT7-12 (Figure S2C). However, theta spectra were altered between sleep deprived $S1/2^{-/-}$ and controls in the time period between ZT7-12 (Figure S2D; 2-way ANOVA, $p = 0.0047$). The increased TPF observed after SD in $S1/2^{-/-}$ mice was not significantly different to the average values obtained for all sleep-deprived and naïve animals during the dark period and thus occurs in the normal physiological range (ZT13-18 and ZT19-24) (Figure S2B).

EEG analyses were complemented by assessing 24 h rest-activity profiles monitored with voluntary wheel running. In this assay, $S1/2^{-/-}$ mice displayed normal entrainment to the LD cycle, but with a reduced wheel activity during D (Figure 1G), which correlates with the increased relative amount of sleep in D (Figure 1B). In L, we observed no significant differences in running wheel activities between the genotypes possibly due to photic masking of voluntary locomotor activity [39] (Figure 1G).

Disturbed activity dependent gene expression

Different vigilance states are characterized by specific cortical gene expression profiles [21]. To identify molecular correlates of the altered sleep-wake behavior and 24 h rest-activity profiles in $S1/2^{-/-}$ mice, we first analyzed cortical gene expression of the circadian marker gene *Per2* and the activity-induced immediate-early gene (IEG) product *Fos* in 4 h bins over a complete 24 h cycle (Figure 1H,I). In line with previous observations [35] the circadian profile of *Per2* in the cortex was grossly normal, however, with a slightly but significantly reduced amplitude in $S1/2^{-/-}$ versus WT mice ($p < 0.001$, 2-way ANOVA) (Figure 1H). In

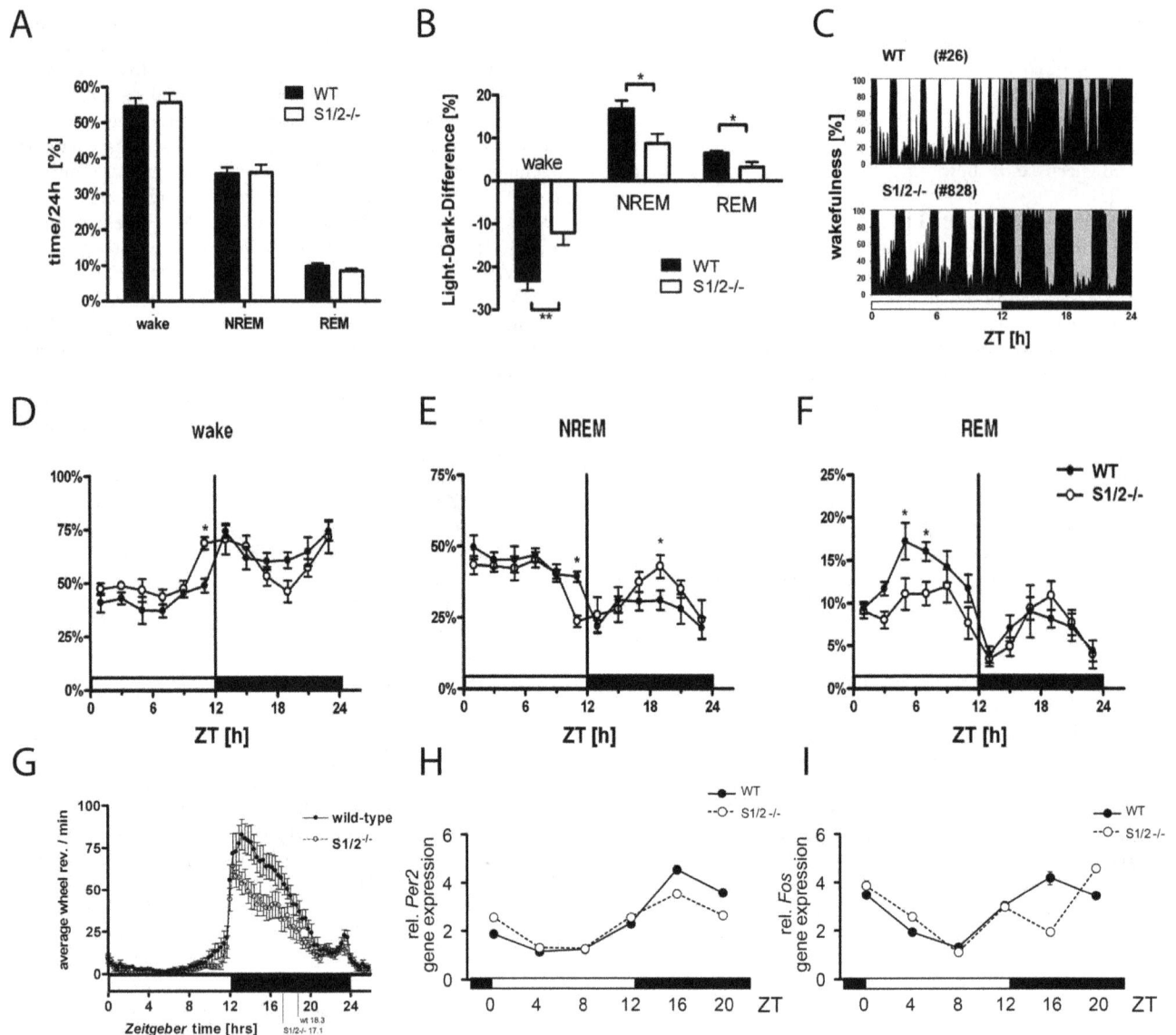

Figure 1. Attenuated sleep-wake amplitude and activity profiles in S1/2$^{-/-}$ mice. A) Group means ($\pm$ SEM) of the total time spend in different vigilance states over 24 h LD periods. The overall time of wake, NREM and REM sleep remained unaltered between genotypes. WT: n = 7, filled bars S1/2$^{-/-}$: n = 8, empty bars. B) Group means of light-dark or amplitude differences for wake, NREM and REM sleep. S1/2$^{-/-}$ animals showed a significantly reduced light-dark amplitude for all vigilance states compared to WT animals ($E_{genotype}$ $F_{(1,\ 39)}$ = 19.87, p<0.0001; $E_{vigilance\ state}$ $F_{(2,\ 39)}$ = 19.39, p<0.0001; $I_{genotype\times vigilance\ state}$ $F_{(2,\ 39)}$ = 1.9, p = 0.16; Post hoc two-tailed T-test: **: p<0.01 *: p<0.05). WT: n = 7, filled bars S1/2$^{-/-}$: n = 8, empty bars. C) 24 h sleep-wake distribution plotted for representative individual WT (#26) and S1/2$^{-/-}$ (#828) mice with black areas given as relative amount of wakefulness obtained from 5 min bins. Note the relative difference in the amount of wakefulness during the light and dark episodes in the WT and the short periods of wakefulness in the light phase. In contrast, the S1/2$^{-/-}$ mouse displayed broadened periods of sleep and wakefulness during the light and dark phases. D-F) Time course of vigilance states wakefulness (D), NREM (E) and REM sleep (F). Curves connect 2 h bin mean values ($\pm$ SEM) expressed as percentage of recording time (E_{time}: NREM: $F_{(11,120)}$ = 9.74, p<0.0001; REM $F_{(11,120)}$ = 9.98, p<0.0001; $E_{genotype}$: NREM n.s.; REM $F_{(1,120)}$ = 7.65, p<0.01 and $I_{genotype\times time}$: Wakefulness $F_{(11,120)}$ = 2.06, p = 0.02; NREM: $F_{(11,120)}$ = 1.82, p = 0.05; REM: $F_{(11,120)}$ = 1.42, p = 0.17; *= p< 0.05 in two-tailed post hoc T-test. WT: n = 7, filled circles S1/2$^{-/-}$: n = 8, empty circles. G) Diurnal wheel-running profiles depicted as accumulated activities of all recordings over a 5-day period plotted as 18 min bins. S1/2$^{-/-}$ mice displayed a significantly altered activity profile in LD compared to wild-type (WT) mice ($I_{genotype\times time}$ $F_{(86,39040)}$ = 1.92, p<0.0001) with reduced half maximal values of nocturnal activities at ZT 17.1 for S12$^{-/-}$ mice compared to WT controls with ZT 18.3. Bonferroni posttest revealed significantly reduced activities between ZT13 and 18 (p_{Bonf}<0.05). n = 12 each genotype. H-I) Daytime dependent gene expression analysis of the circadian marker gene Per2 (H) and the activity-induced gene Fos (I) in the cortex. Daytime dependent cortical expression of the circadian marker gene Per2 was not substantially altered in WT and S1/2$^{-/-}$ mice (H). In contrast, the mRNA expression of the activity regulated marker gene Fos was significantly reduced in S1/2$^{-/-}$ mice at ZT16 compared to WT (I). n = 3 per timepoint and genotype. Data were analyzed with 2-way ANOVA with Bonferroni posttest (p_{Bonf}) and Mann-Whitney test (p_{MW}) for pairwise comparisons. E, effect; I, interaction of factors.

contrast, the diurnal amplitude of cortical mRNA expression of the neuronal-activity marker Fos was preserved; but Fos transcription was strongly reduced at ZT16 in S1/2$^{-/-}$ mice compared to WT animals (p<0.001, 2-way ANOVA; p<0.001 post-hoc test at ZT16) (Figure 1I) correlating with the elevated NREM sleep and reduced running wheel activity in D

(Figure 1E,G). To obtain a more comprehensive insight into the changes in cortical gene expression in S1/2$^{-/-}$ mice, we performed microarray analysis on cortical samples obtained from individual WT and S1/2$^{-/-}$ mice harvested at two opposite time points of the LD cycle (ZT4 – wake phase; and ZT16 – sleep phase; Figure 2A; Table S1 and Table S2) where Fos expression differences were most prominent. This analysis revealed profound sleep-wake differences at the level of gene expression. Most prominently, the number of transcripts upregulated at ZT16 compared to ZT4 was substantially higher in WT (n = 22, corresponding to 21 genes with 2 probe sets detected for preproenkephalin Penk) than in S1/2$^{-/-}$ mice (n = 5) (Table S1 and Table S2, see Table S3 for full gene name descriptions). In accordance with the quantitative (q)RT-PCR analysis (Figure 1H) and based on published results showing an intact circadian clock in S1/2$^{-/-}$ mice [35,36] among the five genes found to be significantly up-regulated in S1/2$^{-/-}$ cortex at ZT16 were three canonical clock genes (Per1, Per2, Cry1)

although at slightly reduced induction levels (Figure 2A and Table S1).

Wake-induced expression of transcripts encoding for neural plasticity genes (i.e. IEG transcription factors such as Fos, Nr4a1, Egr1, Ier1 and Junb and those related to inter- and intracellular signalling such as Tac1, Penk, Dusp1/6, Drd2, Adora2a) was almost completely abolished in the S1/2$^{-/-}$ mutants (Figure 2A and Table S1). Within this cluster of genes were also the oligodendrocyte/myelin markers Enpp2, Plp1 and Cldn11. By qRT-PCR, we validated differential expression of selected genes in independent groups of mice in LD and DD (Figure 2B and Table S1). The analyses under constant darkness (DD) revealed a highly similar attenuated amplitude ruling out potential light masking effects.

Next, we used gene set enrichment analysis (GSEA) to identify cellular processes potentially altered in S1/2$^{-/-}$ mice [40]. Similar to the gene-by-gene analysis, we detected the most profound differences when comparing WT and S1/2$^{-/-}$ array data obtained

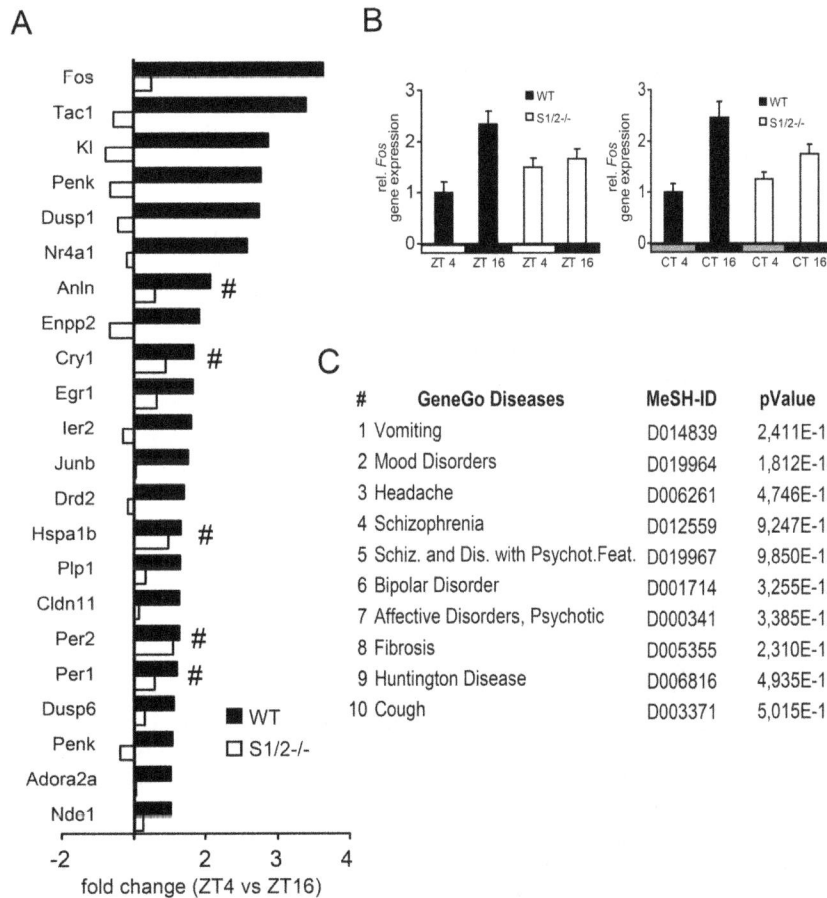

Figure 2. Cortical gene expression signatures correlate with psychiatric disease states. A) Depicted are fold-changes of differentially expressed genes at ZT4 versus ZT16 in the cortex of WT and S1/2$^{-/-}$ mice detected by microarray analyses. In WT mice, several genes were upregulated with a fold-change of at least 1.5 at ZT16 (n = 22, Penk was detected by two independent probe sets) whereas this profile was strongly attenuated in S1/2$^{-/-}$ mice with only 5 genes (marked with #) detected at the same cut-off (among those are 3 canonical clock genes Cry1, Per1 and Per2 as well as Anln and Hspa1b) that follow a normal although reduced 'circadian' profile. Note, that Ttr was for graphical reasons omitted because of its high fold-changes (Table S1). n = 2 per timepoint and genotype. B) Attenuated sleep-wake amplitude of Fos gene expression in the cortex of WT and S1/2$^{-/-}$ mice in LD and DD. At ZT4 and ZT16 (where mice were kept under 12 h light and 12 dark conditions = LD; left panel) and at CT4 and CT16 (where mice were kept under constant darkness = DD; right panel) cortical Fos mRNA expression was analyzed with quantitative RT-PCR. n = 3 for each genotype. C) GeneGo enrichment analysis based on hyper-geometric statistics of the top 10 ranked disease associations of the cortical gene set (deregulated at ZT16 in S1/2$^{-/-}$ cortex compared to WT). This analysis revealed highly significant correlations with neurological and particularly psychiatric disease classifications as indicated. Spelling of classifier 5 'Schizophrenia and Disorders with Psychotic Features' is abbreviated as indicated. MeSH ID, unique Medical Subject Heading disease identifier.

at ZT16. Among the most significantly up-regulated gene sets in WT samples were several involved in cellular metabolism, such as components of the proteasome and ribosome as well as genes associated with oxidative phosphorylation (p-val<0.0001, FDR q-val<0.05) (Figure S3). Again, these molecular adaptations correlated with the attenuated sleep-wake/activity-rest amplitudes observed in S1/2$^{-/-}$ animals. We also analyzed gene expression in cortical samples obtained from WT and S1/2$^{-/-}$ mice after sleep deprivation. mRNA levels of two housekeeping genes, *Atp5b* and *Actb*, as well as *Per2* remained unaltered between WT and S1/2$^{-/-}$ mutants (Figure S4B). In contrast, SD-induced down-regulation of *Per1*, *Fos* and *Egr1* gene expression observed in WT animals was markedly attenuated in S1/2$^{-/-}$ mice correlating with genotype dependent REM sleep alterations at ZT10 (Figure S1C and S4B).

Molecular signatures reveal associations with psychiatric disorders

In an unbiased approach, we applied software tools to detect potential associations of daytime-dependent cortical gene expression signatures (Table S1) in S1/2$^{-/-}$ mice with particular disease classifiers [41]. Among the ten most significant matches were seven neurological medical subject heading (MeSH) classifiers and of those five were related to mood or psychotic disorders, suggesting a potential link between SHARP dysfunction and psychiatric diseases beyond alterations in sleep (Figure 2C). We further extended this analysis by applying pathway modeling algorithms to daytime-regulated genes including SHARP1 and -2 as seed nodes (Figure 3A). This approach aimed at detecting relationships between transcriptionally regulated as well as unregulated but functionally linked gene products to provide a more complete picture [42]. We used the most stringent shortest path algorithm that allows only 1-step indirect connections from curated literature, pathway and protein-interaction databases (see Methods). The corresponding network model predicted close functional interactions of 14 out of 23 gene products (64%) of the cortical gene expression signature (including SHARP1 and -2) and 15 connecting nodes (Figure 3A). Two distinct sub-clusters emerged from the network structure. One cluster connects components involved in neuronal signalling (enkephalin A, substance P, A2A and DRD2) and downstream effectors including negative regulators (DUSP1,6 and HSPs) as well as transcriptional mediators (e.g. FOS, EGR1, JUNB, NR4A1). The second cluster is comprised of central components of the molecular clock (e.g. the core clock transcription factors CLOCK, NPAS2 and BMAL1 as well as clock feedback regulators and modifiers including SHARP1 and -2, PER1 and -2, CRY1 and DBP and Rev-ERBalpha). Remarkably, only SHARP1, PER1 and BMAL1 were detected as connecting nodes between both clusters (Figure 3A). We queried the GeneGo databases with all components of this extended network to reveal associations with particular cellular process and diseases in an unbiased way. Among the top ten ranked disease associations were nine corresponding to psychiatric disorders including depressive, affective and psychotic MeSH classifiers (ranging from major depressive disorder [rank 1, p< 10^{-26}] to BD [rank 4, p<10^{-23}] and SZ [rank 9, p<10^{-16}]) (Figure 3B). Among the top ten ranked GO biological processes are two circadian rhythm related ones (circadian rhythm [rank 1, p<10^{-22}] and rhythmic processes [rank 2, p<10^{-22}]), and several that refer to central metabolic processes most likely reflecting the interaction between circadian clock function and cellular metabolic control [43–45] (Figure 3C).

S1/2$^{-/-}$ mice display endophenotypes of psychiatric disease

EEG recordings revealed a role of SHARP1/2 in the homeostatic control of sleep and unsupervised analysis of cortical gene expression profiles provided a possible link to psychiatric diseases, particularly mood and psychotic disorders. Therefore, we analyzed S1/2$^{-/-}$ mice to assess behavioral aspects that may be relevant in the context of psychiatric diseases: including basic behavior (motivation, exploratory, curiosity and anxiety), working memory performance and sensorimotor gating (Figure 4–5 and Figure S5–S8). In the open field test, we observed a highly significant novelty-induced hyperactivity in an unfamiliar environment (p$_{MW}$ (p value for Mann-Whitney test) <0.0006; Figure 4A), persistent during the entire test (effect of genotype p = 0.0002; 2-way ANOVA, Figure 4B) and most prominent in interval 3, 5 and 10 (p$_{Bonf}$ (p values for Bonferroni post test) <0.01, <0.05 and <0.05, respectively;). S1/2$^{-/-}$ mice spent more time in the center (p$_{MW}$<0.0004) of the test arena than controls possibly indicating reduced anxiety or risk-taking behavior (Figure 4C). Elevated plus maze (Figure 5A) and light-dark preference test (Figure S5B), however, did not reveal alterations of anxiety-related behavior. S1/2$^{-/-}$ mice spent similar time in closed arms in elevated plus maze (p$_{MW}$ = 0.8693) and in the dark compartment during light-dark preference test when compared with WT controls (p$_{MW}$ = 0.1917). On the subsequent day after the open field test, the same test arena was equipped with a 'hole-board' to monitor nose pokes as an indicator of exploratory drive, curiosity-related behavior. Whereas the total travelled distance did not differ between the genotypes under more familiar conditions (Figure 4D), the number of nose pokes (Figure 4E) was significantly reduced in S1/2$^{-/-}$ versus WT mice (p$_{MW}$ = 0.0014). However, motivational behavior as assessed in tail suspension test (p$_{MW}$ = 0.9456; Figure S5C) and in sucrose preference test (p = 0.1719; 2-way ANOVA, Figure S5D) was unaltered.

As impairment of working memory is one of the core symptoms of SZ and BD [46–48], we addressed working memory performance of S1/2$^{-/-}$ mice using the Y-maze test. S1/2$^{-/-}$ animals displayed an increased activity in this novel environment performing more arm choices (p = 0.0022; 2-way ANOVA, Figure 4F), mainly during the first 5 min (p$_{Bonf}$<0.01). Mutants showed less alterations in Y-maze than controls (p = 0.0331; 2-way ANOVA, Figure 4G) with the lower performance during interval 5–10 min (p$_{Bonf}$<0.05). We also observed working memory deficits in a radial arm water maze (Figure 4H–J). In the visible platform task, performance was similar in both genotypes (p = 0.4236; 2-way ANOVA, Figure 4H) but S1/2$^{-/-}$ mice displayed more working errors searching for a hidden platform on the first (p = 0.0524; 2-way ANOVA, interaction genotype× time p = 0.0486; Figure 4I) and on the second day of the experiment (effect of genotype p = 0.0044 and genotype × time p = 0.0422; 2-way ANOVA, Figure 4J) with the most prominent difference during trial 3 (p$_{Bonf}$<0.001; Figure 4J).

To assess sensorimotor gating as an additional endophenotype of several psychiatric diseases [49–51], S1/2$^{-/-}$ mice and WT controls were tested in a prepulse inhibition (PPI) test under normal conditions and after treatment with clozapine. We performed the tests on 3 consecutive days with naïve animals (day 1), injected with vehicle (day 2) and after acute clozapine treatment (3mg/kg; day 3).

To exclude possible effects of multiple testing on PPI, we first exposed naïve wild type animals (age-matched male C57Bl/6) on three consecutive days to PPI (Figure S6). We did not observe effects of multiple testing on PPI (p = 0.1539; 2-way ANOVA;

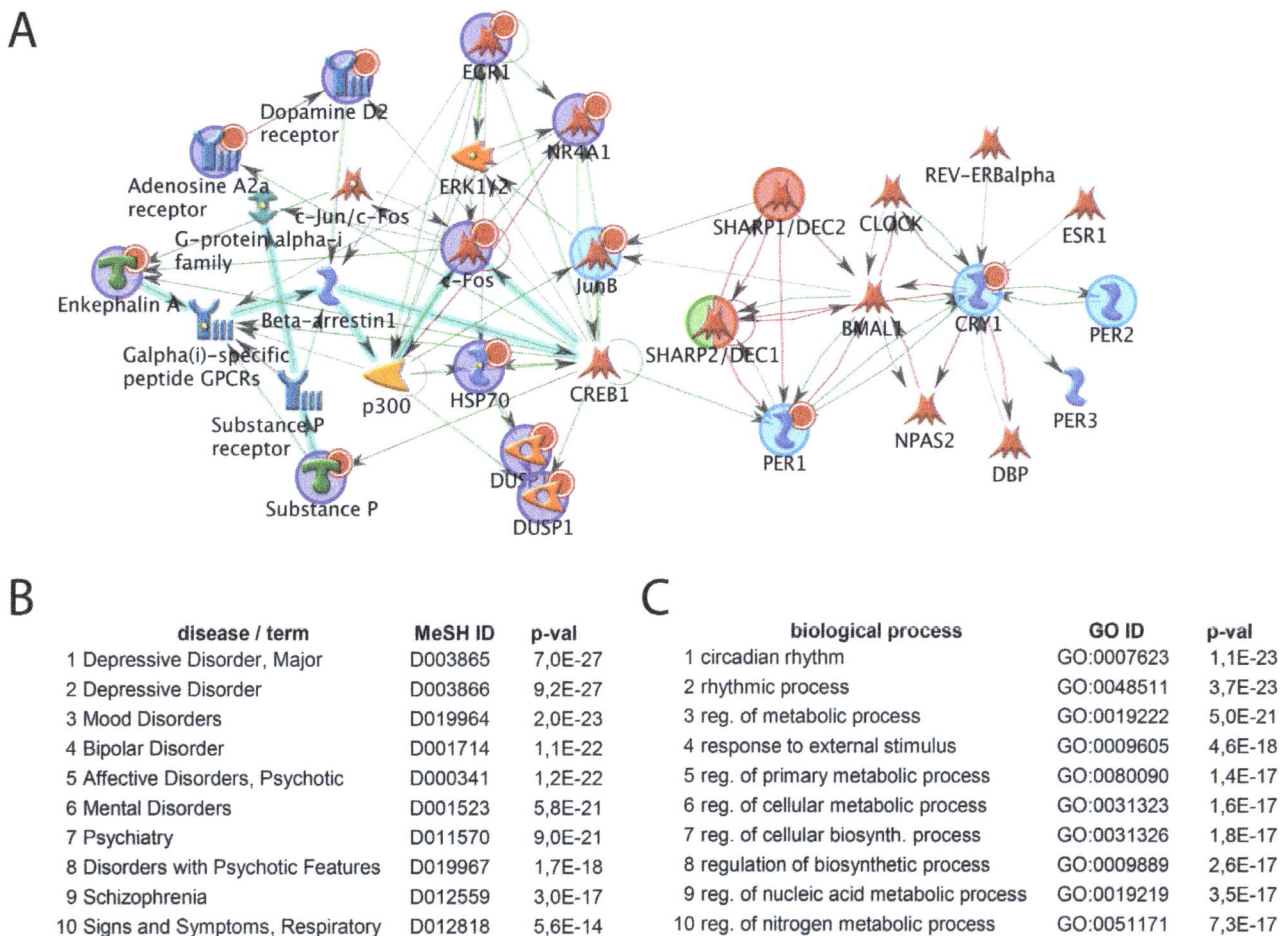

	disease / term	MeSH ID	p-val
1	Depressive Disorder, Major	D003865	7,0E-27
2	Depressive Disorder	D003866	9,2E-27
3	Mood Disorders	D019964	2,0E-23
4	Bipolar Disorder	D001714	1,1E-22
5	Affective Disorders, Psychotic	D000341	1,2E-22
6	Mental Disorders	D001523	5,8E-21
7	Psychiatry	D011570	9,0E-21
8	Disorders with Psychotic Features	D019967	1,7E-18
9	Schizophrenia	D012559	3,0E-17
10	Signs and Symptoms, Respiratory	D012818	5,6E-14

	biological process	GO ID	p-val
1	circadian rhythm	GO:0007623	1,1E-23
2	rhythmic process	GO:0048511	3,7E-23
3	reg. of metabolic process	GO:0019222	5,0E-21
4	response to external stimulus	GO:0009605	4,6E-18
5	reg. of primary metabolic process	GO:0080090	1,4E-17
6	reg. of cellular metabolic process	GO:0031323	1,6E-17
7	reg. of cellular biosynth. process	GO:0031326	1,8E-17
8	regulation of biosynthetic process	GO:0009889	2,6E-17
9	reg. of nucleic acid metabolic process	GO:0019219	3,5E-17
10	reg. of nitrogen metabolic process	GO:0051171	7,3E-17

Figure 3. Unbiased network modeling links cortical signaling with clock components via SHARP1, BMAL1 and PER1. A) Depicted is the network model with the highest significance computed with all genes found to be differentially regulated in the cortex at ZT4 versus ZT16 (see. Figure 2A, Tables S1-S3 and Figure S9 for description of symbols) including SHARP1 and -2. The network connects 14 seed nodes depicted as blue circles (higher expression levels in WT are indicated by associated small red circles) extended by 13 interactors. SHARP1 and -2 are labeled by red circles; all nodes added by the algorithm are not underlined by colored circles. The structure depicts two major clusters and places the circadian regulators SHARP1 and SHARP2 as well as PER1 at central positions. The left cluster (n = 19 objects) is mainly comprised of cellular signaling components (enkephalin A, substance P both encoded by *Penk* and the GPCRs A2A and DRD2) and downstream effectors including negative regulators (DUSP1,6 and HSPs) as well as transcriptional mediators (e.g. FOS, EGR1, JUNB). The right cluster (n = 12) comprises central components of the molecular clock (e.g. the core clock transcription factors CLOCK, NPAS2 and BMAL1 as well as clock feedback regulators and modifiers including SHARP1 and -2, PER1 and -2, CRY1, DBP and NR1D1/Rev-ERBalpha). The extended network gene list was queried against the GeneGo database for enriched correlations with diseases (B) and biological processes (C). Among the ten most significant disease associations were nine mental or mood related disease classifications (B). Among the ten highest ranked biological processes were only circadian rhythm- (rank 1 and 2) and metabolism-associated (rank 3–8) processes (C). MeSH ID, unique Medical Subject Heading disease identifier; GO ID, unique identifier of the gene ontology biological process collection; p-values determined by hypergeometric tests.

Figure S6A) nor on startle response (p = 0.9724, 1-way ANOVA; Figure S6B).

Naïve $S1/2^{-/-}$ mice displayed pronounced impairment of PPI (p = 0.0071; Figure 5A) with most significant difference at prepulse 75 and 80 dB ($p_{Bonf} < 0.01$ and $p_{Bonf} < 0.05$, respectively). Startle response (Figure 5B) was similar in $S1/2^{-/-}$ mice and WT controls (p = 0.9958; 2-way ANOVA) and was not influenced significantly by vehicle injections (p = 0.1434; 2-way ANOVA).

Acute clozapine treatment (3 mg/kg) reduced startle response in both genotypes to similar extend when compared with vehicle injections (p = 0.0009; 2-way ANOVA, Figure 5B). Clozapine diminished PPI in WT mice when compared to vehicle treated animals (p = 0.0025; 2-way ANOVA, Figure 5C). Bonferroni posttest yielded significant difference at 70 dB prepulse ($p_{Bonf} <$

0.01). Clozapine had no effects on PPI in $S1/2^{-/-}$ mice (p = 0.9716; 2-way ANOVA, Figure 5D).

$S1/2^{-/-}$ and control mice showed habituation to 120 dB pulse during PPI assessment (naïve: p<0.0001; Figure S7A; vehicle: p = 0.0006; Figure S7B; clozapine: p = 0.0197; Figure S7C; 2-way ANOVA) which was comparable between the genotypes in all treatment groups (naïve: p = 0.4766; vehicle: p = 0.6974; clozapine: p = 0.6008; 2-way ANOVA).

We also assessed effects of vehicle and clozapine (3 mg/kg) injections in the open field (Figure S8). Vehicle injection reduced hyperactivity in $S1/2^{-/-}$ mutants and increased anxiety in WT and to a lesser extend also in $S1/2^{-/-}$ mutants (p_{MW} = 0.2380, Figure S8A and p_{MW} = 0.2250, Figure S8B). Clozapine treatment dramatically reduced the overall activity (p<0.0001; Figure S8A) and time spent in the center (p = 0.0009; Figure S8B) in both

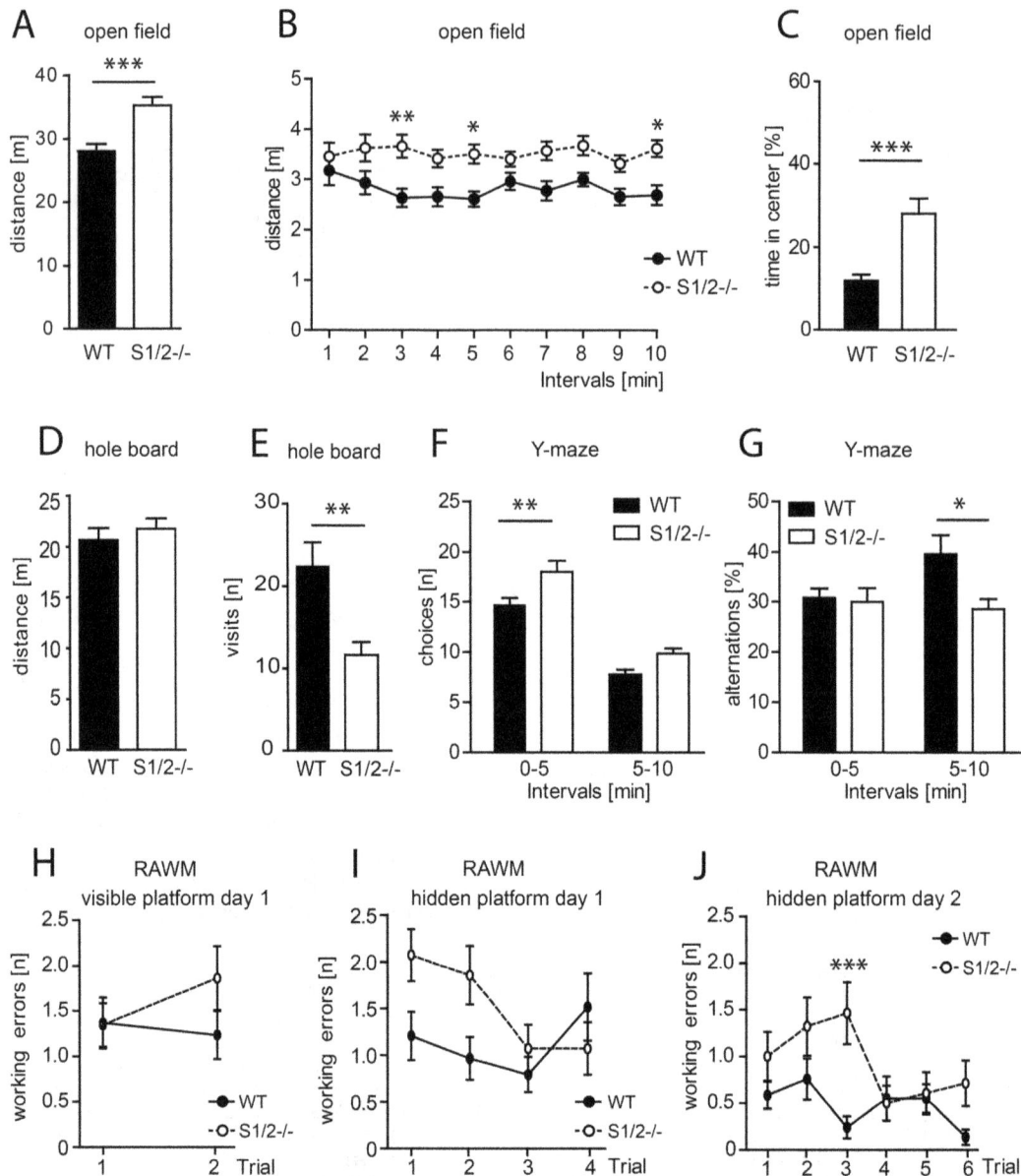

Figure 4. S1/2$^{-/-}$ mice display novelty induced hyperactivity, decreased anxiety and exploratory behavior and working memory disturbances. A–C) Open field test performed in a novel, unfamiliar test arena. WT: n = 24, S1/2$^{-/-}$: n = 26. A) Novelty-induced hyperactivity in S1/2$^{-/-}$ mice as assessed by moving distance in the open field (p$_{MW}$ = 0.0006). B) Analysis in 1 min bins yielded a significant E$_{genotype}$ (F$_{(1,48)}$ = 16.46; p = 0.0002). Moreover, Bonferroni posttest revealed the strongest difference between the genotypes in interval 3, 5 and 10 (p$_{Bonf}$<0.01, p$_{Bonf}$<0.05 and p$_{Bonf}$<0.05, respectively). C) Mutants spent more time in the center (p$_{MW}$ = 0.0004) of the test arena indicating reduced anxiety when compared to controls. D-E) Hole board test performed with a subsequent modification of the open field setup by floor insert with holes. WT: n = 24, S1/2$^{-/-}$: n = 26. D) S1/2$^{-/-}$ mice displayed no alterations in the overall activity measured as total distance travelled. E) S1/2$^{-/-}$ mice performed less nose pokes into holes (p$_{MW}$ = 0.0014) indicating decreased curiosity-related behavior compared to WT. F-G) Y-maze test. WT: n = 23, S1/2$^{-/-}$: n = 20. F) S1/2$^{-/-}$ mice showed increased activity in Y-maze test (E$_{genotype}$ F$_{(1,41)}$ = 10.98; p = 0.0019) most evident in interval 0-5 min (p$_{Bonf}$<0.01). G) Mutant mice performed less alterations in Y-maze than control animals (E$_{genotype}$ F$_{(1,41)}$ = 4.86; p = 0.0331) and p$_{Bonf}$<0.05 for interval 5–10 min. H-J) S1/2$^{-/-}$ mice display impairment of working memory in the radial arm water maze (RAWM). WT: n = 29, S1/2$^{-/-}$: n = 28. H) In the visible platform task, performance was similar in both genotypes (E$_{genotype}$ F$_{(1,55)}$ = 0.65; p = 0.4236). I-J) S1/2$^{-/-}$ mice showed increased number of working errors searching for a hidden platform on the first (I) (E$_{genotype}$ F$_{(1,55)}$ = 3.93; p = 0.0524; I$_{genotype \times time}$ F$_{(3,165)}$ = 2.68; p = 0.0486) and the second (J) day of experiment (E$_{genotype}$ F$_{(1,55)}$ = 9.05; p = 0.0044) and I$_{genotype \times time}$ F$_{(5,275)}$ = 2.34; p = 0.0422). Bonferroni posttest revealed significant difference during the 3rd trial of the second day (p$_{Bonf}$<0.001). WT, black bars/circles. S1/2$^{-/-}$, white bars/circles. Data were analyzed with 2-way ANOVA with Bonferroni posttest (p$_{Bonf}$) and Mann-Whitney test (p$_{MW}$) for pairwise comparisons. ***: p<0.001; **: p<0.01; *: p<0.05. E, effect; I, interaction of factors.

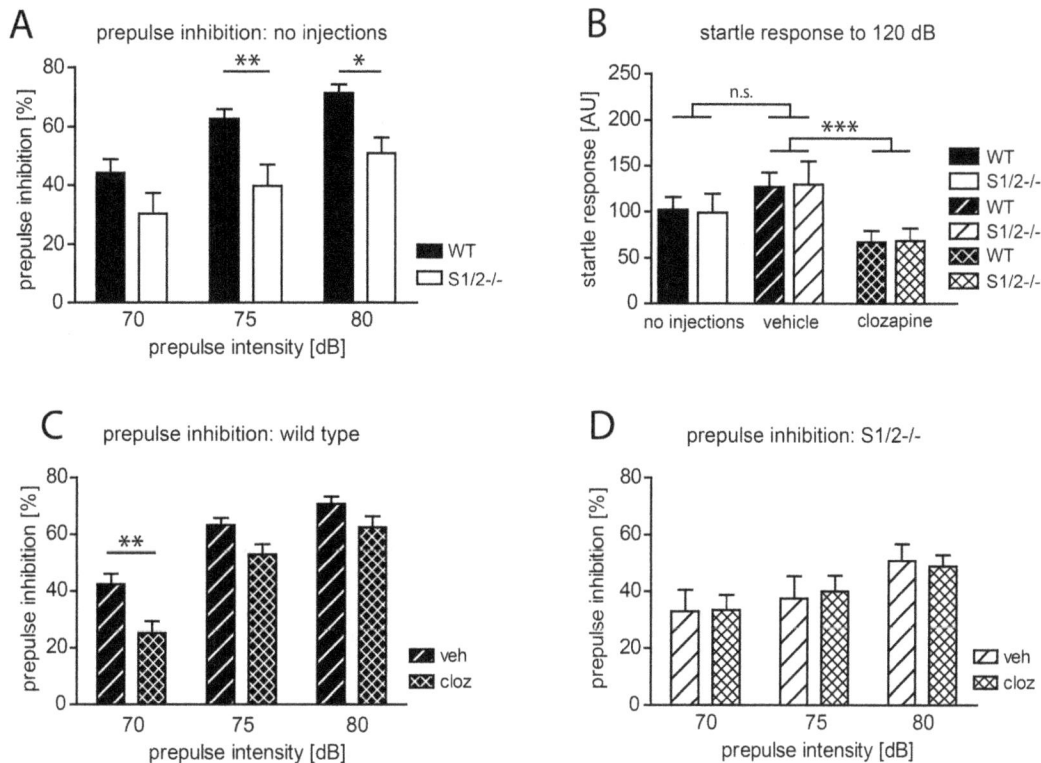

Figure 5. S1/2$^{-/-}$ mice show alterations of prepulse inhibition (PPI) which are resistant to Clozapine treatment. A) S1/2$^{-/-}$ mice display impairment of PPI ($E_{genotype}$ $F_{(1,43)} = 7.99$; $p = 0.0071$). Bonferroni posttest revealed significant difference in prepulse 75 und 80 dB ($p_{Bonf} < 0.01$ and $p_{Bonf} < 0.05$, respectively). WT: n = 24, S1/2$^{-/-}$: n = 21. B) Startle response was similar in S1/2$^{-/-}$ mice and WT controls ($E_{genotype}$ $F_{(1,88)} = 0.00$; $p = 0.9958$) and not influenced significantly by vehicle injections ($E_{treatment}$ $F_{(1,88)} = 2.18$; $p = 0.1434$). Acute clozapine treatment (3 mg/kg) reduced startle in both genotypes to similar extend ($E_{treatment}$ $F_{(1,82)} = 11.83$; $p = 0.0009$ and $E_{genotype}$ $F_{(1,82)} = 0.01$; $p = 0.9030$). 'No injections' and 'vehicle' groups: WT: n = 25, S1/2$^{-/-}$: n = 21; clozapine: WT: n = 20, S1/2$^{-/-}$: n = 20. C) Acute treatment with clozapine (cloz; 3 mg/kg; n = 20) reduced PPI in WT mice when compared to vehicle (veh; n = 24) treated WT animals ($E_{treatment}$ $F_{(1,42)} = 10.33$; $p = 0.0025$). Bonferroni posttest confirmed significant difference when prepulse 70 dB was applied ($p_{Bonf} < 0.01$). D) Acute treatment with clozapine (cloz; 3 mg/kg) did not influence PPI in S1/2$^{-/-}$ mice (n = 20) when compared to vehicle injected mutants (n = 21) ($E_{treatment}$ $F_{(1,39)} = 0.00$; $p = 0.9716$). Data were analyzed with 2-way ANOVA and Bonferroni posttest (p_{Bonf}). ***: $p < 0.001$; **: $p < 0.01$; *: $p < 0.05$. E, effect.

genotypes. However, clozapine effects were stronger on S1/2$^{-/-}$ mice regarding distance (interaction genotype × treatment p = 0.0296, 2-way ANOVA) and time in center (interaction genotype × treatment p = 0.0665, 2-way ANOVA).

Discussion

Altered sleep architecture in S1/2$^{-/-}$ mice

In this study, we have analyzed the sleep architecture, daytime-dependent gene expression in the cortex and behavior in SHARP1 and SHARP2 double deficient (S1/2$^{-/-}$) mice. Our data show that sleep-wake profiles, responses of REM sleep and theta oscillations to sleep deprivation, running wheel behavior and activity-related cortical gene expression are altered in S1/2$^{-/-}$ animals, although the 24 h cumulated total amount of sleep and wakefulness and overall circadian rhythmicity remain unaltered. The alteration of sleep architecture in S1/2$^{-/-}$ mutants, however, does not phenocopy mice that express the human SHARP1/DEC2(P385R) protein which display a reduction in total sleep time [38]. This implies that the P385R mutant SHARP1 protein does not act in a 'simple' dominant-negative fashion interfering with SHARP1/2 repressor functions [38], i.e. by forming heterotypic homo- or heterodimers with 'wild-type' proteins. Since SHARP1 and SHARP2 can homo- and heterodimerize [52] and function in a context dependent fashion either as repressors and co-activators of

CLOCK, NPAS2 as well as other transcriptional regulators [35], it might be possible that the mutant SHARP1/DEC2(P385R) protein could be mechanistically specific e.g. by only affecting discrete repressive functions. This hypothesis should be addressed experimentally and might be helpful in understanding the molecular mechanisms that cause distinct sleep phenotypes in S1/2$^{-/-}$ mice versus those expressing the SHARP1/DEC2(P385R) mutant protein. In addition, S1/2$^{-/-}$ mice display alterations e.g. in REM sleep that have not been observed in SHARP1 single mutants [38]. Moreover, we found that REM sleep associated theta oscillations were altered in S1/2$^{-/-}$ mice upon sleep deprivation. Thus, loss of SHARP function causes an altered adaptability of environmental stressors at the level of neuronal synchronizations which may be of relevance for psychiatric disease related behavior such as anxiety [30,53].

SHARP1/2 mutants display 'mixed-state' endophenotypes of psychiatric diseases

In a novel environment, S1/2$^{-/-}$ mice display locomotor hyperactivity and diminished anxiety comparable to mania-like behavior. Diminished anxiety can be interpreted as increased risk taking [54], one of symptoms of BD [55]. However, alterations in other anxiety tests were absent; possibly because different anxiety tests monitor distinct types of emotional behavior as suggested previously [56,57]. Contrasting anxiety phenotypes have also been found in mice haploinsufficient for the SZ/BD risk gene CACNA1c [58,59] and in mice heterozygous for the BD associated gene *Ank3* showing altered behavior in elevated plus maze and light-dark preference but not in the open field test [60]. However, no hyperactivity was detected in S1/2$^{-/-}$ animals in a more intimate environment resembling the phenotype of mice with a dopamine transporter knockdown where mania-like exploratory behavior is present in novel but diminished in a familiar environment [61]. In S1/2$^{-/-}$ mice, specific exploration measured by nose pokes was diminished resembling more depression-like symptoms. Similarly, when monitored for the 24 h voluntary locomotor activity profile in home cage, S1/2$^{-/-}$ mice displayed hypoactivity during the dark phase (D) which correlates with the observed relative increase of sleep in D. The locomotor hypoactivity, reduced exploratory drive and increased sleepiness in the active phase in S1/2$^{-/-}$ mutants are more reminiscent of a depression-like state. Mixed-state or paradoxical phenotypes of mania- and depression-like behavior have previously been observed when inactivating CLOCK selectively in the hypothalamus [62]. Mouse mutants lacking functional CLOCK or NPAS2 show locomotor hyperactivity and reduced sleep in D [28,29], which has been interpreted as mania-like behavior in CLOCK deficient mice [29]. Therefore, SHARP1/2 mutant mice meet selected 'mixed-state' criteria for face validity towards BD similarly to *Clock* mutants [63]. Nonetheless, it is still unclear which of the mixed-state phenotypes are a direct or indirect consequence of loss of SHARP1/2 functions. It is possible that feedback mechanisms operate at the molecular and behavioral level that cause mutual relationships e.g. between sleep and affective phenotypes seen in S1/2$^{-/-}$ mice.

Altered endophenotypes at the circuitry level

The spectrum of endophenotypes in S1/2$^{-/-}$ mice with relevance for psychiatric diseases is further expanded by the working memory impairments and PPI deficits. Working memory deficits are prominent in SZ and BD [46–48] and corresponding animal models [64–68]. In concordance with published data, acute clozapine treatment reduced PPI in WT [67] but had no further effect on the low PPI levels in S1/2$^{-/-}$ mice. Interestingly, clozapine is also not effective in more than 50% of treatment resistant schizophrenic patients [69]. Although clozapine had differential effects on PPI, it reduced to a similar extend startle amplitude in both S1/2$^{-/-}$ mutant and control mice which has been described in mice [67,68] and human subjects [70]; however, showing stronger sedative effects on S1/2$^{-/-}$ mutants. Resistance of S1/2$^{-/-}$ mice towards clozapine in PPI may be partially related to the blunted DRD2 expression in these mutants [71,72], although other mechanisms might also be involved given the broad pharmacological profile of clozapine. Therefore, S1/2$^{-/-}$ mice may be a valuable model to test novel compounds or therapies to overcome clozapine resistance.

Cortical gene expression profiling reveals associations with psychiatric diseases

We applied unbiased bioinformatic algorithms to identify biological process and disease associations with gene sets obtained from cortical gene expression profiling in WT and S1/2$^{-/-}$ mice [41,42]. These analyses use curator-indexed literature databases and do not provide direct experimental evidence. Nonetheless, these analyses identified several psychiatric diseases (particularly mood- and psychotic disorders) correlating with SHARP1/2 dysfunction-associated cortical gene expression. To substantiate these findings, we scanned the mouse phenotype database

provided by the Jax labs (www.informatics.jax.org/phenotypes. shtml) and found that *Drd2* and *Adora2a* mouse mutants were associated with 'hypoactivity' (mouse phenotype ID MP:0001402) [73,74] and display altered behavioral adaptability to psychostimulants [75,76]. Polymorphisms in *ADORA2A* may modulate psychomotor vigilance and sleep EEG [76] and it has been previously noted that *DRD2* variants are associated with mood disorders [77]. In addition, DRD2 represents an interesting pharmacological target for the treatment of psychosis [78] and ADORA2A has been suggested as a target for the treatment of psychiatric diseases [79]. Moreover, we detected attenuated gene expression of three myelin genes (*Enpp2, Plp1, Cldn11*) in the cortex of S1/2$^{-/-}$ mice. This finding provides an additional link with psychiatric diseases since reduced expression of oligodendrocyte/myelin markers is among the most replicated molecular observations in psychiatric diseases including SZ and major depression, although an underlying mechanistic concept for these observations is still missing [80–82].

Disintegration of activity-dependent and circadian processes

Among the few upregulated genes in the cortex of S1/2$^{-/-}$ mice at ZT16 were three canonical circadian factors (*Per1, Per2* and *Cry1*) indicating a functional clock in agreement with previous observations [35,83]. The sleep-wake amplitude in expression of these circadian genes, however, was attenuated, although not completely abolished, as compared to that of plasticity-related genes. It has been noted before that the expression of clock regulated genes in the cortex is not strictly controlled by circadian mechanisms only [21] which may explain the partially reduced amplitude under LD and DD conditions in S1/2$^{-/-}$ mice. We also detected the genes *Penk* and *Tac* encoding the neuropeptides preproenkephalin and tachykinin as deregulated in the cortex of S1/2$^{-/-}$ mice. These hormones have been associated with anxiety, analgesic effects and altered stress responses [84,85]. It is therefore possible that these and potentially other neuroendocrine factors may have caused or modulated some of the behavioral alterations observed in S1/2$^{-/-}$ mice.

Sleep-wake behavior is regulated by circadian and homeostatic processes [13–15]. Therefore, the attenuated running wheel profile of S1/2$^{-/-}$ mice in L, which is paralleled by increased NREM sleep levels and reduced activity-regulated gene expression, could be driven by disturbance of a thus far unknown homeostatic process. In consequence, an uncoupling of homeostatic and circadian processes could explain the molecular and behavioral alterations seen in S1/2$^{-/-}$ mice. The identification of the postulated homeostatic process(es) altered upon loss of SHARP1 and -2 could help to better understand the link between the disturbed sleep architecture and the molecular and behavioral consequences.

Network modelling of all deregulated genes including SHARP1 and SHARP2 revealed a bipartite assembly of activity/plasticity genes and circadian factors that were connected by SHARP1 and PER1. It may thus be possible that particularly SHARP1 and also PER1 may be key regulators integrating plasticity-related as well as circadian and homeostatic processes in the cortex. As shown in this study, the loss of SHARP function results in a disintegration of both processes consequently leading to psychiatric (endo)phenotypes. Recent observations made with *Sharp1/2* and *Per1* triple null mutant mice, however, revealed a genetic interaction of these factors in the regulation of circadian locomotor activity [37]. In light of our findings presented in this study, it might thus be interesting to characterize sleep and behavior also in *Sharp1/2* and *Per1* triple mutants.

In summary, our findings support the hypothesis that abnormal sleep and certain (endo)phenotypes of psychiatric diseases may be caused by common mechanisms involving components of the molecular clock including SHARP1 and SHARP2. Moreover, genetically defined mouse models of circadian genes with distinct (endo)phenotype profiles, such as S1/2$^{-/-}$ mice, may be useful for pre-clinical treatment trials in the context of psychiatric diseases including sleep and mood disorders.

Materials and Methods

Animal experiments

All animal experiments were conducted in accordance with NIH principles of laboratory animal care and were approved by the Government of Lower Saxony, Germany. The experiments were performed with cohorts of adult male mice aged 3–5 months, respectively. Cohorts of mice within experiments were age matched (±2 weeks). Parental single heterozygous mice were independently backcrossed to C57Bl/6J for more than ten generations as described previously [35]. Wild-type (WT) and *Sharp1* and *-2* double mutant mice (S1/2$^{-/-}$) were obtained from double heterozygous breeding pairs [35,86]. All experimental animals were group housed in the same ventilated sound-attenuated rooms under a 12 h light/12 h dark schedule at an ambient temperature of 21°C with food and water available *ad libitum*. All experiments were performed blinded to genotypes.

Surgical implantation procedures

Surgery was performed under deep intraperitoneal anaesthesia with Ketamine/Xylazine (100 mg/kg; 10 mg/kg). Two stainless steel screws (diameter 0.7 mm; Plastics One) were implanted epidurally in the skull over the right parietal cortex (1.7 mm lateral to midline, 1.0 mm anterior to lambda) and the left frontal cortex (1.7 mm lateral to midline and 1.5 mm anterior to bregma) to derive the electroencephalogram (EEG). A third screw over the left hemisphere served as anchor screw. For electromyographic (EMG) recordings two stainless steel wires were inserted into the neck muscles bilaterally. All electrodes were connected to a mouse-adapted socket (Plastics One), which was fixed with dental acrylic cement.

EEG Recordings

After surgery the animals were allowed to recover for at least 2 weeks before data acquisition. To habituate to recording conditions animals were connected to the recording lead attached to a swivel contact at least 4 days before the start of experiments. Recordings were performed on three consecutive 24 h periods starting at lights-on. Day one was not analyzed, day two served as baseline recordings and on day three animals were sleep deprived by gentle handling. EEG and EMG signals of four animals (two of each genotype) were recorded simultaneously to equally distribute environmental disturbances. EEG and EMG signals were amplified, filtered, analog-digital-converted at 256 Hz and stored on a computer hard disk (Sleep Sign Acquisition, Kissei Comtec). Three vigilance states, wakefulness (W), non rapid eye movement sleep (NREM) and rapid eye movement sleep (REM), were determined offline (Sleep Sign Analysis, Kissei Comtec) in epochs of 4 s by visual assessment of EEG- and EMG-recordings. Epochs containing more than one vigilance state were scored as the prevailing one and epochs containing recording artefacts were omitted from subsequent spectral analysis. The amount of each vigilance state was expressed as percentage of recording time.

Spectral analysis and measurement of slow-wave-activity

For each 4 s epoch scored as NREM or REM sleep, EEG was subjected to a fast Fourier Transformation (FFT) analysis, yielding power spectra between 0.5 and 20 Hz with a 0.5 Hz resolution (Sleep Sign Analysis, Kissei Comtec). Slow wave activity (SWA) in NREM sleep was calculated as the mean power over the frequency range between 0.5 and 4.0 Hz. All SWA measures were expressed as percentage of the individual mean SWA over the last 900 NREM epochs in the baseline light period to correct for individual differences in the absolute power.

Spectral analysis and determination of theta peak frequency

EEG spectral profiles of REM sleep are dominated by frequencies in the Theta band range. To determine the prevailing frequency in REM sleep, the distribution of peak frequency was calculated. Means of FFT spectra of artefact-free 4 s epochs were calculated over two-hour intervals and the frequency of the maximal power in the range between 5 and 10 Hz determined for these mean frequency distributions.

Running wheel analysis of activity profiles

Activity data were recorded and evaluated using the ClockLab data collection and analysis software (Actimetrics) as described previously [35]. To obtain a full activity profile, 24 h accumulated activities of running wheel recordings over a 5 day period were analyzed in 18 min bins.

Tissue Sampling and gene expression analysis

Cortical tissue (bregma 0 to −2 mm) was isolated using a 'rodent brain matrix' 1 mm coronal slicer (ASI Instruments, Warren, MI) from adult WT and S1/2$^{-/-}$ mice harvested at ZT0, ZT4, ZT8, ZT12, ZT16, ZT20 and independent cohorts analyzed at ZT4, ZT16, CT4 and CT16 (n = 3 for each genotype and time point). Animals were kept 24 h under DD (12 h dark, 12 h dark) before being sacrificed under dim red light for the analysis of all CT time points. To analyze gene expression in response to sleep deprivation, cortical samples were collected as described above with a rodent brain matrix and pooled (n = 4 each time point and genotype). RNA was prepared according to the manufacturer's protocols using RNeasy colums (Qiagen, Hilden, Germany) and analyzed for integrity using the Bioanalyzer (Agilent Technologies). The minimal RNA-integrity (RIN) value threshold was 8.5. For microarray analysis, one-round RNA amplification, labeling and hybridization were essentially performed as previously described [87]. Microarrays were scanned and pre-processed according to standard protocols given by the manufacturer (Affymetrix). Array data were analyzed using either R-scripts (www.bioconductor.org) or the Genomics Suite (Partek). Differential gene expression over time was determined using ANOVA and for genotype comparisons by applying moderate T-statistics (using the corresponding bioconductor package). Selection cut-offs were set to fold-changes>1.5 and corrected p-values <0.05. Gene set enrichment analysis (GSEA) of *a priori* defined sets of functionally grouped genes was performed using the GSEA software package downloaded from www.broadinstitute.org/gsea and implemented locally. Analyses were performed with default parameters (permutations set to 1000) and gene sets available in the molecular signature database (MSigDB v3.0) as described previously [87].

Quantitative PCR was performed with an ABI PRISM 7700 detection system (Perkin Elmer), essentially as described [88]. Primers directed against mouse transcripts (Table S4) were designed online at the Roche assay design center (www.roche-applied-science.com/sis/rtpcr/upl/) and used in SYBRgreen assays.

Gene Ontology and network analysis

Gene Ontology (GO) analysis was performed with Genomics Suite (Partek) and MetaCore (GeneGo) using categories provided by the GO consortium (www.geneontology.org). Gene-disease association and network modelling was performed with MetaCore (GeneGo) using manually curated disease databases compiled from RefSeq annotations (http://www.ncbi.nlm.nih.gov/refseq/rsg/) and literature minings listed as interlinked pubmed entries with each gene in the corresponding disease database as implemented in the software (www.genego.com). Dijkstra's shortest path algorithm with a maximum of steps set to 1 was applied for network modeling and hypergeometric tests for GO enrichment and gene/disease associations as implemented in the software.

Behavioral analysis

Mice were tested for free running activity (in home cage), in open field, hole board, elevated plus maze, light-dark preference, tail suspension test, hot plate, Y-maze, radial arm water maze and prepulse inhibition. Behavioral tests monitoring for novelty induced activity, anxiety and curiosity (open filed and hole board), anxiety (elevated plus maze and light-dark preference), pain sensitivity (hot plate), escape motivation and/or depression (tail suspension) and sensorimotor gating (prepulse inhibition test) were essentially performed as described previously [64] Experiments were performed between ZT2-ZT6 during light phase or between ZT 14-18 in the wake-phase and under dim red light where indicated.

Light-dark preference

The light dark preference test was conducted in a box consisting of compartments of the same size: one with black walls (dark) connected by a door with light compartment build of transparent Plexiglas. Mice were placed in the transparent compartment facing the wall and left undisturbed. Latency to enter the dark, the time spent in the dark box and crossings between two compartments were scored for 5 min.

Y-maze

Y-maze was performed using a custom made Y-shaped runway. Mice were put into maze facing the wall and allowed to explore undisturbed the maze for 10 min. The experiment was video recorded and analyzed offline. The number of arm choices (as a measure of activity) and the percent of alterations (choices of a "novel" arm, different than chosen before as a measure of working memory) were scored. The apparatus was cleaned between animals with 70% ethanol p.a. to avoid olfactory cues.

Radial arm water maze

Radial arm water maze (RAWM) was performed following a published protocol [89] with minor changes using an in house built setup based on the authors' specifications containing six arms extending out of a central area. The setup was built out of white plastic and positioned in white painted water so that the walls protruded 20 cm above the water surface. Briefly, mice were trained in RAWM to search for a platform submerged 1 cm below the water surface at the end of the goal arm. On day 1, animals were given two trials to learn to escape from water on a platform tagged with a flag (visible platform task) starting from alternating

arms. Next, the flag was removed, visual cues (contrast-reach graphical forms like a cross, concentric circles, stripes etc.) were fixed on terminal walls of arms and mice were trained during 4 trials to find a platform submerged under water surface (hidden platform task). The duration of each trial (both in visible and hidden task) was 90 s; during this time mice were allowed to swim to the goal arm guided by visual cues. In case of an error defined as choice of a different arm than the goal arm, mice were immediately removed from the wrong arm, put gently again into the start arm and released. Entries into a goal arm, even if the platform was not located, were not counted as errors. If animals entered the wrong arm and after being brought to the start position repeated again the same wrong choice, this was counted as a "working error". The procedure was repeated until mice found a platform (cut off time of 90 s). If mice were not able to find a platform within the given latency, they were gently guided to the proper position and were allowed to stay on the platform for 20 s for information acquisition. Intermittent to all trials, the water was gently mixed to avoid olfactory cues by urination or defecation. Mice were kept on the warm platform (37°C) to avoid body hypothermia between trials.

Sucrose preference test

A sucrose preference test was set up in a standard plastic cage (Makrolon Type II) with normal bedding and with food *ad libitum*. Prior the experiment, two weight balanced water bottles were placed on each cage and weighted 24 hours later to exclude side preferences. On the second day, each cage was equipped with one bottle filled with 4% sucrose solution and one with water prepared freshly every day and provided at the same time point. Position of bottles (left versus right) was changed daily. Liquid intake was measured by weight of consumed water/sucrose solution over 24 h for 4 days.

Drugs

Clozapine was purchased by Sigma-Aldrich (Germany) and dissolved in a drop of 0.1 M HCl, mixed with saline, pH adjusted to 5.3. Mice were injected i.p. with Clozapine (3 mg/kg) or with vehicle (saline pH 5.3) in volume of 10 ml/kg 30 min prior to behavioral testing.

Statistical analysis

EEG and behavioral data are presented as means ± standard error of the mean (SEM) and were compared by ANOVA with Bonferroni (Bonf) post-hoc tests for repeated measurements or Mann-Whitney (MW) tests for genotype comparisons using GraphPad Prism 4 and 5 (GraphPad Software, San Diego, California). p values were indicated as p_{Bonf} or p_{MW}, respectively. Moderate T-statistics and ANOVA were applied for gene expression data (using the corresponding R-packages at www.bioconductor.org and Genomics Suite, Partek). For qRT-PCR analysis the Mann-Whitney test was applied when normality testing failed and the unpaired two-tailed T-test for data showing normal distribution using GraphPad Prism 5. A p-values less than 0.05 were considered significant for all tests applied. Abbreviations for 2way ANOVA in figure legends are as follows: E, effect; I, interaction of factors.

Supporting Information

Figure S1   EEG recordings upon sleep deprivation. A–C) Time course of the vigilance states wakefulness (A), NREM (B) and REM sleep (C) after 6 h of sleep deprivation (SD) performed from ZT0-6. Curves connect 2-h bin mean values (±SEM) expressed as percentage of recording time ($I_{genotype \times time\ of\ day}$: wakefulness $F_{(2, 20)} = 0.23$, p = 0.51; NREM $F_{(2,20)} = 0.41$, p = 0.67; REM $F_{(2,20)} = 0.69$, p = 0.51). WT, n = 7, filled circles. $S1/2^{-/-}$, n = 8, empty circles. Data were analyzed with 2-way ANOVA. *: = p< 0.05 in two-tailed post hoc T-test). I, interaction of factors.

Figure S2   Delta and theta wave oscillations of undisturbed sleep and upon sleep deprivation. A) Baseline slow-wave activity and SD induced rebound sleep in $S1/2^{-/-}$ mice. Slow-wave activity (SWA) was plotted over a 24 h period as percentage of the individual mean SWA over the last 900 NREM epochs in the baseline light period. Using 2-way ANOVA with the factors genotype and time, we detected no significant differences between baseline and SD recordings between WT and $S1/2^{-/-}$ mice. However, a trend towards a higher SWA in $S1/2^{-/-}$ mice was detected. WT: n = 7, $S1/2^{-/-}$: n = 8. B) Group means (±SEM, WT: black bars; $S1/2^{-/-}$: white bars) for mean theta peak frequency (TPF) during REM sleep in consecutive 6-h blocks (L1 = ZT0-6; L2 = ZT7-12; D1 = ZT13-18; D2 = ZT17-24) of baseline recordings (blank bars) and after 6-h SD (hatched bars). TPF varied with time-of-day and was significantly higher in the $S1/2^{-/-}$ group during the 6 h following SD (2-way ANOVA: $E_{genotype}$ $F_{(3,66)} = 2.99$ p = 0.04; E_{time} $F_{(2,66)} = 4.61$; p = 0.01; $I_{genotype \times time}$: $F_{6, 66)} = 0.46$, p = 0.83; asterisks indicate significances between genotypes in post hoc T-test, ** = p<0.01) WT: n = 7, $S1/2^{-/-}$: n = 8. C–D) Power distribution in the 5–10 Hz range comparing fast-fourier transformed (FFT) EEG spectra of WT and $S1/2^{-/-}$ during baseline conditions (C; $I_{frequency \times genotype}$ $F_{(12,117)} = 0.57$, p = 0.8588) and after SD (D; $I_{frequency \times genotype}$ $F_{(12,117)} = 2.57$, p = 0.0047). Note the significant shift of the theta component particularly between 6 and 7 Hz (p<0.05, post-hoc T-test). Data were analyzed with 2-way ANOVA. WT: n = 7, $S1/2^{-/-}$: n = 8. SD, sleep deprivation; base, baseline. E, effect; I, interaction of factors.

Figure S3   Divergent gene expression differences at ZT16 in the cortex of WT and $S1/2^{-/-}$ mice as revealed by gene set enrichment analysis (GSEA). A) P-value versus enrichment plot comparing cortical gene expression of WT with $S1/2^{-/-}$ mice using the GENMAPP gene data sets. With a false-discovery rate (FDR) q-value cut-off set at 0.25 (default of the GSEA algorithm), six gene sets were found to be upregulated in WT samples whereas only two were significantly upregulated in $S1/2^{-/-}$ mice (labeled by a black ellipses). The normalized enrichment score (NES) is plotted versus the FDR q-value (red dots) and the nominal p-value (black dots). B) Statistical parameters of the most significantly deregulated gene sets (FDR q-value <0.25). The most significantly WT versus $S1/2^{-/-}$ upregulated gene sets at ZT16 correspond to molecular machineries involved in protein/RNA synthesis and turnover as well as oxidative phosphorylation, likely reflecting the higher metabolic demand in WT animals at ZT16 due to increased activity and wakefulness. In $S1/2^{-/-}$ cortex, only two (highly similar) gene sets comprising class A and peptide GPCRs were detected as upregulated. SIZE, number of genes; ES, Enrichment score; NES, normalized enrichment score; Nom p-val, nominal p-value; FDR q-val, false discovery rate corrected q-value; FWER p-val, family wise error rate. C-D) Enrichment plots of the top deregulated gene sets encoding for components of proteasome (gene rank order depicted as vertical lines left-shifted = up in WT) and members of the class A GPCR family (gene rank order

depicted as vertical lines right-shifted = up in $S1/2^{-/-}$). n = 2 per timepoint and genotype.

Figure S4   Altered gene expression profiles of control, circadian and activity-regulated genes in the cortex of WT and $S1/2^{-/-}$ mice under baseline and sleep deprivation conditions. A) Schematic drawing of the experimental schedule. WT and $S1/2^{-/-}$ controls (base) and WT and $S1/2^{-/-}$ animals that were sleep deprived from ZT0-6 (SD) were sacrificed at ZT10-12 for cortex preparations and marker gene expression analysis (n = 4 per each condition and genotype). B) Relative gene expression changes of control (*Atp5b*, *Actb*), selected circadian (*Per1*, *Per2*) and immediate early gene products (*Fos*, *Egr1*) in cortex samples plotted as fold changes between baseline and SD values (base/SD) for WT and $S1/2^{-/-}$ groups.

Figure S5 $S1/2^{-/-}$ mice show normal behavior in elevated plus maze, light-dark preference and tail suspension test. A) $S1/2^{-/-}$ mice display normal performance spending similar time in closed arms in elevated plus maze when compared with WT controls ($p_{MW} = 0.8693$). WT: n = 23, $S1/2^{-/-}$: n = 21. B) Time spent in the dark compartment during light-dark preference test was similar between both genotypes ($p_{MW} = 0.1917$). WT: n = 25, $S1/2^{-/-}$: n = 18. C) Tail suspension test did not found significant difference in struggling behavior in $S1/2^{-/-}$ mice ($p_{MW} = 0.9456$). WT: n = 24, $S1/2^{-/-}$: n = 21. D) $S1/2^{-/-}$ mice consume similar volume of sucrose solution as WT controls ($E_{genotype}$ $F_{(1,41)} = 1.93$; p = 0.1719). WT: n = 23, $S1/2^{-/-}$: n = 20. wt: black bars; $S1/2^{-/-}$: white bars. Data were analyzed with 2-way ANOVA or Mann-Whitney test (p_{MW}) for pairwise comparisons. E, effect.

Figure S6   Multiple testing has no significant effects on prepulse inhibition (PPI) in control C57Bl/6 wild type mice. A) C57Bl/6 wild type mice (n = 11) were tested in PPI test on three consecutive days. There are no significant effects of multiple testing on PPI observed (E_{time} $F_{(2,60)} = 1.93$; p = 0.1539). B) Startle response was similar on three testing days (p = 0.9724). Data were analyzed with 2-way ANOVA (A) and 1-way ANOVA (B). E, effect.

Figure S7   SHARP1/2 mutant and control mice show similar habituation to 120 dB pulse. A) Naïve (not injected) $S1/2^{-/-}$ mice and their wildtype littermates showed comparable habituation (E_{time} $F_{(1,44)} = 21.92$; p<0.0001) which was similar between the genotypes ($E_{genotype}$ $F_{(1,44)} = 0.52$; p = 0.4766). WT: n = 25; $S1/2^{-/-}$: n = 21. B) Mice injected with vehicle display habituation (E_{time} $F_{(1,44)} = 13.73$; p = 0.0006) which is not altered in mutants ($E_{genotype}$ $F_{(1,44)} = 0.15$; p = 0.6974). WT: n = 25; $S1/2^{-/-}$: n = 21. C) Animals treated with clozapine (3 mg/kg) habituate to startling pulse (E_{time} $F_{(1,38)} = 5.93$; p = 0.0197) independent of the genotype ($E_{genotype}$ $F_{(1,38)} = 0.28$; p = 0.6008). WT: n = 20; $S1/2^{-/-}$: n = 20. Data were analyzed with 2-way ANOVA. E, effect.

Figure S8 $S1/2^{-/-}$ mice respond stronger to clozapine treatment in the open field than WT controls. A) In a familiar open field box, hyperactivity in vehicle injected $S1/2^{-/-}$ mice was not evident ($p_{MW} = 0.2380$). Clozapine reduced distance travelled ($E_{treatment}$ $F_{(1,38)} = 103.89$; p<0.0001). A 2-way ANOVA yielded a significant $I_{genotype \times treatment}$ ($F_{(1,38)} = 5.11$; p = 0.0296). B) Vehicle treated $S1/2^{-/-}$ mice showed tendency to spend more time in the center of the familiar test arena ($p_{MW} = 0.2250$). Time spent in the center of the open field was reduced by clozapine ($F_{(1,38)} = 13.10$; $p = 0.0009$) in both genotypes. However, clozapine effects were stronger in S1/2$^{-/-}$ mice ($I_{genotype \times treatment}$ $F_{(1,38)} = 3.57$; $p = 0.0665$). Vehicle treated mice: WT: n = 25; S1/2$^{-/-}$: n = 21; clozapine: WT: n = 20; S1/2$^{-/-}$: n = 20. E, effect; I, interaction of factors.

Figure S9 Description of network objects. Graphical symbols describing functional classification of network objects (nodes = genes or functionally grouped genes; edges = connections between nodes) represent default settings by the MetaCore software as depicted.

Table S1 Genes differentially regulated at ZT4 versus ZT16 in cortex samples of WT and S1/2$^{-/-}$ mice. The selection cut-off was set to fold-change (FC) of at least 1.5 and p-value of <0.05 in WT (including all genes/probe sets with yellow and blue background). Note, that *Penk* was detected with two probe sets to be upregulated at ZT16 in the WT cortex and that only one gene (*Chl1*) showed a significant downregulation at ZT16 (indicated by a negative FC). In S1/2$^{-/-}$ mice, five genes were detected to be significantly de-regulated between ZT4 and ZT16 with a p-value <0.05 (blue background), the corresponding FC values were, however, reduced compared to the WT. (n = 4 independent samples per genotype and two replicates per timepoint, p<0.05 was considered significant by ANOVA). We validated the attenuated cortical gene expression in S1/2$^{-/-}$ mice with quantitative RT-PCR (qRT-PCR) for 10 genes in LD and

DD (indicated at the table on the right: ZT4 vs 16 and CT4 vs 16, correspondingly (n = 3 per timepoint per genotype).

Table S2 Normalized expression values of microarray data. Depicted are the means and corresponding standard deviation (SD) of normalized microarray data from ZT4 and ZT16 cortex samples of WT and S1/2$^{-/-}$ mice (n = 2 per timepoint per genotype).

Table S3 List of protein names, gene symbols and synonyms.

Table S4 Table of genes and primer sequences used for gene expression analysis.

Acknowledgments

We like to acknowledge the staff of the MPI-EM's workshop for their support in designing and manufacturing mouse adapted EEG equipment. We also like to thank W. Paulus (UMG, Göttingen) for the access to the EEG setup, K.-A. Nave (Göttingen, MPI-EM) for discussions and support.

Author Contributions

Conceived and designed the experiments: PCB MMB MJR. Performed the experiments: PCB MMB AS LR CK HO MJR. Analyzed the data: PCB MMB AS SPW HO JH MJR. Contributed reagents/materials/analysis tools: RT MCW. Wrote the paper: PCB MMB MJR.

References

1. Toh KL, Jones CR, He Y, Eide EJ, Hinz WA, et al (2001) An hPer2 phosphorylation site mutation in familial advanced sleep phase syndrome. Science 291: 1040–3.
2. Nievergelt CM, Kripke DF, Remick RA, Sadovnick AD, McElroy SL, et al (2005) Examination of the clock gene Cryptochrome 1 in bipolar disorder: mutational analysis and absence of evidence for linkage or association. Psychiatr Genet 15: 45–52.
3. Nievergelt CM, Kripke DF, Barrett TB, Burg E, Remick RA, et al (2006) Suggestive evidence for association of the circadian genes PERIOD3 and ARNTL with bipolar disorder. Am J Med Genet B Neuropsychiatr Genet 141B:234–41. doi:10.1002/ajmg.b.30252.
4. Xu Y, Padiath QS, Shapiro RE, Jones CR, Wu SC, et al (2005) Functional consequences of a CKIdelta mutation causing familial advanced sleep phase syndrome. Nature 434: 640–4. doi:10.1038/nature03453.
5. Shi J, Wittke-Thompson JK, Badner JA, Hattori E, Potash JB, et al (2008) Clock genes may influence bipolar disorder susceptibility and dysfunctional circadian rhythm. Am J Med Genet B Neuropsychiatr Genet 147B: 1047–55. doi:10.1002/ajmg.b.30714.
6. Mansour HA, Talkowski ME, Wood J, Chowdari KV, McClain L, et al (2009) Association study of 21 circadian genes with bipolar I disorder, schizoaffective disorder, and schizophrenia. Bipolar Disord 11: 701–10. doi:10.1111/j.1399-5618.2009.00756.x.
7. Soria V, Martínez-Amorós E, Escaramís G, Valero J, Pérez-Egea R, et al (2010) Differential association of circadian genes with mood disorders: CRY1 and NPAS2 are associated with unipolar major depression and CLOCK and VIP with bipolar disorder. Neuropsychopharmacology 35: 1279–89. doi:10.1038/npp.2009.230.
8. Wulff K, Gatti S, Wettstein JG, Foster RG (2010) Sleep and circadian rhythm disruption in psychiatric and neurodegenerative disease. Nat Rev Neurosci 11: 589–99. doi:10.1038/nrn2868.
9. Coogan AN, Thome J (2011) Chronotherapeutics and psychiatry: setting the clock to relieve the symptoms. World J Biol Psychiatry 12 Suppl 1: 40–3. doi:10.3109/15622975.2011.598389.
10. Wu JC, Kelsoe JR, Schachat C, Bunney BG, DeModena A, et al (2009) Rapid and sustained antidepressant response with sleep deprivation and chronotherapy in bipolar disorder. Biol Psychiatry 66: 298–301. doi:10.1016/j.biopsych.2009.02.018.
11. Nicholas B, Rudrasingham V, Nash S, Kirov G, Owen MJ, et al (2007) Association of Per1 and Npas2 with autistic disorder: support for the clock genes/social timing hypothesis. Mol Psychiatry 12: 581–92. doi:10.1038/sj.mp.4001953.
12. Harvey AG (2008) Sleep and circadian rhythms in bipolar disorder: seeking synchrony, harmony, and regulation. Am J Psychiatry 165: 820–9. doi:10.1176/appi.ajp.2008.08010098.
13. Borbély AA, Achermann P (1999) Sleep homeostasis and models of sleep regulation. J Biol Rhythms 14: 557–68.
14. Scharf MT, Naidoo N, Zimmerman JE, Pack AI (2008) The energy hypothesis of sleep revisited. Prog Neurobiol 86: 264–80. doi:10.1016/j.pneurobio.2008.08.003.
15. Franken P, Dijk D-J (2009) Circadian clock genes and sleep homeostasis. Eur J Neurosci 29: 1820–9. doi:10.1111/j.1460-9568.2009.06723.x.
16. Zhu B, Dong Y, Xu Z, Gompf HS, Ward SAP, et al (2012) Sleep disturbance induces neuroinflammation and impairment of learning and memory. Neurobiology of Disease 48: 348–55. doi:10.1016/j.nbd.2012.06.022.
17. Postuma RB, Gagnon J-F, Montplaisir JY (2012) REM sleep behavior disorder: From dreams to neurodegeneration. Neurobiology of Disease 46: 553–8. doi:10.1016/j.nbd.2011.10.003.
18. Foster RG, Wulff K (2005) The rhythm of rest and excess. Nat Rev Neurosci 6: 407–14. doi:10.1038/nrn1670.
19. Benedetti F, Colombo C (2011) Sleep deprivation in mood disorders. Neuropsychobiology 64: 141–51. doi:10.1159/000328947.
20. Diekelmann S, Born J (2010) The memory function of sleep. Nat Rev Neurosci 11: 114–26. doi:10.1038/nrn2762.
21. Cirelli C, Gutierrez CM, Tononi G (2004) Extensive and Divergent Effects of Sleep and Wakefulness on Brain Gene Expression. Neuron 41: 35–43. doi:16/S0896-6273(03)00814-6.
22. Mackiewicz M, Shockley KR, Romer MA, Galante RJ, Zimmerman JE, et al (2007) Macromolecule biosynthesis: a key function of sleep. Physiol Genomics 31: 441–57. doi:10.1152/physiolgenomics.00275.2006.
23. Colgin LL (2011) Oscillations and hippocampal-prefrontal synchrony. Curr Opin Neurobiol 21: 467–74. doi:10.1016/j.conb.2011.04.006.
24. Franken P, Lopez-Molina L, Marcacci L, Schibler U, Tafti M (2000) The transcription factor DBP affects circadian sleep consolidation and rhythmic EEG activity. J Neurosci 20: 617–25.
25. Franken P, Dudley CA, Estill SJ, Barakat M, Thomason R, et al (2006) NPAS2 as a transcriptional regulator of non-rapid eye movement sleep: genotype and sex interactions. Proc Natl Acad Sci USA 103: 7118–23. doi:10.1073/pnas.0602006103.
26. Naylor E, Bergmann BM, Krauski K, Zee PC, Takahashi JS, et al (2000) The circadian clock mutation alters sleep homeostasis in the mouse. J Neurosci 20: 8138–43.

27. Wisor JP, O'Hara BF, Terao A, Selby CP, Kilduff TS, et al (2002) A role for cryptochromes in sleep regulation. BMC Neurosci 3: 20.

28. Dudley CA, Erbel-Sieler C, Estill SJ, Reick M, Franken P, et al (2003) Altered patterns of sleep and behavioral adaptability in NPAS2-deficient mice. Science 301: 379–83. doi:10.1126/science.1082795.

29. Roybal K, Theobold D, Graham A, DiNieri JA, Russo SJ, et al (2007) Mania-like behavior induced by disruption of CLOCK. Proc Natl Acad Sci U S A 104: 6406–11. doi:10.1073/pnas.0609625104.

30. Dzirasa K, McGarity DL, Bhattacharya A, Kumar S, Takahashi JS, et al (2011) Impaired limbic gamma oscillatory synchrony during anxiety-related behavior in a genetic mouse model of bipolar mania. J Neurosci 31: 6449–56. doi:10.1523/JNEUROSCI.6144-10.2011.

31. Debruyne JP, Noton E, Lambert CM, Maywood ES, Weaver DR, et al (2006) A clock shock: mouse CLOCK is not required for circadian oscillator function. Neuron 50: 465–77. doi:10.1016/j.neuron.2006.03.041.

32. Reick M, Garcia JA, Dudley C, McKnight SL (2001) NPAS2: an analog of clock operative in the mammalian forebrain. Science 293: 506–9. doi:10.1126/science.1060699.

33. Honma S, Kawamoto T, Takagi Y, Fujimoto K, Sato F, et al (2002) Dec1 and Dec2 are regulators of the mammalian molecular clock. Nature 419: 841–4. doi:10.1038/nature01123.

34. Nakashima A, Kawamoto T, Honda KK, Ueshima T, Noshiro M, et al (2008) DEC1 modulates the circadian phase of clock gene expression. Mol Cell Biol 28: 4080–92. doi:10.1128/MCB.02168-07.

35. Rossner MJ, Oster H, Wichert SP, Reinecke L, Wehr MC, et al (2008) Disturbed clockwork resetting in Sharp-1 and Sharp-2 single and double mutant mice. PLoS ONE 3:e2762. doi:10.1371/journal.pone.0002762.

36. Bode B, Rossner MJ, Oster H (2011) Advanced Light-Entrained Activity Onsets and Restored Free-Running Suprachiasmatic Nucleus Circadian Rhythms in Per2/Dec Mutant Mice. Chronobiology International 28: 737–50. doi:10.3109/07420528.2011.607374.

37. Bode B, Shahmoradi A, Rossner MJ, Oster H (2011) Genetic interaction of Per1 and Dec1/2 in the regulation of circadian locomotor activity. J Biol Rhythms 26: 530–40. doi:10.1177/0748730411419782.

38. He Y, Jones CR, Fujiki N, Xu Y, Guo B, et al (2009) The transcriptional repressor DEC2 regulates sleep length in mammals. Science 325: 866–70. doi:10.1126/science.1174443.

39. Mrosovsky N (1999) Masking: history, definitions, and measurement. Chronobiol Int 16: 415–29.

40. Subramanian A, Tamayo P, Mootha VK, Mukherjee S, Ebert BL, et al (2005) Gene set enrichment analysis: A knowledge-based approach for interpreting genome-wide expression profiles. Proceedings of the National Academy of Sciences of the United States of America 102: 15545–50. doi:10.1073/pnas.0506580102.

41. Nikolsky Y, Kirillov E, Zuev R, Rakhmatulin E, Nikolskaya T (2009) Functional analysis of OMICs data and small molecule compounds in an integrated "knowledge-based" platform. Methods Mol Biol 563: 177–96. doi:10.1007/978-1-60761-175-2_10.

42. Dezso Z, Nikolsky Y, Nikolskaya T, Miller J, Cherba D, et al (2009) Identifying disease-specific genes based on their topological significance in protein networks. BMC Syst Biol 3: 36. doi:10.1186/1752-0509-3-36.

43. Rutter J, Reick M, McKnight SL (2002) Metabolism and the control of circadian rhythms. Annu Rev Biochem 71: 307–31. doi:10.1146/annurev.biochem.71.090501.142857.

44. Nikonova EV, Naidoo N, Zhang L, Romer M, Cater JR, et al (2010) Changes in components of energy regulation in mouse cortex with increases in wakefulness. Sleep 33: 889–900.

45. Asher G, Schibler U (2011) Crosstalk between components of circadian and metabolic cycles in mammals. Cell Metab 13: 125–37. doi:10.1016/j.cmet.2011.01.006.

46. Park S, Holzman PS (1992) Schizophrenics show spatial working memory deficits. Arch Gen Psychiatry 49: 975–82.

47. Badcock JC, Michiel PT, Rock D (2005) Spatial working memory and planning ability: contrasts between schizophrenia and bipolar I disorder. Cortex 41: 753–63.

48. Glahn DC, Bearden CE, Cakir S, Barrett JA, Najt P, et al (2006) Differential working memory impairment in bipolar disorder and schizophrenia: effects of lifetime history of psychosis. Bipolar Disord 8: 117–23. doi:10.1111/j.1399-5618.2006.00296.x.

49. Braff DL, Geyer MA (1990) Sensorimotor gating and schizophrenia. Human and animal model studies. Arch Gen Psychiatry 47: 181–8.

50. Perry W, Minassian A, Feifel D, Braff DL (2001) Sensorimotor gating deficits in bipolar disorder patients with acute psychotic mania. Biol Psychiatry 50: 418–24.

51. Braff DL, Geyer MA, Swerdlow NR (2001) Human studies of prepulse inhibition of startle: normal subjects, patient groups, and pharmacological studies. Psychopharmacology (Berl) 156: 234–58.

52. Sato F, Kawamoto T, Fujimoto K, Noshiro M, Honda KK, et al (2004) Functional analysis of the basic helix-loop-helix transcription factor DEC1 in circadian regulation. Interaction with BMAL1. Eur J Biochem 271: 4409–19. doi:10.1111/j.1432-1033.2004.04379.x.

53. Adhikari A, Topiwala MA, Gordon JA (2010) Synchronized activity between the ventral hippocampus and the medial prefrontal cortex during anxiety. Neuron 65: 257–69. doi:10.1016/j.neuron.2009.12.002.

54. Einat H (2007) Different behaviors and different strains: potential new ways to model bipolar disorder. Neurosci Biobehav Rev 31: 850–7. doi:10.1016/j.neubiorev.2006.12.001.

55. Barnett JH, Smoller JW (2009) The genetics of bipolar disorder. Neuroscience 164: 331–43. doi:10.1016/j.neuroscience.2009.03.080.

56. Ramos A, Mormède P (1998) Stress and emotionality: a multidimensional and genetic approach. Neurosci Biobehav Rev 22: 33–57.

57. Trullas R, Skolnick P (1993) Differences in fear motivated behaviors among inbred mouse strains. Psychopharmacology (Berl) 111: 323–31.

58. Casamassima F, Hay AC, Benedetti A, Lattanzi L, Cassano GB, et al (2010) L-type calcium channels and psychiatric disorders: A brief review. Am J Med Genet B Neuropsychiatr Genet 153B:1373–90. doi:10.1002/ajmg.b.31122.

59. Dao DT, Mahon PB, Cai X, Kovacsics CE, Blackwell RA, et al (2010) Mood disorder susceptibility gene CACNA1C modifies mood-related behaviors in mice and interacts with sex to influence behavior in mice and diagnosis in humans. Biol Psychiatry 68: 801–10. doi:10.1016/j.biopsych.2010.06.019.

60. Leussis MP, Berry-Scott EM, Saito M, Jhuang H, de Haan G, et al (2013) The ANK3 bipolar disorder gene regulates psychiatric-related behaviors that are modulated by lithium and stress. Biol Psychiatry 73: 683–90. doi:10.1016/j.biopsych.2012.10.016.

61. Young JW, Goey AKL, Minassian A, Perry W, Paulus MP, et al (2010) The mania-like exploratory profile in genetic dopamine transporter mouse models is diminished in a familiar environment and reinstated by subthreshold psychostimulant administration. Pharmacol Biochem Behav 96: 7–15. doi:10.1016/j.pbb.2010.03.014.

62. Mukherjee S, Coque L, Cao J-L, Kumar J, Chakravarty S, et al (2010) Knockdown of Clock in the ventral tegmental area through RNA interference results in a mixed state of mania and depression-like behavior. Biol Psychiatry 68: 503–11. doi:10.1016/j.biopsych.2010.04.031.

63. Nestler EJ, Hyman SE (2010) Animal models of neuropsychiatric disorders. Nat Neurosci 13: 1161–9. doi:10.1038/nn.2647.

64. Brzózka MM, Radyushkin K, Wichert SP, Ehrenreich H, Rossner MJ (2010) Cognitive and Sensorimotor Gating Impairments in Transgenic Mice Overexpressing the Schizophrenia Susceptibility Gene Tcf4 in the Brain. Biological Psychiatry 68: 33–40. doi:10.1016/j.biopsych.2010.03.015.

65. Brzózka MM, Rossner MJ (2013) Deficits in trace fear memory in a mouse model of the schizophrenia risk gene TCF4. Behav Brain Res 237: 348–56. doi:10.1016/j.bbr.2012.10.001.

66. Castner SA, Goldman-Rakic PS, Williams GV (2004) Animal models of working memory: insights for targeting cognitive dysfunction in schizophrenia. Psychopharmacology (Berl) 174: 111–25. doi:10.1007/s00213-003-1683-8.

67. Duncan GE, Moy SS, Lieberman JA, Koller BH (2006) Effects of haloperidol, clozapine, and quetiapine on sensorimotor gating in a genetic model of reduced NMDA receptor function. Psychopharmacology (Berl) 184: 190–200. doi:10.1007/s00213-005-0214-1.

68. McOmish CE, Burrows E, Howard M, Scarr E, Kim D, et al (2008) Phospholipase C-beta1 knockout mice exhibit endophenotypes modeling schizophrenia which are rescued by environmental enrichment and clozapine administration. Mol Psychiatry 13: 661–72. doi:10.1038/sj.mp.4002046.

69. Porcelli S, Balzarro B, Serretti A (2012) Clozapine resistance: augmentation strategies. Eur Neuropsychopharmacol 22: 165–82. doi:10.1016/j.euroneuro.2011.08.005.

70. Vollenweider FX, Barro M, Csomor PA, Feldon J (2006) Clozapine enhances prepulse inhibition in healthy humans with low but not with high prepulse inhibition levels. Biol Psychiatry 60: 597–603. doi:10.1016/j.biopsych.2006.03.058.

71. Swerdlow NR, Kuczenski R, Goins JC, Crain SK, Ma LT, et al (2005) Neurochemical analysis of rat strain differences in the startle gating-disruptive effects of dopamine agonists. Pharmacol Biochem Behav 80: 203–11. doi:10.1016/j.pbb.2004.11.002.

72. Weber M, Chang W, Breier M, Ko D, Swerdlow NR (2008) Heritable strain differences in sensitivity to the startle gating-disruptive effects of D2 but not D3 receptor stimulation. Behavioural Pharmacology 19: 786–95. doi:10.1097/FBP.0b013e32831c3b2b.

73. Baik JH, Picetti R, Saiardi A, Thiriet G, Dierich A, et al (1995) Parkinsonian-like locomotor impairment in mice lacking dopamine D2 receptors. Nature 377: 424–8. doi:10.1038/377424a0.

74. Chen JF, Beilstein M, Xu YH, Turner TJ, Moratalla R, et al (2000) Selective attenuation of psychostimulant-induced behavioral responses in mice lacking A(2A) adenosine receptors. Neuroscience 97: 195–204.

75. Bello EP, Mateo Y, Gelman DM, Noaín D, Shin JH, et al (2011) Cocaine supersensitivity and enhanced motivation for reward in mice lacking dopamine D2 autoreceptors. Nature Neuroscience 14: 1033–8. doi:10.1038/nn.2862.

76. Bodenmann S, Hohoff C, Freitag C, Deckert J, Rétey JV, et al (2012) Polymorphisms of ADORA2A modulate psychomotor vigilance and the effects of caffeine on neurobehavioural performance and sleep EEG after sleep deprivation. Br J Pharmacol 165: 1904–13. doi:10.1111/j.1476-5381.2011.01689.x.

77. Zou Y-F, Wang F, Feng X-L, Li W-F, Tian Y-H, et al (2012) Association of DRD2 gene polymorphisms with mood disorders: A meta-analysis. J Affect Disord 136: 229–37. doi:10.1016/j.jad.2010.11.012.

78. Allen JA, Yost JM, Setola V, Chen X, Sassano MF, et al (2011) Discovery of β-Arrestin-Biased Dopamine D2 Ligands for Probing Signal Transduction

Pathways Essential for Antipsychotic Efficacy. Proc Natl Acad Sci USA 108: 18488–93. doi:10.1073/pnas.1104807108.

79. Boison D, Singer P, Shen H-Y, Feldon J, Yee BK (2012) Adenosine hypothesis of schizophrenia—opportunities for pharmacotherapy. Neuropharmacology 62: 1527–43. doi:10.1016/j.neuropharm.2011.01.048.

80. Aston C, Jiang L, Sokolov BP (2005)Transcriptional profiling reveals evidence for signaling and oligodendroglial abnormalities in the temporal cortex from patients with major depressive disorder. Mol Psychiatry 10: 309–22. doi:10.1038/sj.mp.4001565.

81. Mabrouk OS, Li Q, Song P, Kennedy RT (2011) Microdialysis and mass spectrometric monitoring of dopamine and enkephalins in the globus pallidus reveal reciprocal interactions that regulate movement. Journal of Neurochemistry 118: 24–33. doi:10.1111/j.1471-4159.2011.07293.x.

82. Takahashi N, Sakurai T, Davis KL, Buxbaum JD (2011) Linking oligodendrocyte and myelin dysfunction to neurocircuitry abnormalities in schizophrenia. Prog Neurobiol 93: 13–24. doi:10.1016/j.pneurobio.2010.09.004.

83. Bode B, Shahmoradi A, Rossner MJ, Oster H (2011) Genetic interaction of Per1 and Dec1/2 in the regulation of circadian locomotor activity. J Biol Rhythms 26: 530–40. doi:10.1177/0748730411419782.

84. Bilkei-Gorzo A, Racz I, Michel K, Zimmer A, Klingmüller D, et al. (2004) Behavioral phenotype of pre-proenkephalin-deficient mice on diverse congenic backgrounds. Psychopharmacology (Berl) 176: 343–52. doi:10.1007/s00213-004-1904-9.

85. Bilkei-Gorzo A, Berner J, Zimmermann J, Wickström R, Racz I, et al. (2010) Increased morphine analgesia and reduced side effects in mice lacking the tac1 gene. Br J Pharmacol 160: 1443–52. doi:10.1111/j.1476-5381.2010.00757.x.

86. Sun H, Lu B, Li RQ, Flavell RA, Taneja R (2001) Defective T cell activation and autoimmune disorder in Stra13-deficient mice. Nat Immunol 2: 1040–7. doi:10.1038/ni721.

87. Fledrich R, Schlotter-Weigel B, Schnizer TJ, Wichert SP, Stassart RM, et al (2012) A rat model of Charcot–Marie–Tooth disease 1A recapitulates disease variability and supplies biomarkers of axonal loss in patients. Brain 135: 72–87. doi:10.1093/brain/awr322.

88. Rossner MJ, Hirrlinger J, Wichert SP, Boehm C, Newrzella D, et al (2006) Global transcriptome analysis of genetically identified neurons in the adult cortex. J Neurosci 26: 9956–66. doi:10.1523/JNEUROSCI.0468-06.2006.

89. Alamed J, Wilcock DM, Diamond DM, Gordon MN, Morgan D (2006) Two-day radial-arm water maze learning and memory task) robust resolution of amyloid-related memory deficits in transgenic mice. Nat Protoc 1: 1671–9. doi:10.1038/nprot.2006.275.

3

Reciprocal Regulation of Epileptiform Neuronal Oscillations and Electrical Synapses in the Rat Hippocampus

Erika R. Kinjo[1,2]*, Guilherme S. V. Higa[1,2], Edgard Morya[3], Angela C. Valle[4], Alexandre H. Kihara[1,2]*, Luiz R. G. Britto[1]

1 Departamento de Fisiologia e Biofísica, Instituto de Ciências Biomédicas, Universidade de São Paulo, São Paulo, São Paulo, Brazil, **2** Núcleo de Cognição e Sistemas Complexos, Centro de Matemática, Computação e Cognição, Universidade Federal do ABC, São Bernardo do Campo, São Paulo, Brazil, **3** Instituto Internacional de Neurociência de Natal Edmond e Lily Safra, Natal, Rio Grande do Norte, Brazil, **4** Laboratório de Neurociências - LIM 01, Departamento de Patologia, Faculdade de Medicina, Universidade de São Paulo, São Paulo, São Paulo, Brazil

Abstract

Gap junction (GJ) channels have been recognized as an important mechanism for synchronizing neuronal networks. Herein, we investigated the participation of GJ channels in the pilocarpine-induced status epilepticus (SE) by analyzing electrophysiological activity following the blockade of connexins (Cx)-mediated communication. In addition, we examined the regulation of gene expression, protein levels, phosphorylation profile and distribution of neuronal Cx36, Cx45 and glial Cx43 in the rat hippocampus during the acute and latent periods. Electrophysiological recordings revealed that the GJ blockade anticipates the occurrence of low voltage oscillations and promotes a marked reduction of power in all analyzed frequencies.Cx36 gene expression and protein levels remained stable in acute and latent periods, whereas upregulation of Cx45 gene expression and protein redistribution were detected in the latent period. We also observed upregulation of Cx43 mRNA levels followed by changes in the phosphorylation profile and protein accumulation. Taken together, our results indisputably revealed that GJ communication participates in the epileptiform activity induced by pilocarpine. Moreover, considering that specific Cxs undergo alterations through acute and latent periods, this study indicates that the control of GJ communication may represent a focus in reliable anti-epileptogenic strategies.

Editor: Stéphane Charpier, University Paris 6, France

Funding: The work was supported by the following funders: FAPESP and CNPq. The funders had no role in study design, data collection and analysis, decision to publish, or preparation of the manuscript.

Competing Interests: The authors have read the journal's policy and have the following conflict: AHK is part of PLOS ONE Academic Board.

* Email: erikareime@gmail.com (ERK); alexandrekihara@gmail.com (AHK)

Introduction

Gap junction (GJ) channels couple adjacent cells, allowing transfer of second messengers, ions, and molecules up to 1 kDa. These channels are composed by a multigene family of integral membrane proteins called connexins (Cx). So far, at least 20 Cx genes were identified in the mouse and human genome [1]. Notably, communication through GJ channels has been recognized as an important mechanism for synchronizing neuronal networks in both physiological and pathological conditions [2–4]. In fact, several evidences from animal models [5–11] and human slices from epileptic patients [12,13] indicate the participation of GJ channels in the generation and maintenance of epileptic seizures. Moreover, specific alterations of Cx expression have been described in tissue from epileptic patients [14–16] and in experimental models [11,17–20].

The aim of this study was to determine the involvement of GJ channels in the epileptiform activity induced by pilocarpine by examining the changes in electrophysiological patterns produced by uncoupling of these channels with carbenoxolone (CBX). After we established the participation of GJ in the ictal discharges, we thoroughly analyzed the regulation of gene expression, changes in protein levels, phosphorylation profile and distribution of the neuronal Cx36 and Cx45 and the glial Cx43, three of the most highly expressed Cxs in the rat hippocampus, [1,18,21–24] during acute seizures and the epileptogenic process. We observed that pharmacological blockade of GJ channels decreases the epileptiform activity, which in turn regulates Cx gene expression, protein levels and phosphorylation. Thus, our results revealed a reciprocal, mutual regulation of Cx-mediated communication and the epileptiform phenomenon.

Methods

Ethics Statement

All experiments were carried out with healthy male Wistar rats (*Rattus norvegicus*) weighing between 270 and 300 g and mean age ranging from 80–90 days. Experiments with animals were conducted in accordance with guidelines of the National Institutes of Health (NIH) and the Brazilian Scientific Society for Laboratory Animals. Experimental protocol (#19, page 67, book 02/2009) was approved by the Ethics Committee in Animal Experimentation of the Institute of Biomedical Sciences/University of São Paulo (ICB/USP). All animals were housed in groups of five in plastic cages under controlled conditions of temperature (22°C±2), relative humidity (45% to 50%) and light/dark cycles (12 hours of light/12 hours of darkness) in a vivarium approved by ICB/USP Ethics Committee in Animal Experimentation. Rats were given *ad libitum* access to a standard rodent maintenance diet (Nuvilab, Curitiba, PR, Brazil) and tap water. Surgeries were performed under diazepam sedation followed by ketamine anesthesia, and all efforts were made to minimize suffering.

Implantation of recording electrodes. Animals underwent sedation with diazepam (6 mg/kg, i.p., União Química, Embu-Guaçu, SP, BRA), anesthesia with ketamine (100 mg/kg, i.p., Parke-Davis, Ann Arbor, MI, USA) and stereotaxic surgery for bilateral electrode implantation. All surgeries were performed in the laboratory in the morning. Bipolar 150-μm-diameter nichrome bipolar electrodes were implanted over neocortical area (AP: −1.5 mm, ML: ±3.0 mm) according to skull references [25].

ECoG recordings and drug administration. Ten days after the surgical procedure, the rats were placed in a Faraday cage and connected to the input panel of a 21-channel Nihon–Koden electroencephalograph (Neurofax EEG 4400) for habituation 1 day before the experiment. In the day of the experiment, which was always performed in the laboratory between 08 AM and 17 PM, after thirty minutes recording of the basal activity, the first group of animals (SE+CBX; n = 6 animals) was submitted to the injection of methyl-scopolamine (1 mg/kg, s.c.; Sigma-Aldrich, USA), used to reduce the peripheral cholinergic effects, followed by pilocarpine hydrochloride (360 mg/kg, i.p.; Sigma-Aldrich, USA) injection thirty minutes later. Thirty minutes after the establishment of *status epilepticus* (SE), the animals were treated with CBX (60 mg/kg, i.p., dissolved in saline; Sigma-Aldrich, USA) and the ECoGs were continuously recorded for two hours at different time points (0, 30, 60, 90 and 120 min). The second group (SE group; n = 5 animals) was treated in a similar way as the first one, except for the approximate volume of sterile saline (i.p.) injected instead of CBX, and the ECoGs were also continuously registered for two hours. The third group (Control CBX; n = 5 animals) received saline instead of pilocarpine, followed by CBX injection. The behavior of the rats was continuously monitored during the ECoG recordings. Recordings were acquired at 512 Hz, notch filter of 60 Hz, low pass of 35 Hz. A Matlab (Mathworks) script run off line ECoG analysis to detect flat periods longer than 250 ms between the on-SE and off-SE raw recordings for each rat, and minimum time interval for each animal to present flat periods were averaged for both groups. ECoG data were sampled in 5 epochs of 10 seconds to represent each period (basal, methyl-scopolamine, SE, t0, t30, t60, t90, t120) with ECoG power spectrum and spectrogram. Power spectrum analysis was performed using Welch's Method, window 128 and overlap 64. Spectrogram used Kaiser window 1024 and overlap 516. The software to run statistical comparisons as analysis of variance and T-test was SPSS. All statistical comparisons considered significance level set at 5%.

SE induction for molecular analysis

Animals were previously treated with methyl-scopolamine nitrate (1 mg/kg, s.c.; Sigma-Aldrich, St. Louis, MO) to reduce peripheral cholinergic effects. Thirty minutes later animals of the experimental group received a single dose of pilocarpine hydrochloride (360 mg/kg, i.p.; Sigma-Aldrich, St. Louis, MO) to induce SE, and control animals received a similar volume of sterile saline. SE induction was always performed in the laboratory between 08 AM and 10 PM.

Euthanasia of animals of the acute group was performed by decapitation 2 hours after the onset of SE. Animals of the latent

group received a single dose of diazepam (10 mg/kg, s.c., União Química, Embu-Guaçu, SP) 2 hours after SE initiation to interrupt seizures, and euthanasia was conducted 3 days after SE induction.

RNA isolation, cDNA synthesis and Real-Time PCR

Hippocampi from control (n = 8), acute (n = 8) and latent (n = 8) animals were directly homogenized in 1–1.5 ml TRIzol reagent (Invitrogen, Carlsbad, CA, USA) and total RNA was extracted following the manufacturer suggested protocol and previously described [26]. Briefly, following two chloroform extraction steps, RNA was precipitated with isopropanol and the pellet washed twice in 70% ethanol. After air-drying, RNA was resuspended in DEPC-treated water and the concentration of each sample obtained from A_{260} measurements. Residual DNA was removed using DNase I (Amersham, Piscataway, NJ, USA) following manufacturer protocol. Quantitative analysis of gene expression was carried out with a Rotor-Gene 6000 Real-Time Rotary Analyzer (Corbett Robotics Inc., San Francisco, CA) with specific primers for rat Cx36 (forward, 5′- GGGGAATGGACCATCT-TGGA-3′; reverse, 5′- TCCCCTACAATGGCCACAAT-3′), Cx 45 (forward, 5′- GGGTAACGGAGGTTCTGGTTACAGGGT-TGTCTACGCCGCC-3′; reverse, 5′- AAGCTCCAACTCAT-GGTGGT-3′) and Cx43 (forward, 5′-ACTTCAGCCTCCAAG-GAGTT-3′; reverse 5′-TGGAGTAGGCTTGGACCTTG-3′). c DNA abundance for cyclophilin A (forward, 5′- GCGTTTT-GGGTCCAGGAATGGC-3′; reverse, 5′- TTGCGAGCAGAT-GGGGTGGG-3′) was determined as internal control. For each 20 μl reverse transcription reaction, 4 μg total RNA was mixed with 1 μl oligodT primer (0.5 μg; Invitrogen) and incubated for 10 min at 65°C. After cooling on ice the solution was mixed with 4 μl 5× first strand buffer, 2 μl of 0.1 M DTT, 1 μl of dATP, dTTP, dCTP and dGTP (each 10 mM), and 1 μl SuperScript III reverse transcriptase (200 U; Invitrogen) and incubated for 60 min at 50°C. Reaction was inactivated by heating at 70°C for 15 min. All PCR assays were performed as follows: after initial activation at 50°C for 2 min and 95°C for 10 min, cycling conditions were 95°C, 10 s and 60°C, 1 min. Dissociation curves of PCR products were obtained by heating samples from 60 to 95°C, in order to evaluate primer specificity. Relative quantification of target gene expression was evaluated using the comparative CT method as previously described in detail [27,28]. Values were entered into one-way ANOVA followed by Tukey's HSD test, with the significance level set at 5%.

Western Blotting

Hippocampi from control (n = 7), acute (n = 7) and latent (n = 7) animals were rapidly dissected, washed with phosphate buffered saline (PBS) and homogenized in RIPA buffer (50 mM Tris, 150 mM NaCl, 0.1% SDS, 0.5% sodium deoxycholate, 1% Triton X-100 and protease inhibitors). Homogenates were centrifuged for 20 min at 14,000 G, 4°C to remove insoluble material. Protein concentration was determined by the BCA method (Thermo Scientific, Rockford, IL, USA) and bovine serum albumin was used as the standard, following manufacturer protocol. Proteins in the membrane preparations were separated by sodium dodecyl sulfate-polyacrylamide gel electrophoresis (SDS-PAGE; 10% gel) and transferred to nitrocellulose membranes. Blots were incubated with 5% non-fat milk in TBST buffer for 2 h at room temperature to block nonspecific binding of the antibodies. After rinsed in TBST, blots were incubated overnight with primary antibodies raised against Cx36 (rabbit polyclonal 36-4600, Zymed/Invitrogen, 1:1000), Cx45 (rabbit polyclonal AB1745, Millipore, Billerica, MA, USA, 1:1000), Cx43 (rabbit polyclonal 71-0700, mouse monoclonal 13-8300, Zymed/Invitrogen, 1:1000) and beta-actin (mouse monoclonal A5316, Sigma-Aldrich, 1:10000) diluted in TBST/3% non-fat milk. After the primary antibody incubation, blots were rinsed in TBST and incubated with the appropriate secondary antibody raised against rabbit or mouse conjugated to horseradish peroxidase (HRP) enzyme (1:5000, Invitrogen, Carlsbad, CA, USA) for 2 h at room temperature. Detection of labeled proteins was achieved by using the enhanced chemiluminescent system (ECLTM kit; Amersham, Piscataway, NJ, USA). Measurements of optical densities (OD) were performed using Alliance 2.7 system (UVItec Limited, Cambridge, United Kingdom). ODs of the bands were normalized using the value found for the beta-actin. Data from the experiments were entered into T-Test analysis with the significance level set at 5%.

Immunohistochemistry

Brains were collected and fixed for 8 hours in 1% paraformaldehyde (PFA) in phosphate buffer 0.1 M pH 7.3 (PB), and cryoprotected in 30% sucrose solution for at least 48 hours at 4°C. Brain coronal sections (12 μm) were obtained on a cryostat. Brain sections containing the hippocampus were incubated overnight with primary antibodies raised against Cx36 (36-4600, Zymed/Invitrogen, 1:100), Cx45 (AB1745, Millipore, Billerica, MA, USA, 1:200), Cx43 (710700, Zymed/Invitrogen, 1:100) and parvalbumin (P3088, Sigma-Aldrich, 1:200) in a solution containing 5% normal goat serum and 0.5% Triton X-100 in PBS at room temperature. After several washes, brain sections were incubated with goat antiserum against rabbit or mouse IgG tagged to Alexa 488 (1:200–1:500, Invitrogen) and 3% normal goat serum diluted in 0.3% Triton X-100 in PBS for 2 hours at room temperature. For double-labeling experiments, secondary antibodies conjugated to Alexa 546 or Alexa 647 (1:200–1:500, Invitrogen) were used. Controls for the experiments consisted of the omission of primary antibodies; no staining was observed in these cases. Counterstaining of brain sections was achieved using 4′,6-diamidino-2-phenylindole (DAPI), diluted in the same 0.3% Triton X-100 of the secondary antibodies. After washing, the tissue was mounted using Vecta Shield (Vector Labs, Burlingame, CA, USA), and analyzed in Nikon TS100F inverted microscope (Nikon Instruments Inc., Melville, NY, USA). Figures were mounted with Adobe Photoshop CS5 (Adobe Systems Inc., San Jose, CA, USA). Manipulation of the images was restricted to brightness and contrast adjustments of the whole image.

Image Quantification. Image analyses were performed with ImageJ software (National Institute of Mental Health, Bethesda, Maryland, USA) and NIS elements (Nikon Instruments Inc.), as previously described [29], employing approximately 30 hippocampal slices from 4 animals (6–8 hippocampal slices from each animal). For Cx36 analyses, after channel separation (RGB) of color images, we performed quantification of the mean pixel intensity, where values correspond to the brightness of the pixels, of Cx36 labeling in the green channel within an area of interest (AOI) defined by the labeling of parvalbumin in the red channel. For analyses of Cx45 and Cx43 images (green channel), we performed quantification of the mean pixel intensity of each AOI (strata oriens, pyramidale, lucidum, radiatum and lacunosum-moleculare). Values were normalized by the mean pixel intensity of the whole image. Mander's colocalization coefficient between Cx36 and parvalbumin was performed. Values from all analyses were entered into one-way analysis of variance (ANOVA), followed by pairwise comparisons in Tukey's HSD test, with the significance level set at 5%. Images and charts were prepared using Adobe Photoshop CS5.

Results

GJ communication is involved in the epileptiform activity

As a first approach, we first verified the contribution of GJ communication in epileptiform electrical activity. For this purpose, we induced SE by injecting pilocarpine in two groups of rats, named SE group and SE+CBX group. After pilocarpine administration, animals experienced a progressive evolution of seizures, and approximately 45 minutes later, 80% of the animals had developed SE, characterized by tonic-clonic generalized seizures [30,31]. Animals treated with CBX without pilocarpine (Control CBX group) did not present behavioral alterations.

Figure 1 (A–H) shows the representative ECoGs of SE+CBX group. During the basal and methyl-scopolamine periods, ECoGs display electrical activity of low frequency and amplitude. After pilocarpine administration, ECoGs exhibited increasing epileptiform potentials characterized by isolated spikes (I, arrows) which evolved to continuous poly-spikes and spike-wave complexes (Ja and Jb, respectively), characterizing the establishment of SE (C). Thirty minutes after the establishment of SE, CBX was injected in the animals of SE+CBX group (D). We observed that CBX treatment induced changes in the epileptiform activity, as illustrated during all analyzed periods (E–H). A prominent aspect of the epileptiform potentials also associated with the signal is the occurrence of low voltage oscillations, which resemble flat periods (K, arrows). While we did not detect differences in the total number or duration of these flat periods, the time frame for the manifestation of these events was significantly reduced in the SE+CBX group compared to the SE group, which received saline instead of CBX (476 ± 116 seconds vs. 2565 ± 881 seconds, respectively; $P<0.01$) (L), demonstrating the effects of the GJ blocker on pilocarpine-induced SE. The Control CBX group, which received saline followed by the CBX injection, did not present any of the above described alterations related to CBX treatment (data not shown).

In addition to the alterations in the epileptiform potentials, we also observed changes in frequency composition. Figure 2 (A–C) shows the frequency composition of ECoGs following 2 hours after CBX or saline injection. (A) The spectrogram of Control CBX group shows greater contribution of low frequencies. On the other hand, the spectrogram of SE group (B) shows high intensity in full range frequencies after saline administration, whereas the spectrogram of SE+CBX group exhibits reduction of intensity of all frequencies that compose the signal (C). In addition, Fig. 2 also shows the representative power spectra of SE+CBX group during all analyzed periods (D–K). We observed that compared with basal and methyl-scopolamine periods (D, E), pilocarpine-induced SE promoted marked changes in the power spectrum (F). Although the potentials observed during the SE period oscillated in the same frequency ranges of the basal and methyl-scopolamine periods (frequencies <5 Hz, 5–11 Hz, 12–35 Hz, known as delta, theta and beta oscillations, respectively), there was a global increase of the power of all frequency ranges. After CBX administration, which occurred 30 minutes after the establishment of SE (G), we visualized changes in the profile of frequency contribution, especially the reduction of the power of frequencies between 15–30 Hz (H–K). Indeed, the time period for the decrease of the power of this frequency band was significantly minor in the SE+CBX group comparing with SE group, which received saline instead of CBX (3925 ± 326 seconds vs. 5599 ± 473 seconds, respectively; $P<0.01$) (L). While CBX administration promoted changes on the above electrophysiological parameters of SE, no behavioral alterations were detected on seizure manifestations.

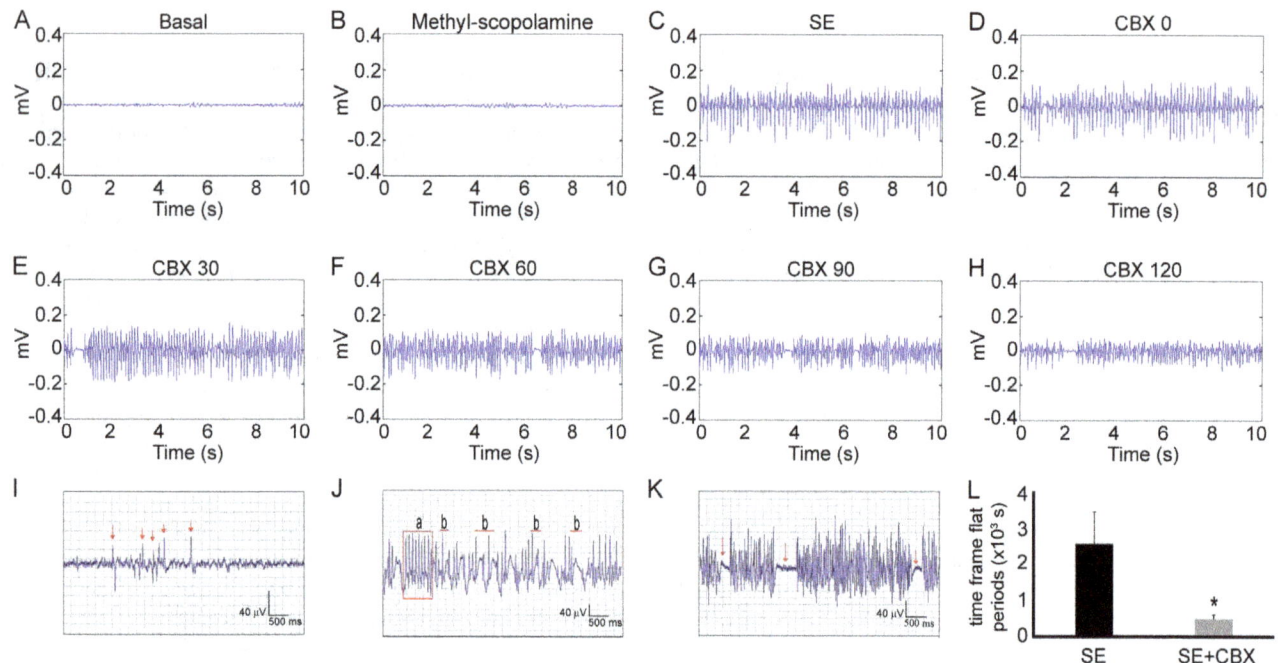

Figure 1. Effects of pharmacological blockade of GJ channels on ECoG. Representative local field potentials of SE+CBX group. (A, B) It is possible to see that basal and methyl-scopolamine periods share similar electrical activity patterns. After pilocarpine injection, we observed increasing epileptiform potentials represented by isolated spikes (I, arrows), poly-spikes (J-a) and spike-wave complexes (J-b), culminating in SE establishment (C). CBX administration 30 minutes after SE establishment (D) was able to induce changes in the epileptiform potentials, which could be seen during the whole analyzed interval post-CBX injection (E–H). We found out that the time frame for occurrence of flat periods (K, arrows) from SE+CBX group was significantly shorter when compared to SE group (L). Bars represent standard errors of mean. *$P<0.01$ in T-Test.

Epileptiform activity changes Cxs gene expression during the latent period

By using primers specifically designed for Cx36, Cx45 and Cx43 we generated amplification plots from cDNA serial dilutions. Dissociation curves of these PCR products were obtained by heating samples from 60 to 95°C. The single peak observed matched to theoretical melting temperature calculated previously, indicating specificity of the primers. Amplification plots indicated that pilocarpine-induced SE did not alter gene expression of any of the analyzed Cxs, as shown in Fig. 3. However, both Cx45 and Cx43 transcript levels have higher expression ($2^2.88 = 7.36$ fold-expression and $2^2.49 = 5.62$ fold expression, respectively; $P<0.001$) in the hippocampus of animals evaluated during the latent period when compared to controls. Cyclophilin A gene expression was used as an internal control (Fig. 3).

Epileptiform activity induces changes in the total and phosphorylated forms of Cx43

In order to verify the protein levels of Cxs in the hippocampi of rats during the acute and latent periods, we performed Western blot analysis. We were not able to detect changes in protein levels of the analyzed Cxs in the acute period (Fig. 4, A–D). During the latent period, Cx36 and Cx45 protein levels did not differ compared with control group (Fig. 4, E–G, respectively). However, both Cx43 total protein levels (phosphorylated and unphosphorylated forms, antibody 71-0700) and one of the unphosphorylated forms (antibody 13-8300) of the protein showed higher levels (193%, $P<0.01$ and 168%, $P<0.001$, respectively) when compared to controls (Fig. 4H).

Cx36 expression in interneurons is not modulated in CA3 by epileptiform activity

Once we determined that GJ communication is involved in the epileptiform activity induced by pilocarpine and that Cxs undergo alterations in gene expression and posttranslational modifications, we focused on Cx distribution in CA3. For this purpose, we conducted double-labeling experiments using parvalbumin (PV), a calcium binding protein which is known to label a subset of GABAergic interneurons that are electrically coupled by Cx36 [32–34]. Indeed, we confirmed the co-expression of Cx36 and PV in the CA3 (Fig. 5, A–D). To determine whether Cx36 amount in PV-positive cells changes in the acute and latent periods, we performed analysis combining pixel intensity profiles and quantification of the mean pixel intensity after RGB decomposition data. We were not able to detect significant differences in pixel quantification analysis (Fig. 5, E–H). Moreover, we did not detect changes in Mander's coefficient from Cx36 and PV signals. Taking together, these results revealed a stable spatial pattern of Cx36 throughout acute and latent periods (Fig. 5, I–L).

Epileptiform activity induces changes in Cx45 spatial pattern within CA3

As we observed widespread Cx45 immunoreactivity in CA3 region, we conducted quantification of the mean pixel intensity in each strata (Fig. 6A) to examine whether Cx45 distribution is altered in the acute and latent periods. We were not able to detect changes in Cx45 distribution during the acute period (Fig. 6B, 6C and data not shown). During the latent period, our quantitative analyses revealed more pronounced labeling in the stratum oriens (119%, $P<0.05$), as well as decreased staining in stratum

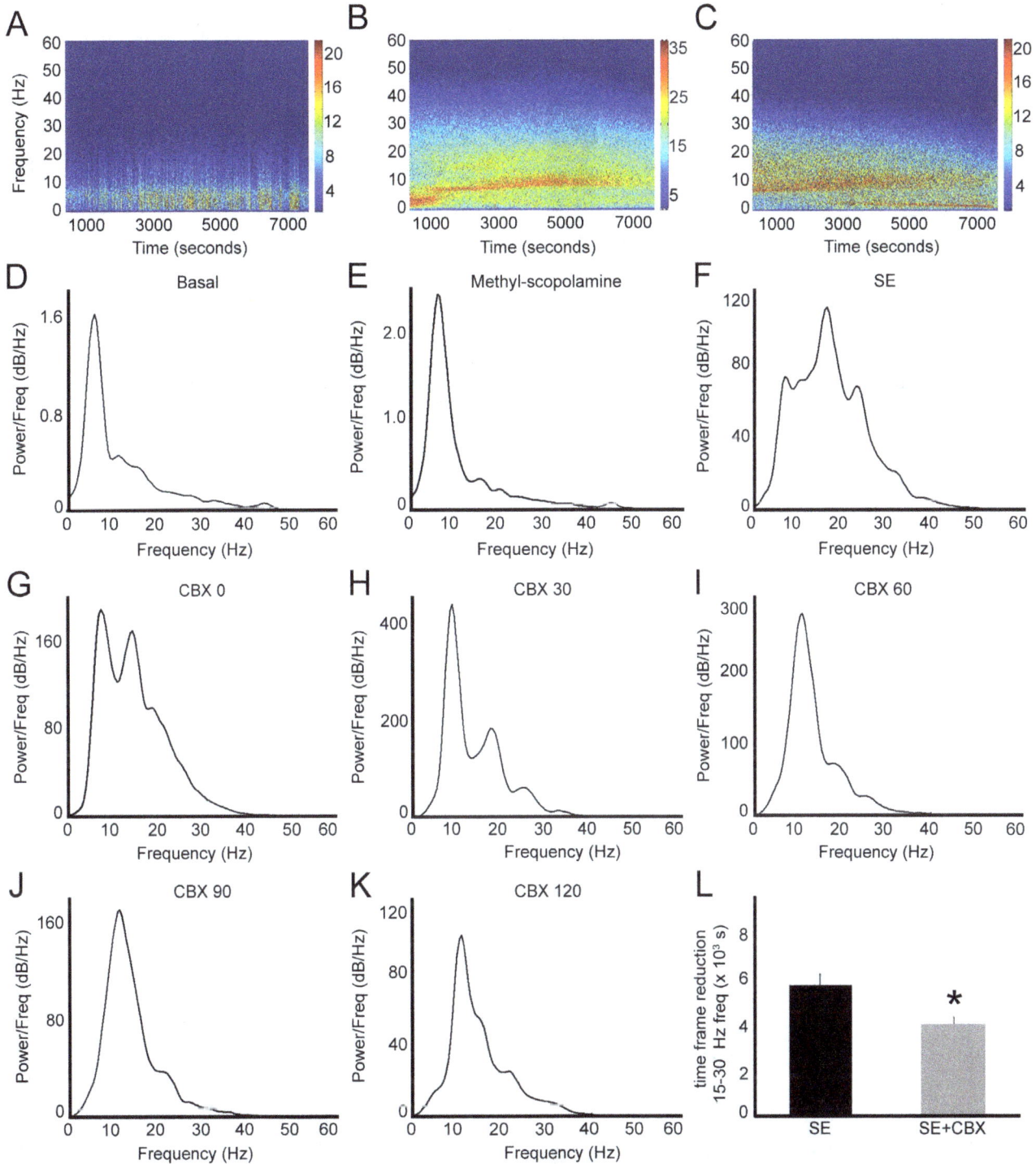

Figure 2. Effects of pharmacological blockade of GJ channels on epileptiform potentials during status epilepticus (SE). (A, B, C) Representative spectrograms of the raw ECoGs from Control CBX, SE and SE+CBX groups, showing the main frequencies, evidenced by the color intensity, which compose the signal during the 2-hour interval after injection of CBX or saline. Note the increase of ECoG power in the SE group (B) and the reduction of color intensity after CBX treatment (C), showing the decrease of power of all frequency bands, especially the beta frequency. Representative power spectra of SE+CBX group. (D, E) Power spectrum of basal and methyl-scopolamine periods shows similar frequency composition. (F) It is possible to observe that pilocarpine-induced SE enhanced the power of all frequency bands, especially at 12–35 Hz range. (G–K) CBX administration 30 minutes after SE establishment caused notable decrease of the power in the beta frequency oscillations observed in the following 2 hours. Since we found that the reduction of beta oscillations occurs during the evolution of SE (data not shown), we tested whether this reduction was significant when compared to the same periods of SE group. (L) We observed that the time period for reduction in the beta frequency range was significantly decreased in the animals that received CBX injection. Bars represent standard errors of mean. *$P < 0.01$ in T-Test.

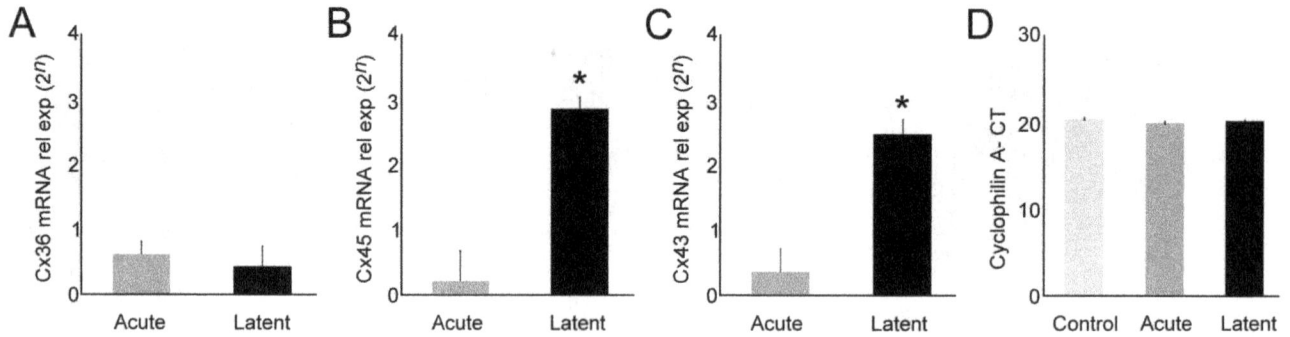

Figure 3. Gene expression levels of Cxs in the rat hippocampus during acute and latent periods. (A) Cx36 gene expression remains stable throughout acute and latent periods. (B) On the other hand, we were not able to detect changes in Cx45 transcript levels in acute period, although increased expression was observed in the latent group. (C) Similar results were observed for Cx43 mRNA levels, since we were not able to detect significant differences in the acute group, but we found increased expression in the latent group when compared to controls. (D) Gene expression of cyclophilin A was used as internal control. Means from acute (n = 8) and latent (n = 8) groups were normalized based on control group (n = 8) expression levels. Bars represent standard errors of mean. $*P < 0.001$ vs. Control group in Tukey's HSD pairwise comparisons after one-way ANOVA.

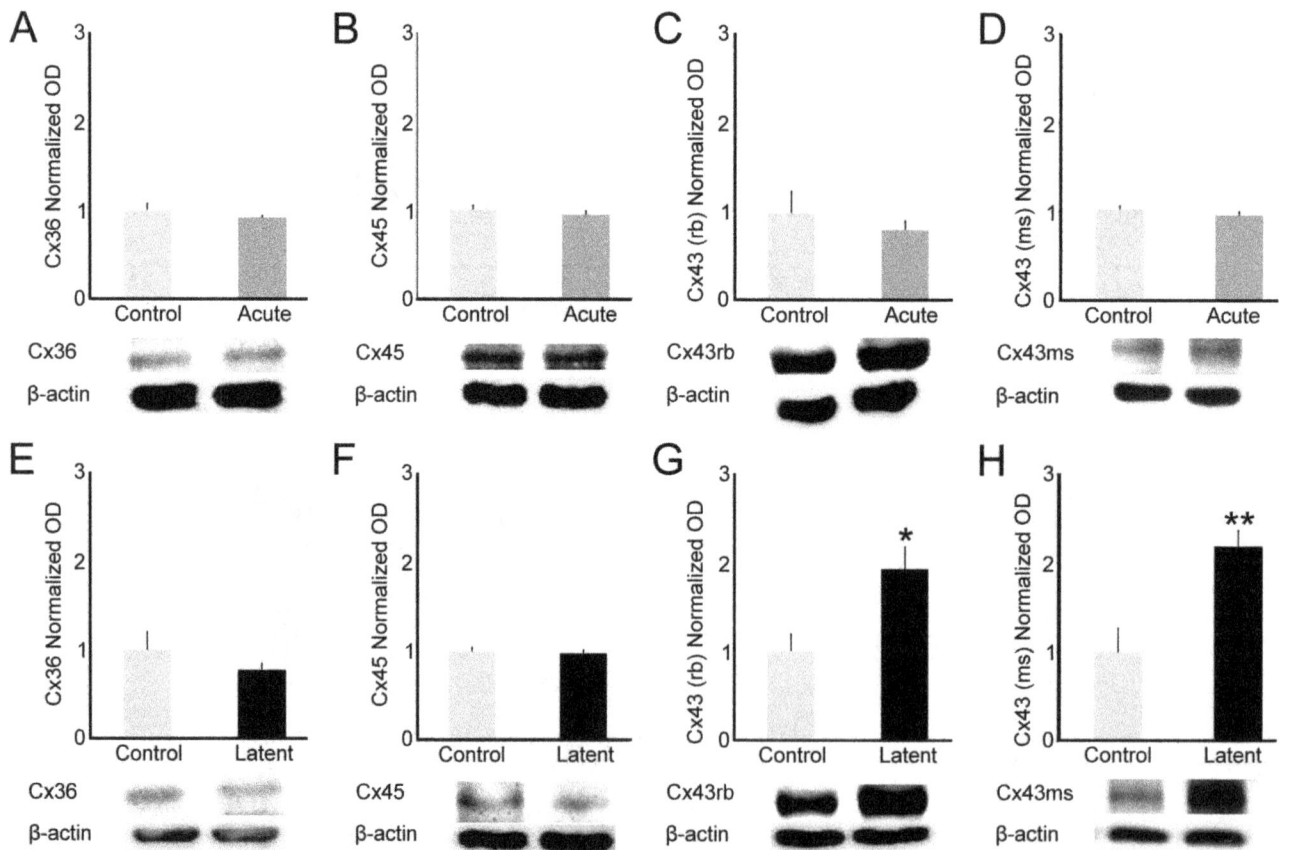

Figure 4. Quantification of Cxs protein levels in the hippocampus during acute and latent periods. (A–D) We observed stable steady levels of Cx36, Cx45, Cx43 protein levels during the acute period. (E–F) Similarly, analysis performed in the latent period showed steady state levels of Cx36 and Cx45 proteins. (G–H) In addition, we observed changes in both Cx43 total protein levels and Cx43 unphosphorylated form, which have higher levels in the latent group when compared to controls. Beta-actin (42 kDa) was used as internal control. Optical densities (OD) from acute (n = 7) and latent (n = 7) groups were normalized by OD from control (n = 7) group in three independent experiments. Bars represent standard errors of mean. $* P < 0.01$; $**P < 0.001$ in T-Test.

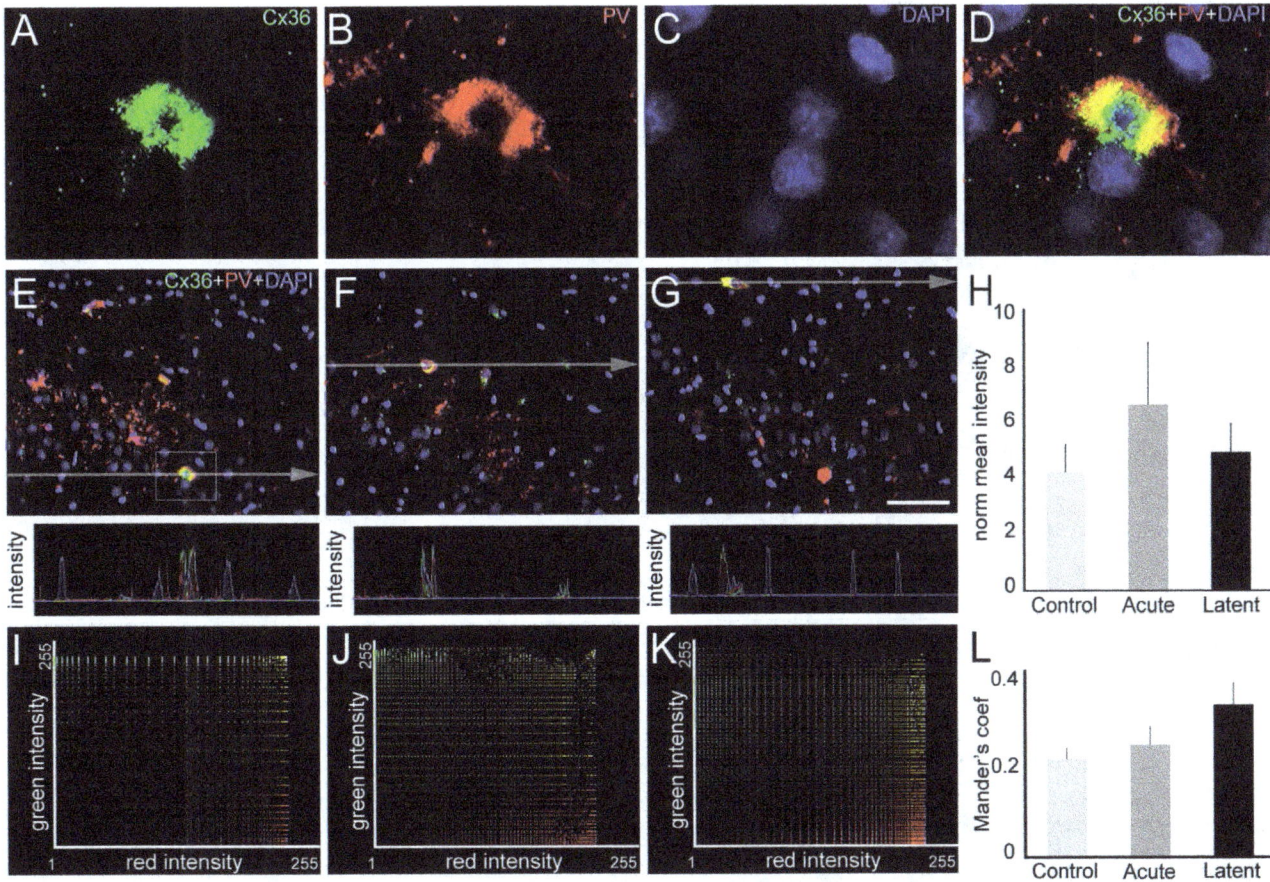

Figure 5. Cx36 expression in parvalbumin (PV)-positive interneurons into CA3. In order to quantify the amount of Cx36 (green) in PV-positive cells (red), we performed double-labeling experiments in coronal sections of rats from control, acute and latent groups counterstained with 4',6-diamidino-2-phenylindole (DAPI, blue). (A–D) High magnification of the selected area highlighted in the control section (E) shows Cx36 (A), PV (B) and DAPI labeling (C). Colocalization of both proteins is evidenced in (D). (E, F, G) In representative images of CA3 area it is possible to visualize that Cx36 remains in PV-positive cells in acute (F) and latent (G) groups. The pixel intensity profile revealed intersection of the green and red signals, supporting the colocalization of both proteins. (H) Pixel intensity analysis showed no significant differences in Cx36 mean intensity in PV-positive cells between the groups. (I–K) Intensity correlation between green (Cx36) vs. red (PV) channels of representative images from control, acute and latent periods, respectively. (L) Quantitative analysis (n = 4 animals per group) revealed that Mander's colocalization coefficient did not change in acute and latent groups. Bars represent standard errors of mean. Scale bar: 50 µm.

lacunosum-moleculare (65%, $P<0.01$) when compared to controls (Fig.6, B–I).

Epileptiform activity induces changes in Cx43 spatial pattern within CA3

To further examine the regulation of specific Cxs within the CA3 region, we evaluated the distribution of Cx43 in CA3 subfields, similarly to the analysis performed for Cx45. The quantification of the mean pixel intensity in each strata (Fig. 7A) revealed that during the acute period, Cx43 immunolabeling was increased in stratum pyramidale (171%, $P<0.05$), whereas reduction of 48% ($P<0.05$) was observed in stratum radiatum (Fig. 7, B–E). In the latent period, we were not able to detect significant changes in Cx43 distribution (Fig. 7, B–D, 7F and data not shown).

Discussion

The main purposes of this work were to demonstrate the involvement of GJ communication in the epileptiform activity and the possible alterations in Cx gene expression, protein levels,

phosphorylation profile and distribution in the hippocampus triggered by pilocarpine. Indeed, our results showed that blockade of Cx channels produced antiepileptiform effects, indisputably correlating the GJ coupling with the epileptiform activity induced by pilocarpine. In spite of previous evidences in the literature regarding the anticonvulsant effects of GJ blockers, based on both in vitro [5–9,35] and in vivo models [10,11], this is the first report addressing this issue in the pilocarpine model, which reproduces most of the characteristics of human temporal lobe epilepsy [30,31,36], such as histopathological features associated with neuronal network reorganization, the occurrence of an initial precipitant injury (the acute phase), a seizure-free interval (latent period), and the occurrence of spontaneous recurrent seizures (chronic phase).

The mechanisms governing oscillations at the cellular and network levels underlie processes related to cognitive and pathological brain states [37,38]. In this study, we were able to detect a marked increase in the power of beta frequency band following pilocarpine administration. Accordingly, a pronounced contribution of 20–80 Hz frequency band was reported in the kainic acid and in the lithium-pilocarpine models of temporal lobe

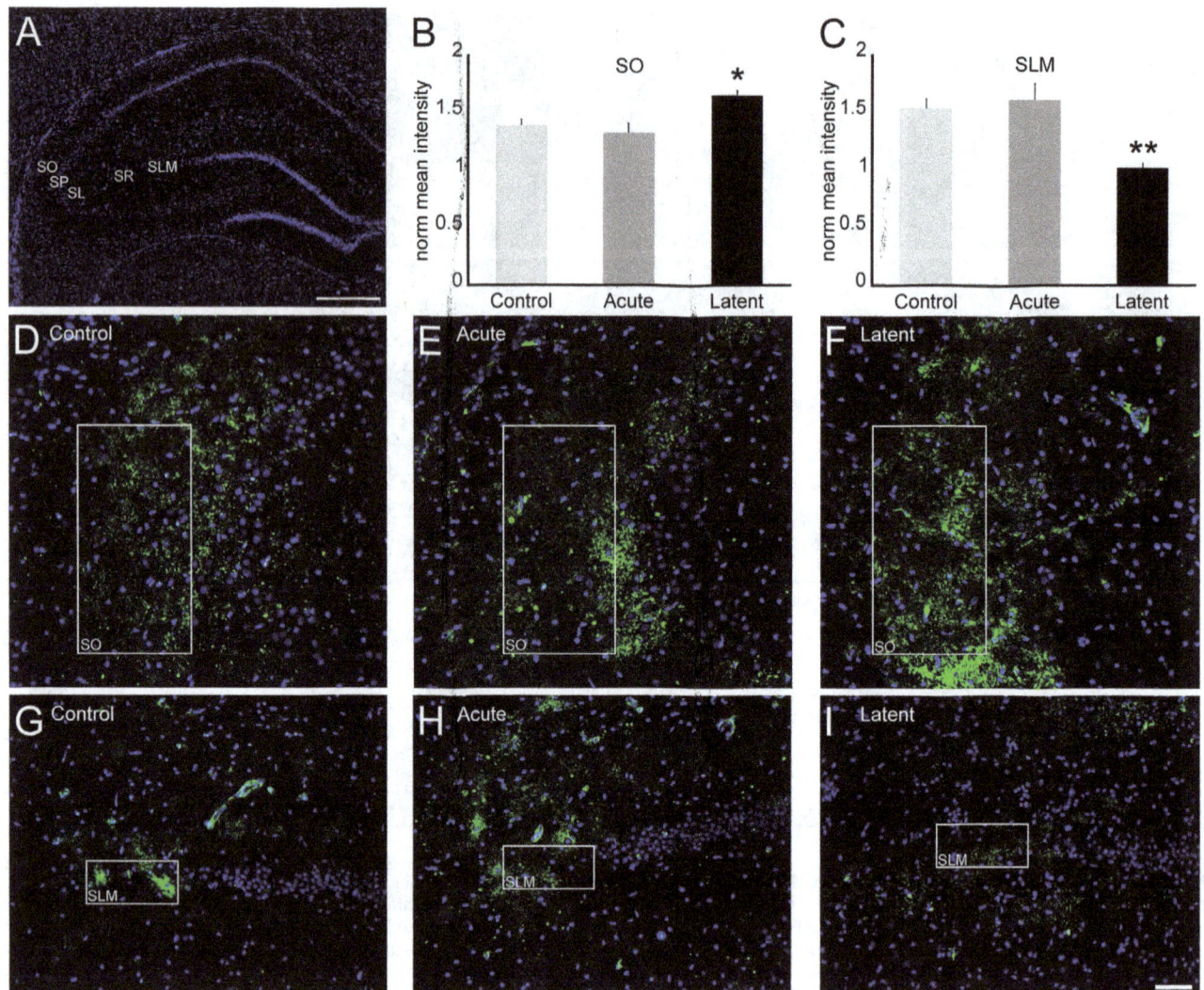

Figure 6. Cx45 distribution in CA3 after epileptiform activity. To examine Cx45 (green) distribution into CA3, we conducted immunofluorescence experiments in coronal sections of rats from control, acute and latent groups counterstained with DAPI (blue). (A) Coronal section labeled with DAPI showing CA3 strata oriens (SO), pyramidale (SP), lucidum (SL), radiatum (SR) and lacunosum-moleculare (SLM). (B, C) Quantification of mean pixel intensity (n = 4 animals per group) showed significant increase in (F) SO and decrease in (I) SLM in the latent period, compared with control animals (D, G). In these subfields, we were not able to detect differences in the acute period (E, H), as well as in the other strata in both acute and latent periods (data not shown). Bars represent standard errors of the mean. *$P < 0.05$, ** $P < 0.01$ *vs.* Control group in Tukey's HSD pairwise comparisons after one-way ANOVA. Scale bar: 50 μm.

epilepsy [39,40]. Furthermore, we also showed that GJ communication participates in this oscillatory activity, since blockade of GJ channels promoted a significant decrease in the power of several frequencies, especially in the beta range.

Another evidence supporting the involvement of GJs in the epileptiform activity presented herein was the anticipation of the low voltage periods after CBX treatment. These events resemble the flat periods previously described [41]. According to that study, flat periods occur in the last two of the five electrographic stages described, namely continuous ictal discharges with flat periods and periodic epileptiform discharges on a flat background, which could be related to the increased inhibitory activity due to the prolonged SE.

Several studies deliberate about the optimal electrographic pattern after management of refractory SE with standard clinical treatments. A number of works point the EEG burst suppression pattern as the model for electrographic pattern (suppression consists of a flat EEG pattern – [42–46]), although others support a flat record pattern, which comprises total suppression of EEG signal background [47]. In spite of these controversies, our results regarding anticipation of flat-like periods after GJ blockade exhibit a certain similarity with the EEG recording expected after SE standard treatment, suggesting that Cx channels could serve as a potential target in refractory SE management.

Moreover, the earlier onset of flat periods after CBX treatment observed in our study could be explained by a hyperpolarization over a large number of cortical neurons [48]. It is known that GABAergic interneurons are important players in the regulation of cortical principal cells discharge. Additionally, synchronized activity of GABAergic interneurons is a mandatory feature that leads to synchronization of action potential of principal cells [49–51]. GJ composed of Cx36 are important structures that participate in the regulation of GABAergic interneuron synchronization [32–34]. In fact, disruption of GJ communication by

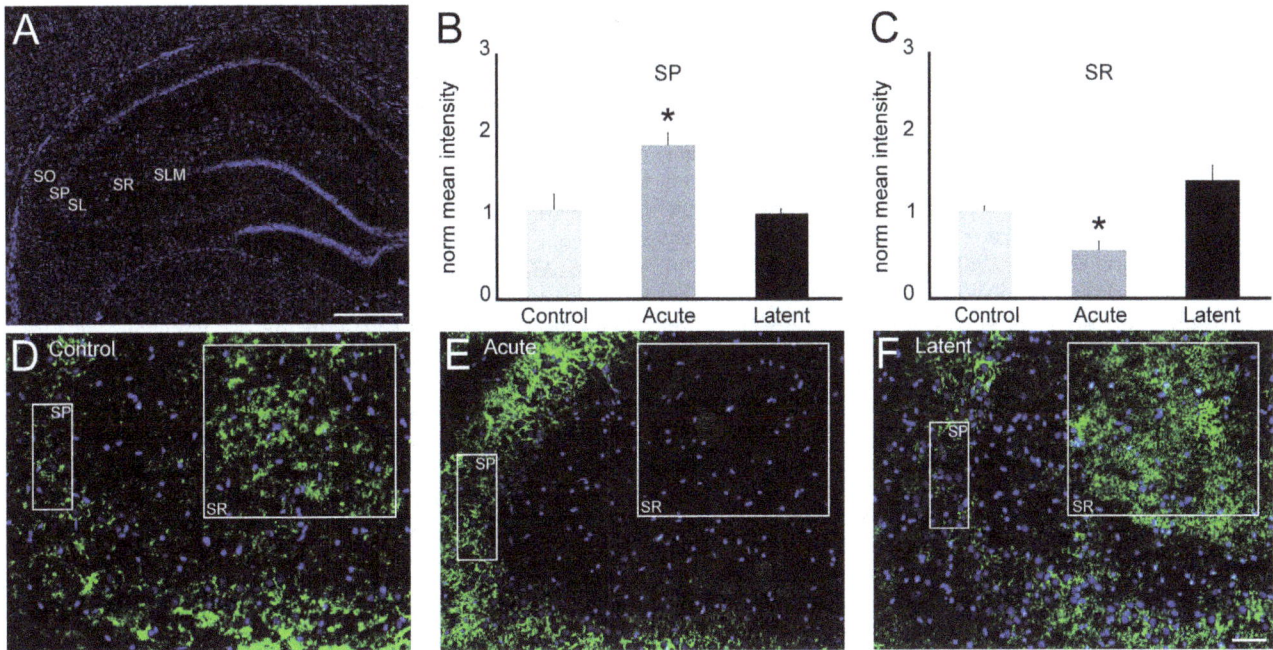

Figure 7. Cx43 distribution in CA3 after epileptiform activity. Immunofluorescence experiments were performed to analyze the distribution of Cx43 (green) in coronal sections of rats from control, acute and latent groups counterstained with DAPI (blue). (A) Coronal section labeled with DAPI showing CA3 strata oriens (SO), pyramidale (SP), lucidum (SL), radiatum (SR) and lacunosum-moleculare (SLM). (B, C) Quantification of mean pixel intensity (n = 4 animals per group) showed significant increase in SP and decrease in SR in the acute period (E) compared to controls (D). In these subfields, we were not able to detect changes in the latent period (F), as well as in the other strata in both acute and latent periods (data not shown). Bars represent standard errors of mean. *$P<0.05$ *vs.* Control group in Tukey's HSD pairwise comparisons after one-way ANOVA. Scale bar: 50 μm.

deletion of Cx36 promotes a higher inhibitory response in neurons during high frequency discharges [52,53]. Therefore, our results obtained with CBX treatment might be due to the desynchronization of GABAergic interneurons following uncoupling, demonstrating an important role of GJ communication in epileptiform potentials.

Although it has been demonstrated that CBX has effects other than on GJ channels, such as on intrinsic neuronal properties [54], antagonism of GABA_A receptors [20], blocking of calcium channels [55] and on endogenous glucocorticoid metabolism [56], there are also evidences that CBX does not affect neuronal excitability and GABA responses [6,57,58], and that the depressed spontaneous epileptiform activity observed in hippocampal slices was not due to the mineralocorticoid agonist action of CBX [59]. In spite of these controversies, CBX has been widely used in GJ studies, where neuroprotective effects were examined [60], often in parallel to the demonstration of its uncoupling properties [35,61,62]. Indeed, the effects of CBX and its analogous on neuronal coupling and synchronization convincingly recapitulated Cx KO models [62,63]. Taken together, these independent evidences from distinct groups allows for the use of CBX in GJ studies [64,65].

In addition to the participation of GJ communication in the epileptiform activity, we also determined several changes in Cx expression during the acute and latent periods. Although there are studies pointing to the participation of Cx36 in epileptiform discharges [19,66–68], we were not able to detect changes in Cx36 mRNA and protein levels. Furthermore, the spatial pattern distribution of Cx36 throughout acute and latent periods remains constant, evidencing the stability of this protein in conditions of epileptiform discharges and subsequent epileptogenesis. However, considering that pilocarpine model induces neuronal loss [69–73],

Cx36 stability might reflect an important role of GJ communication in the networks of GABAergic interneurons and principal cells that express this protein. Moreover, it is possible that even small differences in Cx expression play a significant role in the network coupled by electrical synapses [17], which in turn could participate in the seizure activity and the following process of epileptogenesis.

In agreement with previous studies, we detected the presence of Cx45 in hippocampal neurons [18,23,74]. Moreover, we detected changes in Cx45 distribution in the SO in the latent phase, which is consistent with the enhanced Cx45 transcript levels. Indeed, electronic coupling via GJ was reported between SO interneurons presumably in dendrites [75]. Additionally, the typical low pass filter feature imposed by GJ coupling over of the signal conductance could support synchronization of slow oscillations in the distal dendrites between SO interneurons. Also, it was reported the possible involvement of GABAergic interneurons presumably coupled by GJ in the slow oscillations recorded in hippocampal pyramidal cells [76]. Thus, our data regarding increase of Cx45 in SO could indicate the enhancement of coupling between the interneurons, which might intensify the occurrence of slow oscillations that, in turn, are noticed in a variety of epileptic activities [77,78].

Furthermore, the expression of Cx45 in the SO hippocampal region, as pointed out in our work, could represent a substrate for the GJ coupling between axons of principle cells previously reported in the hippocampus [57,79]. During the latent period, we observed an increased amount of Cx45 in this region. Interestingly, collateral connections from CA3 to CA1 are located within SO, and this is probably the site of occurrence of GJ connections [57]. Taking together, if the axo-axonal coupling that possibly takes place at SO involves Cx45, the upregulation of this protein could account for the generation of high frequency oscillations and the increased excitability observed in epileptic conditions [79].

Contrasting the increased levels in the SO, we noticed a decrease of Cx45 in the SLM during the latent period. It is well established that interneuron-mediated GABAergic synchronous potentials might play an important role in epilepsy [80,81], and that the mechanisms underlying these responses could be mediated by electrical coupling [82,83]. Indeed, propagation of GABAergic synchronized potentials recorded from SLM seems to be under control of electrical coupling [83,84]. Interestingly, the synchronous synaptic release of GABA from interneurons of SLM promoted CA3 pyramidal cell activation [84]. Thus, the reduction of Cx45 could lead to desynchronization of GABA release from the interneurons, consequently decreasing CA3 pyramidal cell activity. Therefore, downregulation of Cx45 in the SLM during the latent period could indicate a plastic homeostatic change of the coupled network in order to restore its activity after the epileptogenic insult, since interneuron networks within SLM could regulate the input from the entorhinal cortex to the hippocampus [85].

Whether modulation of Cx45 expression in SO and SLM remains at later time points (e.g. from the time that animals present spontaneous recurrent seizures) is not known, but it would be worth evaluating the issue.

Interestingly, whereas changes in Cx45 distribution were seen in the latent period, alterations in Cx43 distribution through CA3 layers were observed in the acute period. Astroglial networks provide the supply of glucose and lactate necessary for the maintenance of hippocampal synaptic activity in an activity-dependent manner, and it has been shown that this metabolic network of astrocytes is mediated by GJ composed by Cx43 and Cx30 [86]. Thus, the increase in Cx43 distribution pattern observed in the SP is probably due to the high energetic demand promoted by the sustained epileptic activity. Additionally, the coupled astrocytes could provide an important intercellular pathway for both delivery of metabolites to distant locations during episodes of epileptic discharges and buffering of ions such as potassium [87,88]. Increase of Cx43 in SP could account for two opposite situations: (1) besides providing distribution of metabolites of neurotransmitters and potassium (for review see ref. [89,90]) to distant locations during episodes of epileptic discharges, a Cx43 increase could lead to the formation of GJ hemichannels, a pathway for adenosine release [91], which could also contribute to the local neuroprotective effects; (2) by allowing the propagation of toxic metabolites and death signals to adjacent cells, the increase in astroglial network coupling could amplify the damage to more distant sites, in addition to the possible contribution to the rapid propagation of the electrical signal [15].

Contrary to the observed in SP, we found decreased labeling of Cx43 in the CA3 SR. It has been demonstrated that the contribution of GJ in potassium buffering in the hippocampus is layer-dependent [92]. By comparing the properties of astrocytes from mice with Cx30/Cx43 deficiencies, those authors found that single astrocytes from SR reach larger areas than those from SLM, indicating the unequal size and orientation of astrocytes from those areas. Additionally, they found no impairment of potassium buffering in SR of transgenic mice, in contrast to the observed in the SLM, evidencing the participation of other elements in the potassium redistribution in the SR. Therefore, the reduction of Cx43 labeling noticed here in the SR is unlikely to have a great impact in spatial buffering of potassium during SE; moreover, as CA3 SR is well supplied by a vascular source [93], which in turn accounts for the degree of astrocyte coupling [94], such decrease of Cx43 labeling in this layer during epileptic activity may not have a significant impact in the physiology of CA3 SR cells.

Remarkably, our results disclosed enhancement of the non-phosphorylated form of Cx43 during the latent period, suggesting reduction of astrocyte coupling, since the unphosphorylated form is not related with the assembly into GJ [95,96]. This result is quite in accordance with the immunofluorescence data, once both point to a smaller participation of Cx43-mediated GJ during the latent period, despite the increase in transcript levels at the same period, which could account for upregulation of protein levels in later time points.

In summary, we demonstrated the involvement of GJ channels in a model of temporal lobe epilepsy by describing the antiepileptiform effects of GJ blockade on pilocarpine-induced SE. Additionally, we depicted alterations of specific Cxs genes and protein, and changes in Cx distribution at different sites within the hippocampus throughout acute and latent periods. Taken together, our results revealed a reciprocal regulation of neuronal oscillations and electrical synapses, indicating that the control of Cx-mediated communication may take part in reliable anti-epileptogenic therapies.

Acknowledgments

The authors would like to thank Adilson S. Alves and Ana M. Alves for technical assistance.

Author Contributions

Conceived and designed the experiments: ERK AHK LRGB. Performed the experiments: ERK GSVH ACV. Analyzed the data: ERK GSVH ACV EM. Contributed reagents/materials/analysis tools: ACV AHK LRGB. Wrote the paper: ERK AHK LRGB.

References

1. Sohl G, Maxeiner S, Willecke K (2005) Expression and functions of neuronal gap junctions. Nat Rev Neurosci 6: 191–200.
2. Perez Velazquez JL, Carlen PL (2000) Gap junctions, synchrony and seizures. Trends Neurosci 23: 68–74.
3. Nakase T, Naus CC (2004) Gap junctions and neurological disorders of the central nervous system. Biochim Biophys Acta 1662: 149–158.
4. Bennett MV, Zukin RS (2004) Electrical coupling and neuronal synchronization in the Mammalian brain. Neuron 41: 495–511.
5. Perez-Velazquez JL, Valiante TA, Carlen PL (1994) Modulation of gap junctional mechanisms during calcium-free induced field burst activity: a possible role for electrotonic coupling in epileptogenesis. J Neurosci 14: 4308–4317.
6. Kohling R, Gladwell SJ, Bracci E, Vreugdenhil M, Jefferys JG (2001) Prolonged epileptiform bursting induced by 0-Mg(2+) in rat hippocampal slices depends on gap junctional coupling. Neuroscience 105: 579–587.
7. Traub RD, Bibbig R, Piechotta A, Draguhn R, Schmitz D (2001) Synaptic and nonsynaptic contributions to giant ipsps and ectopic spikes induced by 4-aminopyridine in the hippocampus in vitro. J Neurophysiol 85: 1246–1256.
8. Maier N, Guldenagel M, Sohl G, Siegmund H, Willecke K, et al. (2002) Reduction of high-frequency network oscillations (ripples) and pathological network discharges in hippocampal slices from connexin 36-deficient mice. J Physiol 541: 521–528.
9. Bragin A, Mody I, Wilson CL, Engel J, Jr. (2002) Local generation of fast ripples in epileptic brain. J Neurosci 22: 2012–2021.
10. Szente M, Gajda Z, Said Ali K, Hermesz E (2002) Involvement of electrical coupling in the in vivo ictal epileptiform activity induced by 4-aminopyridine in the neocortex. Neuroscience 115: 1067–1078.
11. Gajda Z, Gyengesi E, Hermesz E, Ali KS, Szente M (2003) Involvement of gap junctions in the manifestation and control of the duration of seizures in rats in vivo. Epilepsia 44: 1596–1600.
12. Gigout S, Louvel J, Kawasaki H, D'Antuono M, Armand V, et al. (2006) Effects of gap junction blockers on human neocortical synchronization. Neurobiol Dis 22: 496–508.
13. Roopun AK, Simonotto JD, Pierce ML, Jenkins A, Nicholson C, et al. (2010) A nonsynaptic mechanism underlying interictal discharges in human epileptic neocortex. Proc Natl Acad Sci U S A 107: 338–343.

14. Aronica E, Gorter JA, Jansen GH, Leenstra S, Yankaya B, et al. (2001) Expression of connexin 43 and connexin 32 gap-junction proteins in epilepsy-associated brain tumors and in the perilesional epileptic cortex. Acta Neuropathol 101: 449–459.

15. Fonseca CG, Green CR, Nicholson LF (2002) Upregulation in astrocytic connexin 43 gap junction levels may exacerbate generalized seizures in mesial temporal lobe epilepsy. Brain Res 929: 105–116.

16. Collignon F, Wetjen NM, Cohen-Gadol AA, Cascino GD, Parisi J, et al. (2006) Altered expression of connexin subtypes in mesial temporal lobe epilepsy in humans. J Neurosurg 105: 77–87.

17. Sohl G, Guldenagel M, Beck H, Teubner B, Traub O, et al. (2000) Expression of connexin genes in hippocampus of kainate-treated and kindled rats under conditions of experimental epilepsy. Brain Res Mol Brain Res 83: 44–51.

18. Condorelli DF, Trovato-Salinaro A, Mudo G, Mirone MB, Belluardo N (2003) Cellular expression of connexins in the rat brain: neuronal localization, effects of kainate-induced seizures and expression in apoptotic neuronal cells. Eur J Neurosci 18: 1807–1827.

19. Beheshti S, Sayyah M, Golkar M, Sepehri H, Babaie J, et al. (2010) Changes in hippocampal connexin 36 mRNA and protein levels during epileptogenesis in the kindling model of epilepsy. Prog Neuropsychopharmacol Biol Psychiatry 34: 510–515.

20. Beaumont M, Maccaferri G (2011) Is connexin36 critical for GABAergic hypersynchronization in the hippocampus? J Physiol 589: 1663–1680.

21. Dere E, Zlomuzica A (2012) The role of gap junctions in the brain in health and disease. Neurosci Biobehav Rev 36: 206–217.

22. Condorelli DF, Belluardo N, Trovato-Salinaro A, Mudo G (2000) Expression of Cx36 in mammalian neurons. Brain Res Brain Res Rev 32: 72–85.

23. Maxeiner S, Kruger O, Schilling K, Traub O, Urschel S, et al. (2003) Spatiotemporal transcription of connexin45 during brain development results in neuronal expression in adult mice. Neuroscience 119: 689–700.

24. Nagy JI, Dudek FE, Rash JE (2004) Update on connexins and gap junctions in neurons and glia in the mammalian nervous system. Brain Res Brain Res Rev 47: 191–215.

25. Timo-Iaria C, Negrao N, Schmidek WR, Hoshino K, Lobato de Menezes CE, et al. (1970) Phases and states of sleep in the rat. Physiol Behav 5: 1057–1062.

26. Kihara AH, Moriscot AS, Ferreira PJ, Hamassaki DE (2005) Protecting RNA in fixed tissue: an alternative method for LCM users. J Neurosci Methods 148: 103–107.

27. Medhurst AD, Harrison DC, Read SJ, Campbell CA, Robbins MJ, et al. (2000) The use of TaqMan RT-PCR assays for semiquantitative analysis of gene expression in CNS tissues and disease models. J Neurosci Methods 98: 9–20.

28. Kihara AH, Paschon V, Akamine PS, Saito KC, Leonelli M, et al. (2008) Differential expression of connexins during histogenesis of the chick retina. Dev Neurobiol 68: 1287–1302.

29. Kinjo ER, Higa GS, de Sousa E, Casado OA, Damico MV, et al. (2013) A possible new mechanism for the control of miRNA expression in neurons. Exp Neurol 248: 546–558.

30. Cavalheiro EA (1995) The pilocarpine model of epilepsy. Ital J Neurol Sci 16: 33–37.

31. Curia G, Longo D, Biagini G, Jones RS, Avoli M (2008) The pilocarpine model of temporal lobe epilepsy. J Neurosci Methods 172: 143–157.

32. Venance L, Rozov A, Blatow M, Burnashev N, Feldmeyer D, et al. (2000) Connexin expression in electrically coupled postnatal rat brain neurons. Proc Natl Acad Sci U S A 97: 10260–10265.

33. Deans MR, Gibson JR, Sellitto C, Connors BW, Paul DL (2001) Synchronous activity of inhibitory networks in neocortex requires electrical synapses containing connexin36. Neuron 31: 477–485.

34. Hormuzdi SG, Pais I, LeBeau FE, Towers SK, Rozov A, et al. (2001) Impaired electrical signaling disrupts gamma frequency oscillations in connexin 36-deficient mice. Neuron 31: 487–495.

35. Chang WP, Wu JJ, Shyu BC (2013) Thalamic modulation of cingulate seizure activity via the regulation of gap junctions in mice thalamocingulate slice. PLoS One 8: e62952.

36. Scorza FA, Arida RM, Naffah-Mazzacoratti Mda G, Scerni DA, Calderazzo L, et al. (2009) The pilocarpine model of epilepsy: what have we learned? An Acad Bras Cienc 81: 345–365.

37. Buzsaki G, Draguhn A (2004) Neuronal oscillations in cortical networks. Science 304: 1926–1929.

38. Uhlhaas PJ, Singer W (2006) Neural synchrony in brain disorders: relevance for cognitive dysfunctions and pathophysiology. Neuron 52: 155–168.

39. Medvedev A, Mackenzie L, Hiscock JJ, Willoughby JO (2000) Kainic acid induces distinct types of epileptiform discharge with differential involvement of hippocampus and neocortex. Brain Res Bull 52: 89–98.

40. Lehmkuhle MJ, Thomson KE, Scheerlinck P, Pouliot W, Greger B, et al. (2009) A simple quantitative method for analyzing electrographic status epilepticus in rats. J Neurophysiol 101: 1660–1670.

41. Treiman DM, Walton NY, Kendrick C (1990) A progressive sequence of electroencephalographic changes during generalized convulsive status epilepticus. Epilepsy Res 5: 49–60.

42. Swank RL, Watson CW (1949) Effects of barbiturates and ether on spontaneous electrical activity of dog brain. J Neurophysiol 12: 137–160.

43. Rashkin MC, Youngs C, Penovich P (1987) Pentobarbital treatment of refractory status epilepticus. Neurology 37: 500–503.

44. Van Ness PC (1990) Pentobarbital and EEG burst suppression in treatment of status epilepticus refractory to benzodiazepines and phenytoin. Epilepsia 31: 61–67.

45. Meierkord H, Boon P, Engelsen B, Gocke K, Shorvon S, et al. (2010) EFNS guideline on the management of status epilepticus in adults. Eur J Neurol 17: 348–355.

46. Parviainen I, Uusaro A, Kalviainen R, Kaukanen E, Mervaala E, et al. (2002) High-dose thiopental in the treatment of refractory status epilepticus in intensive care unit. Neurology 59: 1249–1251.

47. Ramsay RE (1993) Treatment of status epilepticus. Epilepsia 34 Suppl 1: S71–81.

48. Steriade M, Amzica F, Contreras D (1994) Cortical and thalamic cellular correlates of electroencephalographic burst-suppression. Electroencephalogr Clin Neurophysiol 90: 1–16.

49. Kullmann DM, Moreau AW, Bakiri Y, Nicholson E (2012) Plasticity of inhibition. Neuron 75: 951–962.

50. Buzsaki G (1997) Functions for interneuronal nets in the hippocampus. Can J Physiol Pharmacol 75: 508–515.

51. Soltesz I, Deschenes M (1993) Low- and high-frequency membrane potential oscillations during theta activity in CA1 and CA3 pyramidal neurons of the rat hippocampus under ketamine-xylazine anesthesia. J Neurophysiol 70: 97–116.

52. Postma F, Liu CH, Dietsche C, Khan M, Lee HK, et al. (2011) Electrical synapses formed by connexin36 regulate inhibition- and experience-dependent plasticity. Proc Natl Acad Sci U S A 108: 13770–13775.

53. Butovas S, Hormuzdi SG, Monyer H, Schwarz C (2006) Effects of electrically coupled inhibitory networks on local neuronal responses to intracortical microstimulation. J Neurophysiol 96: 1227–1236.

54. Rouach N, Segal M, Koulakoff A, Giaume C, Avignone E (2003) Carbenoxolone blockade of neuronal network activity in culture is not mediated by an action on gap junctions. J Physiol 553: 729–745.

55. Vessey JP, Lalonde MR, Mizan HA, Welch NC, Kelly ME, et al. (2004) Carbenoxolone inhibition of voltage-gated Ca channels and synaptic transmission in the retina. J Neurophysiol 92: 1252–1256.

56. Jellinck PH, Monder C, McEwen BS, Sakai RR (1993) Differential inhibition of 11 beta-hydroxysteroid dehydrogenase by carbenoxolone in rat brain regions and peripheral tissues. J Steroid Biochem Mol Biol 46: 209–213.

57. Schmitz D, Schuchmann S, Fisahn A, Draguhn A, Buhl EH, et al. (2001) Axo-axonal coupling. a novel mechanism for ultrafast neuronal communication. Neuron 31: 831–840.

58. Draguhn A, Traub RD, Schmitz D, Jefferys JG (1998) Electrical coupling underlies high-frequency oscillations in the hippocampus in vitro. Nature 394: 189–192.

59. Ross FM, Gwyn P, Spanswick D, Davies SN (2000) Carbenoxolone depresses spontaneous epileptiform activity in the CA1 region of rat hippocampal slices. Neuroscience 100: 789–796.

60. Paschon V, Higa GS, Resende RR, Britto LR, Kihara AH (2012) Blocking of connexin-mediated communication promotes neuroprotection during acute degeneration induced by mechanical trauma. PLoS One 7: e45449.

61. de Pina-Benabou MH, Szostak V, Kyrozis A, Rempe D, Uziel D, et al. (2005) Blockade of gap junctions in vivo provides neuroprotection after perinatal global ischemia. Stroke 36: 2232–2237.

62. Striedinger K, Petrasch-Parwez E, Zoidl G, Napirei M, Meier C, et al. (2005) Loss of connexin36 increases retinal cell vulnerability to secondary cell loss. Eur J Neurosci 22: 605–616.

63. Volgyi B, Pan F, Paul DL, Wang JT, Huberman AD, et al. (2013) Gap junctions are essential for generating the correlated spike activity of neighboring retinal ganglion cells. PLoS One 8: e69426.

64. Cusato K, Bosco A, Rozental R, Guimaraes CA, Reese BE, et al. (2003) Gap junctions mediate bystander cell death in developing retina. J Neurosci 23: 6413–6422.

65. Kihara AH, Santos TO, Osuna-Melo EJ, Paschon V, Vidal KS, et al. (2010) Connexin-mediated communication controls cell proliferation and is essential in retinal histogenesis. Int J Dev Neurosci 28: 39–52.

66. Pais I, Hormuzdi SG, Monyer H, Traub RD, Wood IC, et al. (2003) Sharp wave-like activity in the hippocampus in vitro in mice lacking the gap junction protein connexin 36. J Neurophysiol 89: 2046–2054.

67. Jacobson GM, Voss LJ, Melin SM, Mason JP, Cursons RT, et al. (2010) Connexin36 knockout mice display increased sensitivity to pentylenetetrazol-induced seizure-like behaviors. Brain Res 1360: 198–204.

68. Gajda Z, Szupera Z, Blazso G, Szente M (2005) Quinine, a blocker of neuronal cx36 channels, suppresses seizure activity in rat neocortex in vivo. Epilepsia 46: 1581–1591.

69. Fujikawa DG (2005) Prolonged seizures and cellular injury: understanding the connection. Epilepsy Behav 7 Suppl 3: S3–11.

70. Fujikawa DG (1996) The temporal evolution of neuronal damage from pilocarpine-induced status epilepticus. Brain Res 725: 11–22.

71. Pitkanen A, Lukasiuk K (2009) Molecular and cellular basis of epileptogenesis in symptomatic epilepsy. Epilepsy Behav 14 Suppl 1: 16–25.

72. Pestana RR, Kinjo ER, Hernandes MS, Britto LR (2010) Reactive oxygen species generated by NADPH oxidase are involved in neurodegeneration in the pilocarpine model of temporal lobe epilepsy. Neurosci Lett 484: 187–191.

73. Weise J, Engelhorn T, Dorfler A, Aker S, Bahr M, et al. (2005) Expression time course and spatial distribution of activated caspase-3 after experimental status

epilepticus: contribution of delayed neuronal cell death to seizure-induced neuronal injury. Neurobiol Dis 18: 582–590.

74. Weickert S, Ray A, Zoidl G, Dermietzel R (2005) Expression of neural connexins and pannexin1 in the hippocampus and inferior olive: a quantitative approach. Brain Res Mol Brain Res 133: 102–109.

75. Zhang XL, Zhang L, Carlen PL (2004) Electrotonic coupling between stratum oriens interneurones in the intact in vitro mouse juvenile hippocampus. J Physiol 558: 825–839.

76. Zhang Y, Perez Velazquez JL, Tian GF, Wu CP, Skinner FK, et al. (1998) Slow oscillations (</ = 1 Hz) mediated by GABAergic interneuronal networks in rat hippocampus. J Neurosci 18: 9256–9268.

77. Gambardella A, Gotman J, Cendes F, Andermann F (1995) Focal intermittent delta activity in patients with mesiotemporal atrophy: a reliable marker of the epileptogenic focus. Epilepsia 36: 122–129.

78. Kirkpatrick MP, Clarke CD, Sonmezturk HH, Abou-Khalil B (2011) Rhythmic delta activity represents a form of nonconvulsive status epilepticus in anti-NMDA receptor antibody encephalitis. Epilepsy Behav 20: 392–394.

79. Traub RD, Whittington MA, Buhl EH, LeBeau FE, Bibbig A, et al. (2001) A possible role for gap junctions in generation of very fast EEG oscillations preceding the onset of, and perhaps initiating, seizures. Epilepsia 42: 153–170.

80. Avoli M (1996) GABA-mediated synchronous potentials and seizure generation. Epilepsia 37: 1035–1042.

81. Taira T, Lamsa K, Kaila K (1997) Posttetanic excitation mediated by GABA(A) receptors in rat CA1 pyramidal neurons. J Neurophysiol 77: 2213–2218.

82. Uusisaari M, Smirnov S, Voipio J, Kaila K (2002) Spontaneous epileptiform activity mediated by GABA(A) receptors and gap junctions in the rat hippocampal slice following long-term exposure to GABA(B) antagonists. Neuropharmacology 43: 563–572.

83. Zsiros V, Aradi I, Maccaferri G (2007) Propagation of postsynaptic currents and potentials via gap junctions in GABAergic networks of the rat hippocampus. J Physiol 578: 527–544.

84. Perkins KL (2002) GABA application to hippocampal CA3 or CA1 stratum lacunosum-moleculare excites an interneuron network. J Neurophysiol 87: 1404–1414.

85. Steward O (1976) Topographic organization of the projections from the entorhinal area to the hippocampal formation of the rat. J Comp Neurol 167: 285–314.

86. Rouach N, Koulakoff A, Abudara V, Willecke K, Giaume C (2008) Astroglial metabolic networks sustain hippocampal synaptic transmission. Science 322: 1551–1555.

87. Giaume C, Koulakoff A, Roux L, Holcman D, Rouach N (2010) Astroglial networks: a step further in neuroglial and gliovascular interactions. Nat Rev Neurosci 11: 87–99.

88. Xu L, Zeng LH, Wong M (2009) Impaired astrocytic gap junction coupling and potassium buffering in a mouse model of tuberous sclerosis complex. Neurobiol Dis 34: 291–299.

89. Theis M, Sohl G, Eiberger J, Willecke K (2005) Emerging complexities in identity and function of glial connexins. Trends Neurosci 28: 188–195.

90. Binder DK, Steinhauser C (2006) Functional changes in astroglial cells in epilepsy. Glia 54: 358–368.

91. Lin JH, Lou N, Kang N, Takano T, Hu F, et al. (2008) A central role of connexin 43 in hypoxic preconditioning. J Neurosci 28: 681–695.

92. Wallraff A, Kohling R, Heinemann U, Theis M, Willecke K, et al. (2006) The impact of astrocytic gap junctional coupling on potassium buffering in the hippocampus. J Neurosci 26: 5438–5447.

93. Coyle P (1978) Spatial features of the rat hippocampal vascular system. Exp Neurol 58: 549–561.

94. D'Ambrosio R, Wenzel J, Schwartzkroin PA, McKhann GM, 2nd, Janigro D (1998) Functional specialization and topographic segregation of hippocampal astrocytes. J Neurosci 18: 4425–4438.

95. Crow DS, Beyer EC, Paul DL, Kobe SS, Lau AF (1990) Phosphorylation of connexin43 gap junction protein in uninfected and Rous sarcoma virus-transformed mammalian fibroblasts. Mol Cell Biol 10: 1754–1763.

96. Hossain MZ, Murphy LJ, Hertzberg EL, Nagy JI (1994) Phosphorylated forms of connexin43 predominate in rat brain: demonstration by rapid inactivation of brain metabolism. J Neurochem 62: 2394–2403.

A Novel Algorithm to Enhance P300 in Single Trials: Application to Lie Detection Using F-Score and SVM

Junfeng Gao[1,5], Hongjun Tian[2], Yong Yang[3], Xiaolin Yu[4], Chenhong Li[1]*, Nini Rao[5]*

1 College of Biomedical Engineering, South-Central University for Nationalities, Wuhan, People's Republic of China, **2** Nanjing Fullshare Superconducting Technology Co., Ltd., Nanjing, People's Republic of China, **3** School of Information Technology, Jiangxi University of Finance and Economics, Nanchang, People's Republic of China, **4** Department of Information Engineering, Officers College of CAPF, People's Republic of China, **5** School of Life Science and Technology, University of Electronic Science and Technology of China, Chengdu, People's Republic of China

Abstract

The investigation of lie detection methods based on P300 potentials has drawn much interest in recent years. We presented a novel algorithm to enhance signal-to-noise ratio (SNR) of P300 and applied it in lie detection to increase the classification accuracy. Thirty-four subjects were divided randomly into guilty and innocent groups, and the EEG signals on 14 electrodes were recorded. A novel spatial denoising algorithm (SDA) was proposed to reconstruct the P300 with a high SNR based on independent component analysis. The differences between the proposed method and our/other early published methods mainly lie in the extraction and feature selection method of P300. Three groups of features were extracted from the denoised waves; then, the optimal features were selected by the F-score method. Selected feature samples were finally fed into three classical classifiers to make a performance comparison. The optimal parameter values in the SDA and the classifiers were tuned using a grid-searching training procedure with cross-validation. The support vector machine (SVM) approach was adopted to combine with an F-score because this approach had the best performance. The presented model F-score_SVM reaches a significantly higher classification accuracy for P300 (specificity of 96.05%) and non-P300 (sensitivity of 96.11%) compared with the results obtained without using SDA and compared with the results obtained by other classification models. Moreover, a higher individual diagnosis rate can be obtained compared with previous methods, and the presented method requires only a small number of stimuli in the real testing application.

Editor: Hans A. Kestler, University of Ulm, Germany

Funding: This work was supported by National Nature Science Foundation of China (No. 81271659, 61262034, 61302011, 81171411 and 30972848), and Academic Team of South Central University for Nationalities: Biomedical Signals Processing (No. XTZ09002). The funders had no role in study design, data collection and analysis, decision to publish, or preparation of the manuscript.

Competing Interests: Dr. Hongjun Tian is employed by Nanjing Fullshare Superconducting Technology Co., Ltd., Nanjing, People's Republic of China. The company had no role in study design, data collection and analysis, decision to publish, or preparation of the manuscript. This does not alter the authors' adherence to all the PLOS ONE policies on sharing data and materials.

* Email: lichen@mail.scuec.edu.cn (CL); raonini@uestc.edu.cn (NR)

Introduction

Research into lie detection has drawn a substantial amount of attention over the past several decades and has found many important applications in the legal, moral and clinical fields [1–3]. Currently, a number of studies that adopt neurophysiological signals have been conducted on lie detection. These methods have used Magnetic Resonance Imaging [4,5] and Event-Related Potentials (ERPs) [6,7]. P300, an endogenous ERP component, has been extensively investigated [8] and has been successfully used for deception detection [9].

Widely used P300-based lie detection methods can be roughly divided into three categories: the bootstrapped amplitude difference (BAD) [10,11], the bootstrapped correlation difference (BCD) [12] and machine learning methods [7,13,14]. For the methods listed above, there are three types of stimuli that are presented to subjects, i.e., Probe (P), Target (T) and Irrelevant (I) stimuli [7].

A good lie detection method should use a small number of stimuli to achieve as high accuracy as possible. To realize this goal for the P300-based lie detection, a critical step is to extract the P300 with a high signal/noise ratio (SNR). Although the P300 is time- and phase-locked to experimental stimuli, the extraction of the P300 with a high SNR is still a challenging task because various types of noise are superimposed seriously on P300 [15]. BAD and BCD use the statistical technique of bootstrapping [16] to generate many different averages of ERP from the same set of stimuli [7]. Using bootstrapping, the SNR of P300 can be increased. However, such a mode involves a large number of stimuli and hence is at the expense of taking a longer time for signal acquisition, which would also increase the fatigue of the subjects. In addition, more recently, a few researchers have investigated single trial-based lie detection methods that were based on machine learning [7,14]. In these methods, some features were extracted from single trials and then were used to train classifiers to differentiate between different brain states. The testing results showed that machine learning methods could achieve a higher detection accuracy than BAD and BCD methods [7]. However, they typically did not remove the noises embedded in single trials, resulting in unsatisfactory detection accuracy.

Consider the noises embedded in single trials for P300 extraction. The EEG recording on one sensor consists of two main parts. One part is extra-skull noise, and the other part is the signal produced by intra-skull neuronal sources at specific brain regions, including ERP and spontaneous EEG. Obviously, the ERP cannot be represented by the signal from the sensor directly. Conventional lie detection methods could not separate P300 from the noise and spontaneous EEG because their time courses and scalp projections usually overlap [17]. Recently, independent component analysis (ICA), a blind source separation (BSS) method [15,18–20], was used to extract stimulus-related ERP into independent components (ICs) [21–24]. The results showed that the decomposed ICs were more distinguishable than the "sensor signals" [22,23]. In our early study [25], we proposed an ICA-based template matching method, topography-template matching (TTM) algorithm, to enhance the SNR of P300, and we achieved promising results. In TTM, we only consider the P300 independent sources affect in Pz site. In addition, one neurophysiologist was employed to select the P300 independent source by his experience. In this study we present a novel spatial denoising algorithm (SDA) to improve that early study. Comparing with our early study, SDA consider more affecting areas including at P3, P4, Pz, Cz and Oz sites. In addition, SDA recognized P300 independent source automatically, not by experience. Hence, the SDA is more reasonable and objective than the early study. The key innovation is how to automatically identify the P300 ICs (i.e., the ICs accounting for the P300), which will be described in the following section.

By removing any redundant features, feature selection can help the original classification system to achieve better classification performance including lower computational costs and higher classification accuracy. Polat et al. indicated that feature selection improves the classification accuracy by using a hybrid system of feature selection and several classifiers [26]. In this study, the F-score [38], a simple but effective technique, was used to select the optimal features from the original extracted features. In addition, to select a suitable classifier, all of the training samples with the selected optimal features were fed into three popular classifiers to compare their performance.

For conventional lie detection like BCD/BAD [10–12] and other some lie detection methods [7,13], a number of stimuli were required to present to the subjects in practical applications, because both of the bootstrapping technique and threshold selection-based classification were based on many stimuli responses. This would limit the real application of lie detection. First, there is often very limited information related to criminal acts. Second, many repeated stimuli with little information would cause two problems. One problem is fatigue, and the other is an increase in the countermeasures [11], because real criminals might be familiar with the stimuli and tend to resist the detection when many stimuli are presented repeatedly. Furthermore, based on the analysis results from a number of stimuli, when the researcher need to make the last judgment, a threshold strategy (see the references [10–12,7,13] for details) was inevitably used, which was a subjective decision on the individual diagnostic rate. The present method aims at using only a small number of stimuli and having no threshold problem.

Materials

Ethics statement

The experiment was approved by Psychology Research Ethical Committee (PREC) of the College of Biomedical Engineering in South-Central University for Nationalities. Thirty healthy subjects (15 females, mean age of 21.5) were recruited from the university. The participants provided their written informed consent according to a human research protocol in this study.

EEG Data Acquisition

Twelve electrodes (Fp1, Fp2, F3, Fz, F4, C3, Cz, C4, P3, Pz, P4, Oz) from an International 10–20 system were used. The vertical EOG (VEOG) signal was recorded from the right eye (2.5 cm below and above the pupil), and the horizontal EOG (HEOG) signal was recorded from the outer canthus. EEG and EOG signals were filtered online with a band pass filter of 0.1–30 Hz, and they were digitized at 500 Hz using Neuroscan Synamps. All of the electrodes were referenced to the right earlobe. Electrode impedances did not exceed 2 kΩ.

Experimental Protocol

The standard three-stimuli protocol [10,12] was employed in this study. The participants were randomly divided into two groups: a guilty group and an innocent group. Six different jewels were prepared, and their pictures served as stimuli during detection. A safe that contained one (for the innocent) or two (for the guilty) jewels was given to each participant. They were instructed to open the safe and memorize the details of the object. We instructed the guilty group to steal only one object which would serve as the P stimulus. The other object in the safe was the T stimulus, and the remaining four pictures were the I stimuli. The object in the safe was not stolen for the innocent, which served as the T stimulus. Then, from the remaining five pictures, one picture was selected randomly and set as the P stimulus, and the remaining four images were set as I stimuli. All of the subjects were instructed to write down the information on the objects in the safe, such as the styles and colors of the jewels.

After the preparation tasks introduced above, the participants began to perform the detection. They were seated in a chair, facing a video screen that was approximately 1 m away from their eyes. The stimuli pictures were presented randomly on the screen. Each item remained for 0.5 s with 30 iterations for one session, and each session lasted for approximately 5 minutes, with 2 minutes of resting time. The inter-stimulus interval was 1.6 s. Each subject was instructed to perform 5 sessions. The stimuli sequence diagram is given in Figure 1. One push button was given to each subject, and he or she was asked to press a "Yes" and "No" button when faced with familiar and unknown items, respectively.

The guilty group was instructed to press the "Yes" and "No" button when faced with the T and I stimuli, respectively. With a P stimulus, they were asked to press the "No" button, attempting to hide the stolen act. In contrast, the innocent group made honest responses to all of the stimuli. All of the subjects had practiced the tasks above before the EEG signals were recorded formally. We planned to exclude any subjects that had more than a 5% clicking error, but none fell into this category. Finally, a sketch map is presented and shown in Figure 2 to describe above protocol.

Methods

General description of method

The present method is separated into the following steps: (1) preprocess the continuous raw EEG recordings, and then, apply SDA on the preprocessed datasets to reconstruct P300 waves that have a higher SNR (from the guilty) and non-P300 waves (from the innocent). For convenience, we hereafter describe the above processed results as reconstructed P300 waves (In fact, the results also contain non-P300 waves); (2) extract original features from the

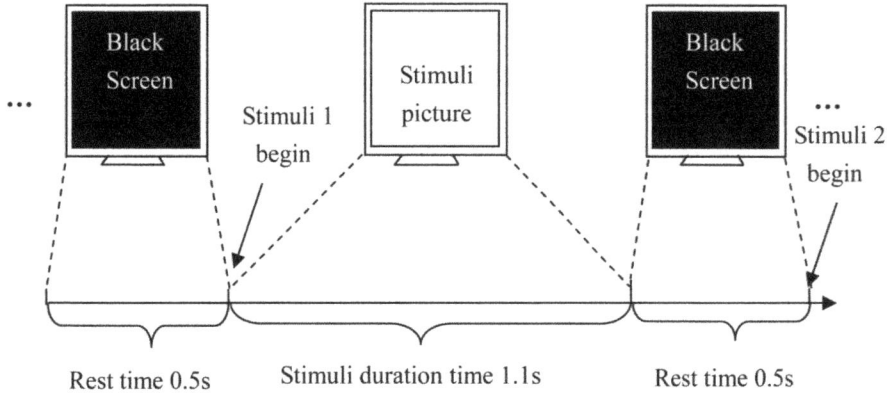

Figure 1. The stimuli sequence diagram.

reconstructed waves; (3) adopt the F-score method to select the optimal features; these features were concatenated as a featured vector and fed into three kinds of typical classifiers; (4) train the classifiers using the two classes of training samples, and then, test the samples using testing samples. By the training procedure, the optimal parameter values including the parameter in SDA and in specific classifier can be determined. During a practical application phase, only several stimuli (Five probe stimuli were needed in this study) are presented to the subjects. The flowchart of the presented CIT system is shown in Figure 3.

Preprocessing

Using EEGLAB toolbox, we segmented the continuous EEG data into epoched datasets, each of which lasted from 0.5 s before to 1.1 s after the stimulus onset. Then, the ocular artifacts [24] in each set were removed by the software SCAN of Neuroscan, i.e., the datasets that contained single trials with the voltage in excess of $\pm 75\mu v$ were discarded. All of the remaining trials were baseline corrected on the pre-stimulus interval. Lastly, the datasets corresponding to **P** responses were selected, and each 5 datasets within each subject was pooled into one average, resulting in 450 averaged datasets for each subject group.

Independent component analysis

Let $\mathbf{X}(t) = [x_1(t), x_2(t), ..., x_C(t)]^T$ denote the observed time series with t varying from 1 to N, where N and C denote the number of samples and sensors, respectively. In ICA method, $\mathbf{X}(t)$ is the result of an unknown mixture of a set of unknown source signals $\mathbf{S}(t)$ $= [s_1(t), s_2(t), ..., s_C(t)]^T$, and the mixture is viewed as linear: $\mathbf{X}(t)$ $= \mathbf{AS}(t)$. Based on the principle of statistical independence [26–27], ICA estimates $\mathbf{S}(t)$ by introducing the unmixing matrix $\mathbf{W}$, i.e., $\mathbf{Z}(t) = \mathbf{WX}(t)$ where $\mathbf{Z}(t)$ (which is the decomposed ICs) is the estimation of signals $\mathbf{S}(t)$. Accordingly, $\mathbf{W}^{-1}$ is referred to as a mixing matrix. Once the signals $\mathbf{S}(t)$ are estimated by an ICA algorithm, a column of the matrix $\mathbf{W}^{-1}$ provides the projection strengths of the corresponding IC onto each electrode.

Spatial denoising algorithm for P300 enhancement

The spatial denoising algorithm, referred to as SDA hereafter, is described in this section. First, each averaged dataset was decomposed by ICA, resulting in mixing matrix $\mathbf{W}^{-1}$ and decomposed ICs $\mathbf{Z}(t)$. The extended infomax algorithm (EICA) was used in ICA because it can allow some sources to have sub-Gaussian distributions [28,29]. By accommodating sub-Gaussian

distributions in the data, EICA could provide a more accurate decomposition of multi-channel EEG signals, especially when various neurophysiological signals follow different distributions.

Many investigators have found that P300 was usually the largest at Pz, the smallest at Fz, and takes intermediate values at Cz [30,32]. They typically acquired the P300 on one of the electrodes listed above [7,9,11,31]. According to the *a priori* physiological knowledge described above and the spatial distribution of an IC, SDA is divided into the following four steps:

(1) Let z_j denote the jth IC in matrix $\mathbf{Z}(t)$. Denote the ith row jth column element in $\mathbf{W}^{-1}$ by W_{ij}^{-1}, and accordingly the jth column by $W_{\bullet j}^{-1}$. First, each matrix $\mathbf{W}^{-1}$ is normalized to the matrix $\mathbf{U}$ by

$$U_{ij} = |W_{ij}^{-1}| \Big/ \max(|W_{\bullet j}^{-1}|), i = 1,2,...,14; \ j = 1,2,...,14 \quad (1)$$

where symbol || denotes an absolute calculation. Let $\mathbf{X}'(t)$ denote a new EEG dataset, which was defined by

$$\mathbf{X}'(t) = \mathbf{UZ}(t) = \begin{bmatrix} u_{11} & \cdots & u_{1j} & \cdots & u_{1n} \\ \vdots & \ddots & \vdots & \ddots & \vdots \\ u_{i1} & \cdots & u_{ij} & \cdots & u_{in} \\ \vdots & \ddots & \vdots & \ddots & \vdots \\ u_{n1} & \cdots & u_{nj} & \cdots & u_{nn} \end{bmatrix} \begin{bmatrix} z_1(t) \\ \vdots \\ z_j(t) \\ \vdots \\ z_n(t) \end{bmatrix} \quad (2)$$

(2) Let Pz, $P3$, $P4$, Cz and Oz equal their respective sequence number in the electrode set (e.g., Pz equals 10 in this study). For the jth column in each matrix $\mathbf{U}$, we calculate a value S_j using the following formula:

$$S_j = U_{Pzj} + k1 * (U_{P3j} + U_{P4j}) + k2 * U_{Czj} + k3 * U_{Ozj}, \quad (3)$$

where the parameters $k1$, $k2$ and $k3$ denote the weighted parameters on different element U_{ij}. A grid-search procedure (see Figure 3) would be used to obtain optimal values of these

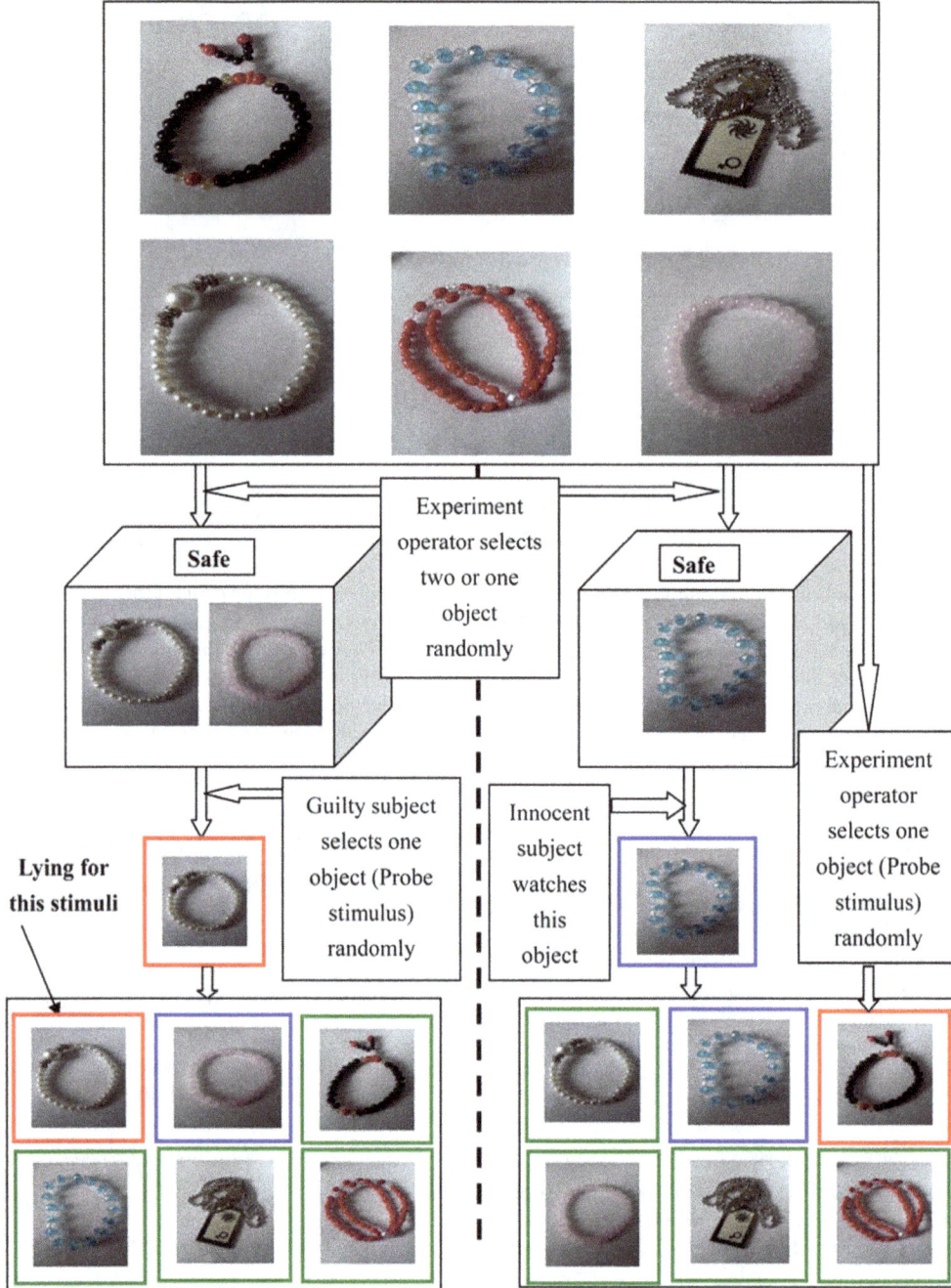

Figure 2. The sketch map of stimuli protocol. The left part and right parts of the dashed line represent the experimental protocol for guilty and innocent subjects, respectively. The pictures with red, blue and green rectangles represents P, T and I stimuli, respectively.

parameters. In this equation, S_j denote the integrated distribution-strength on several interested brain areas from jth IC. The bigger S_j is, the bigger probability jth IC is the P300 ICs.

(3) Sort the 14 values in $\mathbf{S} = \{S_1, S_1, ..., S_{14}\}$ in descending order, resulting in a sorted vector $\mathbf{E}$ and a sorted index vector $\mathbf{F}$, with F_j being the position of the element in vector $\mathbf{S}$.

(4) Back projection: Let m denote how many P300 ICs should be selected to reconstruct the P300 wave. Suppose that $Y_{p_z}(t)$ is the reconstructed P300 wave on the Pz electrode. The procedure of back projection for $Y_{p_z}(t)$ can be given by

$$Y_{p_z}(t) = \sum_{j=1}^{m} W_{P_z F_j}^{-1} \times Z_{F_j}(t), \qquad (4)$$

i.e., only m ICs are considered as P300 ICs and are back projected to the scalp.

A grid-search procedure (see Figure 3) will be used to determine the optimal value of parameter m, which will be discussed later.

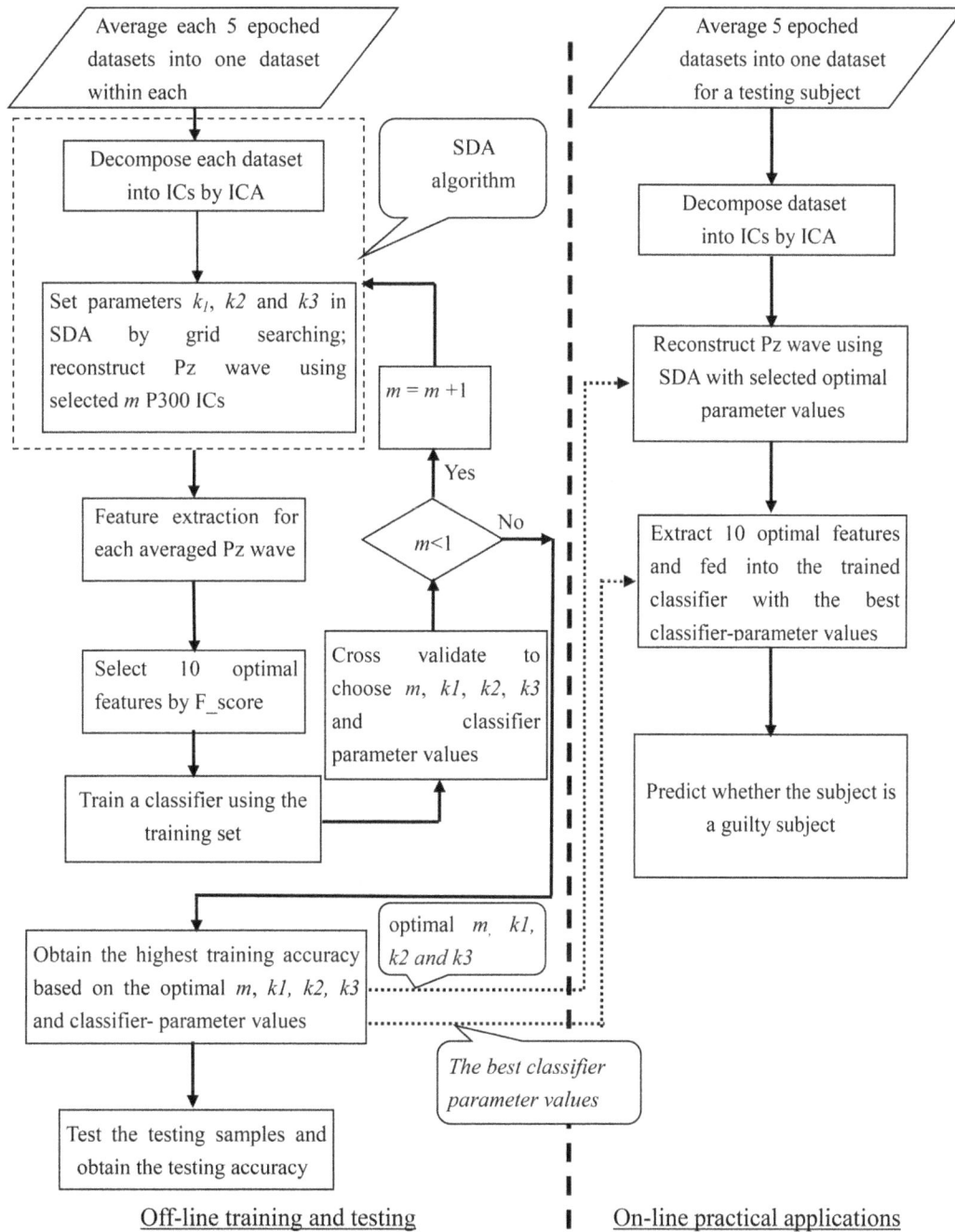

Figure 3. The flowchart of the presented CIT system.

Lastly, for two groups of subjects, two sets of the reconstructed waves can be obtained, respectively. Let **R–G** denote the vector set for the guilty group, and let **R–I** denote for the innocent group. We expect that the SNR of P300 in the set **R–G** would be enhanced compared with the raw ERP signal, using the above SDA.

Feature extraction

Let $\mathbf{Y}(t)$ denote a time wave in the set **R–G** or **R–I**, with t varying from stimulus onset to 1.1 s after the stimulus onset. Time-domain, frequency-domain and wavelet features were selected as

three groups of features in this study. Most of them have been demonstrated to be effective by many researchers [7,25,33–35]. The features are extracted from each signal $\mathbf{Y}(t)$ by the following procedure.

Time-domain features. Four time-domain features are defined as follows:

(1)   Maximum amplitude, which is defined as

$$V_{\max} = \max\{\mathbf{Y}(t)\} \qquad (5)$$

Table 1. Coefficients of the truncated decomposition filters h, g (IIR) and reconstruction filters H, G (FIR) for quadratic spline filters.

e	h(e)	g(e)	H(e)	G(e)
−10	+0.00157	−0.00388		
−9	+0.01909	−0.03416		
−8	−0.00503	+0.00901		
−7	−0.04440	+0.07933		
−6	+0.01165	−0.02096		
−5	+0.10328	−0.18408		
−4	−0.02593	+0.04977		+1/480
−3	−0.24373	+0.42390		−29/480
−2	+0.03398	−0.14034	0.25	+147/480
−1	+0.65523	−0.90044	0.75	−303/480
0	+0.65523	+0.90044	0.75	+303/480
1	+0.03398	+0.14034	0.25	−147/480
2	−0.24373	−0.42390		+29/480
3	−0.02593	−0.04977		−1/480
4	+0.10328	+0.18408		
5	+0.01165	+0.02096		
6	−0.04440	−0.07933		
7	−0.00503	−0.00901		
8	+0.01909	+0.03416		
9	+0.00157	+0.00388		

(2) Latency, which is the time where V_{max} occurs. It takes the form

$$t_{max} = \{t | \mathbf{Y}(t) = V_{max}\} \tag{6}$$

(3) Peak-to-Peak, which is defined as

$$V_{ptp} = V_{max} - V_{min} \tag{7}$$

(4) Positive area, which is the sum of the positive signal values. It can be expressed as

$$A_p = \sum_{t=500}^{1600} 0.5(\mathbf{Y}(t) + |\mathbf{Y}(t)|) \tag{8}$$

Frequency-domain features. The power spectrum density (PSD) is *first* calculated on each $\mathbf{Y}(t)$ by the Bartlett algorithm. Let $p(f)$ be the resultant PSD. Suppose that $p_{max} = \max\{p(f)\}$ denotes the maximum amplitude value of the PSD. Then 3 frequency-domain features can be calculated as follows:

(1) Maximum frequency, i.e.,

$$f_{max} = \{f | p(f) = p_{max}\} \tag{9}$$

(2) Mean frequency, calculated by the weighted average of the frequency. The weighted coefficient is the PSD value. It can be expressed as

$$f_{mean} = \int_0^{250} f \times p(f) df \left/ \int_0^{250} p(f) df \right. \tag{10}$$

(3) The power of the main frequency band that involves the P300, which is calculated by

$$A_{lf} = \int_{0.05}^{5} p(f) df \tag{11}$$

Wavelet features. Many authors have indicated that ERPs are transient signals that include some typical frequency components in a different frequency range, such as delta, theta, alpha, beta and gamma [36]. Recently, the wavelet transform (WT) has been widely used to analyze ERPs [36–38]. The WT is achieved by the breaking up of a signal into shifted and scaled versions of the mother wavelet, which is a waveform that has a limited duration and a zero mean.

In this study, a fast algorithm for the Discrete WT (DWT) was adopted to decompose those averaged single trials [39]. We selected Quadratic B-Spline functions as mother wavelets because they have a near-optimal time-frequency localization property and good similarity with the P300 components [40–41]. The wavelet coefficients were computed by a high-pass filter **h** and a low-pass filter **g**. The coefficients of two filters are given in the first and second columns of Table 1, respectively. The reconstruction filters **H** and **G** can be used to inversely transform the wavelet coefficients to time-domain waveforms. The third and fourth columns of Table 1 give the coefficients of the two reconstruction filters, respectively.

DWT was performed on each wave $\mathbf{Y}(t)$, which resulted in seven sets of wavelet coefficients corresponding to different frequency bands: 0.3–3.9, 3.9–7.8, 7.8–15.6, 15.6–31.2, 31.2–62.5, 62.5–125 and 125–250 Hz. Only the first four bands were useful due to the earlier filtering. Because the *delta* band was the main frequency range for the P300 component, the coefficient set corresponding to the first frequency band was selected as the final wavelet features for each wave $\mathbf{Y}(t)$.

Following the feature extraction, these feature samples were divided into two sample sets: the first set contained all of the *P300 samples* for the guilty group, and the second set contained *non-P300 samples* for the innocent group, with the class label being 1 and −1, respectively.

Feature Selection

In this study, we adopted the F-score method to further select the best subset of features for classification. The F-score method is a very simple but robust feature-evaluating technique. Recently, many researchers have successfully used this method in pattern recognition systems to select the optimal feature subset [42,43].

Given the ith feature vector $\{x_{i1}, x_{i2}, ..., x_{in_+}, ..., x_{iB}\}$ with the number of positive instances n_+ and the number of all of the instances B, the *F-score* value of the ith feature is defined by

$$F(i) = \frac{(\bar{x}_i^{(+)} - \bar{x}_i)^2 + (\bar{x}_i^{(-)} - \bar{x}_i)^2}{\frac{1}{n_+ - 1}\sum_{k=1}^{n_+}(x_{ik} - \bar{x}_i^{(+)})^2 + \frac{1}{B - n_+ - 1}\sum_{k=n_+ +1}^{B}(x_{ik} - \bar{x}_i^{(-)})^2}, \quad (12)$$

where $\bar{x}_i^{(+)}, \bar{x}_i^{(-)}$, and $\bar{x}_i$ are the average of the positive, negative, and whole samples, respectively, and x_{ik} is the kth feature value in the ith feature vector. Positive and negative represent two classes of identification, respectively. A larger *F-score* value indicates that the feature has more discriminative power. For the application of this method, the *F-score* value of all of the features will be sorted. Hence, in this study, those features that have relatively larger F-score values were selected to construct the feature subset.

There are two main methods used to select the appropriate feature subset: the filter method [44] and the wrapper method [45,46]. To obtain simplicity and a lower computation cost, we used the former method to select the feature number for the optimal feature subset.

Classification

The fisher discriminant analysis (FDA) [47], back propagation neural network (BPNN) [48] and support vector machine (SVM) [49,50] were compared in this study to select an optimal classifier. The details of the three classifiers are given in Supporting information files (see Section S1–S3 in File S1). The hybrid models integrating with F-score feature selection is referred to as F-score_FDA, F-score_BPNN and F-score_SVM in this study. Accordingly, three individual classification models (FDA, BPNN and SVM) were also utilized.

A Subject-Wise CV (SWCV) [25,51] was performed on the two classes of optimal feature sample sets. For each set, samples from 14 subjects were grouped into a training set and the samples from the remaining were used as a testing set. Thus by this SWCV, 15

pairs of training sets and testing sets were obtained. For each pair, the training set consisted of the samples from 28 subjects, and the testing set from 2 subjects (i.e., a guilty and an innocent subject). We would like to emphasize the importance of the SWCV procedure. In fact, a statistical classification model that could explain the data for some subjects did not necessarily generalize well to other subjects, even if those were draw from the same distribution. Accordingly, the SWCV procedure was used to assess the generalization ability not only from the different data within one subject but from the data in different subjects. Hence, the advantage of SWCV compared with common CV is that the test accuracy can simulate the generalization performance on other unseen subjects. Accordingly, we can obtain the testing results not only on the level of single-trials, but also on the level of subjects, i.e., to test whether one subject can be recognized correctly.

For each training set yielding by SWCV, the feature samples were mixed to obtain two classes of samples: one is lying group (it was considered as P300 feature samples) and the other is truth-telling group (it was considered as non-P300 feature samples). Subsequently, a common 10-fold CV procedure [52] was performed on each training set, resulting in 10 pairs of sub-training sets and sub-validation sets. Figure 4 shows the schematic diagram of the division of samples and cross validation procedure.

Selection of optimal parameters

For the proposed lie detection method, two groups of parameters must be tuned: 1) The parameters in SDA: m, $k1$, $k2$ and $k3$, and 2) The specific hyperparameters for each classifier. Considering that the parameters in SDA can affect the optimal values of the hyperparameters, the two groups of parameters were tuned together using a multi-dimension grid searching. During the turning, m varied from 1 to 14; and $k1$, $k2$ and $k3$ varied from 0.2 to 1 with a step size of 0.15, by the suggestion of an independent EEG expert. In the tuning procedure above, for BPNN, the number of sigmoid hidden nodes a and the learning rate η were tuned (the control precision was set to be 0.002). For SVM, the penalty parameter C and the radial width σ for radial basis function (RBF) $(K(x,y) = e^{-1/2*(\|x-y\|/\sigma)^2}$, [52]) were tuned. The procedure of training and testing is described as follows:

(1) The classifiers were trained on each sub-training set with different combinations of tuning parameters. By the 10-fold CV, an averaged sensitivity and an averaged specificity can be obtained for the jth training set. Then, the *mean* and *Standard Deviation (SD)* of the 15 sensitivities (15 training

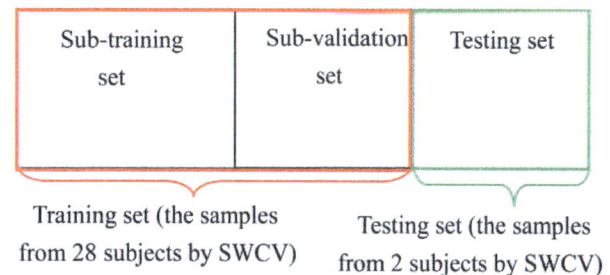

Figure 4. The division of feature samples using SWCV and 10-fold CV. The red rectangle denotes training set, whereas the green rectangle denotes testing set by the division of SWCV; Training set is further divided into sub-training set and sub-validation set by common 10-fold CV.

sets), referred to as M_{asen} and SD_{asen} respectively, are calculated. Similarly, the M_{aspe} and SD_{aspe} for specificity are obtained. Lastly, *balanced accuracy* $BA\_train = \frac{1}{2}(M_{asen} + M_{aspe})$ is calculated for the specific combination of tuning parameters.

(2) Repeat the above steps using a different combination of tuning parameters. Thus, the optimal parameter values were selected when *BA_train* reached the highest value.

(3) On the 15 testing sets, calculate the generalization performance of the trained classifiers with the optimal parameter values. Similar to step 1, M_{tspe} and SD_{tspe} (*mean* and *SD* on the 15 sensitivities), M_{tsen} and SD_{tsen} (on the 15 sensitivities) can be obtained. Finally, calculate the balanced testing accuracy $BA\_test = \frac{1}{2}(M_{tsen} + M_{tspe})$. This accuracy is the final testing measure of the performance evaluation.

Results

Preprocessing

The grand average ERPs on the Fz, Cz, Pz and Oz sites as a function of stimulus type were first calculated within each subject. Figure 5 gives the boxplot of the maximum amplitude at the Pz site for three types of stimuli and the two subject groups, during which 450 samples for each type of stimuli and each group were used to statistical analysis. Using ANOVA on the guilty subject, there is no significant difference ($p > 0.05$) for the maximum amplitude between the P and T stimuli. However, there is a significant difference ($p < 0.001$) between P and I stimuli. In contrast, there is no significant difference ($p > 0.05$) between the P and I stimuli for an innocent subject.

A 2×2 mixed model ANOVA (P vs. I × innocent vs. guilty) was performed on the maximum amplitude at the Pz site. The result shown in Figure 6 revealed significant main effect of innocent versus guilty, $F(1, 28) = 772.467, p < .0005$ and P versus I, $F(1, 28) = 761.201, p < .005$. There is also significant interaction between innocent versus guilty and P versus I, $F(1, 28) = 753.430$, $p < .005$.

More importantly, by a further independent effect analysis of innocent versus guilty when P stimuli was used, the person type effect is significant and yields $F(1,28) = 1514.68, p < .0005$. The amplitude of P300 for the guilty is higher than that for the innocent. In contrast, when using I stimuli, there is no significant person effect ($F < 1$). Hence, P responses at the Pz site were finally selected for further processing to enhance the feature difference of the P300 waves between the two classes of subjects.

SDA

First, the enhancement of the SNR of P300 by SDA is illustrated in Figure 7. A guilty subject's five raw EEG datasets were randomly taken as an example. The raw waves on the Pz with solid thin line and their averaged wave with dashed thick lines are shown in Figure 7A. Similarly, we randomly selected an innocent subject, and the raw waves and averaged wave on Pz are shown in Figure 7B. Applying SDA to the two averaged datasets respectively, the two reconstructed P300 waveforms on Pz are shown in Figure 7C. There is no distinct P300 (dashed lines) in Figure 7A and 7B. As Figure 7C shows, however, there is a clear P300 with a latency of approximately 280 ms for the guilty subject, and the two lines can be differentiated easily. During this evaluation, the parameters m, $k1$, $k2$ and $k3$ were set to 3, 0.9, 0.8, 0.6 by *a priori* knowledge of an independent physiology expert.

Extraction of Wavelet Features

After SDA, the features were extracted from the reconstructed waves for the Pz. Here, we randomly selected a guilty and an innocent subject, and then conducted the wavelet transform on two subjects' denoised P300 signals, respectively. The results of DWT are shown in Figure 8A and 8B respectively. The most distinct difference in the wavelet features and reconstruction waves between the two subjects is in the 0.3–3.9 Hz band (the delta band). For the guilty subject, it can be seen from the bottom row in Figure 8A that there are obvious peaks in the wavelet coefficients and reconstruction waves at approximately 500 ms post-stimulus for this band. This approach is in accordance with the time-domain features of the P300 waveform. In contrast, there are no obviously corresponding features in Figure 8B. The results above suggest that the wavelet coefficients corresponding to the delta band, as a class of P300 features, are suitable for differentiating the P responses between the two groups of subjects.

Result of the feature selection

Table 2 shows the results of the feature selection by the F-score method. W_1–W_{22} denotes 22 WT coefficients. From this table, we can see the *F-score* values of the 29 original features. Those features with relatively larger *F-score* values were selected to construct a feature subset. For simplicity, we directly selected 10 features whose *F-score* values were larger than 0.85 to form the optimal feature subset.

Observing these 10 features, we can see that two optimal time-domain features are closely related to the peak value of P300. Second, one feature (A_{lf}) is related to the main frequency range of P300 (0.3–3.9 Hz). Most importantly, the most of optimal features are selected from the original wavelet features. This indicates the wavelet feature has the better classification capability than the other two kinds of features.

Classification Performance

Using SWCV, *BA_train* reaches the highest value, 96.18%, using the F-score_SVM, and the optimal parameters of m, $k1$, $k2$, $k3$, which are determined by grid searching, are as follows: $m = 2$, $k1 = 0.85$, $k2 = 0.70$ and $k3 = 0.40$. The training accuracies as a function of the parameter m were shown in Figure 9A and 9B for the three hybrid models when $k1 = 0.85$, $k2 = 0.70$ and $k3 = 0.40$. As shown in Figure 9, the accuracy rates increase significantly when m changes from 1 to 2 for all of the models. For example, the increased rate for F-score_SVM is approximately 5%. In addition, the accuracies of F-score_FDA and F-score_SVM reach a maximum when $m = 2$ except for F-score_BPNN, whose accuracy still increases slightly as m varies from 2 to 3. More importantly, the accuracy rates decrease when more than 3 ICs are used in SDA. This result is basically consistent with the report of Lin et al. [53]. Note that the accuracies with $m = 14$ denote the performance without the SDA. For every classification model, those accuracies are distinctly much lower than those when $m = 2$. The results discussed above indicate the remarkable performance of SDA.

Furthermore, Table 3 gives the training accuracies (M_{asen}, M_{aspe}) and testing accuracies (M_{tsen}, M_{tspe}) of the six classification models with the optimal grid searching result. First, the accuracy of the model using FDA is obviously lower than the models using BPNN and SVM. This finding suggests that the data from the two types of subjects in the lie detection cannot be separated linearly. Additionally, the performance of the models that use SVM significantly exceeds those of the models that use FDA and BPNN. Using ANOVA, the statistical results ($F(1, 28) = 7396.689$ and $p < 0.001$) confirm that the testing accuracy for SVM is significantly greater than that for BPNN. The *BA_test* of

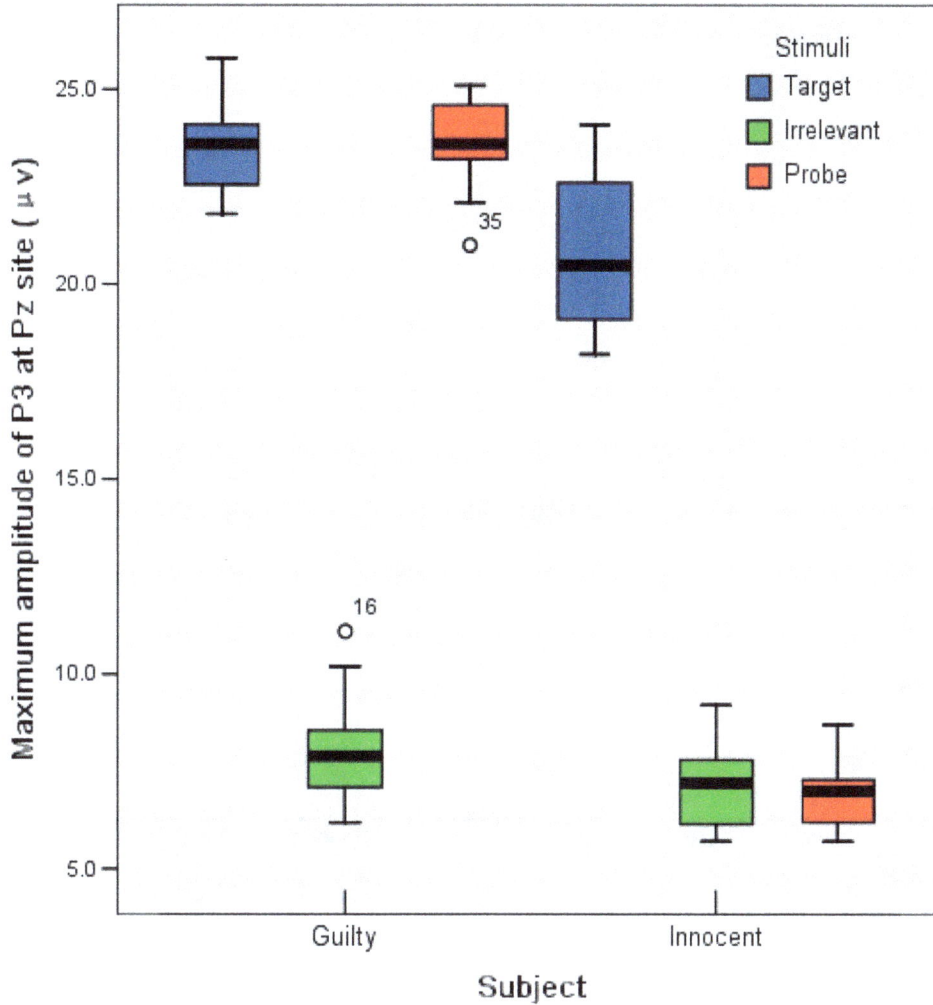

Figure 5. Boxplot of the maximum amplitude of P300 at Pz in different stimuli and subject groups.

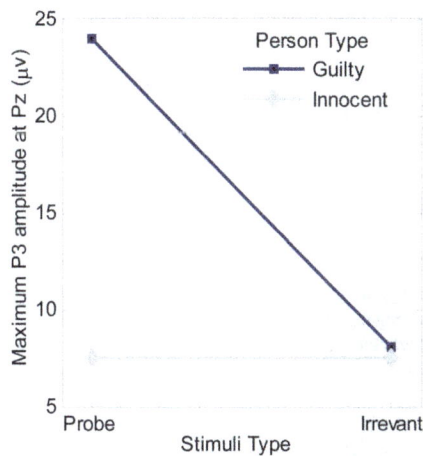

Figure 6. Maximum P300 amplitude at Pz as functions of person type (guilty and innocent) and stimuli type.

96.08% for F-score_SVM strongly suggests that it is suitable for the classification of the two classes of subjects. Additionally, we can see from Table 3 that each hybrid model achieves significantly higher accuracy than the corresponding individual model. For example, on the training sets, SVM reaches a sensitivity and specificity of 91% and 90.98%, respectively. In contrast, F-score_SVM obtains 96.07% and 96.30%, respectively. Based on the above experimental results, the model F-score_SVM reaches the highest classification performance of all of the models.

Comparison with previous methods

The individual diagnostic rates of the presented and previous methods were calculated, and they were compared in this section. In the BAD/BCD method, each 10 waveforms of each type of response on the Pz electrode were selected to average into a waveform, based on the technique of bootstrapping. In the BAD method, the P300 amplitudes of the three types of responses were calculated based on the Peak-to-Peak method [7,13,54]. For the BCD method, the time lag was equal to 0 when the CV was calculated.

For the BAD and BCD methods, we calculated 100 D-values obtained by 100 iterations for each subject. Let N_d denote the times when the D-values were larger than zero. Then N_d and the

(A)

(B)

(C)

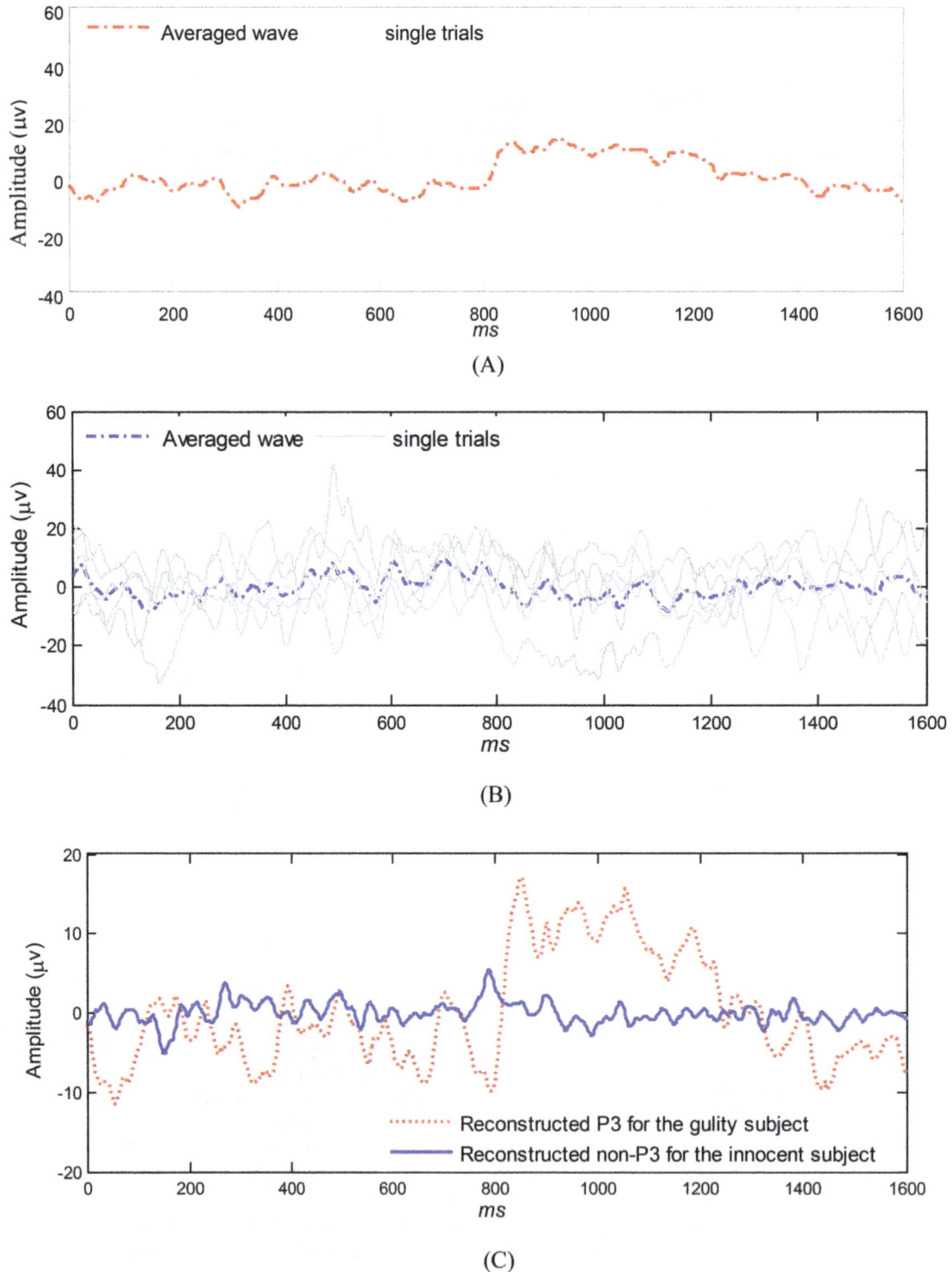

Figure 7. Response waveforms and reconstructed waveforms on Pz after applying SDA for a guilty and an innocent subject. 7A: Single trials (solid lines) and averaged waveform (dashed line) on Pz for a guilty subject before applying SDA. 7B: Single trials (solid lines) and averaged waveform (dashed line) on Pz for a guilty subject before applying SDA. 7C: Reconstructed waveforms (a P300 for the guilty subject and a non-P300 for the innocent subject) by applying SDA on the averaged datasets.

percentage of N_d were calculated for each subject, respectively. If the percentage of N_d was greater than a threshold N_{th}, then this subject would be considered to be a guilty subject [7,12]. Lastly, the error rates of an individual diagnosis as a function of the setting threshold are shown in Figure 10A and 10B, respectively. Considering the equal importance of the detection rates of the two groups of subjects, the individual diagnostic rates of 92% and

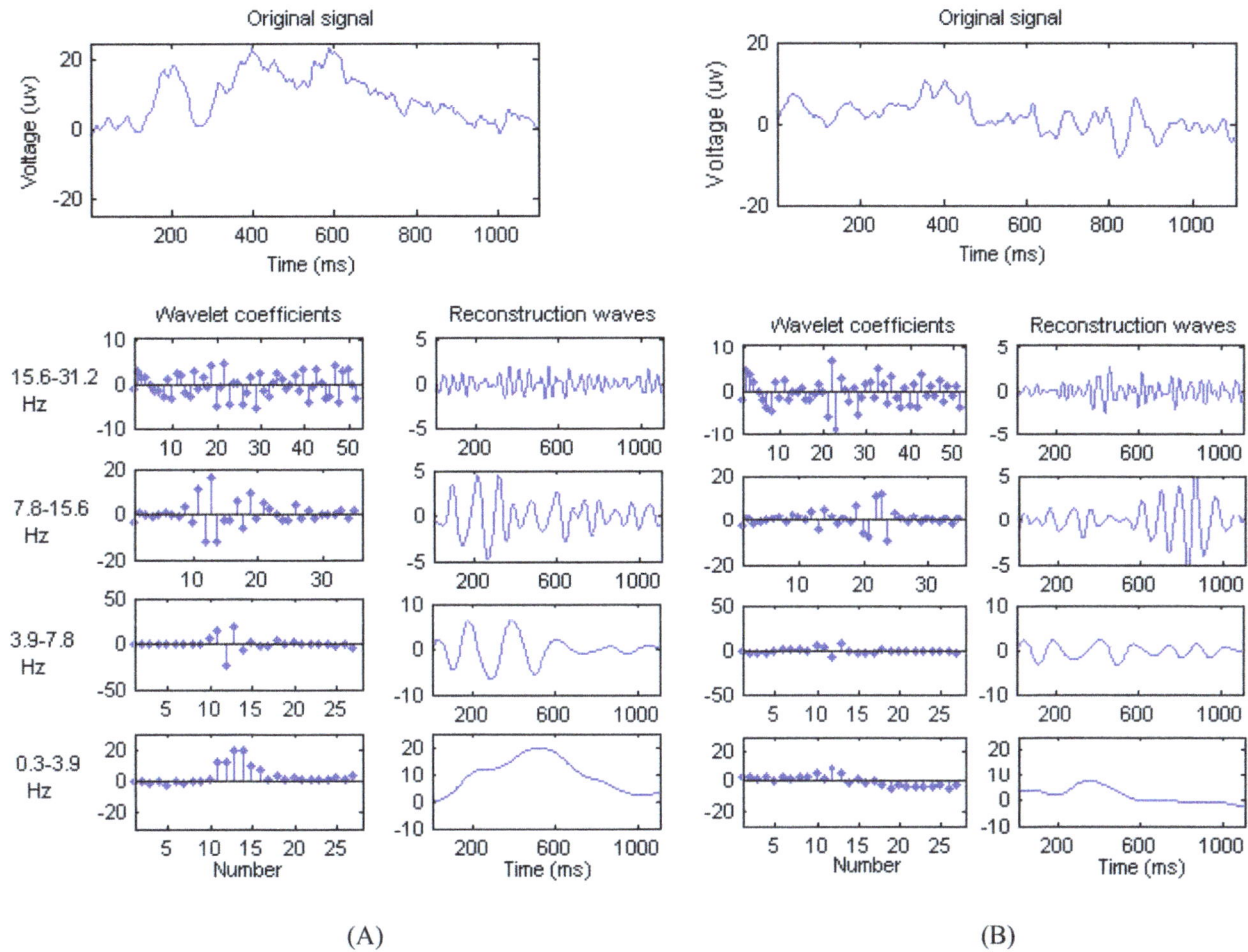

Figure 8. The wavelet coefficients in 4 bands and corresponding reconstructed waveforms. 8A: The original EEG waveforms on Pz for a guilty subject (above panel), its wavelet coefficients (left column) and corresponding reconstruction waves (right column). 8B: The original EEG waveforms on Pz for an innocent subject (above panel), its wavelet coefficients (left column) and corresponding reconstruction waves (right column).

Table 2. The results of feature selection on original 29 features using F-score.

Features	F-score values
V_{max}	0.937
t_{max}	0.567
V_{ptp}	0.877
A_p	0.268
f_{max}	0.049
f_{mean}	0.340
A_{lf}	0.873
W_1–W_5	0.085, 0.005, 0.311, 0.011, 0.099
W_6–W_{10}	0.008, 0.184, 0.106, 0.077, 0.381
W_{11}–W_{16}	0.977, 0.524, 0.255, 0.835, 0.820, 0.947
W_{17}–W_{22}	0.905, 0.937, 0.881, 0.959, 0.871, 0.838

88.71% are reached when the thresholds are set to 83.6% and 85.5% for the BAD and BCD methods, respectively.

Based on the results in the above section, for our method, in fact, the individual diagnostic rate can reach 100% when choosing the test accuracy of 90% as a decision criterion for a subject. That is, one was identified as a liar when the percentage of reconstructed samples classified as P300 was larger than 90%. In contrast, one was a truth-teller if the percentage of reconstructed samples classified as non-P300 was larger than 90%. Obviously, this diagnostic rate is higher than the rates of the BAD and BCD methods, and is also higher than those reported using other machine learning-based methods. For example, Abootalebi et al. [7] reported that the best detection rates are 74%, 80% and 79% for BAD, BCD and the machine learning methods, respectively.

Discussion and conclusions

Lie detection methods using a large number of stimuli suffer from several inherent drawbacks such as more fatigue for subjects, more workload for examiners, increased probability of counter-measure behavior and lower flexibility [25,55]. Obviously, a lie detection method with only a small number of stimuli will be crucial for practical lie detection. The purpose of this study is to develop a novel detection method that uses several stimuli to

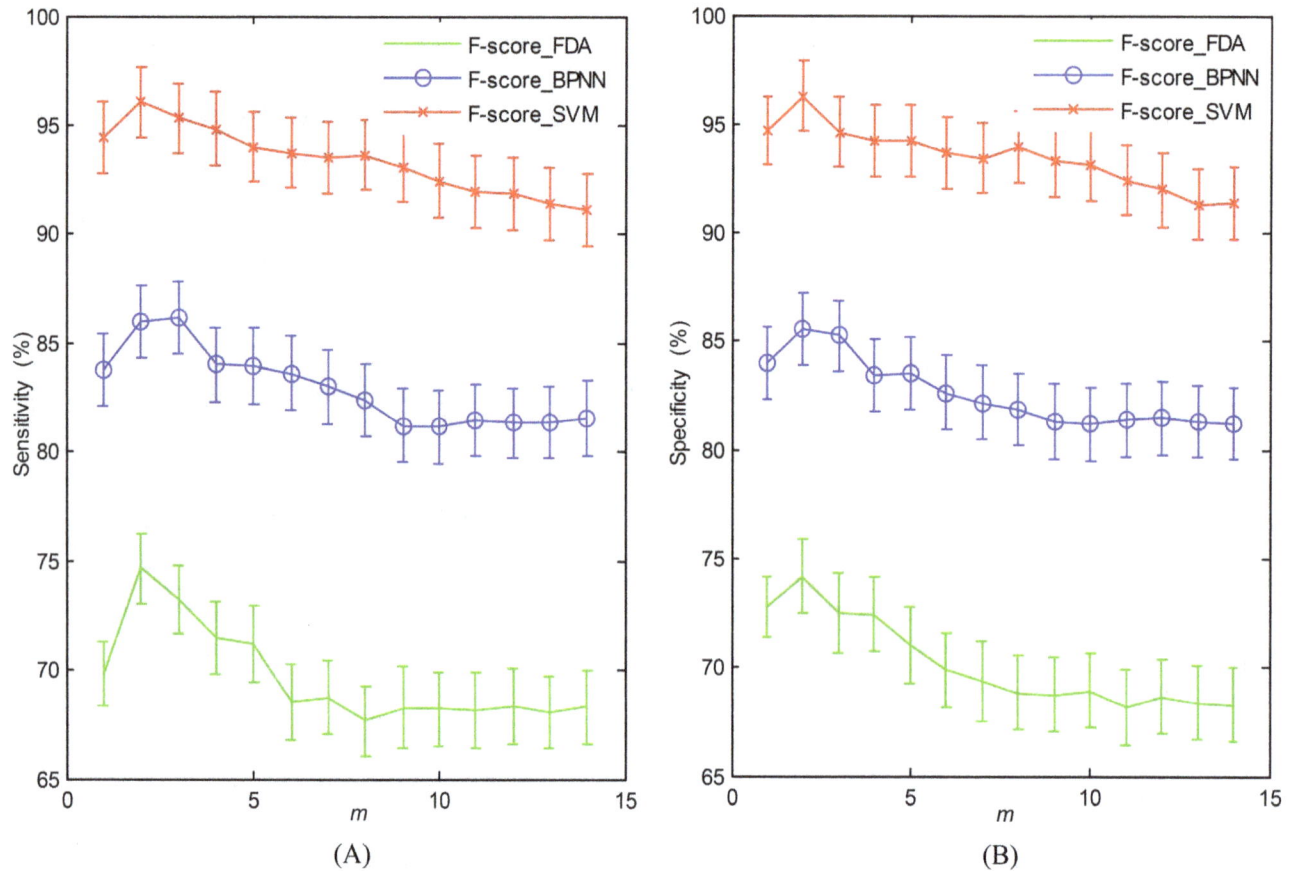

(A)　　　　　　　　　　　　　　(B)

Figure 9. The accuracy (mean ± SD) of classifying P300 (sensitivity) and non-P300 (specificity) for three classification models with different parameter value *m* on training sets (when *k1* = 0.85, *k2* = 0.70 and *k3* = 0.40). 9A: Sensitivity for the training sets. 9B: Specificity for the training sets.

identify the liars, and at the same time, to further increase the individual diagnostic rate and robustness compared to previous studies. For this purpose, we proposed a novel ICA-based SDA to enhance the SNR of P300, and then, we used a machine learning method to distinguish the P300 evoked by guilty subjects from the non-P300 in innocent subjects.

Some recent studies suggested that machine learning-based lie detection methods are more reliable than the BAD and BCD

methods. One advantage is that the investigation of the dynamic variation of single trials might help us to study more cognitive information on lying. The second major advantage lies in that the failure of one trial will not affect the classification results of the other trials. In contrast, for BAD and BCD, the failure will change many bootstrapping averages and hence, the overall result of the lie detection [7]. Third, one can utilize more features of P300 in addition to the time-domain features that are used in the BAD/

Table 3. Sensitivity/specificity on the training and testing sets for different classification models with the optimal parameter combination.

Classifier models	Sensitivity/specificity (%)	
	Training ($M_{asen} \pm SD_{asen} / M_{aspe} \pm SD_{aspe}$)	Testing ($M_{tsen} \pm SD_{tsen} / M_{tspe} \pm SD_{tspe}$)
FDA	68.38±2.13/67.22±1.94	FDA
BPNN	79.27±1.66/78.78±1.72	BPNN
SVM	91.00±1.80/90.98±1.85	SVM
F-score_FDA	74.65±1.57/74.19±1.70(▲)	F-score_FDA
F-score_BPNN	85.97±1.60/85.60±1.66(*)	F-score_BPNN

"▲" denotes that a p-value of <0.001 was obtained by ANOVA between F-score_FDA and F-score_SVM; "*" denotes that a p-value of <0.001 was obtained by ANOVA between F-score_BPNN and F-score_SVM; for BPNN, the number of hidden nodes $a = 5$, and the learning rate $\eta = 0.03$; for SVM, radial $\sigma = 32$, and penalty parameter $C = 2^8$.

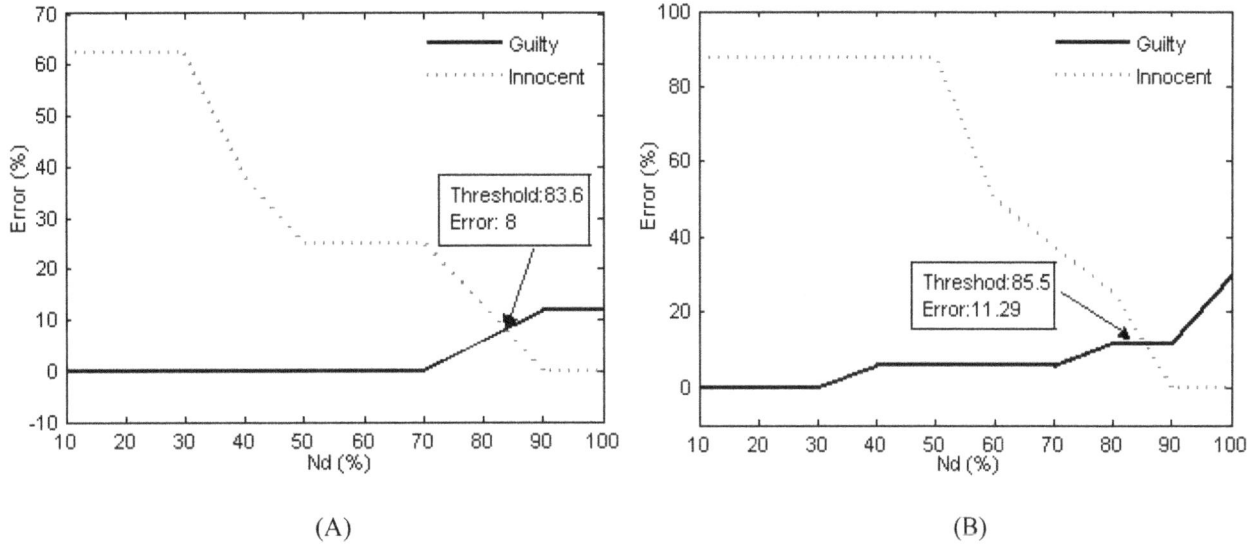

Figure 10. The detection error rates of two groups of subjects. 10A: The detection error rate of the guilty and innocent groups for BAD method. 10B: The detection error rate of the guilty and innocent groups for BCD method.

BCD method. Lastly, note that, in previous methods, it is difficult to decide the related thresholds such as the N_{th} described earlier because this decision involves the tradeoff between the two individual diagnostic rates from the two groups of subjects. In contrast, we can see that this problem does not exist in our method.

In the present study, we assumed that for a P300-based lie detection method, the noise in the single trials could be divided into two categories: one is the ill-assorted responses to a certain type of stimulus, which results from a variation of cognitive state during detection [55]; the other is normal noise such as EOG artifacts and spontaneous EEG. Hence, before applying SAD, we first averaged each 5 raw EEG datasets to decrease the impact of ill-resorted P300's on the SNR of P300, which would increase the robustness of the entire system for lie detection. The efficiency of this preprocessing method for lie detection is not addressed in this study because it has already been proven in the previous report [55]. To reduce the influence of the second type of noise on the performance of the detection to the greatest extent, we proposed a novel SDA to separate the P300 components from the other noise signals, constructing new Pz waves with the more obvious P300 features; this process can be viewed as a spatial filter for the P300.

Previously, we introduced a topography-template matching (TTM) method [25] to reconstruct P300 waveforms that have a higher SNR. TTM was based on correlation theory of the topography of the ICs. SDA differs from the TTM method in the construction algorithm. SDA is computationally efficient to implement. Hence SDA could decrease the training and testing time. In addition, the classification accuracy of the presented method is higher than that in the report [25]. For the sake of brevity, we have not compared the efficiency of these two methods here and the comparison will be addressed in future studies.

For SDA, the experiment results show that the detection accuracy is the highest when 2 (or 3) P300 ICs are selected to reconstruct the Pz waveform. This finding might indicate that 2 or 3 neural sources are responsible for the task of responding to the P stimuli. This inference deserves further study. In addition, we deemed that the physiology meaning of three parameter values of $k1$, $k2$ and $k3$ can be interpreted as follows. A realistic P300 IC

(unknown P300 independent neural source under scalp) should have different distributed weight on different brain scalp areas. Comparing three k values, P300 IC has biggest distributed weight on P3 and P4, medium on Cz and least on Oz scalp areas.

It is worth mentioning that, even though only the waves on the Pz were finally used to extract features, 14 electrodes were still selected to run ICA in order to guarantee the efficiency of the EICA algorithm and SDA. Using ICA has another advantage in that it can help remove the ocular artifacts automatically in the preprocessing phase [24], which few previous studies of lie detection have addressed [56–58]. Using SDA to remove ocular artifacts simultaneously will be investigated in the future.

It should be acknowledged that the procedure for tuning parameters in the present study is complicated and time-consuming. However, once these optimal parameter values were selected by the grid searching method on the training sets, they would be kept stable for the testing and real applications. We assumed, for example, that the parameter m represents the volume conduction feature of the neurons accounting for the P300 on the scalp, which is thought to be relatively stable spatially [31]. Using other parameter optimization methods [52,59] is also possible. We will evaluate this approach in future work.

Using the presented method, only 5 Probe stimuli (together with some Target and Irrelevant stimuli) must be presented to the subject in real applications. This arrangement is attractive and promising for practical applications. Moreover, to increase the reliability of the diagnoses, the examiner could perform our testing procedure multiple times and, then, make a more accurate decision by combining several independent testing results.

The F-score, which is a simple feature-selection method, was combined with classifiers to choose the optimal features. The F-score helps to decrease the feature number and, hence, to decrease the computational burden. More importantly, the experimental results show that it helps to enhance the classification accuracy compared with the individual classification models, indicating the importance of the feature selection for the classification performance. For the sake of simplicity, we remove redundant features by a commonly used threshold strategy. In the future, the wrapper method should be used to improve the proposed method.

Different kernel functions for SVM were not tested in this study. It can be found that the training procedure in this study is very complex. Hence, the selection of kernel functions was not considered for the simplicity of the training procedure. In our early other studies [25,55], we had tested that the radial basis function (RBF) had the best performance than the other kernel functions. Hence, RBF was directly used in SVM method considering the similar lie detection researches.

The proposed method is not specific to research into lie detection and could be extended to other fields of the ERP classification. We believe that more sophisticated feature selection

approaches, such as genetic algorithm [7,60], could further improve the performance of the classifier.

Author Contributions

Conceived and designed the experiments: JFG NNR. Performed the experiments: YY XLY. Analyzed the data: JFG HJT CHL. Contributed reagents/materials/analysis tools: CHL. Wrote the paper: JFG.

References

1. Gamer M, Berti S (2010) Task relevance and recognition of concealed information have different influences on electrodermal activity and event-related brain potentials. Psychophysiology 47(2): 355–364.

2. Ambach W, Bursch S, Stark R, Vaitl D (2010) A Concealed Information Test with multimodal measurement. Int J Psychophysi 75: 258–26.

3. Ito A, Abe N, Fujii T, Ueno A, Koseki Y, et al. (2011) The role of the dorsolateral prefrontal cortex in deception when remembering neutral and emotional events. Neurosci Res 69(2): 121–128.

4. Langleben DD, Loughead JW, Bilker WB, Ruparel K, Childress AR, et al. (2005) Telling truth from lie in individual subjects with fast event-related fMRI. Hum Brain Mapp26(4): 262–272.

5. Phan KL, Magalhaes A, Ziemlewicz TJ, Fitzgerald DA, Green C, et al. (2005) Neural correlates of telling lies: a functional magnetic resonance imaging study at 4 Tesla. Acad Radiol 12(2): 164–172.

6. Rosenfeld JP (2002) Event-related potentials in the detection of deception. Handbook of Polygraph Testing. Academic Press, New York, 265–286.

7. Abootalebi V, Moradi MH, Khalilzadeh MA (2009) A new approach for EEG feature extraction in P300-based lie detection. Comput Methods and Programs in Biomed 94(1): 48–57.

8. Polich J, Herbst KL (2000) P300 as a clinical assay: rational, evaluation, and findings. Int J Psychophysi 38(1): 3–19.

9. Meijer EH, Smulders FTY, Merckelbach HLGJ, Wolf AG (2007) The P300 is sensitive to concealed face recognition. Int J Psychophysi 66(3): 231–237.

10. Rosenfeld JP, Soskins M, Bosh G, Ryan A (2004) Simple, effective countermeasures to P300-based tests of detection of concealed information. Psychophysiology 41(2): 205–219.

11. Rosenfeld JP, Labkovsky E, Winograd M. Lui MA, Vandenboom C, et al. (2008) The Complex Trial Protocol (CTP): A new, countermeasure-resistant, accurate, P300-based method for detection of concealed information. Psychophysiology 45(6): 906–919.

12. Farwell LA, Donchin E (1991) The truth will out: interrogative polygraphy ("lie detection") with event-related potentials. Psychophysiology 28(5): 531–547.

13. Abootalebi V, Moradi MH, Khalilzadeh MA (2006) A comparison of methods for ERP assessment in a P300-based GKT. Int J Psychophysi 62(2): 309–320.

14. Dvatzikos C, Ruparel K, Fan Y, Shen DG, Acharyya M, et al. (2005) Classifying spatial patterns of brain activity with machine learning methods: Application to lie detection. NeuroImage 28(3): 663–668.

15. Jung TP, Makeig S, Humphries C, Lee TW, McKeown MJ, et al. (2000a) Removing electroencephalographic artifacts by blind source separation. Psychophysiology 37(2): 163–178.

16. Wasserman S, Bockenholt U (1989) Bootstrapping: applications to psychophysiology. Psychophysiology 26(2): 208–221.

17. Jung TP, Makeig S, Waterfield M, Townsend J, Courchesne U, et al. (2000b) Removing eye activity artifacts from visual event-related potentials in normal and clinical subjects. Clin Neurophysiol 111(10): 1745–1758.

18. Bell AJ, Sejnowski TJ (1995) An information-maximization approach to blind separation and blind deconvolution. Neural Computation, MIT Press, Cambridge, MA 7(6): 1129–1159.

19. Tang AC, Pearlmutter BA, Zibulevsky M, Carter SA (2000) Blind source separation of multichannel neuromagnetic responses. Neurocomput 32: 1115–1120.

20. Parra L, Sajda P (2003) Blind source separation via generalized eigenvalue decomposition. J Mach Learn Res 4: 1261–1269.

21. Peterson DA, Anderson CW (1999) EEG-based Cognitive Task Classification with ICA and Neural Networks. Engineering Applications of Bio-Inspired Artificial Neural Networks. Springer Berlin Heidelberg, 1999: 265–272.

22. Hung CI, Lee PL, Wu YT, Chen LF, Yeh TCH, et al. (2005) Recognition of Motor Imagery Electroencephalography Using Independent Component Analysis and Machine Classifiers. Ann Biomed Eng 33(8): 1053–1070.

23. Tang AC, Sutherland MT, Wang Y (2006) Contrasting single-trial ERPs between experimental manipulations: Improving differentiability by blind source separation. NeuroImage 29(1): 335–346.

24. Gao JF, Yang Y, Lin P, Wang P, Zheng CX (2010) Automatic Removal of Eye-movement and Blink Artifacts from EEG Signals. Brain Topo 23(1): 105–114.

25. Gao JF, Lu L, Yang Y, Yu G, Na LT, et al. (2012) A Novel Concealed Information Test Method Based on Independent Component Analysis and Support Vector Machine. Clin EEG Neurosci 43(1): 54–63.

26. Comon P (1994) Independent component analysis, a new concept? Signal Process 36(3): 287–314.

27. Makeig S, Bell AJ, Jung TP, Sejnowski TJ (1996) Independent Component Analysis of Electroencephalgraphic Data. Adv Neural Inform Process Systems 8, MIT press, Cambridge MA, 145–151.

28. Jung TP, Humphries C, Lee TW, Makeig S, McKeown MJ, et al. (1998) Extended ica removes artifacts from electroencephalographic recordings. Adv Neural Inform Process Systems, 894–900.

29. Lee TW, Girolami M, Sejnowski EJ (1999) Independent component analysis using an extended informax algorithm for mixed subgaussian and supergaussian sources. Neural Comput 11(2): 409–433.

30. Rosenfeld JP, Ellwanger JW, Nolana K, Wua S, Bermanna RG, et al. (1999) P300 Scalp amplitude distribution as an index of deception in a simulated cognitive deficit model. Int J Psychophysi 33(1): 3–19.

31. Xu N, Gao XR, Hong B, Miao XB, Gao SK, et al. (2004) BCI Competition 2003—Data Set IIb: Enhancing P300 Wave Detection Using ICA-Based Subspace Projections for BCI Applications. IEEE Trans Biomed Eng 51(6): 1067–1072.

32. Polich J (2007) Updating P300: An integrative theory of P3a and P3b. Clin Neurophysiol 118: 2128–2148.

33. Demiralp T, Ademoglu A, Schurmann M, Eroglu CB, Basar E (1999) Detection of P300 waves in single trials by the Wavelet Transform (WT). Brain Lang 66(1): 108–128.

34. Kalatzis I, Piliouras N, Ventouras E, Papageorgiou CC, Rabavilas AD, et al. (2004) Design and implementation of an SVM-based computer classification system for discriminating depressive patients from healthy controls using the P600 component of ERP signals, Comput Meth Prog Biomed 75(1): 11–22.

35. Hsu WY, Lin CC, Ju MS, Sun YN (2007) Wavelet-based fractal features with active segment selection: Application to single-trial EEG data. J Neurosci Meth 163(1): 145–160.

36. Herrmann CS, Knight RT (2001) Mechanisms of human attention: event-related potentials and oscillations. Neurosci and Biobehav Rev 25(6): 465–476.

37. Yong YPA, Hurley NJ, Silvestre GCM (2005) Single-trial EEG classification for brain-computer interface using wavelet decomposition. Eur Signal Process.

38. Mrzagora AC, Bunce S, Izzetoglu M, Onaral B (2006) Wavelet analysis for EEG feature extraction in deception detection Proceedings of the 28th IEEE EMBS Annual International Conference. New York City, USA, Aug 30.

39. Ademoglu A, Micheli-Tzanakou E, Istefanopulos Y (1997) Analysis of pattern reversal visual evoked potentials (PRVEPs) by spline wavelets. IEEE Trans on Biomed Eng 44(9): 881–890.

40. Unser M, Aldroubi A, Eden M (1992) On the asymptotic convergence of B-spline wavelets to Gabor functions. IEEE Trans on Information Theory 38(2): 864–872.

41. Quiroga RQ, Sakowitz OW, Basar E, Schurmann M (2001) Wavelet transform in the analysis of the frequency composition of evoked potentials. Brain Res Protoc 8(1): 16–24.

42. Chen FL, Li FC (2010) Combination of feature selection approaches with SVM in credit scoring. Expert Syst Appl 37: 4902–4909.

43. Polat K, Güneş S (2009) A new feature selection method on classification of medical datasets: Kernel F-score feature selection. Expert Syst Appl 36(7): 10367–10373.

44. Jouve PE, Nicoloyannis N (2005) A filter feature selection method for clustering Foundations of Intelligent Systems. Springer Berlin Heidelberg, 583–593.

45. Kohavi R, John GH (1997) Wrappers for feature subset selection. Arti Intell 97(1): 273–324.

46. Huang CJ, Dian X, Chuang YT (2007) Application of wrapper approach and composite classifier to the stock trend prediction. Expert Syst Appl 34(4): 2870–2878.

47. Chiang L, Russell E, Braatz R (2000) Fault diagnosis in chemical processes using Fisher discriminant analysis, discriminant partial least squares, and principal component analysis. Chemomet Intell Lab Syst 50(2): 243–252.

48. Tarassenko L, Khan YU, Holt MRG (1998) Identification of inter-ictal spikes in the EEG using neural network analysis. IEE Proceedings Science, Measurement & Technology 145(6): 270–278.

49. Kaper M, Meinicke P, Grossekathoefer U, Lingner T, Ritter H (2004) BCI competition 2003-data set IIb: support vector machines for the P300 speller paradigm, IEEE Trans on Biomed Eng 51(6): 1073–1076.

50. Shoker L, Sanei S, Chambers J (2005) Artifact removal from electroencephalograms using a hybrid BSS-SVM algorithm. IEEE Sig Process Letters 12(10): 721–724.

51. Shao SY, Shen KQ, On CJ, Wilder-Smith EPV, Li XP (2009) Automatic EEG artifact removal: A weighted support vector machine approach with error correction. IEEE Trans Biomed Eng 56(2): 336–344.

52. Burges C (1998) A tutorial on support vector machines for pattern recognition. Data Mining and Knowl Discov 2(2): 121–167.

53. Lin CT, Chung IF, Ko LW, Chen YC, Liang SF, et al. (2007) EEG-Based Assessment of Driver Cognitive Responses in a Dynamic Virtual-Reality Driving Environment. IEEE Trans Biomed Eng 54(7): 1394–1352.

54. Soskins M, Rosenfeld J.P, Niendam T (2001) The case for peak-to-peak measurement of P300 recorded at.3 Hz high pass filter settings in detection of deception. Int J Psychophysi 40(17): 173–1800.

55. Gao JF, Yan XG, Sun JC, Zheng CX (2011) Denoised P300 and Machine Learning-based Concealed Information Test Method. Comput Meth Prog Bio 104: 410–417.

56. Matsuda I, Nittono H, Hirota A, Ogawa T, Takasawa N (2009) Event-related brain potentials during the standard autonomic-based concealed information test. Int J Psychophysi 74(1): 58–68.

57. Matsuda I, Nittono H, Ogawa T (2011) Event-related potentials increase the discrimination performance of the autonomic-based concealed information test. Psychophysiology 48(12): 1701–1710.

58. Matsuda I, Nittono H, Ogawa T (2013) Identifying concealment-related responses in the concealed information test. Psychophysiology, 50: 617–626.

59. Friedrichs F, Igel C (2005) Evolutionary tuning of multiple SVM parameters. Neurocomput 24: 107–117.

60. Wu CH, Tzeng GH, Lin RH (2009) A novel hybrid genetic algorithm for kernel function and parameter optimization in support vector regression. Expert Syst Appl 36: 4725–4735.

5

Dissociation of Neural Substrates of Response Inhibition to Negative Information between Implicit and Explicit Facial Go/Nogo Tasks: Evidence from an Electrophysiological Study

Fengqiong Yu[1][9], Rong Ye[1][9], Shiyue Sun[2], Luis Carretié[3], Lei Zhang[1], Yi Dong[5], Chunyan Zhu[1], Yuejia Luo[6], Kai Wang[1,4]*

1 Laboratory of Cognitive Neuropsychology, Department of Medical Psychology, Anhui Medical University, Hefei, China, 2 School of Humanities and Social Sciences, Beijing Forestry University, Beijing, China, 3 Faculty of Psychology, Universidad Autónoma de Madrid, Madrid, Spain, 4 Department of Neurology, the First Affiliated Hospital of Anhui Medical University, Hefei, China, 5 Anhui Mental Health Center, Hefei, China, 6 Institute of Social and affective Neuroscience, Shenzhen University, Shenzhen, China

Abstract

Background: Although ample evidence suggests that emotion and response inhibition are interrelated at the behavioral and neural levels, neural substrates of response inhibition to negative facial information remain unclear. Thus we used event-related potential (ERP) methods to explore the effects of explicit and implicit facial expression processing in response inhibition.

Methods: We used implicit (gender categorization) and explicit emotional Go/Nogo tasks (emotion categorization) in which neutral and sad faces were presented. Electrophysiological markers at the scalp and the voxel level were analyzed during the two tasks.

Results: We detected a task, emotion and trial type interaction effect in the Nogo-P3 stage. Larger Nogo-P3 amplitudes during sad conditions versus neutral conditions were detected with explicit tasks. However, the amplitude differences between the two conditions were not significant for implicit tasks. Source analyses on P3 component revealed that right inferior frontal junction (rIFJ) was involved during this stage. The current source density (CSD) of rIFJ was higher with sad conditions compared to neutral conditions for explicit tasks, rather than for implicit tasks.

Conclusions: The findings indicated that response inhibition was modulated by sad facial information at the action inhibition stage when facial expressions were processed explicitly rather than implicitly. The rIFJ may be a key brain region in emotion regulation.

Editor: Francesco Di Russo, University of Rome, Italy

Funding: This research was supported by the National Natural Science Foundation of China (31000503, 91232717, 31100812, 81301176, and 81300944) and the Ministry of Science and Technology (2011CB707805). The funders had no role in study design, data collection and analysis, decision to publish, or preparation of the manuscript.

Competing Interests: The authors have declared that no competing interests exist.

* Email: wangkai1964@126.com

[9] These authors contributed equally to this work.

Introduction

In social context, appropriately express the negative emotion is important for emotion regulation ability [1–3]. However, in some scenarios, it is necessary to inhibit inappropriate negative emotion in social communication. The negative emotion may influence the current goal-directed behavior and further affect social function [4]. An impairment of this ability has increasingly been suggested to be involved in cognitive neural mechanisms of the etiology, maintenance and relapse of a range of psychiatric disorders, including depression [5–7], anxiety [8] and post-traumatic stress disorder [9].

Sad facial expressions are fundamental negative emotional stimuli that convey important information in social communications [10]. Emotions induced by sad facial expressions influence an individual's ability to inhibit inappropriate behavior. Many psychiatric individuals have disabilities regulating the relationship between sad facial information and response inhibition [11]. For instance, depressed individuals are often characterized by enhanced facilitation and deficient inhibition for sad emotions, which is a stable cognitive vulnerability risk, possibly associated with the occurrence of depression [12]. Moreover, when new mothers had more sad expressions, their infants expressed less joy and spent more time in joint negative affective states [13].

In several neuroimaging studies, neural substrates of facial information interactions with response inhibition have been investigated. ERP studies on emotional Go/Nogo tasks have reported the presence of N2 and P3 components following the onset of emotional Nogo stimuli. These findings are consistent with previous response inhibition studies employing non-emotional stimuli [14–17]. N2 has been suggested to relate to conflict detection and monitoring processes, whereas P3 is responsible for conflict resolution and behavior execution [18,19]. Using a facial go/nogo task, Zhang group detected larger amplitudes and shorter latency at Nogo-P3 stage in both happy and sad conditions which indicated electrophysiological activity was modulated by facial expressions [16]. Todd and colleagues reported that Nogo-N2 was increased after viewing angry faces than happy faces in 4- to 6-year-old children (N = 48) which suggests that facial expressions interact with response inhibition even at early stages [20]. Spatial features were explored with several fMRI and brain injury studies and data indicated that the right inferior frontal cortex (IFC) is a critical brain region involved in general response inhibition [21–25]. Furthermore, many studies indicated the rIFC also plays a crucial role in the neural substrate of response inhibition to negative facial information [26–30]. A recent ERP study combining standardized low-resolution brain electromagnetic tomography (sLORETA) with spatio-temporal principal component analysis, revealed the precise contribution of the anterior cingulated cortex (ACC), specifically in the P3 stage of the interplay of emotion and response inhibition [31]. These findings indicate that combining ERP and source localization techniques may be suitable tools for revealing the temporal and spatial characteristics of the brain systems underlying response inhibition.

Although negative emotion and response inhibition interactions play critical roles in human social life and many studies have explored their neural basis; whether the neural substrates of emotional response inhibition dissociated between explicit and implicit processing of facial expressions has been largely unexplored. In fact, implicit and explicit facial processing may serve different functions and may have distinct neural substrates. Explicit processing means that facial expression is within the voluntary attention scope and is directly processed, whereas implicit processing means that facial expression is within involuntary attention scope, and therefore incidentally processed. Thus, the attention resource for stimuli processing is distinct between the two conditions. In social situations, effortful explicit interpretation of the meaning of facial expressions may be required to guide an individual's social responses. However, in familiar situations, facial expression processed implicitly may also affect behavior without full cognitive awareness. It has been confirmed that facial expression processed explicitly and implicitly induced distinct emotional intensity in subject reports. Rating pictures was associated with significantly less intensity of sadness than passively viewing pictures, likely because the rating task reduced the activation of related brain regions responsible for an emotional experience [32]. In a subsequent ERP study, who found that although enhanced processing of negative facial expression occurred at perceptual stages irrespective of intention in facial expressions, larger amplitudes of a late positive complex was detected when facial expression was explicitly processed compared to when it was implicitly processed. Thus, processing of facial expressions depended on the participant's intentional state at late stage [33]. fMRI studies found that directly focusing on emotional

valence activated more intense neural reactions in the bilateral amygdala and the superior temporal gyrus, both of which are critical for facial processing [34]. Linden and colleague confirmed that implicit expression processing was preserved in schizophrenia patients, but their explicit emotion classification was impaired, and this finding supported a dissociated mechanism between implicit and explicit processing of facial expression [35].

The aim of the present study was to investigate dissociation of the neural substrates of emotional response inhibition between explicit and implicit processing of facial expressions. In previous emotional response inhibition studies, emotional stimuli were either explicitly [27,36] or implicitly [16,28,31] processed, and the attention was not taken into consideration. It is critical to directly determine whether different manipulations of attention levels for negative stimuli processing would bias the validity of response inhibition to negative stimuli. To this end, we developed a modified implicit and explicit emotional Go/Nogo task to investigate how the negative facial information modulates the response inhibition function implicitly and explicitly. Implicit and explicit tasks have been used to manipulate attention resources for facial expression processing [37–39]. In the explicit task, participants were asked to make their Go/Nogo decision based on the recognition of emotional categories, i.e., the emotional information was explicitly processed. In the implicit task, the Go and Nogo trials were defined based on the identification of the gender of the face, i.e., the emotional processing was implicit. Furthermore, the stimuli in the explicit or implicit conditions were identical, which precludes interference due to additional stimuli. A combination of ERP and source localization methods was employed to characterize temporal and spatial characteristics of response inhibition to negative stimuli explicitly and implicitly. Because sad facial expressions are evolutionarily salient emotional stimuli and many psychiatric disorders involve dysfunction in modulating the interaction of inhibition and sad facial emotions [11,40–42], we employed sad and neutral facial stimuli as both Go and Nogo signals using a factorial block design. Based on previous studies that reflected higher emotional intensity in explicit tasks, we hypothesized that significant negative emotional effects would occur in inhibition-related ERP components (N2 and P3) for explicit tasks but not for implicit tasks and within inhibition-related brain areas, such as the rIFC and the ACC.

Materials and Methods

Subjects

The study was approved by the Ethics Committees of Anhui Medical University. All participants signed an informed consent form for the experiment.

Thirty right-handed adults (15 female) aged 23.2±1.54 years (mean ± SD) were paid to participate in the experiment. All participants were screened for current and past psychiatric and neurological disorders, were free of histories of drug use and had normal or corrected-to-normal vision. In addition, all subjects scored within the normal range on the State-Trait Anxiety Inventories [43] and the Beck Depression Inventory [44].

Stimuli

Facial stimuli consisting of 40 sad and 40 neutral faces were selected from the native Chinese Facial Affective Picture System, including 20 female and 20 male faces displaying each emotion type. The faces in the Facial Affective Picture System were assessed with a 9-point scale by 100 college students from two colleges in Beijing. The 9-point scale was used to assess the emotion valence and arousal of each picture in the Facial Affective

Picture System. For the valence dimension, participants were asked to assess the valence of the picture. For both valence and arousal dimensions, higher grades refer to more positive valence and stronger arousal respectively, and vice versa. We selected stimuli for the present experiment in such a way that they differed significantly in valence from one another, $t = 11.65$, $P < 0.001$ (M±SD, sad: 3.11 ± 0.63, neutral: 4.49 ± 0.41), but were similar in arousal ($P > 0.5$). Stimuli were similar to one another in size, background, spatial frequency, contrast grade, brightness, and other physical properties. Each picture was cropped into the shape of an ellipse that incorporated the facial characteristics using Adobe Photoshop 8.0 software. The screen resolution was 72 pixels per inch, and the viewing angle was $5.7 \times 4.6°$. The subjects were seated in a soundproof room with their eyes approximately 100 cm from a 17-in screen. All stimuli were displayed in the center of the screen.

Experimental procedures

The study used the block design method: one block was implicit and the other was explicit. During the implicit task, the participants were instructed to respond immediately after the pictures depicting one gender (Go trials) and to inhibit this response after the other gender (Nogo trial). In the explicit task, the participants were required to respond or inhibit their behavior according to the valence of the facial expression. The participants were asked to complete both of these two tasks separately in two different blocks. The order of the blocks was counterbalanced across participants. Furthermore, each block was sub-divided into two parts in which the facial stimuli were counterbalanced in terms of whether they indicated Go or Nogo trials.

Each block was composed of 480 trials that included 144 Nogo stimuli and 336 Go stimuli (30% vs. 70%). In each block, the Go and Nogo stimuli were presented pseudo-randomly, and the Go trials always preceded the Nogo trials to induce pre-potent motor responses and obvious conflict during response inhibition. At the start of each block, an instruction screen was presented for 2 minutes and prompted the participants to press or refrain from pressing the "J" key with their right hand according to the facial expression or gender. Each trial was initiated by a small grey cross that was displayed for a variable duration (200–400 ms) on the black background. Then, an emotional face was presented at the center of the screen for 1000 ms. Participants were instructed to respond as quickly as possible after the face was presented. Each response was followed by a blank screen, the duration of which varied from 1200 to 1500 ms. The experimental procedure is presented in Figure 1. The individuals in this manuscript have given written informed consent to publish these case details. A training session was included before the formal experiment. All programs were compiled and executed using E-Prime software (Psychology Software Tools, Inc., Pittsburgh, PA).

Event-related potential recording

Electroencephalography (EEG) was performed from 64 scalp sites using tin electrodes mounted on an elastic cap (Neuro Scan, Sterling, Virginia, USA) according to the international 10/20 system. The participants were grounded with a forehead electrode. All EEG channels were referenced to the left mastoid and were re-referenced off-line to the average of the left and right mastoids. Vertical electro-oculogram (EOG) data were recorded supraorbitally and infraorbitally at the left eye. Horizontal EOG data were recorded as the left versus right orbital rim. EEG and EOG activity were amplified with a 0.01–100 Hz bandpass filter and continuously sampled at 500 Hz/channel. All electrode impedances were maintained below 5 ?Ω. Ocular artifacts were removed from the EEG signals using a regression procedure implemented in Neuroscan software [45]. Trials with remaining EOG artifacts (mean EOG voltage exceeding ±100 μV), amplifier clipping artifacts, or peak-to-peak deflections exceeding ±100 μV were excluded from averaging. The EEG activities during correct responses in each condition were aligned and averaged separately. The ERP waveforms were time-locked to the onset of the face stimuli, and the averaging epoch was 1200 ms, including a 200 ms pre-stimulus baseline.

Data analysis

All behavioral and electrophysiological data analyses were conducted using a SPSS software package (Version 16.0; SPSS Inc, Chicago, USA). The degrees of freedom of the F-ratios were adjusted according to the Greenhouse–Geisser epsilon correction in all analyses. Because this study focused on comparing the effects of the emotion of the stimuli on response inhibition during the implicit and explicit tasks, our analyses mainly concentrated on the interactive effects between task, valence and trial type. Post-hoc contrasts were carried out using the Bonferroni procedure ($\alpha < 0.05$).

Behavioral analysis

The error rates, defined as Nogo responses in Go trials and button presses in Nogo trials, and the reaction times to Go stimuli were analyzed. Reaction times above 1500 ms or below 150 ms were omitted from the analyses. Repeated-measures ANOVAs were performed on error rates and reaction times using task (implicit and explicit), valence (sad and neutral) and trial type (Go and Nogo) as within-subject factors.

ERP analysis

With the aim of reliably defining and quantifying N2 and P3 ERP components and increasing the reliability of source analyses, covariance-matrix-based temporal principal component analysis (tPCA) was used in the present study. Albert et al have used this method to analyze N2 and P3 components induced by an emotional Go/Nogo task [31,46]. This technique has been repeatedly used in ERP researches in that the exclusive use of traditional visual inspection of grand averages and on 'temporal windows of interest' for voltage computation may lead to several types of mistake [47–49]. The main advantage of tPCA over traditional methods is that it can get 'clean' ERP components which are free of the influence of adjacent or subjacent components by extracting and quantifying these components. In fact, the brain potentials recorded at an electrode on the head over a time window represents a complex superposition of different overlapping electrical potentials. Such recordings can interfere with visual inspection. In short, the covariance between all ERP time points tends to be high between those time points involved in the same component and low between those belonging to different components. The tPCA computes the covariance between all ERP time points. Therefore the solution is a set of independent factors composed of highly covariant time points, which ideally correspond to ERP components. Temporal factor score, the tPCA derived parameter in which extracted temporal factors may be quantified is linearly related to amplitude.

As signal overlap may also occur at the spatial domain, the spatial principal component analysis (sPCA) was calculated to reliably define the topography for all temporal factors according to the time window of components obtained by tPCA. The temporal factors (TFs) and spatial factors (SFs) were calculated by tPCA and sPCA steps, respectively, for the components of interest (N2 and P3). In the present study, we selected a number of components

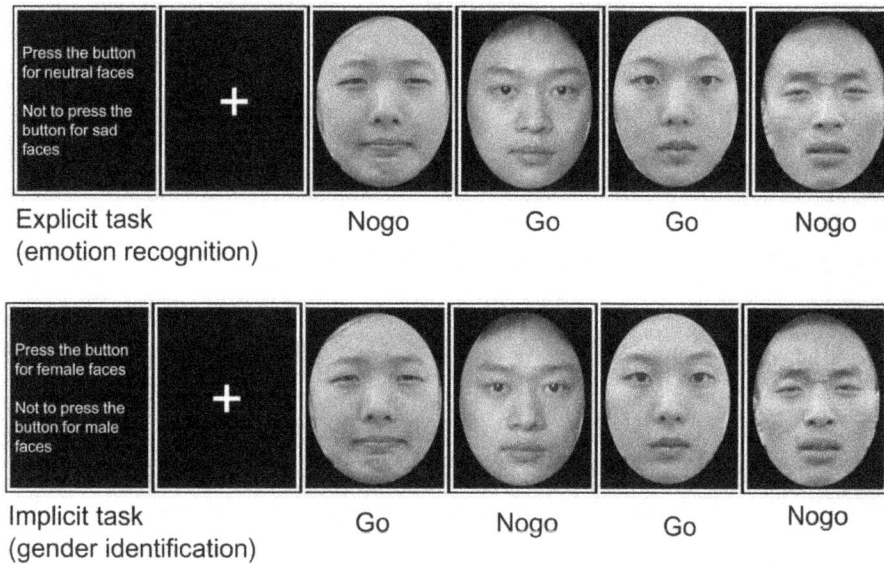

Figure 1. Trial design for (A) an explicit and (B) an implicit emotional Go/Nogo tasks. In explicit task, subjects pressed a response button or inhibit their behavior according to the facial expression (sad/neutral). While in implicit task, subjects made their motor actions based on the facial gender (male/female).

based on a screening test [50]. The promax rotation method was used to extract components [47,48]. Finally, we used repeated measures ANOVAs on these factor scores (linearly related to voltages, as indicated) to analyze the effects of task type, valence and trial type.

Source-localization analysis

In order to three-dimensionally locate the cortical regions that were sensitive to the experimental effects, standardized low-resolution brain electromagnetic tomography (sLORETA) [51] was applied to relevant temporal factor scores. sLORETA is a three-dimensional discrete linear solution that has been frequently used for EEG source analysis. sLORETA is used to estimate current density distributions restricted to the cortical grey matter and the hippocampus in the digitized MNI atlas with 6239 voxels at a spatial resolution of 5 mm. The sLORETA method has been shown to produce results that coincide with those provided by other brain imaging methods during equivalent paradigms [52–55]. Moreover, sLORETA analyses based on temporal factor scores derived from the tPCA method rather than direct voltages have been proven to yield more accurate source-localization results [56]. In addition, the present study employed a relatively large sample size (N = 30) that contributed to reducing the error margin of our EEG-based source analysis.

First, to identify the neural mechanisms underlying response inhibition, voxel-based whole-brain sLORETA images were compared between the Nogo and Go conditions; the sLORETA built-in voxel-wise randomization tests (5000 permutations) based on statistical non-parametric mapping methodology [57] were used. Second, the ROI approach was performed on those regions detected as response inhibition-related in the first step. The current source densities (CSD) of the ROIs were submitted to ANOVA analysis to explore the modulatory effects of task and emotion.

Results

Behavioral data

For our behavioral results, both implicit and explicit tasks were relatively easy to perform. The mean accuracy across subjects in each condition was above 95% (95.3% in the negative Nogo condition, 96% in the negative go condition, 97.2% in the neutral Nogo condition, 96.5% in the neutral go condition using an implicit task, 97.5% in the negative Nogo condition, 95.5% in the negative go condition, 98.2% in the neutral nogo condition, and 98.6% in the neutral go condition using an explicit task). The ANOVA analysis of response time in the Go trial type showed that neither the main effects nor the interaction effects were significant (521.3 ms in the negative go condition, 522.3 ms in the neutral go condition using an implicit task; 526.3 ms in the negative go condition, 5201 ms in the neutral go condition using an explicit task).

ERP data

Figure 2 shows the grand averages at the Fz, Cz and Pz sites. As a result of the tPCA computation, seven temporal factors were extracted from the original ERP waveforms (Figure 3). As previous studies revealed that the time window of Nogo-N2 was 200–400 ms and mainly distributed at frontal-central area and Nogo-P3 occur during 400–600 ms and located at central-parietal area [58,59], we can recognize that TF4 (peak at 284 ms) was associated with the wave labeled N2, and TF2 (peak at 512 ms) was associated with the wave labeled P3 according to factor peak latency and topography characteristics. These labels will be used, henceforth, to make our results easier to understand. The spatial factors extracted by sPCA computations for each temporal factor are shown in Table 1.

As shown in Table 1, multivariate repeated-measures ANOVAs were computed on N2 and P3 spatial factor scores using task, emotion and trial type as within-subject factors. First, these ANOVA analyses detected significant main effects of trial type in N2 and P3 at the fronto-central and posterior areas. The two components showed higher amplitudes in the Nogo condition than

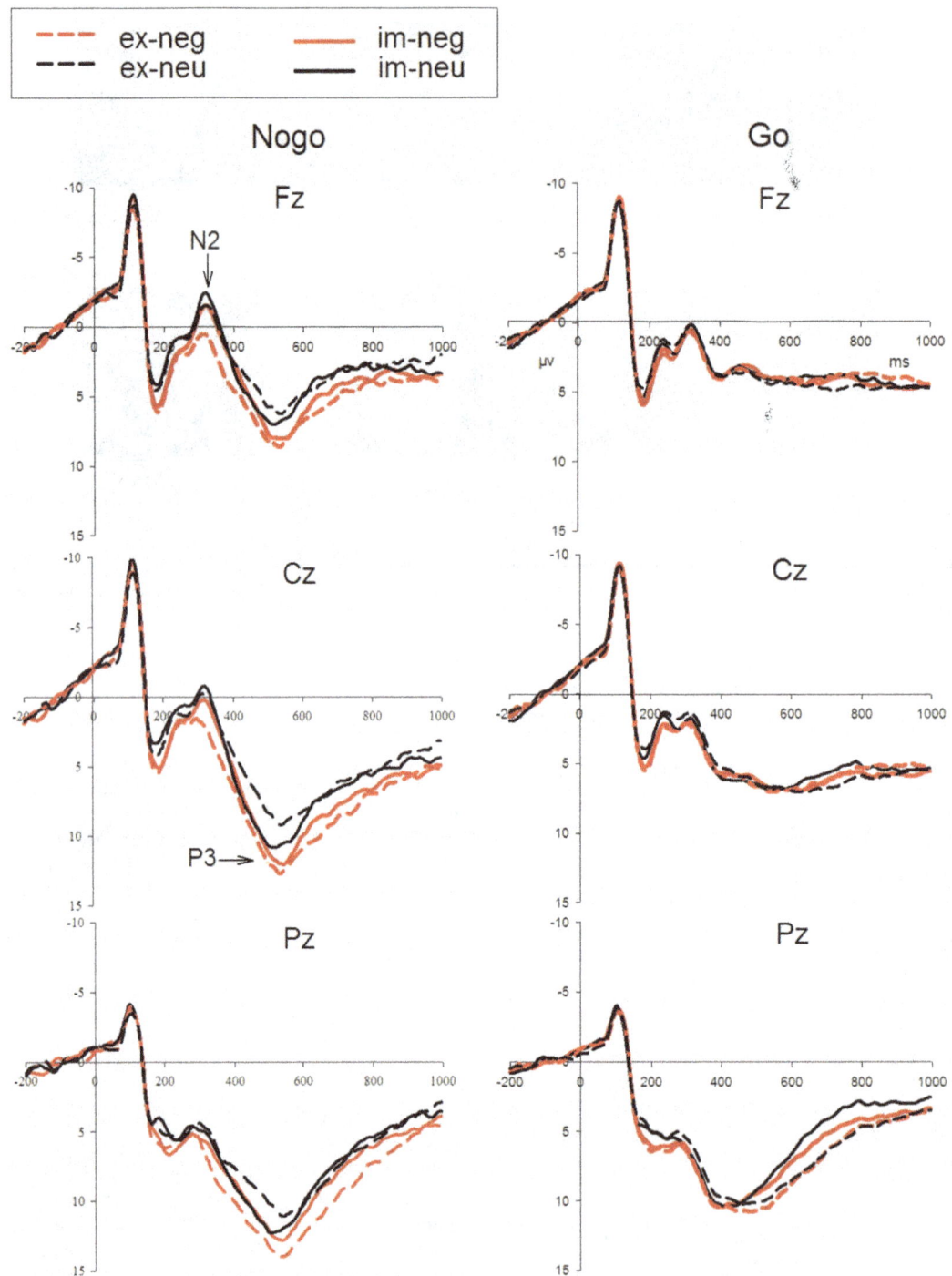

Figure 2. Grand averages evoked by negative (red lines) and neutral (black lines) stimuli in Nogo (left column) and Go trials (right column) under implicit (solid lines) and explicit conditions (dash lines) at Fz, Cz and Pz sites (im: implicit; ex: explicit; neg: negative; neu: neutral).

in the Go condition, which further confirmed that they were associated with response inhibition. In addition, temporal factor score of P3 showed significant emotion and trial type interaction effect. Nogo-P3 amplitudes were higher in negative emotion than in neutral conditions. The amplitudes difference induced by go trials between sad and neutral condition was not significant. Moreover, to testify the modulatory effects of task in the Go and Nogo conditions and its further interaction with trial type and

emotion, the experimental effects of task ×emotion ×trial type were analyzed. We found a significant interaction of these three factors in the centro-posterior and posterior spatial factors of P3. Post-hoc analyses showed that in the explicit task, Nogo-P3 amplitudes elicited by negative signals were larger than those elicited by neutral signals, while this difference was not found in the implicit task. No interaction effects involving task and/or emotion on trial type were observed in N2 spatial factors.

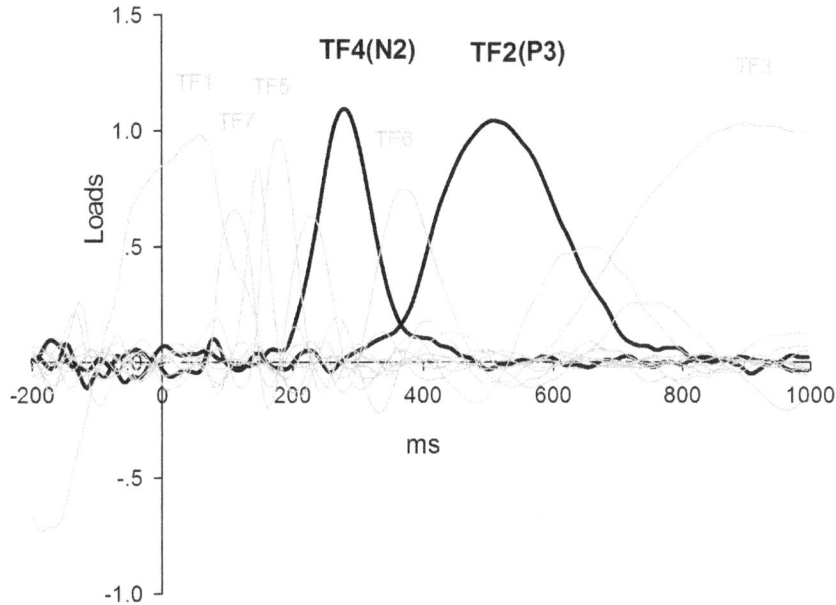

Figure 3. tPCA: factor loadings after promax rotation. TF4 (N2) and TF2 (P3) are drawn in black.

Source-localization data

First, source localization analysis consisted of three-dimensionally localizing the cortical regions that were responsible for the experimental manipulations described above. Based on the ERP results of former steps, which detected significant task × emotion × trial type effects in P3 stage, voxel-based whole-brain sLORETA images were compared between the Nogo and Go conditions during the stage using non-parametric randomization tests.

As illustrated in Figure 4, on P3 stages, Nogo trials compared to Go trials activated the right dorsal lateral prefrontal cortex (rDLPFC, BA 9: max values obtained at x = 50, y = 20, z = 40), the right pre-supplementary motor area (rPre-SMA, BA 6: max values

obtained at x = 55, y = 5, z = 45), and the right frontal eye fields (rFEF, BA 8: max values obtained at x = 50, y = 5, z = 45)), which collectively constitute one junction part coinciding with the typical definition of the right inferior frontal junction (rIFJ) [60–62]. As explained in Data Analysis, the next step was to define ROIs for each of these data-defined areas, to compute their CSD and to submit them to ANOVAs for testing experimental effects. According to the definition of the rIFJ, one ROI was generated using the coordinates from those voxels surpassing the 0.01 threshold for the t value in the previous sLORETA comparison. We observed a significant main effect of trial type [F (1, 29) = 67.82, $P < 0.0001$]. The CSD was higher in the Nogo condition than in the Go condition. More importantly, we detected a

Table 1. Results of the statistical contrasts concerning Trial type (Go and Nogo) ×Emotional condition (negative, neutral) × Task (implicit, explicit) interaction carried out on N2 and P3 extracted spatio-temporal factors.

Temporal factor	Special factor	trial type	emotion×trial type	task×emotion	task×emotion×trial type
		(df = 1, 29)	(df = 1, 29)	(df = 1, 29)	(df = 1, 29)
TF4 (N2)	Frontocentral	$F = 10.25^{**}$	$F = 0.69$, ns	$F = 0.24$, ns	$F = 0.65$, ns
		$P = 0.003$	$P = 0.41$	$P = 0.63$	$P = 0.43$
	Centroposterior	$F = 8.22^{**}$	$F = 0.24$, ns	$F = 0.02$, ns	$F = 1.48$, ns
		$P = 0.008$	$P = 0.63$	$P = 0.89$	$P = 0.23$
TF2 (P3)	Frontocentral	$F = 31.61^{***}$	$F = 15.61^{***}$	$F = 3.36$, ns	$F = 2.53$, ns
		$P < 0.0001$	$P < 0.0001$	$P = 0.08$	$P = 0.12$
	Centroposterior	$F = 17.93^{***}$	$F = 20.48^{***}$	$F = 9.86^{**}$	$F = 4.33^{*}$
		$P < 0.0001$	$P < 0.0001$	$P = 0.004$	$P = 0.046$
	Posterior	$F = 17.17^{***}$	$F = 3.76$	$F = 16.71^{***}$	$F = 7.25^{*}$
		$P < 0.0001$	$P = 0.062$	$P < 0.0001$	$P = 0.012$

TF: temporal factor; df: degrees of freedom; ns: not significant;
*: $P < 0.05$;
**: $P < 0.01$;
***: $P < 0.001$.

significant interaction effect between task and emotion [F (1, 29) = 5.68, P = 0.024]. A simple analysis showed that the CSD was larger in the negative condition than in the neutral condition only during the explicit task.

Discussion

In the present study, we characterized temporal and spatial features of neural substrates of response inhibition to negative faces which were processed explicitly and implicitly. As expected, inhibition-related components, N2 and P3, were successfully induced in the two task sets. The modulatory effect of sad emotion on response inhibition was limited by attention resources during the P3, rather than N2 phase. sLORETA analyses in the P3 stage indicated that—compared to go stimuli—nogo stimuli elicited higher activation in the junctional area of rIFC which consisted of rDLPFC, rPre-SMA and rFEF. ROI analyses confirmed that the three areas were responsible for emotional regulation mechanisms when sad facial emotions interacted with response inhibition explicitly. The implications of these results for understanding emotional response inhibition are discussed below in detail.

Electrophysiological evidence has indicated the diverse functions of N2 and P3 components in response inhibition [19,63,64]. Compared to the aspect of conflict response in the N2 stage, previous studies confirmed the action inhibitory process underlying Nogo-P3 [31,65]. In our study, inhibition related-P3 amplitudes were modulated by sad emotions. Inhibiting sad faces elicited larger P3 amplitudes than neutral faces and these results were consistent with previous studies showing that the capacity of cognitive control could be affected in this predominant fashion when the processing of negative stimuli and emotional significance was sufficient [66–68]. Negative emotion, especially a sad facial expression, is biologically and socially significant in human interaction. Human beings often generate withdrawal-related behaviors to negative stimuli which are perceived as threatening information and remind individuals to keep away from the dangerous situation [69]. Thus, when presented with a sad expression, participants devoted more cognitive resources to inhibiting the negative stimuli and elicited larger Nogo-P3 amplitudes than when presented with neutral faces. However, we detect no effect of task, emotion or trial type on behavioral data, most likely because the stimulus parameters were exactly matched between the manipulated variables and the effort of performing the task was similar and simple.

More importantly, we detected discrepancies of Nogo-P3 amplitudes induced by sad and neutral faces between implicit and explicit tasks. P3 amplitudes were larger with sad conditions than with neutral conditions during explicit tasks, but this was not significant during the implicit tasks. Previous studies suggest that individuals with borderline personality disorders have a pronounced withdrawal propensity with explicit tasks; however, implicit behavioral tendencies, measured by the joystick task, were not altered compared to controls [70]. Our results further indicated that response inhibition to facial expression differently between implicit and explicit tasks at P3 stage. Current data were consistent with a study which revealed that adults with ADHD had smaller P3 amplitudes compared to controls in sad conditions and suggested that Nogo-P3 was related to attention allocation [71]. In the explicit task, participants performed their task according to facial expression, and attention was concentrated on negative emotional aspects of faces. In the implicit task, participants were instructed to respond or to inhibit their response according to facial gender, and their attention was diverted from facial expression. Gross has proposed that the emotional effect on cognition is weakened when attention was disengaged from the emotional aspects of stimuli [72,73]. Thus, our data confirm that the response inhibition to sad faces was modulated by attention resources in the action inhibition stage. This result were also consistent with a previous study in which attention resources modulated facial expression processing and neural activity [32,33,74,75]. McRae group also discovered that the subjective experience and amygdala activity were decreased when attention was diverted from negative emotional pictures to neutral letters [76].

In contrast, Zhang and co-workers reported larger Nogo-P3 amplitudes for emotional conditions than with non-emotional condition [16] in implicit face Go/Nogo tasks. This may be explained by different emotional types used in the study. Happy, fearful, angry faces used in Zhang's work and sad faces have different neural mechanisms and have been reported to have different effects on cognition [27,77,78]. Also, shorter face durations of 100–250 ms used in the study may facilitate distinguishing the effect of emotional and neutral faces on response inhibition. Two factors of emotional type and stimuli duration should be further explored to confirm this. We observed no interaction effect of task and emotion with Nogo-N2. Evidence suggests that N2 subcomponents were sensitive to involuntary attention shifting but not voluntary attention regulation [79,80]. Here, we used block design and participants' responses or response inhibition according to the same instruction presented at the beginning of each task. On this occasion, participants allocated their attention to facial expression or gender voluntarily to perform the task. Thus, the Nogo-N2 was not significantly

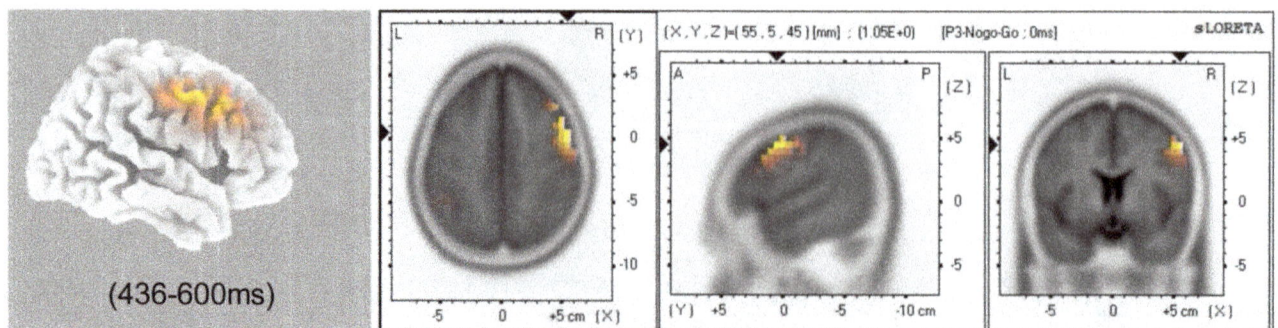

Figure 4. sLORETA solutions to non-parametric randomization tests on P3 temporal factor scores showing voxels in which the Nogo>Go contrast was significant (P<0.01).

different between the tasks. In any case, the present study not only showed sad emotion modulated response inhibition but also that this modulatory effect depended on attention resources in the late processing stage of response inhibition. These findings provide some indications for the use of cognitive behavior modification for individuals with anxiety and depression who are often troubled by negative emotion. For example, we can train these individuals to divert their attention from the negative aspects and deliver more attention resources to neutral and positive aspects of daily events.

Using the factor-score-based sLORETA method, source localization analysis on P3 components detected that the rIFJ showed a higher activation level in the Nogo condition compared to the Go condition. The right inferior frontal junction (rIFJ) (BA 6, 8 and 9) was a posterior component of the rIFC localized at the intersection of the inferior frontal sulcus and the precentral sulcus, which comprises parts of the DLPFC, the pre-SMA and the FEF [60,61]. Consistent results have recently been reported that the rIFJ was the causal source of the top-down modulation underlying selective attention, working memory and response inhibition [81–83]. The rIFJ recruitment in P3 phases of response inhibition in the present study may support the implication that this junction of different brain regions is crucial to the response inhibition [60].

Consistent with our ERP findings, the results of ROI analyses revealed that the rIFJ—the general source of inhibition-related components—was more activated in the negative condition compared to the neutral condition during the context of the explicit task, and not the implicit task in the P3 processing period. Previous papers included discussions about the influence of negative emotions on response inhibition separately under explicit and implicit conditions [16,27,28,31,36]. However, the neural substrate of response inhibition to negative stimuli has been scarcely investigated under the direct manipulation of attention resources. Our results suggested that as the key region of inhibitory processing, rIFJ activity was involved in response inhibition to social sad stimuli. As described above, the rIFJ has recently been reported to be the causal source of the top-down modulation underlying selective attention, working memory, and response inhibition [81–83]. With current explicit tasks, attention was concentrated on sad facial expressions which may increase the required sources for inhibitory processing. Thus, more effort from the rIFJ would be required for behavioral monitoring and action inhibition relative to an implicit task. The IFJ has been reported to be involved in emotion reappraisal processing [84]. Combined with these results, the IFJ may be a critical brain area for emotion regulation.

Our data did differ from that of Piguet and colleagues, who found no activation of inhibition-related specific area such as the rIFJ whereas ACC activation decreased when subjects were asked to inhibit response to sad or happy faces according to an expression or gender switching task [85]. This is likely because the tasks in Piguet's work included not only inhibition but also switching tasks and timing, stimuli and task difficulty were different from our study. A question that arises is why the ACC has not shown trial type by emotion effects in the implicit and/or explicit tasks. Indeed, the ACC has been reported to be sensitive to this interaction in several previous studies also employing implicit tasks [28,31,46]. The nature of the stimuli may contribute to the

explanation of this observed lack of effects. Previous experiments included highly arousing stimuli, such as emotional scenes [31,46] or emotional words specifically selected as being salient for patients included in the experimental sample [28]. Given that the emotional stimuli employed in our study were not especially arousing (sadness is considered a low arousing negative emotion [86]) and that ACC activity has been shown to be sensitive to the intensity/arousal of emotional stimuli [87], these facts may explain the present results.

Our study has several limitations. First, we only used the sad expressions as experimental stimuli and how the six basic emotions interact in response inhibition in implicit and explicit tasks warrants investigation. Second, although the PCA method proved the precision of spatial orientation, the method was still based on the proposition from a mathematical, but not a physiological, standpoint. In addition, there are many sub-cortical areas involved in response inhibition to facial stimuli such as the amygdala, ventral striatum and fusiform gyrus [27,71]. But because of the limitation of electrophysiological source analysis, the sub-cortical areas could not be observed. Further researches employing a wide range of experimental tasks and designs, as well as brain imaging methodologies, such as fMRI, that may improve the spatial resolution, are needed to substantiate and extend these findings.

Conclusions

In summary, using a high temporal resolution of ERPs and recent advances in reconstruction of electrophysiological sources, our data suggest that the neural substrates of response inhibition to sad faces were different between implicit and explicit tasks. The P3 amplitudes were greater in sad compared to neutral conditions in explicit tasks rather than in implicit tasks. Furthermore, the spatial dissociation in brain functions confirmed that the rIFJ was the central node in response inhibition to sad faces. These findings collectively revealed the underlying temporal and spatial characteristics in response inhibition to social negative stimuli explicitly and implicitly, which may have implications for future research concerning the complicated interaction of emotion and cognition and cognitive behavior modification in psychiatry individuals.

Acknowledgments

We thank Long Zhang and Dan Li for data collection.

Author Contributions

Conceived and designed the experiments: FQY RY YJL KW. Performed the experiments: LZ. Analyzed the data: FQY RY SYS LC. Contributed reagents/materials/analysis tools: RY SYS CYZ YD. Wrote the paper: FQY RY KW.

References

1. Taylor GJ, Bagby RM, Parker JD (1991) The alexithymia construct. A potential paradigm for psychosomatic medicine. Psychosomatics 32: 153–164.

2. Mazefsky CA, Herrington J, Siegel M, Scarpa A, Maddox BB, et al. (2013) The role of emotion regulation in autism spectrum disorder. J Am Acad Child Adolesc Psychiatry 52: 679–688.

3. Henry JD, Green MJ, de Lucia A, Restuccia C, McDonald S, et al. (2007) Emotion dysregulation in schizophrenia: reduced amplification of emotional expression is associated with emotional blunting. Schizophr Res 95: 197–204.

4. Dillon DG, Pizzagalli DA (2007) Inhibition of Action, Thought, and Emotion: A Selective Neurobiological Review. Appl Prev Psychol 12: 99–114.

5. Holmes AJ, Pizzagalli DA (2008) Response conflict and frontocingulate dysfunction in unmedicated participants with major depression. Neuropsychologia 46: 2904–2913.

6. Johnstone T, van Reekum CM, Urry HL, Kalin NH, Davidson RJ (2007) Failure to regulate: counterproductive recruitment of top-down prefrontal-subcortical circuitry in major depression. J Neurosci 27: 8877–8884.

7. Pizzagalli D, Pascual-Marqui RD, Nitschke JB, Oakes TR, Larson CL, et al. (2001) Anterior cingulate activity as a predictor of degree of treatment response in major depression: evidence from brain electrical tomography analysis. Am J Psychiatry 158: 405–415.

8. Sehlmeyer C, Konrad C, Zwitserlood P, Arolt V, Falkenstein M, et al. (2010) ERP indices for response inhibition are related to anxiety-related personality traits. Neuropsychologia 48: 2488–2495.

9. Frewen PA, Lanius RA (2006) Toward a psychobiology of posttraumatic self-dysregulation: reexperiencing, hyperarousal, dissociation, and emotional numbing. Ann N Y Acad Sci 1071: 110–124.

10. Luo W, Feng W, He W, Wang NY, Luo YJ (2010) Three stages of facial expression processing: ERP study with rapid serial visual presentation. Neuroimage 49: 1857–1867.

11. Dziobek I, Preissler S, Grozdanovic Z, Heuser I, Heekeren HR, et al. (2011) Neuronal correlates of altered empathy and social cognition in borderline personality disorder. Neuroimage 57: 539–548.

12. Dai Q, Feng Z (2011) Dysfunctional distracter inhibition and facilitation for sad faces in depressed individuals. Psychiatry Res 190: 206–211.

13. Termine NT, Izard CE (1988) Infants' responses to their mothers expressions of joy and sadness. Developmental Psychology 24: 223–229.

14. Chiu PH, Holmes AJ, Pizzagalli DA (2008) Dissociable recruitment of rostral anterior cingulate and inferior frontal cortex in emotional response inhibition. Neuroimage 42: 988–997.

15. Kiss M, Raymond JE, Westoby N, Nobre AC, Eimer M (2008) Response inhibition is linked to emotional devaluation: behavioural and electrophysiological evidence. Front Hum Neurosci 2: 13.

16. Zhang W, Lu J (2012) Time course of automatic emotion regulation during a facial Go/Nogo task. Biol Psychol 89: 444–449.

17. Korb S, Grandjean D, Scherer KR (2010) Timing and voluntary suppression of facial mimicry to smiling faces in a Go/NoGo task—an EMG study. Biol Psychol 85: 347–349.

18. Donkers FC, van Boxtel GJ (2004) The N2 in go/no-go tasks reflects conflict monitoring not response inhibition. Brain Cogn 56: 165–176.

19. Kropotov JD, Ponomarev VA, Hollup S, Mueller A (2011) Dissociating action inhibition, conflict monitoring and sensory mismatch into independent components of event related potentials in GO/NOGO task. Neuroimage 57: 565–575.

20. Todd RM, Lewis MD, Meusel LA, Zelazo PD (2008) The time course of social-emotional processing in early childhood: ERP responses to facial affect and personal familiarity in a Go-Nogo task. Neuropsychologia 46: 595–613.

21. Aron AR, Fletcher PC, Bullmore ET, Sahakian BJ, Robbins TW (2003) Stop-signal inhibition disrupted by damage to right inferior frontal gyrus in humans. Nat Neurosci 6: 115–116.

22. Hampshire A, Chamberlain SR, Monti MM, Duncan J, Owen AM (2010) The role of the right inferior frontal gyrus: inhibition and attentional control. Neuroimage 50: 1313–1319.

23. Wessel JR, Conner CR, Aron AR, Tandon N (2013) Chronometric electrical stimulation of right inferior frontal cortex increases motor braking. J Neurosci 33: 19611–19619.

24. Aron AR, Robbins TW, Poldrack RA (2004) Inhibition and the right inferior frontal cortex. Trends Cogn Sci 8: 170–177.

25. Schulz KP, Bedard AC, Fan J, Clerkin SM, Dima D, et al. (2014) Emotional bias of cognitive control in adults with childhood attention-deficit/hyperactivity disorder. Neuroimage Clin 5: 1–9.

26. Padmala S, Pessoa L (2010) Interactions between cognition and motivation during response inhibition. Neuropsychologia 48: 558–565.

27. Shafritz KM, Collins SH, Blumberg HP (2006) The interaction of emotional and cognitive neural systems in emotionally guided response inhibition. Neuroimage 31: 468–475.

28. Goldstein M, Brendel G, Tuescher O, Pan H, Epstein J, et al. (2007) Neural substrates of the interaction of emotional stimulus processing and motor inhibitory control: an emotional linguistic go/no-go fMRI study. Neuroimage 36: 1026–1040.

29. Ochsner KN, Ray RD, Cooper JC, Robertson ER, Chopra S, et al. (2004) For better or for worse: neural systems supporting the cognitive down- and up-regulation of negative emotion. Neuroimage 23: 483–499.

30. Berkman ET, Burklund L, Lieberman MD (2009) Inhibitory spillover: intentional motor inhibition produces incidental limbic inhibition via right inferior frontal cortex. Neuroimage 47: 705–712.

31. Albert J, Lopez-Martin S, Carretie L (2010) Emotional context modulates response inhibition: neural and behavioral data. Neuroimage 49: 914–921.

32. Taylor SF, Phan KL, Decker LR, Liberzon I (2003) Subjective rating of emotionally salient stimuli modulates neural activity. Neuroimage 18: 650–659.

33. Valdes-Conroy B, Aguado L, Fernandez-Cahill M, Romero-Ferreiro V, Dieguez-Risco T (2014) Following the time course of face gender and expression processing: a task-dependent ERP study. Int J Psychophysiol 92: 59–66.

34. Winston JS, O'Doherty J, Dolan RJ (2003) Common and distinct neural responses during direct and incidental processing of multiple facial emotions. Neuroimage 20: 84–97.

35. Linden SC, Jackson MC, Subramanian L, Wolf C, Green P, et al. (2010) Emotion-cognition interactions in schizophrenia: Implicit and explicit effects of facial expression. Neuropsychologia 48: 997–1002.

36. Hare TA, Tottenham N, Davidson MC, Glover GH, Casey BJ (2005) Contributions of amygdala and striatal activity in emotion regulation. Biol Psychiatry 57: 624–632.

37. Chen CH, Lennox B, Jacob R, Calder A, Lupson V, et al. (2006) Explicit and implicit facial affect recognition in manic and depressed States of bipolar disorder: a functional magnetic resonance imaging study. Biol Psychiatry 59: 31–39.

38. Critchley H, Daly E, Phillips M, Brammer M, Bullmore E, et al. (2000) Explicit and implicit neural mechanisms for processing of social information from facial expressions: a functional magnetic resonance imaging study. Hum Brain Mapp9: 93–105.

39. Gorno-Tempini ML, Pradelli S, Serafini M, Pagnoni G, Baraldi P, et al. (2001) Explicit and incidental facial expression processing: an fMRI study. Neuroimage 14: 465–473.

40. Hummer TA, Hulvershorn LA, Karne HS, Gunn AD, Wang Y, et al. (2013) Emotional response inhibition in bipolar disorder: a functional magnetic resonance imaging study of trait- and state-related abnormalities. Biol Psychiatry 73: 136–143.

41. Gehricke J, Shapiro D (2000) Reduced facial expression and social context in major depression: discrepancies between facial muscle activity and self-reported emotion. Psychiatry Res 95: 157–167.

42. Duerden EG, Taylor MJ, Soorya LV, Wang T, Fan J, et al. (2013) Neural correlates of inhibition of socially relevant stimuli in adults with autism spectrum disorder. Brain Res 1533: 80–90.

43. Silbersweig D, Spielberger CD, Gorsuch RL, Lushene RE (1988) STAI-Manual for the State Trait Anxiety Inventory. Palo Alto (CA): Consulting Psychologists Press.

44. Beck AT, Steer RA, Carbin MG (1988) Psychometric properties of the Beck Depression Inventory: Twenty-five years of evaluation. Clin Psychol Rev 8: 77–100.

45. Semlitsch HV, Anderer P, Schuster P, Presslich O (1986) A solution for reliable and valid reduction of ocular artifacts, applied to the P300 ERP. Psychophysiology 23: 695–703.

46. Albert J, Lopez-Martin S, Tapia M, Montoya D, Carretie L (2012) The role of the anterior cingulate cortex in emotional response inhibition. Hum Brain Mapp33: 2147–2160.

47. Dien J, Beal DJ, Berg P (2005) Optimizing principal components analysis of event-related potentials: matrix type, factor loading weighting, extraction, and rotations. Clin Neurophysiol 116: 1808–1825.

48. Dien J (2010) Evaluating two-step PCA of ERP data with Geomin, Infomax, Oblimin, Promax, and Varimax rotations. Psychophysiology 47: 170–183.

49. Kayser J, Tenke CE (2003) Optimizing PCA methodology for ERP component identification and measurement: theoretical rationale and empirical evaluation. Clin Neurophysiol 114: 2307–2325.

50. Cliff N (1987) Analyzing Multivariate Data San Diego (CA): Harcourt Brace Jovanovich.

51. Pascual-Marqui RD (2002) Standardized low-resolution brain electromagnetic tomography (sLORETA): technical details. Methods Find Exp Clin Pharmacol 24 Suppl D: 5–12.

52. Dierks T, Jelic V, Pascual-Marqui RD, Wahlund L, Julin P, et al. (2000) Spatial pattern of cerebral glucose metabolism (PET) correlates with localization of intracerebral EEG-generators in Alzheimer's disease. Clin Neurophysiol 111: 1817–1824.

53. Mulert C, Jager L, Schmitt R, Bussfeld P, Pogarell O, et al. (2004) Integration of fMRI and simultaneous EEG: towards a comprehensive understanding of localization and time-course of brain activity in target detection. Neuroimage 22: 83–94.

54. Pizzagalli DA, Oakes TR, Fox AS, Chung MK, Larson CL, et al. (2004) Functional but not structural subgenual prefrontal cortex abnormalities in melancholia. Mol Psychiatry 9: 325, 393–405.

55. Vitacco D, Brandeis D, Pascual-Marqui R, Martin E (2002) Correspondence of event-related potential tomography and functional magnetic resonance imaging during language processing. Hum Brain Mapp17: 4–12.

56. Carretie L, Tapia M, Mercado F, Albert J, Lopez-Martin S, et al. (2004) Voltage-based versus factor score-based source localization analyses of electrophysiological brain activity: a comparison. Brain Topogr 17: 109–115.

57. Nichols TE, Holmes AP (2002) Nonparametric permutation tests for functional neuroimaging: a primer with examples. Hum Brain Mapp15: 1–25.

58. Yu F, Yuan J, Luo YJ (2009) Auditory-induced emotion modulates processes of response inhibition: an event-related potential study. Neuroreport 20: 25–30.

59. Yuan J, He Y, Qinglin Z, Chen A, Li H (2008) Gender differences in behavioral inhibitory control: ERP evidence from a two-choice oddball task. Psychophysiology 45: 986–993.

60. Brass M, Derrfuss J, Forstmann B, von Cramon DY (2005) The role of the inferior frontal junction area in cognitive control. Trends Cogn Sci 9: 314–316.

61. Derrfuss J, Brass M, von Cramon DY, Lohmann G, Amunts K (2009) Neural activations at the junction of the inferior frontal sulcus and the inferior precentral

sulcus: interindividual variability, reliability, and association with sulcal morphology. Hum Brain Mapp30: 299–311.

62. Schroeter ML, Vogt B, Frisch S, Becker G, Barthel H, et al. (2012) Executive deficits are related to the inferior frontal junction in early dementia. Brain 135: 201–215.

63. Folstein JR, Van Petten C (2008) Influence of cognitive control and mismatch on the N2 component of the ERP: a review. Psychophysiology 45: 152–170.

64. Ocklenburg S, Gunturkun O, Beste C (2011) Lateralized neural mechanisms underlying the modulation of response inhibition processes. Neuroimage 55: 1771–1778.

65. Bokura H, Yamaguchi S, Kobayashi S (2001) Electrophysiological correlates for response inhibition in a Go/NoGo task. Clin Neurophysiol 112: 2224–2232.

66. Pessoa L (2010) Emotion and attention effects: is it all a matter of timing? Not yet. Front Hum Neurosci 4.

67. Pessoa L, Adolphs R (2010) Emotion processing and the amygdala: from a 'low road' to 'many roads' of evaluating biological significance. Nat Rev Neurosci 11: 773–783.

68. Pessoa L, McKenna M, Gutierrez E, Ungerleider LG (2002) Neural processing of emotional faces requires attention. Proc Natl Acad Sci U S A 99: 11458–11463.

69. Cacioppo JT, Gardner WL (1999) Emotion. Annu Rev Psychol 50: 191–214.

70. Kobeleva X, Seidel EM, Kohler C, Schneider F, Habel U, et al. (2014) Dissociation of explicit and implicit measures of the behavioral inhibition and activation system in borderline personality disorder. Psychiatry Res 218: 134–142.

71. Kret ME, Denollet J, Grezes J, de Gelder B (2011) The role of negative affectivity and social inhibition in perceiving social threat: an fMRI study. Neuropsychologia 49: 1187–1193.

72. Gross JJ (2001) Emotion regulation in adulthhood: timing is everything. Current Directions in Psychological Science 10: 214–219.

73. Ochsner KN, Gross JJ (2005) The cognitive control of emotion. Trends Cogn Sci 9: 242–249.

74. Brassen S, Gamer M, Rose M, Buchel C (2010) The influence of directed covert attention on emotional face processing. Neuroimage 50: 545–551.

75. Rellecke J, Sommer W, Schacht A (2012) Does processing of emotional facial expressions depend on intention? Time-resolved evidence from event-related brain potentials. Biol Psychol 90: 23–32.

76. McRae K, Hughes B, Chopra S, Gabrieli JD, Gross JJ, et al. (2010) The neural bases of distraction and reappraisal. J Cogn Neurosci 22: 248–262.

77. Batty M, Taylor MJ (2003) Early processing of the six basic facial emotional expressions. Brain Res Cogn Brain Res 17: 613–620.

78. Krombholz A, Schaefer F, Boucsein W (2007) Modification of N170 by different emotional expression of schematic faces. Biol Psychol 76: 156–162.

79. Ahveninen J, Kahkonen S, Pennanen S, Liesivuori J, Ilmoniemi RJ, et al. (2002) Tryptophan depletion effects on EEG and MEG responses suggest serotonergic modulation of auditory involuntary attention in humans. Neuroimage 16: 1052–1061.

80. Kahkonen S, Ahveninen J, Pekkonen E, Kaakkola S, Huttunen J, et al. (2002) Dopamine modulates involuntary attention shifting and reorienting: an electromagnetic study. Clin Neurophysiol 113: 1894–1902.

81. Chikazoe J, Jimura K, Asari T, Yamashita K, Morimoto H, et al. (2009) Functional dissociation in right inferior frontal cortex during performance of go/no-go task. Cereb Cortex 19: 146–152.

82. Zanto TP, Rubens MT, Thangavel A, Gazzaley A (2011) Causal role of the prefrontal cortex in top-down modulation of visual processing and working memory. Nat Neurosci 14: 656–661.

83. Levy BJ, Wagner AD (2011) Cognitive control and right ventrolateral prefrontal cortex: reflexive reorienting, motor inhibition, and action updating. Ann N Y A-cad Sci 1224: 40–62.

84. Wager TD, Davidson ML, Hughes BL, Lindquist MA, Ochsner KN (2008) Prefrontal-subcortical pathways mediating successful emotion regulation. Neuron 59: 1037–1050.

85. Piguet C, Sterpenich V, Desseilles M, Cojan Y, Bertschy G, et al. (2013) Neural substrates of cognitive switching and inhibition in a face processing task. Neuroimage 82: 489–499.

86. Russell JA (1989) Affect Grid: A single-item scale of pleasure and arousal. Journal of personality and social psychology 57: 493–502.

87. Gerber AJ, Posner J, Gorman D, Colibazzi T, Yu S, et al. (2008) An affective circumplex model of neural systems subserving valence, arousal, and cognitive overlay during the appraisal of emotional faces. Neuropsychologia 46: 2129–2139.

6

Detection of Olfactory Dysfunction Using Olfactory Event Related Potentials in Young Patients with Multiple Sclerosis

Fabrizia Caminiti[1]*, **Simona De Salvo**[1], **Maria Cristina De Cola**[1], **Margherita Russo**[1], **Placido Bramanti**[1], **Silvia Marino**[1,2], **Rosella Ciurleo**[1]

1 IRCCS Centro Neurolesi "Bonino-Pulejo", Messina, Italy, 2 Department of Biomedical Sciences and Morphological and Functional Imaging, University of Messina, Messina, Italy

Abstract

Background: Several studies reported olfactory dysfunction in patients with multiple sclerosis. The estimate of the incidence of olfactory deficits in multiple sclerosis is uncertain; this may arise from different testing methods that may be influenced by patients' response bias and clinical, demographic and cognitive features.

Aims: To evaluate objectively the olfactory function using Olfactory Event Related Potentials.

Materials and Methods: We tested the olfactory function of 30 patients with relapsing remitting multiple sclerosis (mean age of 36.03 ± 6.96 years) and of 30 age, sex and smoking–habit matched healthy controls by using olfactory potentials. A selective and controlled stimulation of the olfactory system to elicit the olfactory event related potentials was achieved by a computer-controlled olfactometer linked directly with electroencephalograph. Relationships between olfactory potential results and patients' clinical characteristics, such as gender, disability status score, disease-modifying therapy, and disease duration, were evaluated.

Results: Seven of 30 patients did not show olfactory event related potentials. Sixteen of remaining 23 patients had a mean value of amplitude significantly lower than control group ($p < 0.01$). The presence/absence of olfactory event related potentials was associated with dichotomous expanded disability status scale ($p = 0.0433$), as well as inversely correlated with the disease duration ($r = -0.3641$, $p = 0.0479$).

Conclusion: Unbiased olfactory dysfunction of different severity found in multiple sclerosis patients suggests an organic impairment which could be related to neuroinflammatory and/or neurodegenerative processes of olfactory networks, supporting the recent findings on neurophysiopathology of disease.

Editor: Steven Jacobson, National Institutes of Health, United States of America

Funding: The authors have no support or funding to report.

Competing Interests: The authors have declared that no competing interests exist.

* Email: fabriziacaminiti@tiscali.it

Introduction

Olfactory dysfunction is often an early important manifestation of neurodegenerative diseases, such as Parkinson's disease [1–4], Alzheimer's disease [5–6], Huntington's disease [7], motor neuron disease [8], and its evaluation can be useful for diagnosis. The olfactory impairment in Multiple Sclerosis (MS) has also been reported [9–11], but to date, there are considerable disputes about. Moreover, it remains unclear whether olfactory loss occurs as an early symptom of MS. It has been suggested that some neurotropic viruses are involved in the development of neurodegenerative diseases. The olfactory loss in MS seems to be associated with the passage of human herpervirus-6 (HHV-6) into the central nervous system (CNS). Recently, HHV-6 has been detected in the olfactory bulbs and tracts and frequently in the nasal cavities of MS patients, supporting the hypothesis that this virus uses olfactory pathways as a route to enter into the CNS and then trigger the MS [12].

The incidence of olfactory dysfunction in MS is highly variable. Originally, it has been reported that the olfactory pathways (nerves and tracts) were spared in MS [13], with an estimation of incidence of olfactory changes by 1% [14]. Later, trials investigating the olfactory function in MS patients reported that these subjects had worse performances of 15% [15], 22% [16] and 38.5% [17] than healthy controls. This variability may arise from differences related to olfactory function testing methods and/or in study design, but it can also be related to corticosteroid treatment and to different MS subtypes. The smell function may improve during periods of disease remission and worsen during relapses. In addition, the olfactory dysfunction may also be an early indicator of disease progression in MS [18]. Several studies showed in MS patients a deterioration in the ability to detect odor threshold as well as in the ability to identify and discriminate the odors. Moreover, it has been suggested that the threshold detection is impaired in the early stage of disease, whereas the ability to identify and discriminate the odors is related to disability progression which is often associated with a cognitive impairment [11,19]. Other authors highlighted that olfactory dysfunction in MS is related to the number of active plaques in the frontal and temporal lobes [9,17,19,20], symptoms of anxiety and depression [9] and disability progression [7].

The studies evaluating the relationship between MS and the three olfactory abilities used psychophysical tests [11,17,19–23], such as the Sniffin' Sticks Test [24,25] and the University of Pennsylvania Smell Identification Test (UPSIT) [26]. However, the psychophysical tests of identification and discrimination require complex cognitive functions and high attention levels which could be compromised also in the early stage of MS [27,28].

Olfactory Event-Related Potentials (OERPs) are a valid electrophysiological technique for the study of olfactory system. This method allows to observe changes in olfactory function in an objective way. Indeed, it is independent from patients' response bias. OERP presence is a strong indicator of good olfactory function; conversely, the OERP absence suggests an olfactory loss.

OERPs are the result of sequential activation of different brain areas that begins from olfactory bulbs and tracts and involves the orbitofrontal and insular cortices, along with rostrum-medial regions of the temporal lobe [29]. The trasmission of olfactory sensory input travels from the olfactory neuroepithelium located into the nasal cavities towards the olfactory bulbs through the first cranial nerves, which here makes contact with the second order neurons (dendrites of mitral and tufted cells within glomeruli). From here, the postsynaptic fibers that form the olfactory tracts project to the primary olfactory areas, which comprise the anterior olfactory nucleus, tenia tecta, olfactory tubercole, piriform cortex, amygdale, anterior cortical amygdaloid nucleus, periamygdaloid and entorhinal cortices. The piriform cortex is connected to thalamus, hypothalamus and orbitofrontal cortex (OFC), and the entorhinal cortex is connected to hippocampus. The thalamus has connections towards secondary olfactory areas, as the OFC and insular cortex [30].

The OERPs consist of a large negative component, called N1, followed by a large positive component, called P2. Three scalp electrodes placed along the midline (Fz, Cz, and Pz) allow to identify the relative cortical fronto-centro-parietal regions activated by olfactory stimuli and then to detect the OERP topography. Indeed, N1 and P2 components have maximal amplitudes over the Cz and Pz positions [31]. Other components, P1 and N2, are often undetectable. The early OERP components (N1 and P1) reflect the exogenous cortical activity related to sensory input detection and primary sensory processing. On the other hand, the later OERP components, such as P2, reflect endogenous cortical activity related to secondary cognitive processing [32,33]. Latency and amplitude are the main parameters of OERP components. Latency of N1 and P2 components is a measure of the time required for sensory and cognitive processing of odor stimuli, respectively. Amplitude reflects the significance of the stimulus and its amount of information [33]. The latency of P2 has reached high reliability and is observed approximately from 530 to 800 ms after stimulus onset. The amplitude of N1-P2 is observed approximately between 4 and 20 μv [31].

Currently, few published studies used an objective method, such as OERPs, to evaluate the olfactory function in MS [22,23].

The purpose of our study is to evaluate the olfactory function in a group of Relapsing Remitting (RR) MS patients by using OERP technique, in order to verify objectively if the olfactory pathways are involved in neuroinflammatory and/or neurodegenerative impairment.

Materials and Methods

Study population

Thirty patients (19 females and 11 males) with diagnosis of RRMS according to the revised McDonald criteria [34] (mean age of 36.03±6.96 years and mean Expanded Disability Status Scale (EDSS) score of 2.08±1.07) and 30 age, sex and smoking–habit matched health controls, without neurological or psychiatric disorders, (18 females and 12 males; mean age of 35.83±8.74 years) were recruited from June to October 2013 at IRCCS Centro Neurolesi "Bonino-Pulejo" of Messina, (Italy). The disease duration ranged from 2 to 13 years with a mean duration of 5.87±3.29 years. A more detailed description of patients' and controls' characteristics is showed in Table 1.

A careful medical history was obtained from all participants in order to exclude diseases of nasal and paranasal cavities or other causes of smell impairment. An otorhinolaryngoiatric evaluation, by using upper airway rhinoscopy, assured the patency of nasal cavities and excluded anatomic abnormalities. We excluded the subjects treated with drugs that may affect olfactory function and/ or OERP recording such as antispasmodics, antidepressants, hypnotic-sedatives and steroids. For this reason, we excluded patients who have had MS relapses treated with steroids in 3 months prior to enrollment. Other exclusion criteria were pregnancy or lactation. Relationships between OERP results and patients' clinical characteristics, such as gender, disability status (EDSS score), disease-modifying therapy (DMT), and disease duration, were evaluated.

Olfactory evaluation

All subjects underwent an OERP examination to evaluate their olfactory function. A selective and controlled stimulation of the olfactory system to elicit the OERPs was achieved by a computer-controlled Olfactometer (Olfactometer OM2S - Burghart, Medical Instruments), linked directly with an electroencephalograph (Micromed Brain Quick 32 Ch) [35]. Olfactometer is a complex instrument which generates olfactory stimuli of rapid onset and precisely controlled in terms of time, duration and intensity, without inducing the simultaneous activation of different sensory systems (tactile, termica). During the recording two odorants were presented: phenyl ethyl alcohol (PEA, 40% v/v; Labochem Science S.r.l., Italy) and H_2S/N_2 (4 ppm; Rivoira, Italy). These odorants, used in appropriate concentrations, do not give any problems of toxicity and trigeminal activation. The use of the Olfactometer allows the elicitation of OERP components more easily than other methods, because the odorants do not mix and their concentration remains constant. The flow of air (8 l/min) that carries the odorants had constant temperature (36.5°C) and humidity (80%) to inhibit irritation of the nasal mucosa. The subjects did not present problems or side effects.

Subjects were asked to breath normally through their mouth. A constant level of vigilance were maintained by asking subjects to avoid eyes blinking. The teflon outlet nose (4 mm lumen tube) piece was placed in the nasal vestibulum. Stimulation was presented while subjects were lying down in a well-ventilated room. A succession of 40 randomized olfactory stimuli was presented in two blocks of 20 stimuli, alternating right and left nostril. The duration of each stimulus was 200 ms and time between stimuli (interstimulus interval, ISI) was 40 s. The change of nostril was made during ISI between twentieth and twenty-first stimulus, without interruption of the electroencephalographic

Table 1. Description of patients' and normal control subjects' characteristics.

	MS patients			Normal controls		
	Females	Males	All	Females	Males	All
Participants	19 (63.33%)	11 (36.67%)	30 (100%)	18 (60%)	12 (40%)	30 (100%)
Age (mean ± SD)	35.21±8.20	37.45±4.04	36.03±6.96	33.55±9.39	39.25±6.62	35.83±8.74
EDSS (mean±SD)	2.13±1.21	2.00±0.84	2.08±1.07			
DD (mean±SD)	5.31±3.04	6.82±3.63	5.87±3.29			
DMT						
None	5 (16.67%)	4 (13.33%	9 (30%)			
Copaxone	1 (3.33%)	2 (6.67%)	3 (10%)			
Avonex	3 (10%)	1 (3.33%)	4 (13.33%)			
Rebif 22	2 (6.67%)	0 (0%)	2 (6.67%)			
Rebif 44	2 (6.67%	2(6.67%)	4 (13.34%)			
Gylenia	1 (3.33%)	0 (0%)	1 (3.33%)			
Tysabri	3 (10%)	1 (3.33%)	4 (13.33%)			
Extavia	2 (6.67%)	1 (3.33%)	3 (10%)			
N1 (Cz) presences	16 (53.33%)	7 (23.33%)	23 (76.66%)	18 (60%)	12 (40%)	30 (100%)
Latencies (mean ± SD)	632.69±13.03	648.14±38.12	637.39±23.77	630.39±18.96	641.33±19.42	634.7±19.59
P2 (Cz)presences	16 (53.33%)	7 (23.33%)	23 (76.66%)	18 (60%)	12 (40%)	30 (100%)
Latencies (mean ± SD)	720.44±16.80	743.00±11.59	727.30±18.49	711.67±20.91	728.58±20.17	718.43±21.95
Amplitudes (mean ± SD)	4.50±1.99	3.64±1.03	4.24±1.77	7.28±1.82	6.57±1.77	6.99±1.81

DD = Disease Duration; DMT = Disease Modifying Therapy; SD = Standard Deviation; EDSS = Expanded Disability Status Scale.
Latency values are in ms. Amplitude values are in μV.

(EEG) recording. EEG was recorded from three scalp electrodes placed along the midline (Fz, Cz, and Pz positions of the 10–20 International System). The references electrode was placed on the earlobe (A2) and the ground on the forehead [31]. Eye movements and blinks (electro-oculogram) were monitored by an electrode above the right eyebrow. Other muscle artifacts were monitored and discarded. The data were filtered with a band-pass 0.01–30 Hz and a notch filter was used. The EEG activity was averaged from 500 ms in the pre-stimulus period until 2000 ms in the post-stimulus period. The OERPs were obtained by averaging of artifact-free EEG epochs. The latencies were measured to the first negative peak (N1) and to the second positive peak (P2). Amplitude was measured from the peak of N1 to that of P2. OERPs were considered absent when it has not been possible to identify clear responses from background noise in an artifact free recording. The subjects who showed N1 and P2 wave presence, with normal latency and amplitude, have been considered normosmic. Conversely, the absence of N1 and P2 waves indicated a severe olfactory dysfunction. Finally, N1 and P2 wave presence with an alteration in latency and/or amplitude has been considered as a condition of slight alteration of smell (borderline).

Statistical analysis

Statistical analysis was performed by using the 2.15.3 version of the open-source software R.

Wilcoxon rank sum test, independent Student's t-test, and X^2 test were used to compare patient and control groups where appropriate.

In order to assess the statistical relationship between presence/absence of OERPs and disability degree, the EDSS score was first converted into a dichotomous variable according to its mean value. Then, the Fisher's exact test on the contingence table was applied.

The Kruskall-Wallis test was performed to compare the different therapeutic treatments, considering three categories: none therapy, first-line drug administered (i.e. Copaxone, Avonex, Rebif 22, Rebif 44, Extavia), second-line drug administered (i.e. Tysabri, Gylenia). Linear correlations between variables were computed by Pearson's coefficient, or the point-biserial correlation coefficient when one variable was dichotomous. For all statistical tests, a $p < 0.05$ was considered as significance level.

Ethical considerations

The study was conducted in accordance with the Declaration of Helsinki and was approved by Ethic Committee of IRCCS Centro Neurolesi "Bonino-Pulejo"; all subjects gave written informed consent before any study-related procedures were performed.

Results

Table 1 summarizes the demographic and clinical characteristics of patients and controls, and the main parameters of OERP components.

All control subjects had amplitude values in the normal range [31]. Seven of 30 MS patients (3 women and 4 men) did not show OERP presence (Figure 1c). The mean age of such subgroup was slightly higher (37.71±4.96 years) than in the remaining 23 patients (35.52±7.49 years), but in a no statistically significant way (p = 0.6229). The comparisons of OERP parameters between the remaining 23 patients and the control group showed no significant differences in terms of latency of N1 and P2 components. On the contrary, very significant differences for amplitude values in each canal were observed (Fz: p<0.0001; Cz: p<0.0001; Fz: p<0.001)

(Figure 2). The highest difference was observed for Fz, for which it would seem that MS women suffered of a slightly more significant reduction of N1-P2 amplitude than men ($p<0.001$ and $p<0.01$, respectively) who, instead, presented a higher difference of Pz ($p = 0.0044$) than women ($p = 0.0159$). In the light of MS group response reduction only in amplitude parameter, we also compared the mean amplitudes (computed on Fz, Cz and Pz for any subject) between two groups by considering a reference value of 3.67 μV, which was the minimum value obtained from control subjects (Table 2). Sixteen of 23 of MS patients (subjects who showed the OERP presence) had a mean value of amplitude lower than control group. (Figure 1a and 1d). In fact, we observed a very significant difference ($p<0.01$) by comparing mean amplitudes of MS patients with controls. The remaining 7 MS patients showed normal OERP amplitude (Figure 1b).

No significant difference in amplitude and latency values of OERP components between the 23 MS patients and the 30 controls depending on gender was found ($X^2 = 0.18$, $p = 0.67$). A positive correlation between gender and P2 latencies in MS group ($r = 0.5742$, $p<0.01$) was found. Comparing OERPs of MS patients with gender, we observed a significant reduction of P2 latencies on Cz ($p<0.01$) and Pz ($p = 0.0223$) positions in the MS female group. In addition, an association between EDSS and presence/absence of OERPs was noted ($p = 0.0433$). From these results it is emerged a negative correlation between the presence/absence of OERPs and the disease duration ($r = -0.36409$, $p = 0.04793$): a longer disease duration was related to a higher probability of recording OERP absence. We did not observe significant differences in OERPs of MS patients when compared to DMTs.

Discussion

This study evaluated the olfactory function by using OERPs in a group of RRMS patients. Unbiased olfactory dysfunction of different severity was found. In particular, a strong impairment of olfactory function was found in 7 of 30 MS patients (23%), which no showed OERPs (Figure 1c), while 23 MS patients showed OERP responses. Of these latter, 16 (69.56%) had a marked reduction in N1-P2 amplitude, but normal latency (borderline

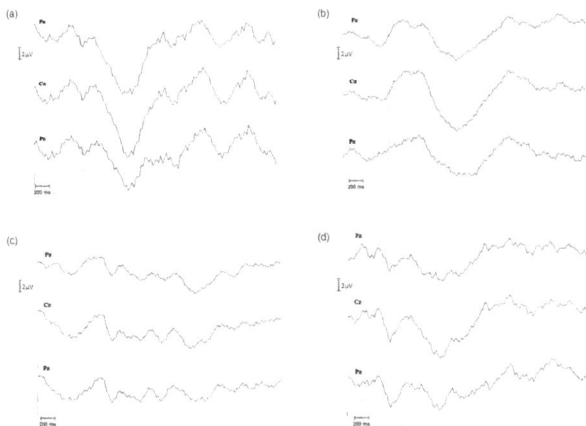

Figure 1. Averaged OERP traces. Filter band-pass 0.01–30 Hz. EEG averaging from 500 ms pre-stimulus to 2000 ms post-stimulus. (a) OERPs of healthy control subject; (b) OERPs of MS patient with normal latency and amplitude; (c) OERPs of MS patient without olfactory responses; (d) OERPs of MS patient with reduced N1-P2 amplitude and normal latency.

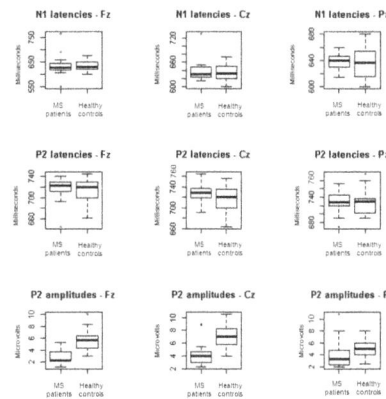

Figure 2. Box-plots comparing the parameters of OERP components of MS patients and healthy controls on Fz, Cz, Pz electrodes. Box-plots represent the distribution of latency and amplitude of N1 and P2 components for both MS patients and controls in Fz, Cz, Pz canals. Significant differences emerged only in P2 amplitude values, which were lower in MS patients than in controls (Fz: $p<0.0001$; Cz: $p<0.0001$; Pz: $p<0.001$).

olfactory function) (Figure 1d), and the remaining 7 patients had normal latency and amplitude of N1 and P2 components (Figure 1b).

Hawkes et al. [22] reported a OERP study where the 25% of 45 MS patients showed an impaired smell function. In particular, a statistically significant increase of N1 and P2 latency and decrease of amplitude for MS patients were found. In our study, 16 MS patients with borderline smell function reported only a significant reduction of amplitude, but not an increase of latency. These different results could be due to clinical heterogeneity of patients and to experimental conditions in which the studies have been performed. Dahlslett et al. [23] reported a study performed on 21 MS patients where the 23.8% showed hyposmia. In this study, the hyposmia or normosmia condition was based on the detection of olfactory potentials in one side or both, respectively. In our study, hyposmia diagnosis required an alteration in both latency and amplitude of main OERP components, independently from the stimulated side. A trend towards reduced P2 latency in MS female group found in our study confirms how reported from literature in healthy subjects. Indeed, several studies reported that OERPs elicited in women subjects are of shorter latency and greater amplitude than in men, suggesting an hormonal modulation of the sense of smell and sex-related differences in high levels of neural processing of odors [31,33,36]. In 7 patients the absence of OERPs was associated with higher EDSS scores and longer disease duration than the other 23 patients. This result corroborates how is emerged from previous studies, in which the olfactory dysfunction correlated positively with disability level [8,9,23].

The neuro-inflammatory processes in MS involve either the cerebral white matter, causing demyelination, and the grey matter, leading to axonal damage. In addition to the inflammation, the widespread neuronal degeneration is currently considered a central component of MS pathology [37]. Whether neurodegeneration occurs as a consequence of the inflammatory attack (secondary neurodegeneration) or as a distinct phenomenon (primary neurodegeneration) is a matter of controversy. Components of the immune/inflammatory response, such as lymphocytes, pro-inflammatory cytokines and activated macrophages, are found in close proximity to degenerating neurons, suggesting that

Table 2. Mean OERP values computed on Fz, Cz, Pz for each MS patient and normal control.

MS patients			Normal controls		
N1 latency (mean of Fz.Cz.Pz)	P2 latency (mean of Fz.Cz.Pz)	P2 amplitude (mean of Fz.Cz.Pz)	N1 latency (mean of Fz.Cz.Pz)	P2 latency (mean of Fz.Cz.Pz)	P2 amplitude (mean of Fz.Cz.Pz)
617.67	719.33	1.98	608.67	705.33	8.07
655.67	716.00	3.20	622.67	720.67	6.63
603.33	699.00	4.65	631.33	672.00	5.33
626.00	684.67	3.83	619.00	694.67	4.80
651.67	723.33	8.37	665.67	746.33	4.87
644.00	734.33	3.00	645.67	718.67	4.93
626.67	725.00	2.17	646.33	690.33	5.27
629.00	711.00	4.53	647.67	744.67	6.90
628.00	708.67	3.57	663.00	751.33	6.33
622.50	710.00	2.15	641.67	709.33	4.43
642.33	720.00	3.63	644.33	750.00	6.27
626.67	740.67	2.77	667.33	733.33	6.67
646.67	726.33	4.00	655.00	740.67	7.07
641.00	737.00	2.00	620.00	723.33	7.40
627.33	740.00	3.03	644.33	728.00	4.83
685.33	727.33	2.37	664.67	723.00	6.70
670.33	729.33	2.50	637.67	700.00	6.53
613.00	734.67	3.57	667.33	762.67	3.67
641.67	730.33	5.17	630.67	698.33	6.27
621.33	720.67	7.30	636.67	691.67	5.90
643.33	745.00	2.97	627.00	700.00	8.60
625.33	731.67	3.10	618.33	705.00	4.33
656.33	752.67	3.33	610.00	731.67	4.33
-	-	-	613.33	690.00	4.83
-	-	-	604.67	730.00	5.90
-	-	-	616.67	730.00	5.27
-	-	-	606.67	713.33	9.33
-	-	-	615.00	721.67	4.43
-	-	-	653.33	738.67	6.07
-	-	-	630.00	728.33	6.33

Latency values are in ms. Amplitude values are in μV. Minimum and maximum values are underlined.

neurodegeneration is secondary to the inflammation and that it may be considered as an underlying cause for permanent and progressive disability in MS [37,38]. On the other hand, there is evidence that axonal transection and neuronal damage occur early supporting a primary neurodegenerative course [39]. Immune-mediated inflammation may affect the olfactory pathways. In fact, MS plaques have been found in the olfactory tracts and bulbs of MS patients [40]. Moreover, it is likely that, similar to the initial frequent involvement of the optic nerve in MS, neurodegeneration may occur in the myelin-free olfactory nerves in the early stages of disease. Several studies reported that in MS there is a relationship between smell loss and lesion load in the inferior frontal- and temporal-lobe regions, the areas involved in processing of olfactory stimuli [9,17,20,21].

Our findings showed a clear correlation of olfactory dysfunction with disability degree and disease duration. This suggests that the abnormal olfactory function found in 7 MS patients could be associated with an inflammatory lesion load and also with a neurodegenerative process of olfactory networks. Conversely, the borderline olfactory function found in 16 MS patients could be associated only with a primary neurodegenerative course not yet engaging demyelination of olfactory networks. Indeed, an inflammatory demyelination of the olfactory pathways would lead to reduced conduction and inhibition in the transmission of electrophysiological impulses, and thus to a delay in latency, which has not been found in our study.

It could be postulated that the heterogeneity of olfactory dysfunction found in our patients is due to different demyelination/neurodegeneration severity in different olfactory structures. Indeed, the 7 MS patients, who did not show OERPs, could have a severe impairment of central olfactory pathways (bulbs and traits) and cortical areas. On the other hand, 16 MS patients with borderline olfactory function could have a slight impairment of olfactory central networks and/or of peripheral structures (cranial nerves I). These results could be confirmed by future MRI study, in order to analyze lesion load, plaque distribution and axonal damage in olfactory structures of MS patients in relation to degree of olfactory deficit and disability.

The MS patients present different symptoms related to different temporal-spatial distribution of the lesions. However, some symptoms are more frequent than others, such as motor impairment, dizziness, visual deficits, and urinary disorder, and some of these are more disabling and with a higher impact on quality of life than a possible impairment of smell. In fact, smell reduction is a symptom frequently ignored by patients and the enrolled subjects did not report olfactory problems. The lack of awareness of olfactory deficit in MS patients could lead to an underestimation of this disorder, which instead may be indicative of subclinical neurodegenerative process.

The close relationship between MS and olfactory dysfunction has been confirmed by several studies performed by using psychophysical tests. However, these results must be refined from all the variables that can affect the subjective tests such as the cultural factors of examined subjects, the clinical findings, mood and cognitive functions. Despite the great difficulty of OERP elicitation, which hinders their frequent use in clinical practice, in recent years this electrophysiological technique showed an important development, especially in the diagnosis of neurode-generative diseases. In addition, to date, it reached high reliability and represents an objective method for discriminating the reduced olfactory perception.

According to our findings, we believe that the olfactory examination may be an objective marker of neuroinflammatory or neurodegenerative process in MS. However, given the rather small sample of MS patients we considered, the results must be interpreted with caution. To achieve a confirmation of results the study should be extended to a large population. Since longitudinal studies have not been still performed, they could give new information about the changes of subjects' OERPs over time and could help to monitor the possible associations among smell impairment and disease progression.

Author Contributions

Analyzed the data: FC SDS MCDC. Wrote the paper: FC SM RC. Design of study and experiments: FC SM RC. Execution of experiments: FC SDS RC. Enrollment of subjects: MR. Critical revision of the manuscript: PB.

References

1. Doty RL (2012) Olfaction in Parkinson's disease and related disorders. Neurobiol Dis 46: 527–552.
2. Haehner A, Hummel T, Reichmann H (2009) Olfactory dysfunction as a diagnostic marker for Parkinson's disease. Expert Rev Neurother 9: 1773–1779.
3. Wattendorf E, Welge-Lüssen A, Fiedler K, Bilecen D, Wolfensberger M, et al. (2009) Olfactory impairment predicts brain atrophy in Parkinson's disease. J Neurosci 29: 15410–15413.
4. Singh S, Schwankhaus J (2009) Olfactory disturbance in Parkinson disease. Arch Neurol 66: 805–806.
5. Kjelvik G, Sando SB, Aasly J, Engedal KA, White LR (2007) Use of the Brief Smell Identification Test for olfactory deficit in a Norwegian population with Alzheimer's disease. Int J Geriatr Psychiatry 22: 1020–1024.
6. Bahar-Fuchs A, Moss S, Rowe C, Savage G (2011) Awareness of olfactory deficits in healthy aging, amnestic mild cognitive impairment and Alzheimer's disease. Int Psychogeriatr 23: 1097–1106.
7. Moberg PJ, Pearlson GD, Speedie LJ, Lipsey JR, Strauss ME, et al. (1987) Olfactory recognition: differential impairments in early and late Huntington's and Alzheimer's diseases. J Clin Exp Neuropsychol 9: 650–664.
8. Hawkes CH, Shephard BC (1998) Olfactory evoked responses and identification tests in neurological disease. Ann N Y Acad Sci 855: 608–615.
9. Zorzon M, Ukmar M, Bragadin LM, Zanier F, Antonello RM, et al. (2000) Olfactory dysfunction and extent of white matter abnormalities in multiple sclerosis: a clinical and MR study. Mult Scler 6: 386–390.
10. Fleiner F, Dahlslett SB, Schmidt F, Harms L, Goektas O (2010) Olfactory and gustatory function in patients with multiple sclerosis. Am J Rhinol Allergy 24: e93–97.
11. Lutterotti A, Vedovello M, Reindl M, Ehling R, DiPauli F, et al. (2011) Olfactory threshold is impaired in early, active multiple sclerosis. Mult Scler 17: 964–969.
12. Harberts E, Yao K, Wohler JE, Maric D, Ohayon J, et al. (2011) Human herpesvirus-6 entry into the central nervous system through the olfactory pathway. Proc Natl Acad Sci U S A 108: 13734–13739.
13. Lumsden CE (1983) The neuropathology of multiple sclerosis. In: Vinken PJ, Bruyn GW, eds. Handbook of clinical neurology. New York: Elsevier 9: 217.
14. Heberhold C (1975) Evaluating function and disorders of smell. Arch Otorhinolarynngol 210: 67–164.
15. Hawkes CH, Shephard BC (1998) Olfactory evoked responses and identification tests in neurological disease. Ann N Y Acad Sci 855: 608–615.
16. Zivadinov R, Zorzon M, Monti Bragadin L, Pagliaro G, Cazzato G (1999) Olfactory loss in multiple sclerosis. J Neurol Sci 168:127–30.
17. Doty RL, Li C, Mannon LJ, Yousem DM (1998) Olfactory dysfunction in multiple sclerosis. Relation to plaque load in inferior frontal and temporal lobes. Ann N Y Acad Sci 855: 781–786.
18. Silva AM, Santos E, Moreira I, Bettencourt A, Coutinho E, et al. (2012) Olfactory dysfunction in multiple sclerosis: association with secondary progression. Mult Scler 18: 616–621.
19. Rolet A, Magnin E, Millot JL, Berger E, Vidal C, et al. (2013) Olfactory dysfunction in multiple sclerosis: evidence of a decrease in different aspects of olfactory function. Eur Neurol 69: 166–170.
20. Doty RL, Li C, Mannon LJ, Yousem DM (1999) Olfactory dysfunction in multiple sclerosis: relation to longitudinal changes in plaque numbers in central olfactory structures. Neurology 53: 880–882.
21. Doty RL, Li C, Mannon LJ, Yousem DM (1997) Olfactory dysfunction in multiple sclerosis. N Engl J Med 336: 1918–1919.
22. Hawkes CH, Shephard BC, Kobal G (1997) Assessment of olfaction in multiple sclerosis: evidence of dysfunction by olfactory evoked response and identification tests. J Neurol Neurosurg Psychiatry 63: 145–151.
23. Dahlslett SB, Goektas O, Schmidt F, Harms L, Olze H, et al. (2012) Psychophysiological and electrophysiological testing of olfactory and gustatory function in patients with multiple sclerosis. Eur Arch Otorhinolaryngol 269: 1163–1169.
24. Kobal G, Klimek L, Wolfensberger M, Gudziol H, Temmel A, et al. (2000) Multicenter investigation of 1.036 subjects using a standardized method for the assessment of olfactory function combining tests of odor identification, odor discrimination, and olfactory thresholds. Eur Arch Otorhinolaryngol 257: 205–211.
25. Hummel T, Kobal G, Gudziol H, Mackay-Sim A (2007) Normative data for the "Sniffin'Sticks" including tests of odor identification, odor discrimination, and olfactory thresholds: an upgrade based on a group of more than 3.000 subjects. Eur Arch Otorhinolaryngol 264: 237–243.
26. Doty RL, Shaman P, Kimmelmann CP, Dann MS (1984) University of Pennsylvania Smell identification test: a rapid quantitative olfactory function test for the clinic. Laryngoscope 94: 176–178.
27. Amato MP, Razzolini L, Goretti B, Stromillo ML, Rossi F, et al. (2013) Cognitive reserve and cortical atrophy in multiple sclerosis: a longitudinal study. Neurology 80: 1728–1733.
28. Amato MP, Goretti B, Ghezzi A, Lori S, Zipoli V, et al. (2010) Cognitive and psychosocial features in childhood and juvenile MS: two-year follow-up. Neurology 75: 1134–1140.
29. Barresi M, Ciurleo R, Giacoppo S, Foti Cuzzola V, Celi D, et al. (2012) Evaluation of olfactory dysfunction in neurodegenerative diseases. J Neurol Sci 323 16–24.
30. Giessel AJ, Datta SR (2014) Olfactory maps, circuits and computations. Curr Opin Neurobiol 24: 120–132.
31. Rombaux P, Mouraux A, Bertrand B, Guerit JM, Hummel T (2006) Assessment of olfactory and trigeminal function using chemosensory event-related potentials. Clin Neurophysiol 36: 53–62.
32. Pause BM, Sojka B, Krauel K, Ferstl R (1996) The nature of the late positive complex within the olfactory event-related potential (OERP). Psychophysiology. 33: 376–384.
33. Olofsson JK, Nordin S (2004) Gender differences in chemosensory perception and event-related potentials. Chem senses. 29: 629–37.
34. Polman CH, Reingold SC, Banwell B, Clanet M, Cohen JA (2011) Diagnostic criteria for multiple sclerosis: 2010 revisions to the McDonald criteria. Ann Neurol 69: 292–302.
35. Olfaktologie und Gustologie of the German Society for Ear, Nose and Throat Medicine, Head and Neck Surgery (http://www.hno.org/olfaktologie).
36. Stuck BA, Frey S, Freiburg C, Hörmann K, Zahnert T, et al. (2006) Chemosensory event-related potentials in relation to side of stimulation, age, sex, and stimulus concentration. Clin Neurophysiol 117: 1367–1375.

37. Trapp BD, Stys K (2009) Virtual hypoxia and chronic necrosis of demyelinated axons in multiple sclerosis. Lancet Neurol; 8: 280–291.

38. Trapp BD, Peterson J, Ransohoff RM, Rudick R, Mörk S, et al. (1998) Axonal transection in the lesions of multiple sclerosis. N Engl J Med 338: 278–85.

39. Racke MK (2009) Immunopathogenesis of multiple sclerosis. Ann Indian Acad Neurol; 12: 215–20.

40. McDonald WI (1986) The mystery of the origin of multiple sclerosis. J Neurol Neurosurg Psychiatry 49: 113–123.

7

Mismatch Negativity (MMN) in Freely-Moving Rats with Several Experimental Controls

Lauren Harms[1,2,3,4]*, **W. Ross Fulham**[2,3,4,5], **Juanita Todd**[1,2,3,4], **Timothy W. Budd**[1,2,3,4], **Michael Hunter**[1,2,4], **Crystal Meehan**[1,2,3], **Markku Penttonen**[6], **Ulrich Schall**[2,3,4,5], **Katerina Zavitsanou**[7,8], **Deborah M. Hodgson**[1,2,3,4], **Patricia T. Michie**[1,2,3,4]

1 School of Psychology, University of Newcastle, Callaghan, NSW, Australia, 2 Priority Centre for Translational Neuroscience and Mental Health Research, University of Newcastle, Newcastle, NSW, Australia, 3 Schizophrenia Research Institute, Darlinghurst, NSW, Australia, 4 Hunter Medical Research Institute, Newcastle, NSW, Australia, 5 School of Medicine and Public Health, University of Newcastle, Callaghan, NSW, Australia, 6 Department of Psychology, University of Jyvaskyla, Jyvaskyla, Finland, 7 School of Psychiatry, Faculty of Medicine, University of New South Wales, Sydney, NSW, Australia, 8 Neuroscience Research Australia, Randwick, NSW, Australia

Abstract

Mismatch negativity (MMN) is a scalp-recorded electrical potential that occurs in humans in response to an auditory stimulus that defies previously established patterns of regularity. MMN amplitude is reduced in people with schizophrenia. In this study, we aimed to develop a robust and replicable rat model of MMN, as a platform for a more thorough understanding of the neurobiology underlying MMN. One of the major concerns for animal models of MMN is whether the rodent brain is capable of producing a human-like MMN, which is not a consequence of neural adaptation to repetitive stimuli. We therefore tested several methods that have been used to control for adaptation and differential exogenous responses to stimuli within the oddball paradigm. Epidural electroencephalographic electrodes were surgically implanted over different cortical locations in adult rats. Encephalographic data were recorded using wireless telemetry while the freely-moving rats were presented with auditory oddball stimuli to assess mismatch responses. Three control sequences were utilized: the *flip-flop* control was used to control for differential responses to the physical characteristics of standards and deviants; the *many standards* control was used to control for differential adaptation, as was the *cascade* control. Both adaptation and adaptation-independent deviance detection were observed for high frequency (pitch), but not low frequency deviants. In addition, the *many standards* control method was found to be the optimal method for observing both adaptation effects and adaptation-independent mismatch responses in rats. Inconclusive results arose from the *cascade* control design as it is not yet clear whether rats can encode the complex pattern present in the control sequence. These data contribute to a growing body of evidence supporting the hypothesis that rat brain is indeed capable of exhibiting human-like MMN, and that the rat model is a viable platform for the further investigation of the MMN and its associated neurobiology.

Editor: Manuel S. Malmierca, University of Salamanca- Institute for Neuroscience of Castille and Leon and Medical School, Spain

Funding: This project was funded by a National Health and Medical Research Council of Australia Project Grant, ID 1026070. The contents of this article are solely the responsibility of the authors and do not reflect the views of the NHMRC (http://nhmrc.gov.au). Support was received from the University of Newcastle Near Miss grant, CAPEX funding and travel fellowship schemes (http://www.newcastle.edu.au). Further support was provided by the Hunter Medical Research Institute (http://www.hmri.com.au) and the Schizophrenia Research Institute (http://www.schizophreniaresearch.org.au), which are supported by infrastructure funding from NSW Health. The funders had no role in study design, data collection and analysis, decision to publish, or preparation of the manuscript.

Competing Interests: The authors have declared that no competing interests exist.

* Email: lauren.harms@newcastle.edu.au

Introduction

One of the most commonly reported and replicable electrophysiological abnormalities observed in people with schizophrenia is the reduction in the amplitude of the mismatch negativity (MMN) in response to deviations in the acoustic environment [1–3]. In adult humans, MMN is evident as a negative shift in the auditory event-related potential (ERP) elicited by a rare, unexpected stimulus (the *deviant*) when it interrupts a train of common, expected stimuli (the *standards*), and typically occurs 100–200 ms after stimulus onset [4,5]. A meta-analysis reported that persons with schizophrenia exhibit reductions in the size of the MMN with an overall effect size of 0.99 [3]. MMN responses can be observed in different states of consciousness and in the absence of attention to the stimuli, leading to its characterisation as an automatic, pre-attentive process [4]. MMN is primarily generated in the auditory cortex, with some contribution from the frontal cortex and other areas [6,7]. It has been observed in neural activity measured using electroencephalography (EEG) [8], magnetoencephalography [9] and optical imaging [10]. MMN is typically measured using *oddball* sequences of auditory stimuli, in which a repeated train of standards is unexpectedly interrupted by a low-probability deviant. MMN is commonly elicited by presenting deviants that differ from the standards in some simple characteristic feature, such as frequency or duration [8].

In recent years, the MMN research community has begun to focus on developing animal models of MMN, in order to investigate the neurobiological mechanisms underlying the MMN, such as the role of specific neurotransmitter systems, contributions from different cortical layers or brain regions to the surface potential, and relationship to upstream effects that appear to be related to MMN such as stimulus specific adaptation (SSA) [11,12]. Several models in rats, mice and non-human primates have been studied with varied results (for detailed review, [2]). There are two important factors that need to be examined and controlled when identifying an animal homologue of the human MMN: first is the possibility of differential responses to the physical characteristics of the stimuli used as the standards and deviants. This is addressed in *flip-flop* sequences, where two oddball sequences are presented with the identity of the standard and deviant reversed (e.g. a particular tone is the deviant in one sequence and the standard in the other). This permits the response to a stimulus when it is a deviant to be compared to the same stimulus when it is a standard (Figure 1A). The second factor is the role of *adaptation* versus *'true' deviance detection*, which, within some theoretical frameworks, is considered to be a memory-based or a predictive coding error signal [13–15]. Several studies in both humans and animals have shown that with repeated exposure to a stimulus, the neural populations responding to that stimulus undergo *adaptation*, in which their responses are dampened with higher probabilities of stimulation [12,16–23]. This means that a larger response to a deviant stimulus may simply be due to lower levels of adaptation of neural populations responding to a rare stimulus (the deviant) compared to a frequent stimulus (the standard). Note that while the term *adaptation* is used here, other terms are often used to describe similar, but not exactly synonymous phenomena (the reduction of a response to a stimulus with repeated exposure), such as habituation, refractoriness, and stimulus-specific adaptation. This is addressed in several studies by using a *many-standards control* sequence (Figure 1B). In this sequence, the deviant tone from the oddball sequence is presented with the same probability as it is presented within the oddball sequence, but it is nested within many other equally-probable tones. The tones are presented pseudo-randomly (without repetition) so that no pattern of regularity is established. This lack of regularity ensures that no specific 'prediction' is set that can be violated. Comparing the response to the same physical stimulus when it is a deviant within the oddball sequence, to when it is the control stimulus within the many standards sequence, provides a measure of the adaptation-independent comparison process contribution that is thought to underlie MMN.

Using these approaches, MMN in humans has been found to comprise two 'elements' after controlling for the physical characteristics of the stimulus using the flip-flop control method: an adaptation element ('sensorial' element, represented by the difference between the rare control stimulus and the common standard stimulus), and a prediction error-like element ('cognitive' element, represented by the difference between the rare control stimulus and the rare deviant stimulus) [19,20,24–26]. While this feature of MMN has several designations: memory-based MMN [27,28], prediction error [29], cognitive (versus sensory) MMN [19,20], and deviance detection [21,30–32] to name a few, for the purposes of clarity in the remainder of the paper, *adaptation-independence* and/or *deviance detection* will be used to describe the element of MMN that remains when adaptation is controlled for.

While the two elements comprising MMN (adaptation and adaptation-independent deviance detection) are not commonly disentangled in human studies (for exceptions, [19,20]), it is important for animal models to test for both. This is because a) it is unknown whether a given species is capable of generating an adaptation-independent response as humans do, and b) these two elements likely have diverging neural mechanisms and signatures. If the aim of establishing an animal model of MMN is to investigate the underlying neural mechanisms of MMN, then the MMN elements being investigated should be identified.

The many standards control sequence, as mentioned, controls for the effects of stimulus presentation probability so that differential adaptation can be observed in the absence of the established models of regularities. However, this control has been subject to two criticisms [33]. First, it may be overly conservative, because the variety (usually frequency range) of stimuli presented in the many standards sequence is substantially larger than that in the oddball paradigm. It has been demonstrated using local field potential and multiunit activity recordings that many standards sequences using a broad range of frequencies produce larger responses than those from narrow sequences, regardless of presentation rate [21]. This would indicate that potentially, the control response in the many standards sequence is not affected as much by adaptation and therefore is increased in amplitude. However, the deviant response from the oddball sequence (containing a narrow range of stimuli) would presumably undergo *more* adaptation than the control response, and consequently be reduced in size. This possible imbalance in the amount of adaption undergone by the control and deviant responses could result in an underestimation of the difference between the control and deviant responses (deviance detection). Second, in the oddball paradigm, deviants are presented within a repetitive, predictable sequence, but no such repetition is established within the many standards control sequence. To avoid these issues, a cascade control sequence has been proposed [33]. In this method, firstly, there are a small number, nominally five, stimuli that vary from low to high frequency, with the highest frequency stimulus corresponding to the deviant, and the second highest frequency stimulus corresponding to the standard within an ascending oddball sequence (Figure 1C,D). Secondly, the stimuli are presented in a regular pattern from low to high frequency, then back down to low frequency, repetitively (Figure 1D). The high-frequency stimulus at the upper extreme of the stimulus range is used as a control for high-frequency deviants in the ascending oddball task. An equivalent sequence can be adapted for low-frequency deviants in a descending oddball sequence. Within the cascade sequence, the variety of stimuli presented is more comparable to that in the oddball task, and the control stimulus is always preceded by a stimulus that is physically identical to the standard within the oddball task. This can improve the estimation of adaptation effects. In addition, the cascade control incorporates a background regularity, albeit a more complex one than oddball sequences, but where the occurrence of the high (and low) frequency tones at the extremes of the cascade sequence are predictable, in contrast to the equivalent high (and low) frequencies of oddball sequences. Therefore, the cascade control provides the opportunity to observe adaptation-independent deviance detection in the context of unpredictable deviants vs. predictable deviants, assuming of course that the rat brain is able to model the regularity of the cascade sequence.

In a recent review of animal models of MMN [2], several important trends were identified. First, mismatch responses (MMR) in animals typically occur earlier than in humans, likely due to the smaller brain size. Second, the difference between the deviant and the standard can be either negative or positive in polarity (positive shifts are far more common in recordings in anaesthetised animals, particularly when anaesthetised with

A) Oddball Sequences – Flip-Flop Design
Used in: Study 1, Study 2

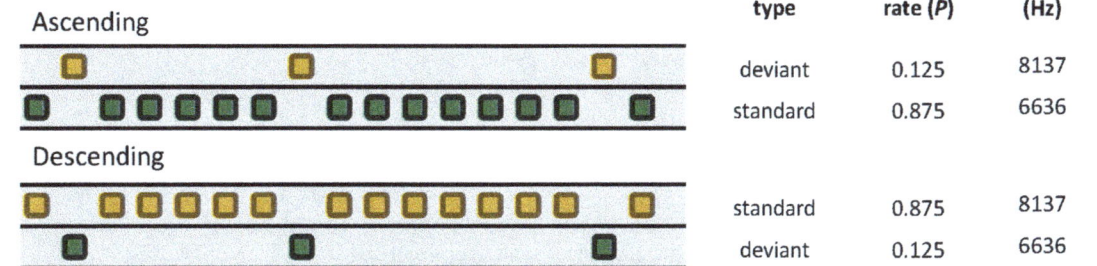

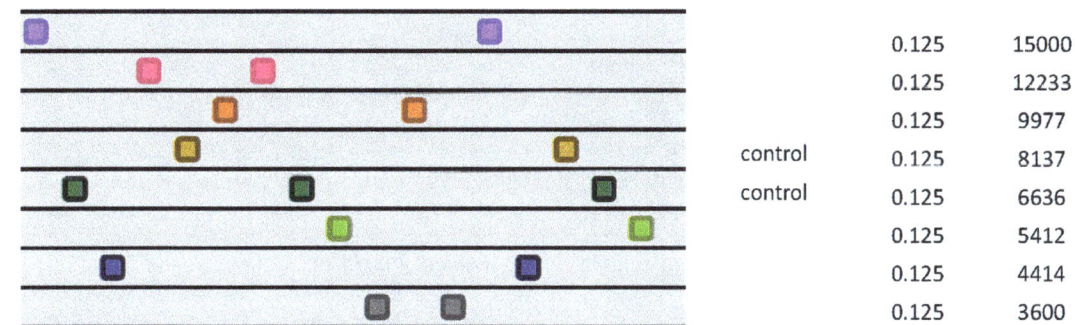

Ascending

Descending

Stimulus type	Presentation rate (P)	Frequency (Hz)
deviant	0.125	8137
standard	0.875	6636
standard	0.875	8137
deviant	0.125	6636

B) Control Sequence – Many-Standards Design
Used in: Study 2

Stimulus type	Presentation rate (P)	Frequency (Hz)
	0.125	15000
	0.125	12233
	0.125	9977
control	0.125	8137
control	0.125	6636
	0.125	5412
	0.125	4414
	0.125	3600

C) Oddball sequences – Cascade Design
Used in: Study 3

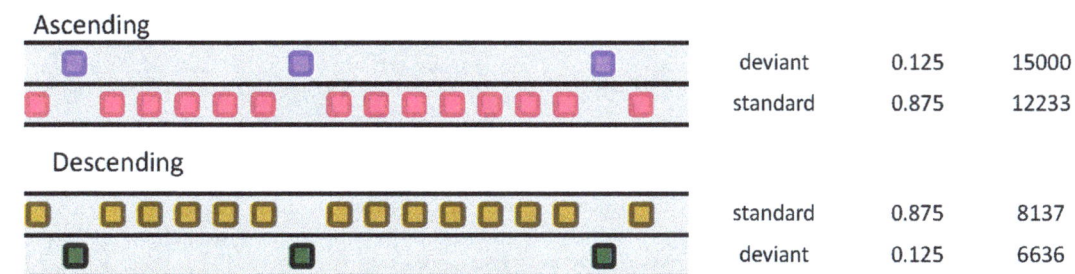

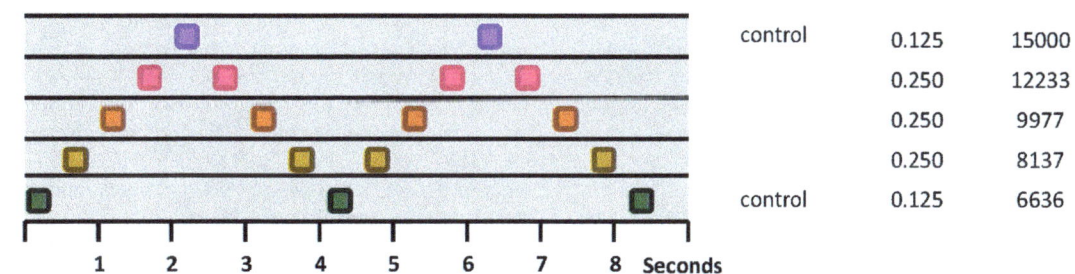

Ascending

Descending

Stimulus type	Presentation rate (P)	Frequency (Hz)
deviant	0.125	15000
standard	0.875	12233
standard	0.875	8137
deviant	0.125	6636

D) Control Sequence – Cascade Design
Used in: Study 3

Stimulus type	Presentation rate (P)	Frequency (Hz)
control	0.125	15000
	0.250	12233
	0.250	9977
	0.250	8137
control	0.125	6636

1   2   3   4   5   6   7   8   Seconds

Figure 1. Control sequence designs used in the current investigation. (A) Both Study 1 and Study 2 used a flip-flop design for oddball sequences. This design allows for the comparison of the response to a stimulus when it is a rare, unexpected deviant to the same tone when it is a common, expected standard, controlling for differences in responses to the physical characteristics of the stimuli, but not for differential adaptation. **(B)** The many-standards control sequence was used in Study 2 to test responses to stimuli that would have prompted the same level of adaptation as the deviant stimulus. Comparing the responses to the deviant used in the oddball sequence, where it defies established stimulus regularity predictions, to the control in the many-standards sequence, which does not defy regularity predictions (there is no established regularity) yields a measure of adaptation-independent deviance detection. Comparing the responses to the control (presented rarely) in the many-standards sequence to the standard (presented often) in the oddball sequence yields a measure of adaptation to a rare stimulus vs. a common stimulus. **(C)** The cascade sequence designs were used for Study 3. The oddball sequences are similar to those used in Study 1 and Study 2, except that a flip-flop design was not used, and the stimuli presented in the ascending and descending sequences are respectively on the upper and lower end of the range of sequences used in the control sequence. (**D**) The control sequence (like the many-standards sequence) presents the stimuli used as deviants in the oddball sequences at the same probability as they are when deviants in a context where they do not defy established patterns in regularity, thus enabling the control of differential adaptation.

urethane). Finally, deviance detection that is independent of the effects of differential adaptation is rarely observable in small-field recordings (e.g. local field potentials, multiunit activity) from primary auditory cortex [17,18,21], but are more often observed with epidural electrodes [28,29,34–38]. This is in agreement with emerging studies suggesting that non-primary areas of the auditory cortex are involved in adaptation-independent MMN [20]. Indeed a recent study has demonstrated that while non-MMN components of the auditory ERP are localised to primary (core) auditory cortical areas and can be tonotopically mapped, adaptation-independent MMN is highly distributed over the auditory cortex, including secondary auditory 'belt' regions and are not tonotopically localised [32]. All of the studies that instituted a control method for adaptation effects used either a deviant-alone control (another method for controlling for adaptation) or the many standards control sequence. To our knowledge, the cascade control method has not been tested in an animal model thus far.

Our laboratory has previously published one of the aforementioned animal model studies [35], in which adaptation-independent deviance detection was observed in awake rats to deviants in stimulus frequency. These were only observed for high-frequency deviants (3600 Hz), not low-frequency deviants (2500 Hz), in agreement with similar findings in anaesthetised rats [28], indicating a possible enhanced salience for increments in frequency, compared to decrements. Another possible reason for why rats in our previous study exhibited deviance detection to high but not low frequency stimuli could be the frequency of the tones that were tested (2500 and 3600 Hz), which were at the lower end of the rats' frequency sensitivity [39,40]. Examining whether deviance detection can be elicited to higher-frequency tones that are closer to the peak of rats' frequency sensitivity (e.g. ~16000 Hz) will determine if the preference for high-frequency deviants was an artefact resulting from the use of low frequency sounds.

Many previous studies in animal models have only investigated MMRs in single locations, typically over auditory cortex. However, it is possible that MMRs in rats are more readily observed at other locations depending upon the orientation and location of generators. In humans for example, the major generators of MMN are located in auditory cortex, yet the largest response is seen over frontal areas even though there may be only a small contribution from frontal generators [7,41]. Therefore, an examination of the effect of recording location on the amplitude of MMRs is warranted.

In the current investigation, we aimed to replicate our laboratory's previous evidence of adaptation-independent deviance detection in the rat, with the overall aim of determining which conditions produce the most robust adaptation responses and adaptation-independent deviance detection responses. In Study 1, we used the same recording system previously used in our laboratory [35], to determine if MMRs are produced to tones of higher frequencies (closer to the rats' peak frequency sensitivity). In Study 2, we used a new system allowing multichannel recordings, to characterize the morphology at different locations of adaptation and adaptation-independent deviance detection using the many standards control. Finally, in Study 3, we investigated the utility of the cascade control method for recording MMRs in rats.

Methods

2.1 Ethics Statement

All experiments were performed under strict adherence to the National Health and Medical Research Council's Australian code of practice for the care and use of animals for scientific purposes and were approved by the University of Newcastle's Animal Care and Ethics Committee (Approval number A-2009-108). Surgical procedures were performed under well-maintained anaesthesia and all efforts were made to reduce the number of animals used and alleviate pain and discomfort following surgery through use of analgesics.

2.2 Animals and Surgery

2.2.1 Study 1. Nine male Wistar rats (sourced from the University of Newcastle's Central Animal House) were used for Study 1. All rats were on a 12 h light/dark cycle with lights on at 06:30 h. The surgery was performed when the animals were on average 96 days old (89–111 days old). The average weight of the animals was 456.9 g (381–513 g) on the day of surgery. Animals were anaesthetised with fentanyl (300 μg/kg i.p.) and medetomidine (300 μg/kg i.p.), and/or isoflurane and the rat was fixed onto a stereotaxic frame (Stoelting, IL, USA) and placed on a heating pad during surgery. A battery operated biotelemetric radio-transmitter (model # TA11CA-F40, Data Sciences International, St. Paul, MN, USA) was implanted in the peritoneal cavity. Insulated biopotential leads from the transmitter were passed subcutaneously to the base of the skull. The skin over the skull was exposed and 2 small burr holes were drilled in the skull, one hole for the active electrode over the right auditory cortex (4.5 mm posterior to Bregma and 3.5 mm lateral to the midline) and the other for the reference electrode in the left cerebellum (2 mm posterior to the lambda and 2 mm lateral to the midline). These locations are based on previous research demonstrating MMN-like epidural responses in the rat [37]. The leads were fixed with dental acrylic. Carprofen (5 mg/kg s.c.) and buprenorphine (0.05 mg/kg s.c.) were administered pre-operatively as analgesics. The animals were allowed to recover for at least 6 days after surgery before the first ERP recordings.

Testing occurred within an experimental chamber covered with grounded copper mesh acting as a Faraday cage. The rat was placed in a partition (internal dimensions: length 23.5 cm, width 12.0 cm, height 24.0 cm) within the experimental chamber. EEGs were recorded using custom acquisition software written in LabVIEW (version 8.2.1). Two channels of data were continuously digitised (1000 Hz): a single EEG channel, and an analogue trigger pulse generated by the PC sound card in parallel with the auditory stimulus. Stimulus event codes were logged with the EEG data. The bandwidth of the data acquisition system was 0.2–150 Hz and the input voltage range was ±10 mV.

2.2.2 Studies 2 and 3. Eighteen male Wistar rats were used for Study 2, 15 of which were also used for Study 3. These rats were on a 12 h light/dark cycle with lights on at 00:00 h (midnight) and were used as controls for another study investigating the role of developmental exposure to immune activation on electrophysiological measures. Seven female Wistar rats (sourced from the University of Newcastle's Central Animal House) were time-mated with three male Wistar breeders. The day of positive sperm detection was designated as gestational day (GD) 0. Four pregnant females were injected with saline on GD10 and three were injected with saline on GD19, resulting in nine male offspring exposed to prenatal saline injection at GD10 and nine at GD19, all of which were used for Study 2. For Study 3, only eight rats exposed to GD10 injection and seven exposed at GD19 were used. Pregnant females were anesthetised with isoflurane, and given an intravenous administration (via the lateral tail vein) of 0.1 M phosphate buffered saline (at 1 mL/kg body weight).

The surgery to implant electrodes was performed on the male offspring of these pregnant animals when they were, on average, 108 days old (76–137 days) and weighed on average 481.76 g (370–593 g). Rats were anaesthetised with isoflurane, placed on a heating pad, and fixed to a stereotaxic frame (Stoelting, IL, USA). The dorsal surface of the skull from +4.00 mm to −12.00 mm relative to Bregma and 4–5 mm lateral from the midline was exposed and the periosteum was removed. A custom-made electrode connector was implanted onto the rat's skull. The connector consisted of a 10-pin male-female socket (BD075-10-A-1-L-D from Global Connector Technology, Lawrence, MA, USA), with the pins soldered to magnet wire (8057 from Belden, St Louis, MO, USA) and embedded in epoxy resin (RS 1991402, RS Components, Sydney, Australia). Seven wires from the connector were soldered to stainless steel screws (B002SG89S4, Amazon Supply, USA). Seven 0.9 mm burr holes were made into the skull of the rat, penetrating all the way through the skull, but not through the dura. The screw electrodes were implanted into these holes until they were fixed in place. Five screws were used as recording electrodes and were placed above the left and right auditory cortices (LAC and RAC, 5.00 mm posterior to Bregma and 4.00 mm lateral to the midline), the left and right frontal cortices (LFC and RFC, 2.00 mm anterior to Bregma and 2.00 mm lateral to the midline), and a location to the left of the midline (LML, 3.50 mm posterior to Bregma and 1.00 mm left of the midline). The ground screw was placed over the right posterior cortex (2.0 0 mm anterior to Lambda and 2.50 mm right of the midline), and the reference screw over the cerebellum (1.00 mm posterior to Lambda and 1.00 mm to the right of the midline). The wire connecting the screw electrodes to the connector was wound around their respective screws and the wires, screws and socket were fixed to the animal's head using dental cement (Dentsply, Mount Waverly, VIC, Australia). Carprofen (5 mg/kg s.c.) and buprenorphine (0.05 mg/kg s.c.) were administered pre-operatively as analgesics. The animals were allowed to recover for at least 4 days after surgery before the first ERP recordings.

Immediately prior to testing, a wireless telemetric 8-channel headstage from Multi Channel Systems (Reutlingen, Germany) was connected to a battery using reusable adhesive, and then attached to the electrode connector previously implanted on the rat's head. Testing occurred within an expanded PVC sound-attenuating chamber (ENV-018V, Med Associates, St. Albans, VT USA) with the interior covered with sound-absorbing foam. The awake rat was placed in a 32 cm diameter plastic bucket, containing pressed-paper bedding, where it was free to roam. EEG data were recorded using Multi Channel Systems MCRack software. Each channel of EEG data was digitised at 200 0 Hz (high pass filter 0.1 Hz; low pass filter 5000 Hz; voltage range ±12.4 mV). Event code markers and a trigger pulse generated by the sound card in parallel with the auditory stimuli were recorded as digital signals at the same sampling rate.

2.3 Sound Generation

2.3.1 Study 1. Auditory stimuli were generated with a custom program written in Presentation (version 14.1, Neurobehavioral

Systems, Inc.), amplified and delivered through a speaker (50 Hz–19000 Hz frequency response) mounted at an approximate height of 1 m above the floor of the experimental chamber. Sound intensity was calibrated with a sound meter (Brüel & Kjær Model 2260) using a linear weighting to an average of 78 dB_L SPL across locations within the chamber for the sounds in the 6636 and 8137 Hz range used in this study.

2.3.2 Studies 2 and 3. Auditory stimuli were generated with a custom program written in Presentation (version 14.1, Neurobehavioral Systems, Inc.), amplified and delivered through a speaker (1 kHz–30 kHz frequency response) mounted at an approximate height of 50 cm above the floor of the experimental chamber. Sound intensity was calibrated with a sound meter (Brüel & Kjær Model 2260) using a linear weighting to an average of 70 dB_L SPL across locations within the chamber for the sounds in the 3600 and 15000 Hz range used in these studies.

2.4 Experiment Design and Stimuli

2.4.1 Study 1 – Flip-flop Control. Rats were tested for one half-hour session each day, for three days. The awake rat was placed in the experimental chamber for 15 min before each session to acclimatise. Each session consisted of an ascending and a descending oddball sequence separated by a 3 min break. The order of the two sequences alternated for each rat across test sessions, and was balanced across rats.

Two sequences were presented in Study 1. These were oddball sequences where the roles of the deviant and standard were reversed (flip-flop condition) resulting in either an ascending deviant sequence (low frequency standard and high frequency deviant) or a descending deviant sequence (high frequency standard and low frequency deviant) (Figure 1A). In the ascending and descending oddball sequences, 87.5% of the tones were standards and 12.5% deviants. Previous findings have demonstrated that certain components of the deviant response were sensitive to the recent stimulus history of standards, in that it increased in amplitude as the number of preceding standard increased from 1 to 5 or more [35]. In order to maximise MMRs, the oddball sequences of Studies 1–3 reported here were designed to have at least 3 standards prior to each deviant. For all sequences, tones had a 10 ms rise and fall time and a stimulus onset asynchrony (SOA) of 500 ms. Two tones of 100 ms duration were used: a low frequency tone of 6636 Hz and a high frequency tone of 8137 Hz, equivalent to a 0.29 octave difference or normalised frequency difference (or Δf) of $(f_2-f_1)/(f_2 \times f_1)^{1/2} = 0.20$ where $f_1 = 6636$ Hz and $f_2 = 8137$ Hz [12]. Each of the sequences consisted of 1600 tones and ran for 13.33 min.

2.4.2 Study 2 – Many-Standards Control. Rats were tested for MMRs on one 62 min session a day for three days, and were exposed to three different testing orders for each of the three days. The rat was placed in the experimental chamber with bedding for 5 min before each session to acclimatise. The rat did not have access to food or water during the session but was free to explore the testing chamber during the recordings. On each of the three testing days, the rat was also tested in separate sessions on two other auditory paradigms that are not reported here.

Each session in Study 2 consisted of four types of sequences each presented twice, resulting in eight sequences per session. Two of the four types of sequence were the ascending and descending oddball sequences described for Study 1 (Figure 1A). The other sequences were many-standards control sequences in which tones equivalent to the deviants in the ascending and descending oddball sequences were presented at the same probability as in the oddball sequences (12.5%) but randomly interspersed with six other tones (also presented at 12.5%), ensuring that a pattern of regularity in the auditory stimuli was not established [11,24] (Figure 1B).

The two many-standards control sequences were subtly different in order to accommodate the pseudo-random stimulus orders within the ascending and descending oddball sequences. For all sequences, tones had a 10 ms rise and fall time, a duration of 100 ms and a SOA of 500 ms. Eight frequencies (each of 100 ms duration) differing on a logarithmic scale were presented: 3600 Hz, 4414 Hz, 5412 Hz, 6636 Hz (equivalent to oddball low frequency deviant), 8137 Hz (equivalent to high frequency oddball deviant), 9977 Hz, 12233 Hz and 15000 Hz. In the first of the control sequences, the 8137 Hz stimulus was presented in exactly the same temporal location (relative to the beginning of the sequence) as in the ascending oddball deviant sequence. In the second of the control sequences, the 6636 Hz stimulus was presented in the same temporal location as in the descending oddball deviant sequence, but neither of the sequences controlled for the tone preceding the deviant. The remaining tones were presented in pseudorandom order except that no tone was ever repeated. In order to avoid the possibility of an MMN being elicited by tones at the extremes of a range for either the frequency control conditions, known as the extreme substandard effect [24,26,42], the standard and deviant used in the ascending and descending sequences were the fourth and the fifth highest frequencies (Figure 1B).

Within each session, sequences were presented in one of four orders, and repeated in that same order. Blocks of sequences began with one oddball sequence, followed by the two control sequences (with two order combinations), and ending with the other oddball sequence. Within a block, sequences were separated by 1 min silent breaks and a 3 min silent break separated the two blocks. Each sequence contained 800 stimuli and ran for 6.67 minutes, and each session ran for 62 min.

2.4.3 Study 3 – Cascade control.
The same animals used for Study 2 were also used in Study 3. Rats were tested for one recording session using the cascade control sequences. The rat was placed in the experimental chamber for 5 min before the commencement of the session and was free to explore during recordings. Three types of sequence were presented, and similar to Study 2, each sequence consisted of 800 tones, each played with 100 ms duration, 10 ms rise and fall time and SOA of 500 ms. Similar to Studies 1 and 2, Sequences 1 and 2 were ascending and descending oddball sequences (Figure 1C). The ascending sequence consisted of a low-frequency standard (12233 Hz, 87.5%) and a high frequency deviant (15000 Hz, 12.5%), and the descending sequence consisted of a high-frequency standard (8137 Hz, 87.5%) and a low-frequency deviant (6636 Hz, 12.5%). Sequence 3 was a cascade control sequence (Figure 1D). Five tones were presented in this sequence: 6636 Hz, 8137 Hz, 9977 Hz, 12233 Hz and 15000 Hz, played in order from lowest frequency to highest frequency, back to lowest frequency in a 'cascading' order, similar to Ruhnau et al. [33]. In this sequence, the two tones used as deviants in ascending and descending oddball sequences are presented with the same probability as in the oddball sequences (12.5%), whereas the other tones are presented at a probability of 25%. Within a session, sequences were presented in one of two orders: either 1) Ascending, Control, Descending; or 2) Descending, Control, Ascending. Each of these blocks was presented twice within a session with a 3 min silent break between the two blocks and 1 min silent breaks between each sequence within a block. The total session time was approximately 49 min.

2.5 Data Extraction

Data processing was performed off-line with EEGDisplay 6.3.12 [43]. Intervals of gross artefacts in the continuous EEG record were excluded using an automated algorithm that rejected signals exceeding ±1400 µV. Epochs were extracted from the continuous EEG consisting of a 100 ms pre-stimulus baseline and a 400 ms post-stimulus interval. The first 25 tones at the start of each tone sequence were excluded from analysis to allow for transitory effects associated with switching between different types of sequences or the beginning of the session. Within oddball sequences, the first standard following each deviant was excluded from the analysis to allow for recovery of a stable response to standards. Following these pre-processing steps, epochs were averaged off-line for each animal and session separately and ERPs extracted for each of the stimulus types, including the responses to deviants and standards, as well as their respective controls for each of the studies. ERPs were baseline corrected over a 50 ms pre-stimulus interval for Study 1 and a 100 ms pre-stimulus interval for Studies 2 and 3.

The ERPs recorded in these studies exhibited distinct components over the first 200 ms, although the amplitudes of these components differed according to the type and frequency of the stimulus. For Study 1, they were characterised by a negative component peaking at approximately 22 ms (denoted as N22), followed by a positive peak at 37 ms (P37) and a second broad negative component with a peak latency of approximately 60–100 ms (N80). For Studies 2 and 3 (using different EEG recording and acoustic delivery), the components were identified to occur slightly earlier with an additional early positive component being identified, and a clear separation of the broad late negative shift into two distinct peaks. The ERP was characterised by an initial positive peak at 13 ms (P13), a negative peak at 18 ms (N18), followed by a positive peak at 30 ms (P30) and a broad negative component with two discernible peaks from approximately 45–65 ms (N55) and 65–105 ms (N85).

For Study 1, three mean amplitude measures were extracted over latency windows corresponding to the ERP peaks: a 15 ms window from 15–30 ms for N22, an 8 ms window from 35–43 ms for P37 and a 40 ms window from 60–100 ms for N80. A wide window was used to assess N22 because there were relatively large individual differences in the latency of the peak, which was far more variable across animals than P37 (Figure 2). For Studies 2 and 3, five mean amplitude measures were extracted over the following latency windows: a 4 ms window from 11–15 ms (P13), a 7 ms window from 15–22 ms for N18, a 21 ms window from 22–43 ms for P30, a 23 ms window from 43.5–65.5 ms for N55 and a 40 ms window from 65.5–105.5 ms for N85.

2.6 Statistical Analysis

All analyses were performed controlling for stimulus identity. That is, only responses to stimuli of the same frequency were compared. For example, although the 8 kHz deviant in Study 2 was presented in an ascending oddball sequence with a 6 kHz standard, all analyses performed on the 8 kHz deviant involved comparisons with the 8 kHz standard (used in the descending oddball sequence) and the 8 kHz control (used in the many-standards control sequence). Therefore, for this study, when referring to a Deviant vs. Standard comparison, we do not refer to the Deviant and Standard tones within an individual sequence, rather we refer to the deviant tone of a certain frequency and its respective flip-flop controlled standard tone of the same frequency.

Mean amplitudes of the ERP components were analysed using Analysis of Variance (ANOVA) with one or more repeated measures factors depending upon the study. Within-subjects factors were *Stimulus Type* (Study 1: Deviant and Standard,

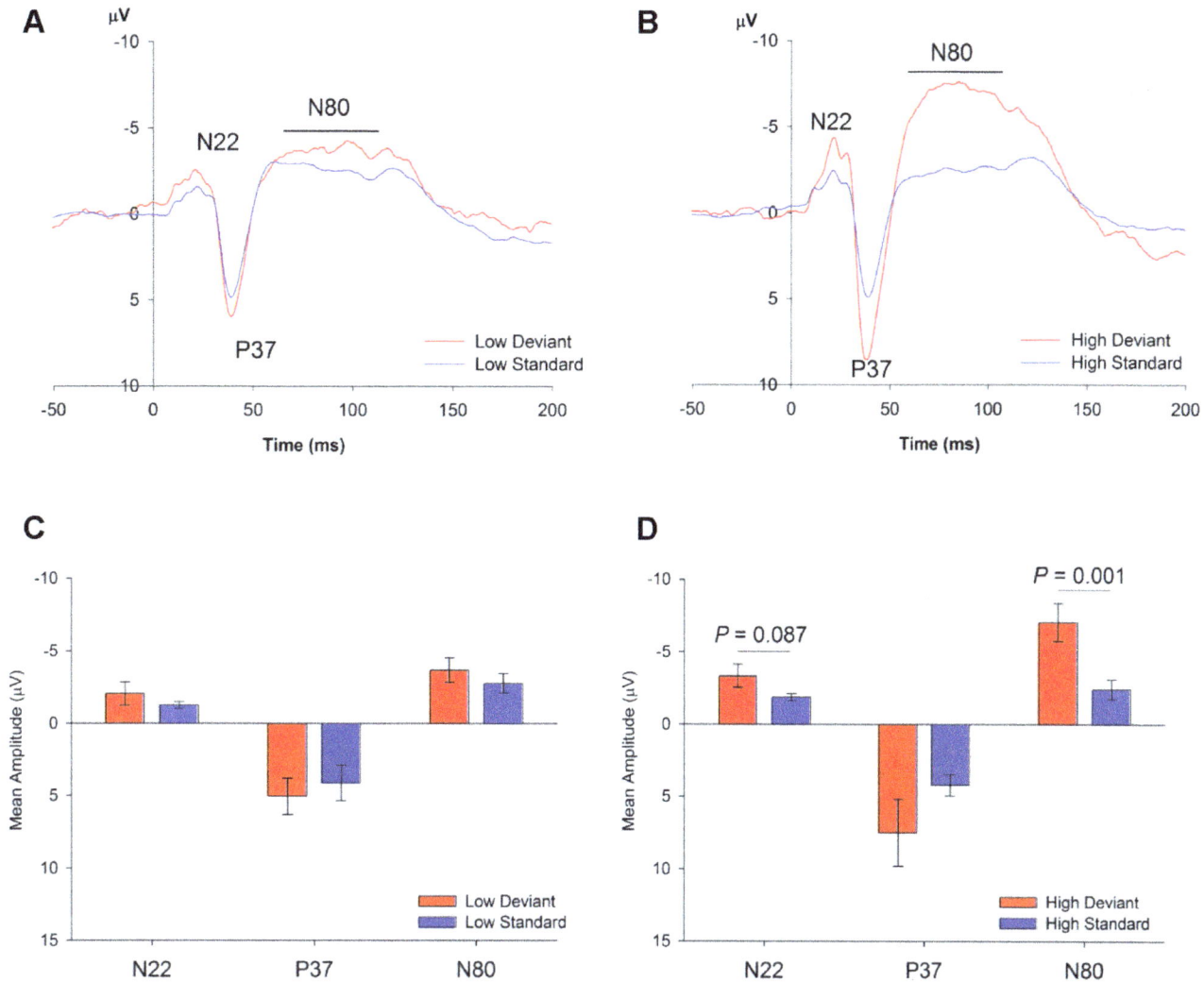

Figure 2. Rat ERPs in Study 1. (A,B) ERPs to the oddball deviant (red) and the standard (blue) for the low (**A**) and high (**B**) frequency stimuli. All stimuli show a similar pattern with the same components (N22, P37, N80): responses to deviants are larger in amplitude in comparison to standards. (**C,D**) Mean amplitudes (± standard error, SE) of N22, P37 and N80 generated by oddball deviants (red) and standards (blue), showing that responses to the deviant compared to the standard were larger for the N80 component ($P = 0.001$), and the N22 (although not significantly, $P = 0.087$).

Study 2: Deviant, Control and Standard, Study 3: Deviant and Control), Stimulus Frequency (Studies 1 and 2: 6636 Hz, 8137 Hz; Study 3: 6636 and 15000 Hz) and electrode location (in the case of Studies 2 and 3, left and right auditory cortices, LAC and RAC; left and right frontal cortices, LFC and RFC; and left of the midline, LML). Each ERP component was analysed separately. Gestational age of maternal treatment (for Studies 2 and 3 only) with saline was also used as a between-subjects factor to ensure that the different gestational day of treatment did not impact findings in this group of animals. In instances where sphericity was violated, Huynh-Feldt adjusted degrees of freedom were used to determine significance levels.

Given the large number of regions and components analysed in Study 2 and 3, significance levels for the first-pass, omnibus ANOVA were set at P<0.01, to reduce the likelihood of Type 1 errors. Once an effect was identified in this first ANOVA, follow-up ANOVAs and *post-hoc* comparisons used a significance level of P<0.05. *Post hoc* pairwise comparisons were made using Bonferroni correction and *P* values will be expressed as the Bonferroni-corrected value, P_b. These pairwise comparisons were

used to determine whether *oddball effects*, *deviance detection* or *adaptation* were present to a statistically significant degree. *Oddball effects* occur when the amplitude of the response to the deviant is significantly larger than that to the standard stimulus (i.e. more positive for positive components and more negative for negative components) and these were assessed in Studies 1 and 2 (designs in which deviants and standards of the same frequency were presented). This measure of MMN, while controlling for different stimulus frequencies, does not comprise a control for different levels of adaptation to the standard and deviant stimuli. Therefore, two other comparisons were made. In Studies 2 and 3, the amplitude response to the deviant was compared to the control to determine the level of *deviance detection*, and in Study 2, the amplitude response to the control was compared to the standard to determine the level of *adaptation*. The magnitude of these oddball, adaptation and deviance detection effects were expressed as effect sizes measured by Cohen's *d*.

2.6.1 Incomplete data. In Studies 2 and 3, some animals did not have a complete dataset. This was caused by poor-quality, noisy EEG traces from particular electrodes that caused certain regions to be removed from analysis.

For Study 2, only two rats had incomplete data (both were missing data for three regions). These rats were removed from the analysis, resulting in a final sample size of 16 for Study 2.

For Study 3, on the other hand, there were a large number of animals with incomplete data: no regions produced usable data in all animals. A total of seven rats had incomplete data, but none were missing data for more than three regions. The data for Study 3 were initially analysed without the seven animals with incomplete data. However, removing so many from the analysis could result in a dramatic loss of useful information and reduced power. For instance, only one animal had missing data from each of the frontal cortex sites. Therefore, in order to still utilize the full dataset from Study 3, automatic imputation was used to impute the missing data for the incomplete samples. Five data imputations were made in SPSS for variables with missing data points. Data were imputed using linear regression separately for each component, after which, analyses were performed as described above for the original (incomplete) dataset and the five datasets containing imputations. Effects will be reported as significant if they are present in the majority of datasets (>4 of 6), and statistics (F and P values) will be reported for the most conservative change (lowest F value).

Results

3.1 Study 1 – Flip-flop Control

Raw mean amplitude data for Study 1 are available in Data S1. In Study 1, the early components, N22 and P37 were larger in response to deviant stimuli (Stimulus Type: N22 $F_{1,8} = 11.22$, $P = 0.010$; P37, $F_{1,8} = 13.11$, $P = 0.007$; Figure 2). The later component, N80, in addition to main effects of Stimulus Type ($F_{1,8} = 37.05$, $P<0.001$) and frequency ($F_{1,8} = 8.08$, $P = 0.022$), also exhibited a Stimulus Type×Frequency interaction ($F_{1,8} = 11.06$, $P = 0.010$) due to the deviant producing a larger N80 than the standard only for high frequency stimuli ($P_b = 0.001$; $d = 1.74$). No other significant changes in the response to the deviant were identified although a similar trend-level effect was observed for N22 to the high frequency deviant ($P_b = 0.087$; $d = 0.65$).

3.2 Study 2 – Many-standards Control

Raw mean amplitude data for Study 2 are available in Data S2.

3.2.1 Effects of GD of Saline Treatment. In order to ensure that the pool of animals used in this study was relatively homogenous and not differentially affected by the developmental intervention at different GDs, GD was included as a between subjects factor in all statistical analyses. The only effect of GD was seen for the P30 component to high frequencies. For the P30 component, a main effect of GD ($F_{1,14} = 5.01$, $P = 0.042$) and a Stimulus Type×GD interaction ($F_{2,28} = 3.53$, $P = 0.043$) were observed. There was a significant effect of Stimulus Type for GD19 rats ($F_{2,16} = 5.88$, $P = 0.012$), but not for GD10 rats ($F_{2,12} = 2.51$, $P = 0.122$). Although not significant, the mean values for the deviant, control and standard P30 responses for the GD10s followed the expected pattern, with largest values for the response to the deviant and smallest values for the response the standard (Deviant = 7.60, Control = 6.22, Standard = 5.83). However, GD19 rats had a larger control response than both deviant and standard (Deviant = 3.72, Control = 5.02, Standard = 2.98). However, with the exception of the P30 component, overall, GD had little effect on component amplitudes and conditions. Half of the rats in Study 2 (the GD19 rats) having unexpectedly large control

P30 responses relative to deviant responses may result in an overestimation of adaptation effects (Control vs. Standard) and an underestimation or reversal of deviance detection (Deviant vs. Control). This will be considered when interpreting and discussing results for P30.

3.2.2 Overall Effects of Region. Figure 3 shows the ERPs generated for each of the different frequencies in the many-standards control condition over each of the different sites, as well as for all of the sites averaged together (Figure 3F). Analysis of the effects of region were only performed on deviant and standard stimuli from the oddball sequences and the 6636 Hz and 8137 Hz (low- and high-frequency) stimuli from the many-standards control sequence. There were significant region effects for all five components. For the earliest component, P13, amplitudes were largest at the midline and auditory cortex sites and smallest at the frontal sites ($F_{3.25,21.47} = 9.47$, $P<0.001$). N18 amplitudes, on the other hand, were largest at auditory sites compared to frontal and midline sites ($F_{2.85,39.94} = 5.33$, $P = 0.004$). The later components (P30, N55 and N85) were largest at frontal cortex sites (P30: $F_{4,56} = 25.73$, $P<0.001$; N55: $F_{1.90,26.63} = 7.50$, $P = 0.003$; N85: $F_{2.05,28.75} = 7.92$, $P = 0.002$). P30 was smallest at the midline site, but both N55 and N85 exhibited equal amplitudes over auditory cortex and midline sites.

3.2.3 Effects of Stimulus Type and Frequency. Figures 4A and 4B illustrate the ERPs to deviant, control and standard stimuli for low, and high frequency stimuli, respectively. The components P13, N18 and N55 had similar Type and Frequency effects regardless of the region recorded from. That is, while there were main effects of Region on component amplitudes, there were no interactions between Region and Frequency or Type. Therefore, the effect of Type and Frequency on these component amplitudes pooled over regions was analysed. These effects are represented in Figures 4C and 4D. A Type×Frequency effect was present for the P13 component ($F_{1.31,18.37} = 7.16$, $P = 0.010$). The effect of type was limited to high frequencies $F_{1.33,18.56} = 10.36$, $P = 0.003$. The P13 amplitude to deviant stimuli was larger than control stimuli (deviance detection, $P_b = 0.028$; $d = 0.73$; Figure 4B,D) and standard stimuli (oddball effect, $P_b = 0.014$; $d = 0.85$; Figure 4B,D) for high frequency stimuli, but not low frequency stimuli. In addition, P13 amplitude was larger to high-frequency control stimuli than to high-frequency standards (adaptation, $P_b = 0.035$; $d = 0.76$; Figure 4B,D).

A similar Type×Frequency effect was observed for N18 amplitudes ($F_{2,28} = 20.90$, $P<0.001$), and again, the effect of Type was limited to the high-frequency stimuli ($F_{1.59,22.23} = 17.30$, $P<0.001$), for which N18 amplitudes to both control and deviant stimuli were larger compared to those to standard stimuli (adaptation and oddball effects, respectively; Adaptation $P_b<0.001$; $d = 1.33$; Oddball $P_b = 0.001$; $d = 1.24$; Figure 4B,D). Unlike the P13 component, deviance detection to the high-frequency stimuli did not reach significance for the N18 component ($P_b = 0.072$; $d = 0.66$; Figure 4B,D).

The strongest effects of Stimulus Type were observed to high-frequency stimuli for the N55 component (Type×Frequency $F_{1.68,23.53} = 52.12$, $P<0.001$), where statistically-significant oddball ($P_b<0.001$; $d = 2.04$; Fig. 5B,D), deviance detection ($P_b = 0.010$; $d = 0.87$; Fig. 5B,D) and adaptation effects ($P_b<0.001$; $d = 1.99$; Fig. 5B,D) were observed. Such effects on the N55 component were not seen for low-frequency stimuli (Figure 4A,C).

For the remaining ERP components in Study 2 (P30 and N85), the recording site played a significant role in the expression of MMN-like responses (indicated by Type×Frequency×Region interactions). These effects are represented in Table 1 for all

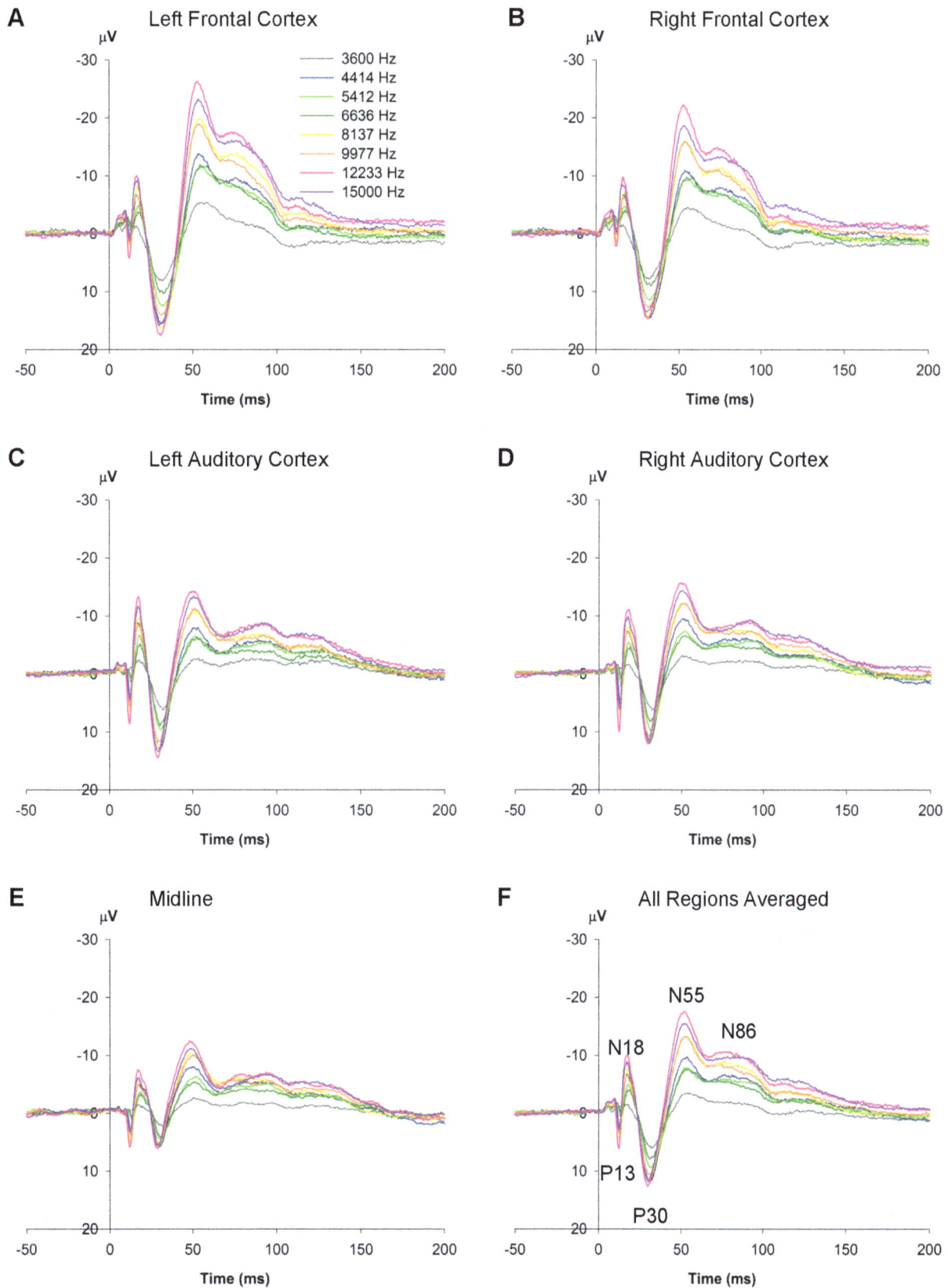

Figure 3. Rat ERPs in the many-standards control sequence (Study 2). ERPs recorded from electrodes implanted into the skull above the left frontal cortex (**A**), right frontal cortex (**B**), left auditory cortex (**C**), right auditory cortex (**D**), midline (**E**), and averaged over all of the regions (**F**).

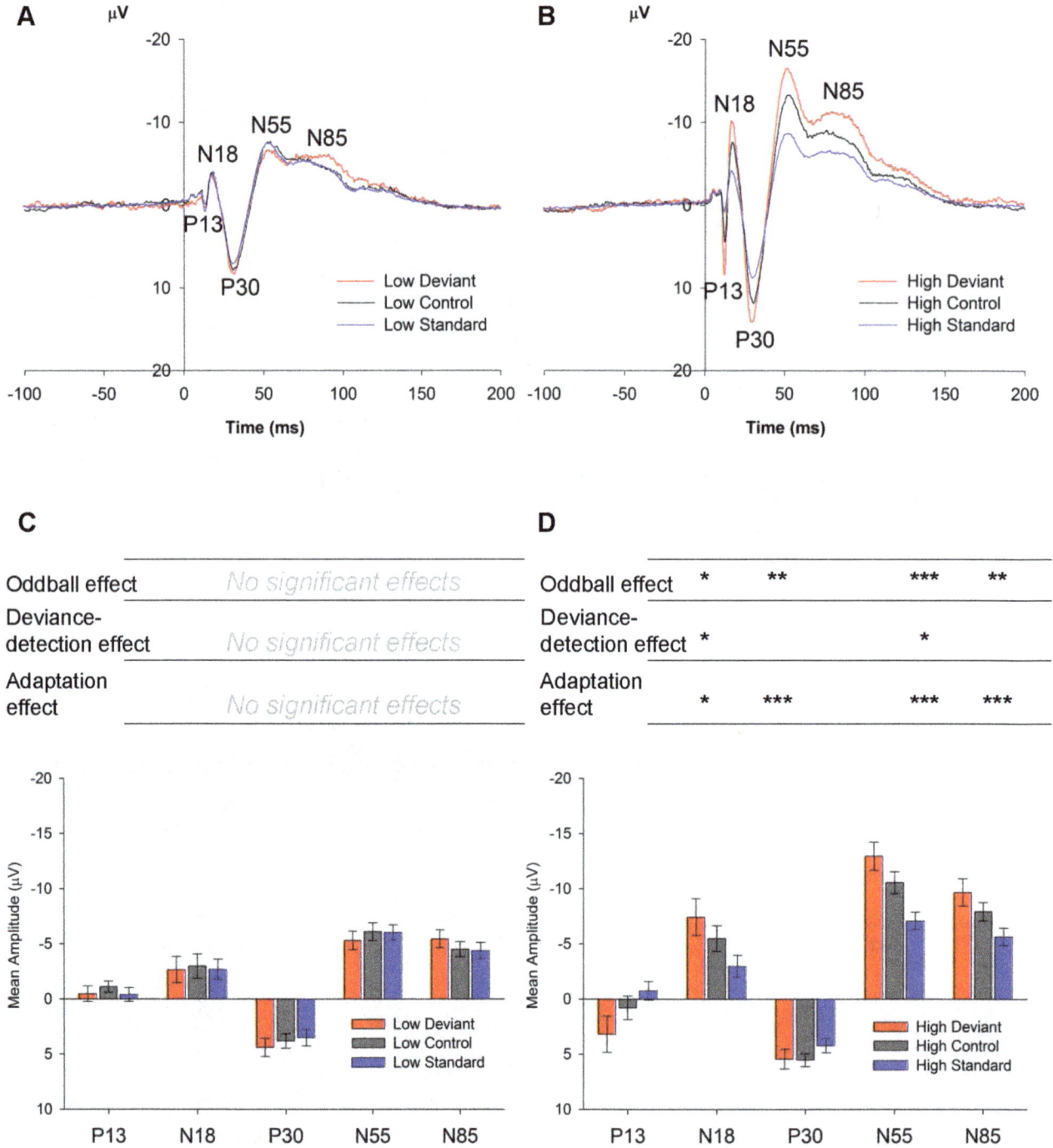

Figure 4. Rat ERPs in Study 2, averaged over all regions. (**A,B**) ERPs (averaged over all five regions) to the oddball deviant (red), the many-standards control (black) and the standard (blue) for the low (**A**) and high (**B**) frequency stimuli. All stimuli show a similar pattern with the same components (P13, N18, P30, N55 and N85): responses to deviants are larger in amplitude in comparison to the controls for high frequency, but not low frequency stimuli for P13 ($P_b = 0.023$, $d = 0.73$) and N55 ($P_b = 0.010$, $d = 0.87$). (**C,D**) Mean amplitudes ($\pm$ standard error, SE) of P13, N18, P30, N55 and N85 generated by oddball deviants (red), many-standards controls (grey) and standards (blue), averaged over all five regions. Significance levels for statistical comparisons between stimulus types for each component are shown above the bars for their respective components. Asterisks indicate statistical significance under 0.05, with * $0.050 < P > 0.010$, ** $0.010 < P > 0.001$, *** $P < 0.001$.

components (even though in the omnibus analysis, Region interactions were not identified for the other components, P13, N18 and N55, these are included in Table 1 for consistency).

A Type × Frequency × Region effect was identified for P30 ($F_{3.76, 52.63} = 5.96$, $P = 0.001$). MMN-like effects were present over

several regions for both high- and low-frequency stimuli. As illustrated in Table 1, the majority of MMRs for the P30 component occur over the left and right frontal sites (Deviance Detection in the RFC $P_b = 0.043$, $d = 0.72$; Adaptation in the LFC $P_b = 0.001$, $d = 1.22$; Oddball effects in the LFC $P_b = 0.004$,

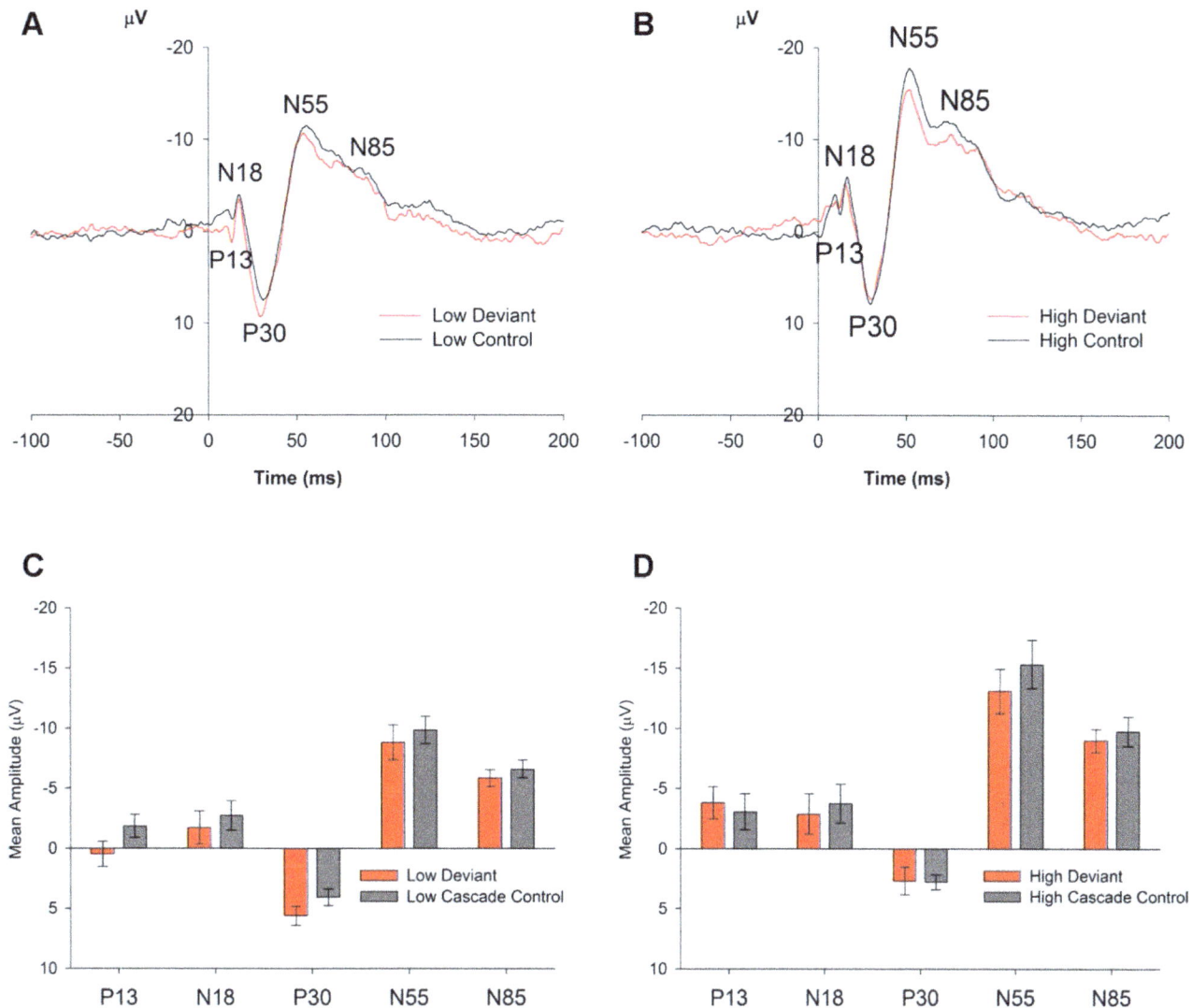

Figure 5. Rat ERPs in Study 3, averaged over all regions. (A,B) ERPs (averaged over all five regions) to the oddball deviant (red) and the cascade control (black) for the low (**A**) and high (**B**) frequency stimuli. As in Study 2, all stimuli show a similar pattern with the same components (P13, N18, P30, N55 and N85), however in this case, responses to deviants were not larger in amplitude in comparison to the controls and the standards. **(C,D)** Mean amplitudes ($\pm$ standard error, SE) of P13, N18, P30, N55 and N85 generated by oddball deviants (red) and the cascade controls (grey), averaged over all five regions.

$d = 0.98$, and RFC $P_b = 0.033$, $d = 0.42$). No significant MMRs were observed over the midline site. At auditory sites, an adaptation effect (P30 amplitude to control > standard, $P_b = 0.002$, $d = 1.01$) was observed for the RAC, but this was accompanied by a *reversed* deviance detection effect (i.e. amplitude to control > deviant, $P_b = 0.009$, $d = 0.85$), and no oddball effect. These puzzling results may be driven by the interaction with GD noted in 3.2.1, where it was found that half of the rats (the rats exposed to saline at GD19), had unusually high P30 amplitudes to control stimuli. Similar to P30, N85 amplitudes were also affected by a Type×Frequency×Region interaction ($F_{5.49, 76.90} = 5.60$, $P < 0.001$). Oddball and adaptation effects were observed in most regions for high frequency stimuli (Table 1), but deviance detection was only observed to a statistically significant degree over the left ($P_b = 0.004$, $d = 1.01$) and right frontal sites ($P_b = 0.008$, $d = 0.90$) and the left auditory site ($P_b = 0.039$, $d = 0.61$).

3.3 Study 3 – Cascade Control

Raw mean amplitude data for Study 3 are available in Data S3. Contrary to Study 2, no effects of stimulus type (deviant vs. control) or stimulus type interactions were identified for Study 3 (Figure 5). GD of saline treatment did not affect responses for any of the components extracted in Study 3 (no significant main effects or interactions with GD in ANOVAs). The most prominent effects observed in Study 3 were that of region, with main effects of region being present for all components. The regional effects for each component from Study 2 were replicated in Study 3. As in Study 2, the P13 component in Study 3 was largest at the midline site and smallest at frontal cortex sites (Effect of Region $F_{4, 24} = 5.12$, $P = 0.004$, observed in original data and 5/5 imputations of missing data). Similar trends were observed for the other components, all of which showed the same regional distribution of responses as in Study 2 (N18: $F_{4, 52} = 3.78$, $P = 0.009$ for original data and 4/5 imputations; P30: $F_{4, 24} = 5.88$, $P = 0.002$ for original data and 5/5 imputations; N55: $F_{4, 24} = 13.008$, $P < 0.001$ for

Table 1. Oddball effects, Deviance detection and adaptation for each frequencies and component combination in Study 2.

		Low Frequency					High Frequency				
	Component	P13	N18	P30	N55	N85	P13	N18	P30	N55	N85
Oddball effect (deviant>standard)	LFC			**	*			**	**	***	**
	RFC			*						***	**
	LAC						*	**		***	**
	RAC					*	*	*		***	**
	LML						*	*		***	**
	Pooled						*	**		***	**
Deviance detection (deviant>control)	LFC				†					*	**
	RFC				†				*		**
	LAC						*			*	*
	RAC								††		
	LML						*			*	
	Pooled						*			*	
Adaptation (control>standard)	LFC							**	*	***	**
	RFC							*		***	*
	LAC							**		***	**
	RAC								**	***	***
	LML							**		***	***
	Pooled						*	***		***	***

Levels of significance for the statistical difference between responses to deviant and standard stimuli (Oddball effect), deviant and control stimuli (Deviance detection) and control and standard stimuli (Adaptation) are shown for individual components and frequency conditions. Significant levels of oddball effects, deviance detection and adaptation were rarely observed for the low frequency stimuli. By contrast, high frequency stimuli often elicited both deviance detection and adaptation responses. Significance levels are indicated as: * or 0.05>P>0.01, ** 0.01>P>0.001, *** P<0.001. In the large majority of cases, the changes were in the expected direction for MMN-like effects (i.e. deviant>control>standard), indicated by unformatted asterisks. Dagger symbolss (†) indicate that the change was in the opposite direction to expected (i.e. standard>control>deviant).

original data and 5/5 imputations; N85 $F_{4,52} = 6.68$, $P<0.001$ for original data and 5/5 imputations).

When the imputed data were analysed for the later components (P30, N55 and N85), significant effects of Frequency were revealed for all three components. The P30 component was larger for low frequency compared to high frequency stimuli ($F_{1,13} = 16.81$, $P< 0.001$ for 5/5 imputations) and the N55 and N85 components were larger for the high frequency stimuli (N55: $F_{1,13} = 25.79$, $P< 0.001$; N85: $F_{1,13} = 21.34$, $P<0.001$; both for 5/5 imputations).

Discussion

The overall aim of the current investigation was to determine optimal conditions with which to observe robust human-like MMRs in rats, with a particular focus on the type of sequence used to control for potential contributions to the size of MMR in rats. The flip-flop sequences controlled only for differences in the physical characteristics of deviant and standard stimuli but not differential adaptation. The "many controls standards" sequence (i) controlled for the probability of presentation and hence adaptation; (ii) it precluded the development of a predictive model and therefore (iii) no stimulus including the control deviant violated predictions. The cascade control sequence (i) controlled for the probability of presentation and adaptation; (ii) it provided the basis for a predictive model but (iii) the control deviant did not violate that predictive model. Significant MMRs were observed for high frequency deviants with the flip-flop design of Study 1, which as noted, did not include a control for differential adaptation. The many-standards control for adaptation, used in Study 2, replicated findings from Study 1, suggesting that the MMRs observed were due to both deviance detection and adaptation, but use of a cascade control design in Study 3, did not replicate these effects, although this control did not allow extraction of adaptation effects.

4.1 Oddball effects, deviance detection and adaptation

Both Study 1 and Study 2 confirmed the presence of oddball effects, that is, significant increases in ERP amplitudes in response to deviant stimuli compared to standard stimuli. While in Study 1, oddball effects were only observed to a statistically significant degree for the later negative component (N80), Study 2 using a different sound generation and recording system revealed that these oddball effects can also be observed at earlier components (P13, N18, P30), in addition to the later negative components N55 and N85. In Study 2, a many-standards control sequence was used to separate oddball effects into separate elements: an *adaptation* index, a measure of the degree of reduction in peak amplitudes to frequent standard stimuli versus control stimuli, and adaptation-independent *deviance detection* index, a measure of the degree of enhancement of peak amplitudes to deviant stimuli versus control stimuli. We therefore can separate two processes that contribute to the oddball effect: (i) deviance detection, the difference between stimuli that conform to patterns of regularity and those that defy predicted patterns and (ii) adaptation, the difference between frequently- and rarely-presented stimuli. In Study 2, by far the strongest oddball effect on peak amplitude to deviant stimuli was observed for the late N55 component, but significant effects were also observed for the earlier P13 and N18 components as well as the later N85 component. Significant levels of deviance detection and adaptation were identified for the N55 component (Figure 4D), indicating that the oddball effect on this component was driven by both adaptation-independent and –dependent processes. Similar effects were found for P13 and N85, where both deviance detection and adaptation contributed to the oddball effect, but not for N18, where only adaptation effects were observed. These

findings indicate that the rat brain is capable of generating human-like MMN, and that like human MMN, these effects are in-part, independent of adaptation and driven by memory-based or prediction error signalling processes.

4.2 The role of frequency for MMR in rats

Studies 1 and 2 replicated the results of previous investigations in our lab [35], where deviance detection was observed for high, but not low frequency deviants when all tone frequencies were selected from a relatively low frequency range (2500–3600 Hz). In Study 1, while control for differential adaptation was not employed in this flip-flop only design, we observed similar increases in the response to the deviant, compared to the standard when tone frequencies were selected from higher frequency range (6636–8137 Hz), and closer to the optimum auditory sensitivity range of rats. The morphology of ERPs was similar to those described previously in Nakamura et al. [35], with a negative peak at approximately 20–30 ms, and a positive peak at approximately 30–40 ms (Figure 2A). Two additional negative components were identified in Nakamura et al. [35]: a negative peak at 42 ms, and a late negative difference between the deviant and the control stimuli from 50–70 ms after stimulus onset. In the current Study 1, however, these two components were replaced by a broad, and much larger negative peak from 60–100 ms. It was hypothesised that by increasing the frequency range used in Study 1 compared to Nakamura et al. [35], MMRs would also be observed for low frequency deviants. However, as in Nakamura et al., increased responses to low frequency deviants were not observed (Figure 3A and C), indicating that the lack of observable MMRs for low frequency deviants is not due to the relative sensitivity of the rat's auditory system to low frequencies, but perhaps associated with a lower salience for unexpected decreases in frequency compared to frequency increases [44]. A similar effect was also evident in Study 2. When differential adaptation was controlled for, both adaptation and deviance detection were observed in several ERP components from several sites for high-frequency deviants, but rarely occurred for low-frequency deviants. Table 1 illustrates this dramatic difference between high and low frequencies in terms of capacity to elicit oddball, deviance detection and adaptation effects. Other researchers using anesthetised rats have observed similar effects, namely evidence of MMRs to high-frequency, but not low-frequency deviants [28]. The same effect has also been observed previously for human MMN [45], as well as for changes in evoked potentials to alterations in tone frequency (increases in frequency were associated with larger ERP changes) [46]. These findings indicate an overall trend towards a higher sensitivity of the rat brain to increments in frequency rather than decrements. A possible explanation for such a trend may be that the ultrasonic vocalizations that rats use to communicate with each other are of a much higher frequency and range from 22 kHz (alarm/distress call) to 50 kHz (reward, appetitive call) [44]. The auditory system of the rat may therefore be somewhat 'primed' to perceive high frequency noises. Future studies could examine this by measuring MMRs to low frequency alarm (22 kHz) calls and high frequency appetitive (50 kHz) calls in a flip-flop condition. It should be noted that adaptation to low frequency changes was not observed in Study 2. While adaptation has been shown to occur for low frequency changes in other rat models [17,21,47], it has been found that neural populations in the rat inferior colliculus exhibit less adaptation to low frequency tones compared to high frequency tones [47].

Effects of stimulus frequency were seen for ERPs in the many standards condition (Figure 3), with increments in frequency producing larger responses (except for one frequency, 4414 Hz, which produced a larger response compared to the 5412 and 6636 Hz stimuli). As all stimuli were presented at the same intensity (70 dB$_L$), the altered responses to the different frequencies could possibly be due to the sensitivity of the rat's auditory system to different frequencies. Rats exhibit low sensitivity to tones at low frequencies (<1 kHz), but this increases with increasing frequency until peak sensitivity is reached at 8 [39] to 16 kHz [40]. The current data indicate a similar effect, with responses to the 3600 Hz stimulus being relatively low amplitude, but with responses increasing in magnitude with increasing frequency, and a peak response seen to the stimuli presented at 12233 Hz, indicating that this may be the peak sensitivity range for the rats in our study. This dramatic effect of frequency on the response to different stimuli highlights the importance of controlling for stimulus identity and only comparing deviant stimuli to their respective standards and controls of the same frequency.

4.3 Effects of the cascade control method

Deviance detection was not observed in Study 3, which used the same recording system, electrode array and animals as Study 2, but instituted a different control method, the cascade control. Such results would indicate that contrary to Study 2, Study 3 did not find evidence of 'true' adaptation-independent MMN in rats. There could be a number of reasons for this lack of replication of MMRs using this method.

Firstly, the cascade control necessitated the use of a higher frequency deviant for the ascending oddball condition, in comparison to Studies 1 and 2 (15000 Hz vs. 8137 Hz). At face value, the findings from Study 3 do not conform to the suggestion proposed above, that rats are most sensitive to increments in frequency – if this is the case, one would expect to observe evidence of deviance detection for frequency increments of 12233 to 15000 Hz. It is unlikely that the lack of deviance detection to 15000 Hz stimuli is due to a lack of auditory sensitivity to the tone, because the frequency is well within the rat's frequency sensitivity range, if not at the peak of the auditory sensitivity for the rat [40]. Indeed, this peak sensitivity may be the reason why deviance detection is not observed to tones of 15000 Hz. Study 2 results revealed that in the many standards control condition (where tones from 3600–15000 Hz were presented), by far the largest ERP amplitudes (for every recording site) were observed for stimuli presented at 12233 and 15000 Hz (Figure 3), the two frequencies used as standards and deviants respectively for the ascending oddball sequence of Study 3. Therefore, perhaps the lack of deviance detection observed for deviants of 15000 Hz can be explained by a ceiling effect: the exogenous evoked potentials to both the standard and deviant tones are so large that any deviance-associated increase in the ERP simply cannot be observed. By contrast, ERP amplitudes to frequencies used as deviants and standards in Studies 1 and 2 (6636 and 8137 Hz) sit closer to the middle of the amplitude response range to differing frequencies (Figure 3), such that any amplitude changes related to deviance or adaptation are more readily observable. If indeed a ceiling effect is occurring that 'masks' possible effects of deviance in the cascade control condition, such effects could be minimized by shifting the range of frequencies used for the cascade control condition down (e.g. 3000 Hz–9000 Hz) so that the tones used as standards and deviants are not at the peak level of auditory sensitivity for the rat. In addition, the sound intensity of stimuli could be reduced.

Secondly, while it was suggested that the wide range of stimuli used in the many standards condition may result in an overestimation of adaptation effects [33], it has also been suggested that stimuli at the extreme ends of a range in control sequences (as

used for the control deviants in the cascade control sequence) may result in control stimuli at the outer ends being perceived as deviants and again, an overestimation of adaptation in the oddball sequences [24,42]. Therefore, the use of the cascade control sequence, with the stimuli used as deviants sitting at the outer extremes of the range of stimuli, may result in an underestimation of deviance detection. This issue would be trivial in human studies, as the pattern of regularity used in the control sequence would negate this. The third explanation for why deviance detection may not have been observed using the cascade control method is therefore that it is unknown whether the pattern of regularity established by the cascade sequence can be modelled by the rat brain. If not, higher order expectations based on these more complex statistical regularities within the environment cannot be generated and therefore, the frequencies at the extremes of the cascade sequence are as unexpected as any other of the cascade frequencies. In fact, given that the extreme frequencies occur with a lower probability than other cascade frequencies (12.5% vs. 25%), in the absence of a rule that governs the cascade sequence regularity, they will appear to be aberrant (rare) and therefore generate deviance detection in their own right. In addition, without data from a flip-flop control standard being measured, it is not known whether the animals in Study 3 are even exhibiting any oddball response (a larger response to the deviant vs. the standard). The results from Study 3 therefore remain somewhat inconclusive. Future studies should include four oddball sequences for the cascade control method – the two used in the current study, as well as flip-flop controls for each of them. In addition, further examination of the cascade control, how it compares to the many standards control, and the ability of the rat brain to model such complex regularities is warranted.

4.4 Relationship of these data to MMRs in humans

The results from Study 2 revealed that MMRs (both adaptation and deviance detection) can be observed in the late, negative components, N55 and N85, which most closely resemble human MMN in their polarity (negative) and their relative latency (it is expected for ERP components to occur with a reduced latency in the rat brain [48]). However, oddball effects were also observed on earlier components such as P13 and N18 (and P30 to a lesser degree). This may seem at variance with the human MMN literature that has focussed on late effects. However, recent research has shown evidence of adaptation-independent deviance detection on human middle latency responses (MLRs). In human investigations of MMN, a bandpass filter (e.g. 0.1–35 Hz) is typically applied, which filters out early high frequency midlatency ERP components, but allows the slower MMN component to be observed. However, when a suitable bandpass filter is applied so that early ERPs can be detected (e.g. 15–200 Hz), additional MLR components can be observed [49]. These include positive peaks at approximately 12 and 30 ms (P0 and Pa) and negative peaks at approximately 22 and 40 ms (Na and Nb) [49]. Several human studies have now confirmed evidence of deviance detection in MLRs, notably Na peaking at 20 ms [50], Pa at 30 ms [51], and Nb peaking at 40 ms [49]. The bandpass filters associated with our data acquisition system permitted the detection of a series of early responses that exhibited adaptation and/or deviance detection. These early components might be homologues for the human MLR components that show deviance detection, although further research is required to support this view.

This study also highlights the importance for including controls for differential adaptation in human studies, which rarely occurs (for review, see [2]). While it is known that MMN in healthy subjects includes an adaptation-independent deviance detection component, we thus far do not know if observed reductions in MMN (for example, in patients with schizophrenia, or in subjects given NMDAR antagonists [2]), are due to reductions in adaptation or deviance detection, a very important question for future research into the functional importance of MMN in disease states [2].

4.5 The role of recording site in component amplitudes and the expression of adaptation and deviance detection

Studies 2 and 3 recorded ERPs from five separate sites over the rat cortex: over left and right auditory cortices (LAC and RAC), left and right frontal cortices (LFC and RFC) and another at the midline, similar to the vertex in human recordings (due to the bone suture at the exact midline the electrode was placed just left of the midline, LML). Marked effects of site were found for the amplitudes of all ERP components in Studies 2 and 3 (Figure S1). P13, the earliest component, was largest at the midline and auditory sites and smallest at frontal sites. This pattern of scalp topography contrasts with the later components, which were smallest at the midline site. N18 was largest at the auditory sites and the remaining later components (P30, N55 and N85) were maximal at frontal sites.

The site of the recording electrode also had a significant impact on the expression of rat MMRs for P30 and N85, but not P13, N18 and N55. MMRs were rarely observed for P30, but tended to be over the frontal cortex and auditory cortex sites, not midline sites (where P30 was smallest). Similarly, deviance detection at N85 was observed only for the sites where N85 was largest (both frontal sites and LAC site). These findings do not necessarily indicate that MMRs can only be observed at particular locations, but rather suggest that the capability of detecting statistically significant changes at a particular recording site or region is reliant on that site producing a strong signal. Since deviance detection was strongest for the N55 and N85 components, and these components are largest at frontal cortex sites, recording from frontal sites is most likely the best choice for observing human-like deviance detection in the rat.

4.6 Conclusions

This study presents a careful characterisation of different control paradigms, stimulus frequencies and recordings sites and how readily they detect MMN-like responses in the rat brain. The data presented in this study contribute to a growing body of evidence [28,29,32,34–38] supporting the conclusion that the rat brain is quite capable of producing MMRs that are similar to the human MMN and are not entirely dependent on neural adaptation but rather are in part, contributed to by a more complex deviance detection process. This model can now be used to investigate the neurobiology of both adaptation and adaptation-independent deviance detection, using different pharmacological, developmental and neurobiological manipulations.

for each region. ERPs for each of the five regions recorded from to the oddball deviant (red), the many-standards control (black) and the standard (blue) for the low (left) and high (right) frequency stimuli. All stimuli show a similar pattern with the same components (P13, N18, P30, N55 and N85).

Data S1   Mean amplitude data from Study 1. Data values are mean amplitudes (in µV) of the components N22, P37 and N80, measured in Study 1. 'High' or 'Low' in the variable name refers to whether the ERP response was to the high frequency or low frequency stimulus. 'Dev' or 'Std' refers to whether the ERP response was to a deviant or standard stimulus, respectively.

Data S2   Mean amplitude data from Study 2. Data values are mean amplitudes (in µV) of the components P13, N18, P30, N55 and N85, measured in Study 2. 'High' or 'Low' in the variable name refers to whether the ERP response was to the high frequency or low frequency stimulus. 'Con', 'Dev' or 'Std' refers to whether the ERP response was to a control, deviant or standard stimulus, respectively. 'GD' is the gestational day of saline exposure. Recording sites are identified in the variables by the following abbreviations: AvReg – "Averaged region", mean amplitude averaged over all regions; LAC, Left auditory cortex; LFC, Left frontal cortex; LML, midline (slightly to the left of); RAC, Right auditory cortex; RFC, Right frontal cortex.

Data S3   Mean amplitude data from Study 3. The data for the mean amplitudes (in µV) of each component of the ERPs from Study 3 (P13, N18, P30, N55, N85) are represented on separate sheets of the spreadsheet file. Incomplete, original data are labelled as imputation = 0, the imputed data are labelled as imputations 1–5. 'High' or 'Low' in the variable name refers to whether the ERP response was to the high frequency or low frequency stimulus. 'Con', 'Dev' or 'Std' refers to whether the ERP response was to a control, deviant or standard stimulus, respectively. 'GD' is the gestational day of saline exposure. Recording sites are identified in the variables by the following abbreviations: AvReg – "Averaged region", mean amplitude averaged over all regions; LAC, Left auditory cortex; LFC, Left frontal cortex; LML, midline (slightly to the left of); RAC, Right auditory cortex; RFC, Right frontal cortex.

Acknowledgments

We thank Tama Nakamura for Study 1 data collection and Tony Kemp, Gavin Cooper and Jason Nolan for technical assistance.

Author Contributions

Conceived and designed the experiments: PTM DMH LH WRF JT TWB MH MP US KZ. Performed the experiments: LH CM. Analyzed the data: LH WRF PTM. Contributed reagents/materials/analysis tools: WRF MP DMH PTM. Wrote the paper: LH WRF TWB MH CM MP US KZ DMH PTM.

References

1. Michie PT (2001) What has MMN revealed about the auditory system in schizophrenia? Int J Psychophysiol 42: 177–194.
2. Todd J, Harms L, Schall U, Michie PT (2013) Mismatch Negativity: Translating the Potential. Front Psychiatry 4: 171.
3. Umbricht D, Krljes S (2005) Mismatch negativity in schizophrenia: a meta-analysis. Schizophr Res 76: 1–23.
4. Näätänen R (1992). Attention and brain function. Hillsdale, NJ: Lawrence Erlbaum Associates.
5. Picton TW, Alain C, Otten L, Ritter W, Achim A (2000) Mismatch negativity: different water in the same river. Audiol Neurootol 5: 111–139.
6. Molholm S, Martinez A, Ritter W, Javitt DC, Foxe JJ (2005) The neural circuitry of pre-attentive auditory change-detection: an fMRI study of pitch and duration mismatch negativity generators. Cereb Cortex 15: 545–551.

7. Alho K (1995) Cerebral generators of mismatch negativity (MMN) and its magnetic counterpart (MMNm) elicited by sound changes. Ear Hear 16: 38–51.

8. Naatanen R, Escera C (2000) Mismatch negativity: clinical and other applications. Audiol Neurootol 5: 105–110.

9. Hari R, Hamalainen M, Ilmoniemi R, Kaukoranta E, Reinikainen K, et al. (1984) Responses of the primary auditory cortex to pitch changes in a sequence of tone pips: neuromagnetic recordings in man. Neurosci Lett 50: 127–132.

10. Rinne T, Gratton G, Fabiani M, Cowan N, Maclin E, et al. (1999) Scalp-recorded optical signals make sound processing in the auditory cortex visible? Neuroimage 10: 620–624.

11. Nelken I, Ulanovsky N (2007) Mismatch Negativity and Stimulus-Specific Adaptation in Animal Models. Journal of Psychophysiology 21: 214–223.

12. Ulanovsky N, Las L, Nelken I (2003) Processing of low-probability sounds by cortical neurons. Nat Neurosci 6: 391–398.

13. Friston K (2005) A theory of cortical responses. Philosophical Transactions of the Royal Society of London - Series B: Biological Sciences 360: 815–836.

14. Winkler I, Karmos G, Naatanen R (1996) Adaptive modeling of the unattended acoustic environment reflected in the mismatch negativity event-related potential. Brain Res 742: 239–252.

15. Fishman YI (2014) The mechanisms and meaning of the mismatch negativity. Brain Topogr 27: 500–526.

16. Eriksson J, Villa AE (2005) Event-related potentials in an auditory oddball situation in the rat. Biosystems 79: 207–212.

17. Farley BJ, Quirk MC, Doherty JJ, Christian EP (2010) Stimulus-specific adaptation in auditory cortex is an NMDA-independent process distinct from the sensory novelty encoded by the mismatch negativity. J Neurosci 30: 16475–16484.

18. Fishman YI, Steinschneider M (2012) Searching for the mismatch negativity in primary auditory cortex of the awake monkey: deviance detection or stimulus specific adaptation? J Neurosci 32: 15747–15758.

19. Maess B, Jacobsen T, Schroger E, Friederici AD (2007) Localizing pre-attentive auditory memory-based comparison: magnetic mismatch negativity to pitch change. Neuroimage 37: 561–571.

20. Opitz B, Schroger E, von Cramon DY (2005) Sensory and cognitive mechanisms for preattentive change detection in auditory cortex. Eur J Neurosci 21: 531–535.

21. Taaseh N, Yaron A, Nelken I (2011) Stimulus-specific adaptation and deviance detection in the rat auditory cortex. PLoS ONE 6: e23369.

22. Ulanovsky N, Las L, Farkas D, Nelken I (2004) Multiple time scales of adaptation in auditory cortex neurons. J Neurosci 24: 10440–10453.

23. von der Behrens W, Bauerle P, Kossl M, Gaese BH (2009) Correlating stimulus-specific adaptation of cortical neurons and local field potentials in the awake rat. J Neurosci 29: 13837–13849.

24. Jacobsen T, Schroger E (2001) Is there pre-attentive memory-based comparison of pitch? Psychophysiology 38: 723–727.

25. Jacobsen T, Schröger E (2003) Measuring duration mismtach negativity. Clin Neurophysiol 114: 1133–1143.

26. Jacobsen T, Schröger E, Horenkamp T, Winkler I (2003) Mismatch negativity to pitch change: varied stimulus proportions in controlling effects of neural refractoriness on human auditory event-related brain potentials. Neurosci Lett 344: 79–82.

27. Astikainen P, Ruusuvirta T, Wikgren J, Penttonen M (2006) Memory-based detection of rare sound feature combinations in anesthetized rats. Neuroreport 17: 1561–1564.

28. Astikainen P, Stefanics G, Nokia M, Lipponen A, Cong F, et al. (2011) Memory-based mismatch response to frequency changes in rats. PLoS ONE 6: e24208.

29. Jung F, Stephan KE, Backes H, Moran R, Gramer M, et al. (2013) Mismatch responses in the awake rat: evidence from epidural recordings of auditory cortical fields. PLoS ONE 8: e63203.

30. Grimm S, Escera C (2012) Auditory deviance detection revisited: evidence for a hierarchical novelty system. Int J Psychophysiol 85: 88–92.

31. Imada A, Morris A, Wiest MC (2012) Deviance detection by a P3-like response in rat posterior parietal cortex. Front Integr Neurosci 6: 127.

32. Shiramatsu TI, Kanzaki R, Takahashi H (2013) Cortical mapping of mismatch negativity with deviance detection property in rat. PLoS ONE 8: e82663.

33. Ruhnau P, Herrmann B, Schroger E (2012) Finding the right control: the mismatch negativity under investigation. Clin Neurophysiol 123: 507–512.

34. Ahmed M, Mallo T, Leppanen PH, Hamalainen J, Ayravainen L, et al. (2011) Mismatch brain response to speech sound changes in rats. Front Psychol 2: 283.

35. Nakamura T, Michie PT, Fulham WR, Todd J, Budd TW, et al. (2011) Epidural Auditory Event-Related Potentials in the Rat to Frequency and duration Deviants: Evidence of Mismatch Negativity? Front Psychol 2: 367.

36. Ruusuvirta T, Penttonen M, Korhonen T (1998) Auditory cortical event-related potentials to pitch deviances in rats. Neurosci Lett 248: 45–48.

37. Tikhonravov D, Neuvonen T, Pertovaara A, Savioja K, Ruusuvirta T, et al. (2008) Effects of an NMDA-receptor antagonist MK-801 on an MMN-like response recorded in anesthetized rats. Brain Res 1203: 97–102.

38. Tikhonravov D, Neuvonen T, Pertovaara A, Savioja K, Ruusuvirta T, et al. (2010) Dose-related effects of memantine on a mismatch negativity-like response in anesthetized rats. Neuroscience 167: 1175–1182.

39. Kelly JB, Masterton B (1977) Auditory sensitivity of the albino rat. J Comp Physiol Psychol 91: 930–936.

40. Mazurek B, Haupt H, Joachim R, Klapp BF, Stover T, et al. (2010) Stress induces transient auditory hypersensitivity in rats. Hear Res 259: 55–63.

41. Alho K, Woods DL, Algazi A, Knight RT, Naatanen R (1994) Lesions of frontal cortex diminish the auditory mismatch negativity. Electroencephalogr Clin Neurophysiol 91: 353–362.

42. Winkler I, Paavilainen P, Alho K, Reinikainen K, Sams M, et al. (1990) The effect of small variation of the frequent auditory stimulus on the event-related brain potential to the infrequent stimulus. Psychophysiology 27: 228–235.

43. Fulham WR (2012) EEG Display. 6.3.12 ed. Newcastle, Australia: The University of Newcastle.

44. Brudzynski SM (2013) Ethotransmission: communication of emotional states through ultrasonic vocalization in rats. Curr Opin Neurobiol 23: 310–317.

45. Peter V, McArthur G, Thompson WF (2010) Effect of deviance direction and calculation method on duration and frequency mismatch negativity (MMN). Neurosci Lett 482: 71–75.

46. Pratt H, Starr A, Michalewski HJ, Dimitrijevic A, Bleich N, et al. (2009) Auditory-evoked potentials to frequency increase and decrease of high- and low-frequency tones. Clin Neurophysiol 120: 360–373.

47. Duque D, Perez-Gonzalez D, Ayala YA, Palmer AR, Malmierca MS (2012) Topographic distribution, frequency, and intensity dependence of stimulus-specific adaptation in the inferior colliculus of the rat. J Neurosci 32: 17762–17774.

48. Bickel S, Javitt DC (2009) Neurophysiological and neurochemical animal models of schizophrenia: focus on glutamate. Behav Brain Res 204: 352–362.

49. Grimm S, Escera C, Slabu L, Costa-Faidella J (2011) Electrophysiological evidence for the hierarchical organization of auditory change detection in the human brain. Psychophysiology 48: 377–384.

50. Grimm S, Recasens M, Althen H, Escera C (2012) Ultrafast tracking of sound location changes as revealed by human auditory evoked potentials. Biol Psychol 89: 232–239.

51. Slabu L, Escera C, Grimm S, Costa-Faidella J (2010) Early change detection in humans as revealed by auditory brainstem and middle-latency evoked potentials. Eur J Neurosci 32: 859–865.

8

Upregulation of GPR109A in Parkinson's Disease

Chandramohan Wakade[1]*, Raymond Chong[1]*, Eric Bradley[1], Bobby Thomas[2], John Morgan[3]

1 Department of Physical Therapy, Georgia Regents University, Augusta, Georgia, United States of America, **2** Department of Pharmacology & Toxicology and Neurology, Georgia Regents University, Augusta, Georgia, United States of America, **3** Department of Neurology, Georgia Regents University, Augusta, Georgia, United States of America

Abstract

Background: Anecdotal animal and human studies have implicated the symptomatic and neuroprotective roles of niacin in Parkinson's disease (PD). Niacin has a high affinity for GPR109A, an anti-inflammatory receptor. Niacin is also thought to be involved in the regulation of circadian rhythm. Here we evaluated the relationships among the receptor, niacin levels and EEG night-sleep in individuals with PD.

Methods and Findings: GPR109A expression (blood and brain), niacin index (NAD-NADP ratio) and cytokine markers (blood) were analyzed. Measures of night-sleep function (EEG) and perceived sleep quality (questionnaire) were assessed. We observed significant up-regulation of GPR109A expression in the blood as well as in the substantia nigra (SN) in the PD group compared to age-matched controls. Confocal microscopy demonstrated co-localization of GPR109A staining with microglia in PD SN. Pro and anti-inflammatory cytokines did not show significant differences between the groups; however IL1-β, IL-4 and IL-7 showed an upward trend in PD. Time to sleep (sleep latency), EEG REM and sleep efficiency were different between PD and age-matched controls. Niacin levels were lower in PD and were associated with increased frequency of experiencing body pain and decreased duration of deep sleep.

Conclusions: The findings of associations among the GPR109A receptor, niacin levels and night-sleep function in individuals with PD are novel. Further studies are needed to understand the pathophysiological mechanisms of action of niacin, GPR109A expression and their associations with night-sleep function. It would be also crucial to study GPR109A expression in neurons, astrocytes, and microglia in PD. A clinical trial to determine the symptomatic and/or neuroprotective effect of niacin supplementation is warranted.

Editor: Michelle L. Block, Indiana School of Medicine, United States of America

Funding: The National Parkinson's Foundation, CSRA Augusta chapter provided the funding for this study (20000-01080000-12100-64076-PSG00028) and the NIH grant NS060885 paid for the human brain samples which were obtained from the NICHD Brain and Tissue Bank University of Maryland School of Medicine. The funders had no role in study design, data collection and analysis, decision to publish, or preparation of the manuscript.

Competing Interests: The authors have declared that no competing interests exist.

* Email: cwakade@gru.edu (CW); rchong@gru.edu (RC)

Introduction

Inflammation is thought to play a central role in Parkinson's disease (PD) pathology [1]. After the initial report that demonstrated the presence of microglia in the substantia nigra in post mortem samples [2], further research have demonstrated the role of activated microglia and cytokines in clinical and animal studies [3]. In addition, the use of non-aspirin non-steroidal anti-inflammatory drugs was found to reduce the risk of PD [4].

GPR109A (also known as hydroxycarboxylic acid receptor 2 (HCAR2), niacin receptor 1 (NIACR1), HM74a in humans and PUMA-G in mice) is a G protein-coupled anti-inflammatory receptor. It is present in macrophages and neutrophils, at higher levels of expression than other human organs and tissues [5]. Its anti-inflammatory role is well-established in in-vivo and in-vitro studies [6–9]. The physiological ligand of GPR109A is beta-hydroxy butyrate (BHB). However, BHB levels are generally not high enough in inflammatory conditions to elicit an anti-inflammatory response. GPR109A has a high affinity for niacin

(also known as vitamin B3 or nicotinic acid) which also acts as its agonists and help suppress inflammation [10,11]. We propose that GPR109A is a crucial part of the chronic inflammation and microglia activation in PD in the substantia nigra and this inflammatory state correlates with GPR109A levels in the blood macrophages. Although macrophages are crucial in inflammation [12–14], it remains unknown how they engage and remain engaged with microglia in PD. GPR109A up-regulation both in macrophages and microglia is an indication for anti-inflammatory therapy. Niacin supplementation may reduce the participation of these activated microglia and macrophages in ongoing neuroinflammation.

Niacin is a precursor of nicotinamide adenine dinucleotide (NAD) that is regulated by the oscillating sleep-wake circadian cycle, thereby influencing the oxidative pathways in the mitochondria [15]. Impaired NAD levels may thus be negatively impacted by abnormal sleep function and/or low niacin levels [16–19]. As a pharmacologic ligand, Niacin but not nicotinamide, acts through GPR109A. However, the dose of niacin as a vitamin supplement (and precursor of nicotinamide and NAD) is much less than what is needed to affect GPR109A as an anti-inflammatory agent.

It is plausible to visualize the effects of neuroinflammation systemically in PD because the blood brain barrier is compromised. Cytokines such as interferon gamma are known to stimulate GPR109A in murine macrophages, producing a pro-inflammatory cascade of events. GPR109A agonists, in contrast, suppress lipopolysaccharide (LPS)-induced inflammation via nuclear factor-κB (NFkB) pathway in the gut. GPR109A is present in a variety of human tissues including the brain. GPR109A plays an anti-inflammatory role in the retinal pigment epithelium [20]. BHB is used by neurons as an alternative energy source and was shown to be protective in mesencephalic neurons against 1-methyl-4-phenylpyridinium (MPP+) toxicity [21]. It should be noted that this effect of BHB is attributed to mitochondrial energy generation and likely to be independent of GPR109A. The role of GPR109A in neurological diseases has never been established. Here we demonstrate for the first time, evidence of elevated GPR109A levels and decreased niacin levels in PD patients compared to age-matched controls and their associations with night-sleep function.

Methods

Subjects

Fifty-seven subjects participated in the study approved by the Institution's review board. Twelve subjects were in the Young control group (6 men, 25 ± 1 years old) and 23 in the age-matched control group (13 men, 69 ± 7 years old). The remaining 22 subjects were individuals diagnosed with idiopathic PD [22] (15 men, 71 ± 8 years old, duration of disease $= 10 \pm 6$ years, H&Y $= 2.3 \pm 0.7$, median $= 2$).

Ethics

Participants gave written informed consent under protocols approved by the Institutional Review Boards of the Georgia Regents University. Lab personnel accessed only de-identified data.

Blood sample collection

Subjects who took any form of over-the-counter anti-inflammatory drugs and/or vitamin B3 supplement were instructed to skip them for at least 48 hours before the morning blood draw. No subject was taking high-dose pain prescription drugs at the time of the study. Approximately 8 ml of whole blood was collected from the subjects in purple-top ethylenediaminetetraacetic acid (EDTA) tubes and kept on ice. Whole blood was spun at $2,000 \times g$ for 15 minutes in 15 ml tubes. Plasma was separated and stored at $-80°C$. White blood cells (WBCs) were then collected and placed into fresh tubes, re-suspended in phosphate buffered saline (PBS) and spun at $300 \times g$ for 10 minutes. RBCs were collected and stored at $-80°C$. Supernatant was suctioned out from WBCs. One ml of ACK Lysing Buffer (Lonza cat # 10-548E) was added to the WBC pellet to lyse any existing RBCs and spun again at $300 \times g$ for 10 minutes. Supernatant was discarded from the clean WBC pellet. 200 μl of PBS was used to re-suspend the WBCs and aliquots of 50 μl were then stored at $-80°C$ until further analyses.

Western blot analysis

Western blotting was performed as detailed by Wakade et al. [23]. WBCs were lysed using Sample Buffer Laemmli 2x Concentrate (Sigma-Aldrich Cat # S3401). Samples were vortexed and heated to $100°C$ for 10 minutes and centrifuged at 14,000 RPM to collect undissolved material. Protein was measured using RC DC Protein Assay Kit (BioRad Cat # 500-0122) according to the manufacturer's guidelines. An equal amount of protein was loaded for each sample based on concentration into 10% Mini-Protean TGX Precast Gels (BioRad Cat # 456-1036). Samples were run on the gel for 10 minutes at 80 V for and then 50 minutes at 100 V for the length of the gel. Then samples were transferred to nitrocellulose membrane for 1 hour at 100 V. Blots were then blocked with 5% dry milk solution in TBST for 1 hour. Primary antibody from HM74/GPR109A (Bioworld Technologies Cat # BS2605) was then added in fresh 5% dry milk solution in a 1:1000 ratio and incubated overnight. Blots were washed three times for 5 minutes each in TBST. HRP-conjugated goat anti-rabbit secondary antibody (Jackson Immuno Research Cat # 111-035-003) was diluted in a 1:1000 ratio in fresh 5% dry milk TBST solution and incubated for 1 hour at room temperature. Blots were then washed three times with TBST for 5 minutes. HRP was detected using GE Amersham ECL western blotting detection reagent (GE Amersham Cat # RPN2106) on autoradiography film (Denville Scientific Cat # E3012). Primary antibody for b-Actin (Sigma-Aldrich Cat # A5441) was used to confirm loading equality.

GPR109A analyses

White blood cells (WBCs) from PD patients and controls were used to probe for GPR109A expression. Cell lysates were prepared as described above and protein levels were estimated. GPR109A protein was probed using the antibody from Bioworld Technologies.

Niacin index

Niacin index is calculated as NAD/NADP X 100. RBCs were lysed as described in the Methods outlined in the following kit manuals. To obtain the niacin index (NAD/NADP), the NAD/NADH quantification kit (Sigma-Aldrich Cat # MAK037) and NADP/NADPH quantitation kit (Sigma-Aldrich Cat # MAK038) were used in tandem. 10 μl of RBC samples were used for each kit according to manufacturer's guidelines in a 96-well plate with included standards. Samples were filtered using a 10 kda MW cut off spin filter (ABCAM Cat # ab93349) spun at $20,000 \times g$ for 30 minutes. All colorimetric detection were accomplished using spectrophotometer absorbance at $A = 450$ nm. The niacin index and the NAD/NADH ratio were then calculated for each sample.

Total plasma metabolites by HPLC/MS

Fasting blood samples were collected in the purple-top EDTA tubes from nine PD patients and nine age-matched controls ($N = 18$). Plasma portions were separated and analyzed for niacin metabolites (nicotinic acid, niacinamide and niacinuric acid). Samples were then sent to NMS Labs with a decoder. Detection level was set to 10 ng/ml for each metabolite; less than 10 ng/ml were not detected. The quantitative analysis for niacin and metabolites was performed at NMS Labs (Willow Grove, PA) using LC-MS/MS, liquid chromatography with tandem mass spectrometer detector. Twenty-five μl of deuterated internal standard was added to 0.20 ml aliquot of serum/plasma samples. Samples were pH-adjusted and extracted by solid phase extraction where samples were eluted with basic methanol, dried, and reconstituted with formic acid in water solution, and transferred to vials for instrumental analysis. Analysis was performed on Waters ACQUITY LC system with an Aquasil C18, 2.1×100 mm, 5.0 micron, part number 77505-102130, or equivalent USP L1 column, and TQ MS/MS detector. Quantitation was achieved by monitoring two transition ions following LC separation with positive-ion electrospray tandem mass spectrometry (LC-MS/MS) for each analyte and standard. Each analytical run was independently calibrated at concentrations of 10, 20, 50, 100, 400 and 500 ng/ml. Two levels of control were run in each analytical batch. This LC-MS/MS method has a LLOQ of 10 ng/ml and current between run % CV of 11.40%, and 6.59% at 20 and 400 ng/ml, respectively for nicotinic acid, % CV of 5.61%, and 6.00% at 20 and 400 ng/ml, respectively for nicotinamide, and % CV of 11.40%, and 6.00% at 20 and 400 ng/ml, respectively for nicotinuric acid.

Beta-hydroxybutyrate (BHB) analyses

Serum samples were filtered using a 10 kda MW cut-off spin filter(ABCAM Cat # ab93349) spun at 14,000 RPM for 30 minutes. BHB was detected on a 96-well plate according to manufacturer's guidelines (BHB Assay Kit, ABCAM, cat # ab83390).

Night-sleep EEG test

A subset of 28 subjects from the blood experiment participated in the overnight EEG sleep study: 12 in the Young group (6 men, 25 ± 1 years old), nine in the Older age-matched control group and (one man, 68 ± 6 years old) and seven in the PD group (six men, 73 ± 5 years old, median H&Y = 2). PD subjects' disease profiles are summarized in Table 1. The Older group comprised mostly live-in spouses of the PD subjects in order to warrant comparable dietary intake and sleep environment. Worse motor symptoms were strongly associated with rating of disease severity and increased prescription of Carbidopa.

The Zeo portable sleep EEG monitor was used to assess the quality of night-sleep. It is a validated, unobtrusive, easy and convenient dry wireless 2-channel EEG system. The monitor is embedded in a headband which contains a lightweight recharge-able battery that lasts 16 hours on a full charge. Subjects wore the headband to sleep on the night after the morning blood draw in

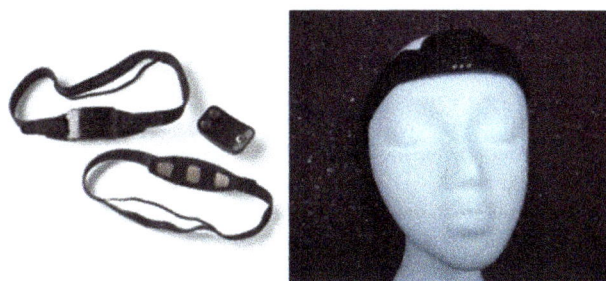

Figure 1. Illustration of the EEG sleep monitor.

which the activities of the day was considered to be routine, i.e. not unduly tired and not preparing or returning from a long trip (Figure 1). The headband has a 12-bit analog-to-digital converter that samples EEG signals at 128 Hz and filters with a second order band-pass of 2–47 Hz. The processed signal was then transmitted via a 2.4 GHz wireless protocol to a receiver station (typically placed on the nightstand). Numeric and graphical results were automatically generated which provided details of the sleep including time to fall asleep, number of times awoken during sleep, and time during dream sleep (REM) and deep sleep. Sleep efficiency (refreshing versus disruptive sleep) were then derived. Sleep efficiency was calculated as the ratio of actual time spent sleeping divided by the total attempted sleep, which is the sum of time taken to fall asleep + actual sleep + time spent awake during night-sleep multiplied by 100. A low percentage value is undesirable because it indicates that the subject either took a long time to fall asleep, awoke in the middle of the night-sleep for a relatively long duration, or both. On the other hand, a high percentage value is desirable as it indicates that the subject fell asleep relatively quickly and did not or rarely woke up in the middle of the night.

Table 1. PD characteristics.

	Mean ± SD	Range
Age (years)	73±5	66–80
Disease duration (years)	8±7	2–22
UPDRS total	29±19	7–55.5
UPDRS brady	6±5	0–15.5
H&Y	2.4±1.0	1–4
MMSE	28±2	23–30
PDQ total	12±7	4–25
RAPID1	5±4	1–12
RAPID2	5±3	1–10
RAPID3	21±33	0–90
Symptoms rating	8±3	1–10

UPDRS total, sum of section 3 of the Unified PD Rating Scale [62].
UPDRS brady, sum of UPDRS section 3 last five items assessing body bradykinesia [26].
H&Y, Hoehn & Yahr disease rating scale [63].
MMSE, mini-mental status examination [64].
PDQ total, sum of PD Quality of Life questionnaire [65,66].
RAPID1 (Rapid Assessment of Postural Instability in PD item 1), difficulty in performing activities of daily living (0 = no difficulty; 1 = difficulty) [67,68].
RAPID2, fear of falling (ranging from 1 = "no fear" to 10 "very fearful").
RAPID3, number of falls over the last three months (including near falls).
Symptoms rating, self-reported rating of PD symptoms, ranging from 1 to 10: 1 = "very bad day" - symptoms are the worse compared to a typical day; 10 = "very good day" - symptoms are absent or minimal compared to a typical day).

Scoring the individual's sleep stages was based on analyzing each 2-second interval using a 2-minute moving average smoothing algorithm. The resulting signal that contained the majority of a particular sleep stage every 30 seconds was reported. The wireless system has been shown to have excellent overall agreement in scoring the various sleep states when compared to the 'gold standard' described by Rechtschaffen and Kales in 1968 [24]. The validity of the EEG sleep monitor in scoring the various sleep stages has been compared to a polysomnography in a sleep laboratory. The percent agreement between the two methods was found to range between 74.7% and 95.8%.

Statistics

A two-sample multivariate t-test (Hotelling's T-square) was used to analyze for differences among the NAD/NADH ratio, NAD/NADP ratio, GPR109A and BHB levels between the Older and PD groups. EEG sleep data were analyzed with 1-way ANOVA followed by Tukey's test for significant main effects. Cohen's d was used to determine the effect size for significant results [25]. The Spearman correlation test was also used to determine the associations among the PD subjects' disease profiles, NAD/NADH ratio, NAD/NADP ratio, GPR109A, BHB levels, sleep function and quality of life. Data from the Young group are shown to enable visualization of normative values and were not included in the multivariate or correlation analyses. $p < 0.05$ was considered to be statistically significant for all analyses.

Results

GPR109A, NAD/NADH and BHB analyses

The correlations among the blood dependent variables (NAD/NADH ratio, GPR109A and BHB) for the combined Older age-matched control and PD data ranged from -0.125 to 0.205 ($p > 0.05$). The Group main effect was significant, Wilks's lambda $= 0.729$, F $(3, 42) = 5.20$, $p = 0.0038$. Follow-up discriminant function and univariate analyses revealed that GPR109A was the most sensitive variable in differentiating the PD group from the Older age-matched control group (total-sample standardized canonical co-efficient $= 0.92$), followed by NAD/NADH (-0.75) and BHB (0.36). The 1-tailed univariate analyses corroborated the discriminant function for GPR109A ($p = 0.009$, $d = 0.68$), NAD/NADH ($p = 0.033$, $d = 0.50$) and BHB ($p = 0.072$, $d = 0.48$).

Within the PD group, NAD/NADH levels were positively correlated with BHB levels ($r = 0.943$, $p = 0.017$).

A representative western blot of GPR109A is shown in figure 2A. The GPR109A was detected at around 45 KD. The densitometry scan shown in figure 2B demonstrates the relative densities of the western blot bands. Twenty out of 22 PD subjects showed up-regulation of GPR109A ($p = 0.009$ between the Older age-match control and PD groups). This may indicate either an active and/or chronic inflammatory state. Whether this is reflective of neuroinflammation is speculative at this point. Beta-actin was used as the housekeeping protein.

The NAD/NADH ratio was significantly reduced in the PD group compared to the Older age-matched controls ($p = 0.033$). Reduced NAD indicates poor mitochondrial function, lethargic Kreb's cycle and/or increased oxidative state (Figure 2C).

A trend approaching significance in increased levels of BHB in the plasma of PD patients compared to age-matched controls was observed ($p = 0.071$, Figure 2D). BHB is known to fluctuate in a variety of conditions including starvation, diabetes mellitus and other co-morbidities.

The strength of association between the independent variable (Group) and the linear combination of the dependent variables,

eta-squared η^2 was 0.27, indicating that 27% variance in the dependent variables (NAD/NADH ratio, GPR109A and BHB) was attributed to group differences.

Reduced niacin index (NAD/NADP ratio) in RBCs

We observed that NAD/NADP ratio was reduced in the PD group compared to the Older age-matched controls ($p = 0.038$). (Figure 3A).

Total plasma metabolites by HPLC/MS

Fasting blood samples in the PD group demonstrated lower total niacin metabolites (nicotinic acid, niacinamide and niacinuric acid) than their age-matched controls. ($p = 0.025$). The majority of the samples did not detect nicotinic acid and nicotinuric acid (Figure 3B).

Increased expression of GPR109A in the substantia nigra of PD brains

We demonstrate here for the first time the up-regulation of GPR109A in the substantia nigra of PD patients compared to the Older age-matched controls (Figure 4). Three out of the four PD patients showed robust increase in GPR109A expression. Patient PD1 showed an outlier GPR109A level (Grubb's critical Z = 1.48, $p < 0.05$). It is possible that the GPR109A was degraded. It is also possible that the patient was taking niacin supplements or anti-inflammatory drugs. The medical records of these individuals are no longer available.

Co-localization of GPR109A and microglia in PD and control brain

Paraffin embedded brain human samples (post-mortem) 20 µm in thickness were stained for GPR109A and microglia. Confocal microscopy images showed that the majority of the microglial marker, CD11b (green) were co-localized with GPR109A (red). Control samples showed less microglia and GPR109A+ cells. Note that in the control samples, not all the GPR109+ cells were co-localized with the CD11b maker. Few neuronal nuclei (blue) are seen (Figure 5).

Sleep quality

Compared to the Older age-matched group, PD subjects had decreased sleep efficiency. They slept less hours, and spent less than half the amount of time in REM and light sleep (Figure 6). As a percentage of sleep time, the groups were similar. The more severe the level of bradykinesia, the longer it took them to fall asleep ($r = -0.76$, $p = 0.028$).

Severity of body bradykinesia [26] captured problems with quality of life and sleep function better than overall motor symptom assessment. Worse bradykinesia were associated with less duration of actual night-sleep, increased difficulty with activities of daily living, fear of falling, feeling of depression, higher frequencies of painful muscle cramps, restlessness of legs and higher frequency of falls (Table 2).

Association between quality of night-sleep and blood analyses

The PD characteristics and sleep correlation analyses are summarized Table 1 and 2 respectively. Higher BHB levels were marginally associated with higher NAD/NADH ratios ($r = 0.750$, $p = 0.066$). Lower NAD/NADH ratio and BHB levels were associated with higher frequency of painful muscle cramps in the extremities and higher frequency of painful posturing of the extremities. Conversely, higher NAD/NADH levels were

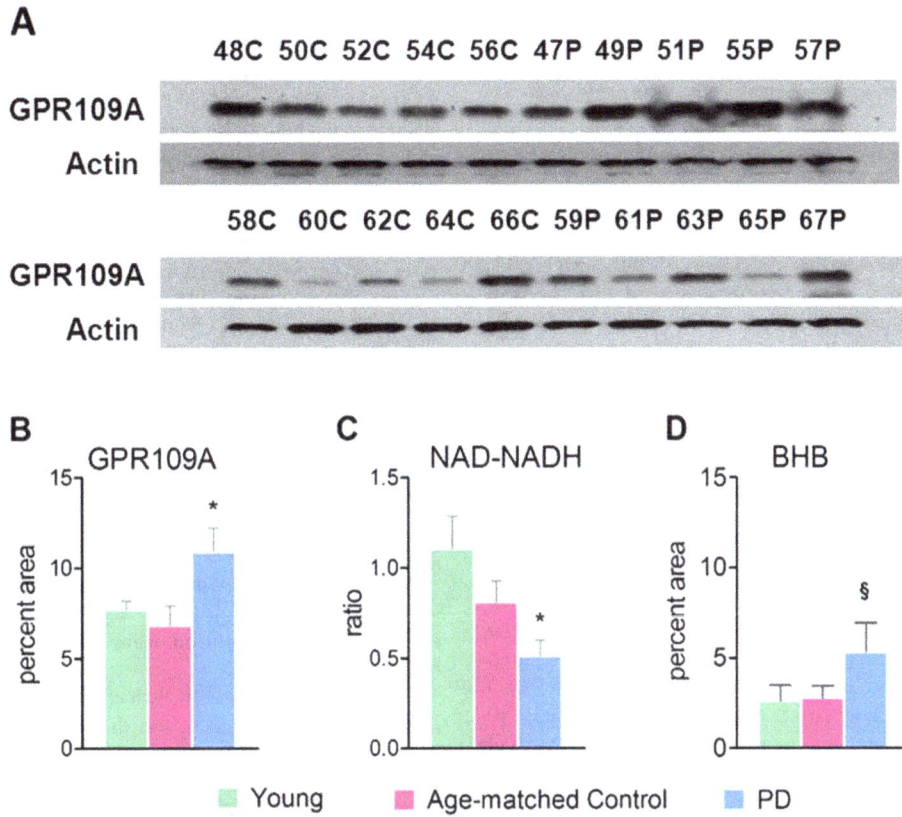

Figure 2. GPR109A expression, NAD/NADH ratio and BHB levels in blood. (A) Representative GPR109A western blots (B) GPR109A densitometry, (C) NAD/NADH ratio and (D) BHB levels. GPR109A expression and NAD/NADH ratio were tested in the WBCs. The BHB levels were tested in the sera. Young, n = 6; Older, n = 23, PD, n = 22. $*p = 0.009$ between Age-matched control and PD groups. $**p = 0.033$ between Age-matched control and PD groups. $§p = 0.071$ between Age-matched control and PD groups.

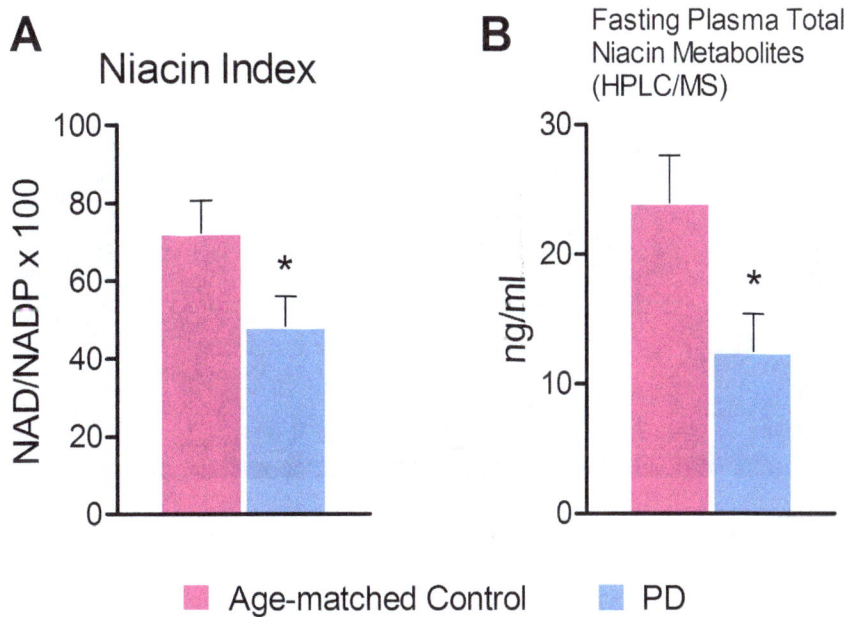

Figure 3. A, Reduced Niacin index (NAD/NADP ratio) in RBCs and B, Total plasma metabolites by HPLC/MS. A. NAD/NADP ratio was significantly reduced in the PD patients compared to age-matched controls (n = 18, p = 0.038). B. Total niacin metabolites from PD patient's samples were significantly lower than that of their age-matched controls (p = 0.025). This data is in unison with our niacin factor (NAD/NDAP ratio) data.

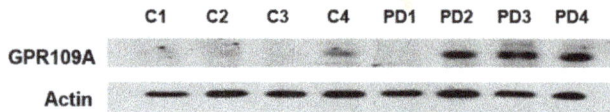

Figure 4. Up-regulation of GPR109A in the substantia nigra of PD patients.

associated with a longer duration of deep sleep while higher levels of BHB were associated with lower frequency of tiredness and sleepiness in the morning (Table 3).

Discussion

Role of GPR 109A and PD

We are the first to report here the up-regulation of GPR109A expression in the blood and the substantia nigra of PD patients. It is an additional indication of an ongoing inflammatory process in PD, and potentially opens novel avenues of detection and treatment [27,28]. Up-regulation of GPR109A in the WBCs and microglia (substantia nigra) of PD patients suggests the need for GPR109A agonist therapy such as niacin. It is possible that different dosages and durations of niacin therapy will be required in combatting inflammation via GPR109A and increase NAD levels to boost anti-oxidative mechanisms. Although it remains to be seen whether niacin supplementation or other agonists of GPR109A help ameliorate PD symptoms, we have demonstrated a novel proof of concept which warrants further investigation. A "cross-talk" between peripheral macrophages and CNS microglia may be pivotal in keeping the neuroinflammation ongoing. GPR109A may play an important role in this crosstalk.

Niacin index (NAD/NADP ratio) and PD

NAD/NADP ratio in erythrocytes is an indirect way to indicate the niacin index in the body. Altered NAD/NADP ratio has been implicated in pellagra and other neurological conditions. These

levels are also known (especially NAD) to respond to niacin treatment. There are multiple roles of NAD in cellular metabolism. It's a critical co-enzyme for three rate limiting steps in the TCA cycle. The role of NAD in the longevity of mitochondria and efficient mitochondrial function through silent information regulator 2 (SIRT2) pathway has been shown [29,30]. Other studies have also raised the potential therapeutic role of other NAD precursors [31–33]. Exogenous application of NAD precursors, such as nicotinic acid mononucleotide, nicotinamide mononucleotide, and nicotinamide riboside protected against axonal degeneration after axotomy [34]. These studies suggest that maintenance of cellular bioenergetic homeostasis and NAD levels are crucial to support the NAD-dependent enzymes, such as enhancing SIRT1 activities, and for protection against excitotoxicity [32]. Altered NAD-NADP ratio (niacin index) has been implicated in ATP depletion and mitochondrial dysfunction, causing aging [35–37] and neuronal death in neurodegenerative diseases like PD [32].

Sleep disorders in PD

NAD levels are shown to couple mitochondrial bioenergetics with light-dark cycle in mice [15]. Lower NAD levels were associated with impaired mitochondrial function in clock mutant mice.

REM sleep, the majority of which takes place in the later part of night-sleep, was reduced by less than half the duration of that in the Older controls. It has been suggested that this phase of night-sleep may be an important non-motor symptom of PD including those in the early stages of the disease [38–41]. The disordered REM phase is manifested in the lack of inhibition of the neuromuscular system. However, patients may not always experience daytime sleepiness. It is possible that the night-sleep disruptions are not severe enough [42] and therefore patients may not seek medical advice. REM abnormalities may thus be under-reported [43].

Although it is well-known that many PD patients have abnormal REM sleep patterns, our study also indicates that they

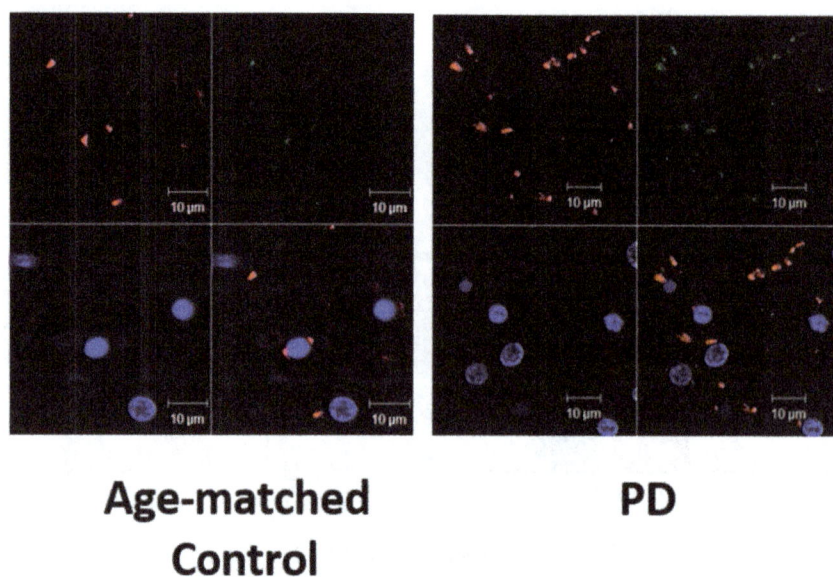

Age-matched Control   **PD**

Figure 5. Co-localization of GPR109A and microglia in PD and control brain. Confocal microscopy image of SN of human brain samples showing the glial marker, CD11b (green) co-localized with GPR109A (red). Control sample shows less microglia and GPR109A + cells. Note that all the GPR109+ cells are not co-localized with CD11b maker in control sample. Few neuronal Nuclei (blue) are seen.

Table 2. Subject characteristics.

	UPDRS total	UPDRS brady
UPDRS total		
UPDRS brady	0.893	
H&Y	0.982	0.873
Sleep4	−0.891	−0.746
PDQ1	0.899	0.973
PDQ3	0.879	0.805
PDQ7	0.786	0.879
PDQ total	0.821	0.786
Times woken	-	−0.771
Actual sleep (min)	-	−0.821
Light sleep (min)	-	−0.821
Carbidopa (mg/day)	0.973	0.826
RAPID1	-	0.901
RAPID2	-	0.821
RAPID3	-	0.778

Values represent good to excellent coefficient of correlations ($p<0.05$ for all). Empty cells indicate moderate or low correlations ($p>0.05$).
Abbreviations are the same as Table 1.
*Sleep4 (PD Sleep questionnaire item 4), restlessness of legs or arms at night or in the evening causing disruption of sleep [69].
§PDQ1 (PD Quality of Life questionnaire item 1), difficulty getting around in public.
§PDQ3, feeling depressed.
§PDQ7, painful muscle cramps or spasms.
Times woken, number of times woken during EEG night-sleep assessment.
Actual sleep, sum of EEG light sleep, deep sleep and REM sleep durations.
Carbidopa, prescribed with dopamine (as Sinemet) to minimize breakdown of levodopa before it crosses the blood brain barrier.
*High scores indicate less problems.
§High scores indicate more problems.

do not get enough of it as well. Abnormal REM sleep combined with inadequate deep sleep in subjects with low levels of niacin produced an overall low quality of night-sleep.

Relationship between decreased niacin levels, body pain and abnormal sleep in PD

Our discovery of the associations between niacin deficiency and frequent pain in the body and decreased sleep efficiency in PD are novel. These associations may be related to loss of nuclear SIRT1 activities, which is known to produce abnormal sleep cycles [44].

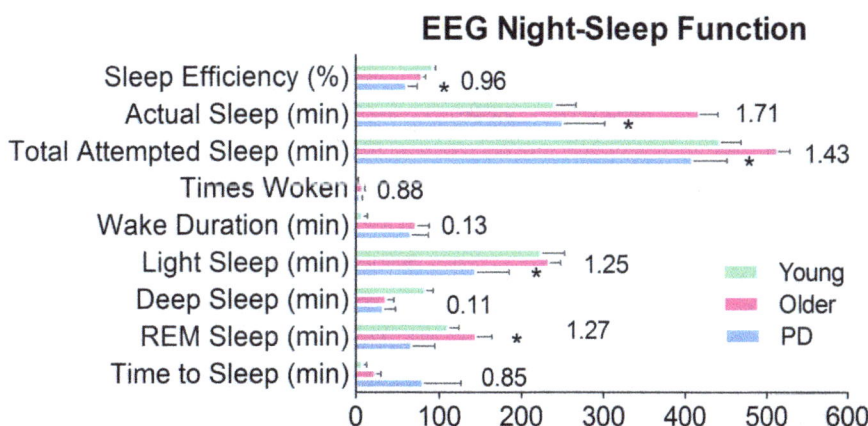

Figure 6. Sleep in PD. Sleep Efficiency, ratio of actual sleep divided by total attempted sleep. Actual Sleep, total duration spent sleeping (not including Wake and Time to Z). Total Attempted Sleep, from time to bed to morning rise. Times Woken, number of times subject awaken during night-sleep. Wake Duration, total duration of time spent awake during night-sleep. Light Sleep, light sleep stage. Deep Sleep, deep sleep stage. REM Sleep, rapid eye movement sleep stage. Time to Sleep, the time it takes to fall asleep (a.k.a. sleep latency). *$p<0.05$ between the PD and Older groups. (Young group's data are shown in order to visualize normative values.) Numbers are the effect sizes between the Older and PD groups, based on Cohen's d using averaged standard deviation [25].

Table 3. Associations among PD NAD/NADH ratio, GPR109A, BHB and sleep quality.

	NAD/NADH	GPR109A	BHB
Sleep11	0.793	-	0.901
Sleep12	0.775	-	0.955
Sleep14	-	-	0.927
EEG deep sleep (min)	0.786	-0.75	-

Values represent good to excellent coefficient of correlations (p<0.05 for all). Empty cells indicate moderate or low correlations (p>0.05).
*Sleep11, painful muscle cramps in arms or legs while sleeping at night.
*Sleep12, wake up early in the morning with painful posturing of arms or legs.
*Sleep14, feel tired and sleepy after waking in the morning.
*High scores indicate less problems.

Treatment of moderately old mice (first-phase OXPHOS defects) with nicotinamide mononucleotide (NMN) (NAD precursor) increased oxidative phosphorylation activity and other markers of mitochondrial function in the skeletal muscle within one week without altering muscle strength [45]. The cellular mechanisms of how low NAD levels are associated with sleep disorders in the development and progression of PD remains to be determined [46–49].

General discussion: GPR 109A agonists for reduction of inflammation

There are multiple agonists of GPR109A that might be useful as anti-inflammatory agents, including BHB, niacin, and Na butyrate [50]. Alisky et al. [51] reported an account of a man with PD who was initially given 500 mg of niacin daily to treat his high triglyceride level. The treatment appeared to work and a higher dose of 1000 mg was subsequently attempted. Three months later, during a follow-up primary care visit, the patient's family reported an unexpected positive side-effect of the niacin treatment in the form of an increase in his physical functioning. They included the ability to rise from a chair (which he previously was unable to do without assistance) and being able to walk faster (which he previously was very slow to execute due to freezing). These improvements were thought to be attributed to a noticeable decrease in his rigidity and bradykinesia, the classical symptoms of PD. The niacin dosing however, was too high, which may explain the nightmares and skin reactions. A lower dose that can elicit similar symptomatic relief without side effects would be noteworthy [28]. It needs to be further clarified whether the above-mentioned effect of niacin was due to its metabolic effects or its effects on GPR109A or the combination thereof.

Similarly, two case-control studies found that those who consumed a niacin-rich diet had a decreased risk of developing the disease, after correcting for occupational and environmental factors [52]. In addition, the carbidopa medication that PD patients take depletes niacin levels in the body [53]. Thus, niacin depletion may worsen PD prognosis.

The neuroprotective role of niacinamide is documented in MPTP and other models of PD in mice [54,55]. The role of NAD, decreased apoptosis (by blocking PARP pathway), decreased oxidative stress and inhibition of NOS have been implicated as possible mechanisms involved in neuroprotection by niacinamide [32]. Niacin has been shown to be neuroprotective in animal

stroke models [56]. Niacin was thought to be involved in vascular and axonal remodeling of the animals. However, there is no published data that demonstrates the neuroprotection of niacin in any PD animal model. Both niacin and niacinamide are sources of NAD. Niacin but not niacinamide acts as an agonist of GPR109A. Therefore, although both niacin and niacinamide are neuroprotective, their mechanisms appear to be different. Multiple second messenger pathways are associated with GPR109A which are helpful for cell survival. Their pathways and cell types involved in PD pathology are still unknown.

Butyrates (GPR109A agonists) are also known to inhibit inflammation through inhibiting NFκB in Crohn's disease [57]. Butyrates decrease pro-inflammatory cytokine (TNFα, IL-6 and IL-1β) expression via inhibition of NFκB activation and IκB degradation [58]. Butyrates also inhibit NFκB activation via GPR109A and increases IκB levels in-vitro in intestinal epithelial cell lines [59].

It would be interesting to see if and how up-regulation of GPR109A modulates the homing of microglia in the substantia nigra. GPR109A appears to be a new plausible prognostic marker and a pharmaceutical target in the treatment of PD. Niacin supplementation may not only serve as an anti-inflammatory agent but also replenishes NAD levels which are essential for healthy mitochondrial function as well as dopamine synthesis [60,61]. The effects of niacin on the NAD/NADH ratio, GPR109A levels and functional recovery in PD patients need to be studied in a clinical trial with tight control on drug intake and dietary habits [28].

Acknowledgments

We thank 1) the National Parkinson's Foundation, CSRA Augusta chapter for funding the study, 2) the NICHD Brain and Tissue Bank University of Maryland School of Medicine and the New York Brain Bank at Columbia University for the human brain samples. NIH grant NS060885 paid for the human brain samples, and 3) Paula Jackson, Cindy Haley, and Farrow Buff for their administrative support.

Author Contributions

Conceived and designed the experiments: CW RC. Performed the experiments: CW RC EB. Analyzed the data: CW RC. Contributed reagents/materials/analysis tools: CW RC BT JM. Contributed to the writing of the manuscript: CW RC BT. Neurological scoring: JM RC. Sleep function and patients assessments: RC. Western blots, biochemichal analyses: EB CW. PD substantia nigra samples: BT.

References

1. Barnum CJ, Tansey MG (2010) Modeling neuroinflammatory pathogenesis of Parkinson's disease. Progress in Brain Research 184: 113–132.

2. Banati RB, Daniel SE, Blunt SB (1998) Glial pathology but absence of apoptotic nigral neurons in long-standing Parkinson's disease. Movement Disorders 13: 221–227.

3. Crotty S, Fitzgerald P, Tuohy E, Harris DM, Fisher A, et al. (2008) Neuroprotective effects of novel phosphatidylglycerol-based phospholipids in the 6-hydroxydopamine model of Parkinson's disease. European Journal of Neuroscience 27: 294–300.

4. Gagne JJ, Powers MC (2010) Anti-inflammatory drugs and risk of Parkinson's disease: A meta-analysis Neurology 74: 995–1002.

5. Maciejewski-Lenoir D, Richman JG, Hakak Y, Gaidarov I, Behan DP, et al. (2006) Langerhans cells release prostaglandin D2 in response to nicotinic acid. Journal of Investigative Dermatology 126: 2637–2646.

6. Digby JE, McNeill E, Dyar OJ, Lam V, Greaves DR, et al. (2010) Anti-inflammatory effects of nicotinic acid in adipocytes demonstrated by suppression of fractalkine, rantes, and mcp-1 and upregulation of adiponectin. Atherosclerosis 209: 89–95.

7. Digby JE, Martinez F, Jefferson A, Ruparelia N, Chai J, et al. (2012) Anti-inflammatory effects of nicotinic acid in human monocytes are mediated by GPR109A dependent mechanisms. Arteriosclerosis, Thrombosis, and Vascular Biology 32: 669–676.

8. Digby JE, Martinez FO, Jefferson A, Ruparelia N, Wamil M, et al. (2011) Anti-inflammatory effects of nicotnic acid: Mechanisms of action in human monocytes. Circulation Supplement 124: A14830.

9. Ganji SH, Qin S, Zhang L, Kamanna VS, Kashyap ML (2009) Niacin inhibits vascular oxidative stress, redox-sensitive genes, and monocyte adhesion to human aortic endothelial cells. Atherosclerosis 202: 68–75.

10. Offermanns S (2006) The nicotinic acid receptor GPR109A (HM74A or PUMA-G) as a new therapeutic target. Trends in Pharmacological Sciences 27: 384–390.

11. Taggart AK, Kero J, Gan X, Cai TQ, Cheng K, et al. (2005) (D)-beta-Hydroxybutyrate inhibits adipocyte lipolysis via the nicotinic acid receptor PUMA-G. Journal of Biological Chemistry 280: 26649–26652.

12. Kigerl KA, Gensel JC, Ankeny DP, Alexander JK, Donnelly DJ, et al. (2009) Identification of two distinct macrophage subsets with divergent effects causing either neurotoxicity or regeneration in the injured mouse spinal cord. Journal of Neuroscience 29: 13435–13444.

13. Lawrence T, Natoli G (2011) Transcriptional regulation of macrophage polarization: enabling diversity with identity. Nature Reviews Immunology 11: 750–761.

14. Hasan D, Chalouhi N, Jabbour P, Hashimoto T (2012) Macrophage imbalance (M1 vs. M2) and upregulation of mast cells in wall of ruptured human cerebral aneurysms: preliminary results. Journal of Neuroinflammation 9: 222.

15. Peek CB, Affinati AH, Ramsey KM, Kuo HY, Yu W, et al. (2013) Circadian clock NAD+ cycle drives mitochondrial oxidative metabolism in mice. Science 342: 1243417.

16. Imai S (2010) "Clocks" in the NAD World: NAD as a metabolic oscillator for the regulation of metabolism and aging. Biochimica et Biophysica Acta 1804: 1584–1590.

17. Reimund E (1991) Sleep deprivation-induced neuronal damage may be due to nicotinic acid depletion. Medical Hypotheses 34: 275–277.

18. Sancar G, Brunner M (2014) Circadian clocks and energy metabolism. Cellular and Molecular Life Sciences.

19. Yoshino J (2013) [Importance of NAMPT-mediated NAD-biosynthesis and NAD-dependent deacetylase SIRT1 in the crosstalk between circadian rhythm and metabolism]. Nihon Rinsho Japanese Journal of Clinical Medicine 71: 2187–2193.

20. Martin PM, Ananth S, Cresci G, Roon P, Smith S, et al. (2009) Expression and localization of GPR109A (PUMA-G/HM74A) mRNA and protein in mammalian retinal pigment epithelium. Molecular Vision 15: 362–372.

21. Kashiwaya Y, Takeshima T, Mori N, Nakashima K, Clarke K, et al. (2000) D-beta-hydroxybutyrate protects neurons in models of Alzheimer's and Parkinson's disease. Proceedings of the National Academy of Sciences of the United States of America 97: 5440–5444.

22. Hughes AJ, Daniel SE, Kilford L, Lees AJ (1992) Accuracy of clinical diagnosis of idiopathic Parkinson's disease: a clinico-pathological study of 100 cases. Journal of Neurology, Neurosurgery and Psychiatry 55: 181–184.

23. Wakade C, Sukumari-Ramesh S, Laird MD, Dhandapani KM, Vender JR (2010) Delayed reduction in hippocampal postsynaptic density protein-95 expression temporally correlates with cognitive dysfunction following controlled cortical impact in mice. Journal of Neurosurgery 113: 1195–1201.

24. Shambroom JR, Fabregas SE, Johnstone J (2011) Validation of an automated wireless system to monitor sleep in healthy adults. Journal of Sleep Research.

25. Cohen J (1988) Statistical power analysis for the behavioral sciences. Hillsdale, NJ: Lawrence Erlbaum Associates.

26. Stebbins GT, Goetz CG, Lang AE, Cubo E (1999) Factor analysis of the motor section of the unified Parkinson's disease rating scale during the off-state. Movement Disorders 14: 585–589.

27. Han M, Nagele E, DeMarshall C, Acharya N, Nagele R (2012) Diagnosis of Parkinson's disease based on disease-specific autoantibody profiles in human sera. PloS One 7: e32383.

28. Wakade C, Chong RK, Bradley E, Morgan J (2014) Niacin supplementation modulates GPR109A levels and NAD-NADH ratio and ameliorates PD symptoms. Submitted.

29. Piper PW, Harris NL, MacLean M (2006) Preadaptation to efficient respiratory maintenance is essential both for maximal longevity and the retention of replicative potential in chronologically ageing yeast. Mechanisms of Ageing and Development 127: 733–740.

30. Belenky P, Racette FG, Bogan KL, McClure JM, Smith JS, et al. (2007) Nicotinamide riboside promotes Sir2 silencing and extends lifespan via Nrk and Urh1/Pnp1/Meu1 pathways to NAD+. Cell 129: 473–484.

31. Jia H, Li X, Gao H, Feng Z, Zhao L, et al. (2008) High doses of nicotinamide prevent oxidative mitochondrial dysfunction in a cellular model and improve motor deficit in a Drosophila model of Parkinson's disease. Journal of Neuroscience Research 86: 2083–2090.

32. Arduino DM, Esteves AR, Oliveira CR, Cardoso SM (2010) Mitochondrial metabolism modulation: a new therapeutic approach for Parkinson's disease. CNS & Neurological Disorders Drug Targets 9: 105–119.

33. Khan NA, Auranen M, Paetau I, Pirinen E, Euro L, et al. (2014) Effective treatment of mitochondrial myopathy by nicotinamide riboside, a vitamin B3. EMBO Molecular Medicine 6: 721–731.

34. Sasaki Y, Araki T, Milbrandt J (2006) Stimulation of nicotinamide adenine dinucleotide biosynthetic pathways delays axonal degeneration after axotomy. Journal of Neuroscience 26: 8484–8491.

35. Ban N, Ozawa Y, Inaba T, Miyake S, Watanabe M, et al. (2013) Light-dark condition regulates sirtuin mRNA levels in the retina. Experimental Gerontology 48: 1212–1217.

36. Chang HC, Guarente L (2013) SIRT1 mediates central circadian control in the SCN by a mechanism that decays with aging. Cell 153: 1448–1460.

37. Jung-Hynes B, Reiter RJ, Ahmad N (2010) Sirtuins, melatonin and circadian rhythms: Building a bridge between aging and cancer. Journal of Pineal Research 48: 9–19.

38. Boeve BF (2013) Idiopathic REM sleep behaviour disorder in the development of Parkinson's disease. Lancet Neurology 12: 469–482.

39. Chahine LM, Daley J, Horn S, Colcher A, Hurtig H, et al. (2013) Questionnaire-based diagnosis of REM sleep behavior disorder in Parkinson's disease. Movement Disorders 28: 1146–1149.

40. Poewe W (2006) The natural history of Parkinson's disease. Journal of Neurology 253 Suppl 7: VII2–6.

41. Postuma RB, Lang AE, Gagnon JF, Pelletier A, Montplaisir JY (2012) How does parkinsonism start? Prodromal parkinsonism motor changes in idiopathic REM sleep behaviour disorder. Brain 135: 1860–1870.

42. Peerally T, Yong MH, Chokroverty S, Tan EK (2012) Sleep and Parkinson's disease: a review of case-control polysomnography studies. Movement Disorders 27: 1729–1737.

43. Sixel-Doring F, Trautmann E, Mollenhauer B, Trenkwalder C (2011) Associated factors for REM sleep behavior disorder in Parkinson disease. Neurology 77: 1048–1054.

44. Ramsey KM, Affinati AH, Peek CB, Marcheva B, Hong HK, et al. (2013) Circadian measurements of sirtuin biology. Methods in Molecular Biology 1077: 285–302.

45. Mendelsohn AR, Larrick JW (2014) Partial reversal of skeletal muscle aging by restoration of normal NAD(+) Levels. Rejuvenation Research 17: 62–69.

46. Asher G, Schibler U (2011) Crosstalk between components of circadian and metabolic cycles in mammals. Cell Metabolism 13: 125–137.

47. Bellet MM, Sassone-Corsi P (2010) Mammalian circadian clock and metabolism - the epigenetic link. Journal of Cell Science 123: 3837–3848.

48. Ghosh S, George S, Roy U, Ramachandran D, Kolthur-Seetharam U (2010) NAD: A master regulator of transcription. Biochimica et Biophysica Acta 1799: 681–693.

49. Sassone-Corsi P (2012) Minireview: NAD(+), a circadian metabolite with an epigenetic twist. Endocrinology 153: 1–5.

50. Gille A, Bodor ET, Ahmed K, Offermanns S (2008) Nicotinic acid: Pharmacological effects and mechanisms of action. Annual Review of Pharmacology and Toxicology 48: 79–106.

51. Alisky JM (2005) Niacin improved rigidity and bradykinesia in a Parkinson's disease patient but also caused unacceptable nightmares and skin rash–a case report. Nutritional Neuroscience 8: 327–329.

52. Fall PA, Fredrikson M, Axelson O, Granerus AK (1999) Nutritional and occupational factors influencing the risk of Parkinson's disease: A case-control study in southeastern Sweden. Movement Disorders 14: 28–37.

53. Bender DA, Earl CJ, Lees AJ (1979) Niacin depletion in Parkinsonian patients treated with L-dopa, benserazide and carbidopa. Clinical Science 56: 89–93.

54. Hoane MR, Tan AA, Pierce JL, Anderson GD, Smith DC (2006) Nicotinamide treatment reduces behavioral impairments and provides cortical protection after fluid percussion injury in the rat. Journal of Neurotrauma 23: 1535–1548.

55. Anderson DW, Bradbury KA, Schneider JS (2008) Broad neuroprotective profile of nicotinamide in different mouse models of MPTP-induced parkinsonism. European Journal of Neuroscience 28: 610–617.

56. Chen J, Cui X, Zacharek A, Jiang H, Roberts C, et al. (2007) Niaspan increases angiogenesis and improves functional recovery after stroke. Annals of Neurology 62: 49–58.

57. Segain JP, Raingeard de la Bletiere D, Bourreille A, Leray V, Gervois N, et al. (2000) Butyrate inhibits inflammatory responses through NFkappaB inhibition: implications for Crohn's disease. Gut 47: 397–403.

58. Chai JT, Digby JE, Choudhury RP (2013) GPR109A and vascular inflammation. Current Atherosclerosis Reports 15: 325.

59. Canani RB, Costanzo MD, Leone L, Pedata M, Meli R, et al. (2011) Potential beneficial effects of butyrate in intestinal and extraintestinal diseases. World Journal of Gastroenterology 17: 1519–1528.

60. Birkmayer JG, Vrecko C, Volc D, Birkmayer W (1993) Nicotinamide adenine dinucleotide (NADH)–a new therapeutic approach to Parkinson's disease.

Comparison of oral and parenteral application. Acta neurologica Scandinavica Supplementum 146: 32–35.

61. Pearl SM, Antion MD, Stanwood GD, Jaumotte JD, Kapatos G, et al. (2000) Effects of NADH on dopamine release in rat striatum. Synapse 36: 95–101.

62. (2003) The Unified Parkinson's Disease Rating Scale (UPDRS): Status and recommendations. Movement Disorders 18: 738–750.

63. Goetz CG, Poewe W, Rascol O, Sampaio C, Stebbins GT, et al. (2004) Movement Disorder Society Task Force report on the Hoehn and Yahr staging scale: Status and recommendations. Movement Disorders 19: 1020–1028.

64. Folstein MF, Folstein SE, McHugh PR (1975) "Mini-mental state". A practical method for grading the cognitive state of patients for the clinician. Journal of Psychiatric Research 12: 189–198.

65. Jenkinson C, Fitzpatrick R, Peto V, Greenhall R, Hyman N (1997) The Parkinson's Disease Questionnaire (PDQ-39): Development and validation of a Parkinson's disease summary index score. Age Ageing 26: 353–357.

66. Jenkinson C, Fitzpatrick R (2007) Cross-cultural evaluation of the short form 8-item Parkinson's Disease Questionnaire (PDQ-8): Results from America, Canada, Japan, Italy and Spain. Parkinsonism and Related Disorders 13: 22–28.

67. Chong RK, Morgan J, Mehta SH, Pawlikowska I, Hall P, et al. (2011) Rapid assessment of postural instability in Parkinson's disease (RAPID): A pilot study. European Journal of Neurology 18: 260–265.

68. Chong RK, Lee KH, Morgan J, Mehta SH, Hall P, et al. (2012) Diagnostic value of the rapid assessment of postural instability in Parkinson's disease (RAPID) questionnaire. International Journal of Clinical Practice 66: 718–721.

69. Chaudhuri KR, Pal S, DiMarco A, Whately-Smith C, Bridgman K, et al. (2002) The Parkinson's disease sleep scale: A new instrument for assessing sleep and nocturnal disability in Parkinson's disease. Journal of Neurology, Neurosurgery, and Psychiatry 73: 629–635.

9

Attentional Modulation of Auditory Steady-State Responses

Yatin Mahajan*, Chris Davis, Jeesun Kim

The MARCS Institute, University of Western Sydney, Penrith, New South Wales, Australia

Abstract

Auditory selective attention enables task-relevant auditory events to be enhanced and irrelevant ones suppressed. In the present study we used a frequency tagging paradigm to investigate the effects of attention on auditory steady state responses (ASSR). The ASSR was elicited by simultaneously presenting two different streams of white noise, amplitude modulated at either 16 and 23.5 Hz or 32.5 and 40 Hz. The two different frequencies were presented to each ear and participants were instructed to selectively attend to one ear or the other (confirmed by behavioral evidence). The results revealed that modulation of ASSR by selective attention depended on the modulation frequencies used and whether the activation was contralateral or ipsilateral. Attention enhanced the ASSR for contralateral activation from either ear for 16 Hz and suppressed the ASSR for ipsilateral activation for 16 Hz and 23.5 Hz. For modulation frequencies of 32.5 or 40 Hz attention did not affect the ASSR. We propose that the pattern of enhancement and inhibition may be due to binaural suppressive effects on ipsilateral stimulation and the dominance of contralateral hemisphere during dichotic listening. In addition to the influence of cortical processing asymmetries, these results may also reflect a bias towards inhibitory ipsilateral and excitatory contralateral activation present at the level of inferior colliculus. That the effect of attention was clearest for the lower modulation frequencies suggests that such effects are likely mediated by cortical brain structures or by those in close proximity to cortex.

Editor: Manuel S. Malmierca, University of Salamanca- Institute for Neuroscience of Castille and Leon and Medical School, Spain

Funding: The study was supported by MARCS Institute research fund. The funders had no role in study design, data collection and analysis, decision to publish, or preparation of the manuscript.

Competing Interests: The authors have declared that no competing interests exist.

* Email: y.mahajan@uws.edu.au

Introduction

A listener in a typical everyday situation receives multiple auditory inputs some of which may be relevant and others not. As such, the listener has to selectively attend to particular inputs and sustain this attention over time. It is through sustained selective attention that a listener is able to enhance task-relevant processing and suppress irrelevant processing [1,2].

The neurophysiological mechanisms underlying selective auditory attention and its neural correlates have been studied using various electrophysiological methods (EEG, MEG and electrocorticography). Early research on the attentional modulation of cortical responses typically examined event-related potentials (ERPs) and paralleled the early behavioral work on aural discrimination by using simple transient stimuli, such as tone bursts and tone pips. Use of these stimuli provided a high degree of control over stimulus properties and presentation times. Results showed larger auditory P1, N1 and T-complex responses to attended stimuli [3,4] and reduced activity to unattended stimuli [1,5].

Recently, another neurophysiological measure, the auditory steady state response (ASSR) has been used to examine the effect of attention on neurophysiological responses underlying selective auditory attention. The ASSR consists of evoked responses from central auditory pathway and auditory cortex when presented with

rapid periodic/rhythmic auditory stimuli that lead to synchronization of cortical oscillations to its frequency and phase [6]. The ASSR can be generated by modulating an auditory input (carrier signal: white noise or pure tones) either in an amplitude (AM) or frequency (FM) domain or both [7].

One benefit of using ASSR is that the modulating frequency of the auditory stream will be represented in the neural response, and multiple modulation frequencies can be used in a single stimulus paradigm to record ASSR simultaneously. Since the modulation frequencies used to record ASSR are predefined, precise frequency analyses can be performed at those frequencies. When the modulating auditory streams are attended, the attention typically influences the activity of neurons that match the temporal structure of the input and so neural responses will be tied to the timing of the attended events. These properties of ASSR enable the researchers to study the neural correlates of auditory selective attention such that the cortical responses (ASSR) are 'tagged' to the multiple modulation frequencies used that may be attended or unattended in a stimulus paradigm called 'frequency tagging'.

Frequency tagging for ASSR was first introduced in a binaural interaction experiment to study the contribution of ipsilateral and contralateral pathways at the level of human auditory cortex [8]. Frequency tagging when used to evaluate auditory selective attention typically involves presentation of different auditory input in each ear with each ear modulated by a particular modulation frequency. The listener attends to sounds in one ear while ignoring the stimulus from the other ear. The ASSR is tagged for both the attended and unattended modulation frequencies from each ear. The effects of selective attention can be investigated from the resultant power of the ASSR. Furthermore, the effect of attention at different levels of auditory system can be probed with the frequency tagging paradigm by using a number of modulation frequencies. That is, the effects of attention can be assessed at different loci along central auditory pathway because such are activated by differing modulation frequencies, e.g., primary and secondary auditory cortices responsive to 4–16 Hz, the medial geniculate body of upper brainstem to 16–32 Hz and lower brainstem and other brainstem regions to 32–256 Hz AM frequency [9–11].

There have been only a handful of studies investigating the effect of selective attention on ASSR that have used frequency tagging. A summary of the findings and methods used in these studies is presented in Table 1. With the exception of [8,12], all the studies shown in Table 1 employed an active attention task in which either a change in modulation frequency or carrier frequency was to be detected while paying attention to a particular ear and simultaneously ignoring the auditory stream from the other. Three general results can be drawn from these studies. First, the power of the ASSR was modulated by the deployment of attention. That is, apart from two studies [13,14], the power of the ASSR was increased for the stream of rhythmic auditory stimuli

that was attended compared to the stream that was unattended or ignored.

Second, it appears that the enhancement of ASSR by attention is clearest in the hemisphere contralateral to the stimulated ear. Müller et al. [15] reported that attention enhanced the power of contralateral ASSR tagged to 20 Hz and suppressed ipsilateral 20 Hz ASSR. Bharadwaj et al. [16] found significantly increased ASSR in the hemisphere contralateral to attended sound source and only a trend of enhancement in the ipsilateral one. Ross et al. [17] also reported increased 40 Hz ASSR amplitude on attention in the contralateral hemisphere during monaural stimulation. The other studies did not report results as a function of contralateral and ipsilateral activations per se, but rather in terms of attention effects in the left or right hemisphere. Of these studies all but one [14] reported an effect of attention in left hemisphere; Lazzouni et al. [14] reported modulation of ASSR in the right hemisphere. A reason why attention might have a more potent effect contralaterally than ipsilaterally is there are more neurons and connections from subcortical structures to contralateral cortical ones [18]. It should be noted, however, that although the suppression of ipsilateral responses compared to contralateral responses is reported in a number of frequency tagging paradigms [8,12,14], these studies either had no attention related task or did not alternate the modulation frequencies across the ears. Alternating the frequencies and attentional load across the ears allows for the ipsilateral and contralateral auditory pathways to potentially contribute equally for each frequency providing a fairer

Table 1. A summary of research on attentional modulation of ASSR using the frequency tagging paradigm.

Study	Number of participants/ Carrier Signal	Modulation frequencies	Effect of Attention on ASSR	Hemispheric lateralization	Task (Listening)
Linden et al., 1987	10 (5 females)/500 Hz	37 and 41 Hz	No effect	NR	Active (Change in carrier) frequency)
Fujiki et al., 2002	12 (5 females)/1000 Hz	26.1 and 20.1 Hz	NR	Left hemisphere laterality; suppression of ipsilateral responses in right hemisphere	Active (No task)
Kaneko et al., 2003	10 (4 females)/1000 Hz	39.1 and 41.1 Hz	NR	Binaural suppression of ipsilateral responses; contralateral hemisphere dominance	Active (No task)
Bidet-Caulet et al., 2007	12 (8 females)/659–784 Hz	21 and 29 Hz	Increased responses when attending; decreased when unattended	Left hemisphere laterality	Active (Target detection and localization)
Müller et al., 2009	15 (6 females)/500 Hz	20 and 45 Hz	Contralateral responses enhanced and ipsilateral responses suppressed only for 20 Hz	Left hemisphere laterality	Active (Target detection, change in modulation frequency)
Xiang et al., 2010	28 (15 females)/250–500 Hz	4 and 7 Hz	Responses enhanced by attention for each frequency tested	NR	Active (Deviant tone detection)
Lazzouni et al., 2010	15 (8 females)/1000 Hz	39 and 41 Hz	No effect of attention on ASSR power but increased ASSR amplitude (time-domain)	Right Hemisphere laterality; Binaural suppression of ipsilateral responses	Active (Target detection, change in carrier)
Bhardwaj et al., 2014	10 (2 females)/Vowels	35 and 45 Hz	Increased responses for attended frequencies	Larger responses in contralateral hemisphere	Active (Target detection)
Current Study	23 (10 females)/White noise	16, 23.5, 32.5 and 40 Hz	Contralateral responses enhanced for 16 and 23.5; ipsilateral responses suppressed for 16 Hz	No hemispheric laterality	Active (Target detection, change in modulation frequency)

Note: NR = Not Relevant.

assessment of hemispheric dominance related to attention. Indeed, in this regard, only one study [15] has employed a suitable design to properly assess the effect of attention on ASSR as a function of ipsilateral and contralateral responses in a frequency tagging paradigm.

Third, the Table 1 suggests that the modulation of ASSR by attention may depend on the modulation frequencies used; however the results are inconsistent. Müller et al. found significant attentional modulation only for 20 Hz and not for 45 Hz ASSR. Other studies have found significant attentional modulation of ASSR when tagged to 35–45 Hz modulation frequencies [14,16]. Moreover, using an active listening oddball paradigm with 20 Hz and 40 Hz AM frequencies, Skosnik et al. [19] found increased ASSR amplitude for attended 40 Hz targets compared to 20 Hz ones. Although the existing data suggests that attentional modulation of ASSR might depend on the modulation frequencies being used in the paradigm, such a conclusion may not be appropriate as it relies on cross experiment comparisons that often involve the change of many factors. In our view then, to resolve the apparent inconsistencies in the existing research an experiment is required that systematically examines multiple modulation frequencies. Furthermore, examining multiple modulation frequencies in a single experiment is worthwhile, since no previous study has ever used more than two modulation frequencies to evaluate the effect of attention on ASSR.

In sum, attention has been found to modulate the ASSR, with the strength (direction) of this activation influenced by the stimuli input, i.e., activation in the hemisphere contralateral to the attended ear produces increased amplitude and reduced amplitude in the ipsilateral hemisphere. Further, the left hemisphere is reported to be more sensitive to attentional modulation than right. The findings are inconsistent on how different modulation frequencies may interact with the attention effect.

The purpose of the present research was to build on the above research that has used a frequency tagging paradigm with the aim of determining how selective sustained attention modulates cortical responses (ASSR) as a function of contralateral/ipsilateral activations across different modulation frequencies. The results will contribute to the growing body of literature evaluating the neural correlates of selective auditory attention by frequency tagging.

Materials and Methods

Ethics Statement
The methods of the present research were approved by the human research ethics committee at the University of Western Sydney. Written informed consent was obtained from each participant before the experiment.

Participants
Twenty three participants (10 females), aged 22–35 years were recruited using notice board advertisements around the university campus. All the participants were right handed as assessed by Edinburgh handedness inventory and reported no significant neurological and psychological history. All the participants had normal hearing bilaterally with hearing thresholds of ≤15 dB HL at 500 Hz, 1000 Hz and 2000 Hz determined by screening audiometry.

Experimental stimuli
The experimental stimuli consisted of four 'standard' 30 second long white noise stimuli amplitude modulated at 16 Hz, 23.5 Hz, 32.5 Hz and 40 Hz with 100% modulation depth sampled at the rate of 44,100 Hz. The stimuli were ramped with 20 ms rise time at the onset and 20 ms fall time at the offset to avoid clicks. The white noise was used as a carrier signal in order to evoke reliable and robust ASSR. The broadband signal when used to elicit ASSR, produces larger magnitude of ASSR as compared to pure tone and band-limited noise as carrier signals [20]. The stimuli were created using the signal processing toolbox of MATLAB and were presented at a comfortable level around 70–75 dB SPL for all the participants. The experiment was completed in two sessions. In one session, the participants were presented with 16 Hz and 23.5 Hz AM stimuli and in the other session the 32.5 Hz and 40 Hz AM stimuli. The two sessions of recording were counterbalanced between the participants.

During each session the participants were presented each of the two stimuli in each of their two ears dichotically such that the one ear was stimulated by 16 Hz or 32.5 Hz and other ear by 23.5 Hz or 40 Hz modulated white noise. The ear of stimulation was counterbalanced equally between the two sets of stimuli such that a particular amplitude modulated stimulus was presented equally to both left and right ears and at the same time the opposite ear was stimulated with a different stimulus.

The experiment also consisted of 'target' stimuli, in which the modulation frequency changed multiple times during 30 seconds of stimulation (based on paradigm used by Müller et al.). The stimuli with 16 Hz and 23.5 Hz amplitude modulation changed to 40 Hz modulation for 2 seconds, either two, three or four times within 30 seconds of stimulation for target stimuli before returning to original modulation rate. The target stimuli with 32.5 Hz and 40 Hz amplitude modulation changed to 12.5 Hz modulation frequency. The target stimuli were also counterbalanced equally between ears in two sessions of recording. The two frequencies using as stimulus pairs were selected so that there was a relatively small difference between them; this was done to minimize involuntary switching of attention to one of the frequencies. That is, as part of a pilot study conducted to determine the best combination of modulation frequencies, we found that when the difference in frequencies was large (e.g., 16 and 40 Hz) then participants' attention involuntarily switched to higher modulation frequency (i.e. the 40 Hz). Further, even if the stimulus intensity was equalized across all the modulation frequencies, the perceived loudness of the higher modulation rate stimulus was greater than the lower one and this plausibly would induce an involuntary attention switch towards the high modulation frequency. To minimize this possible effect, we selected modulation frequencies pairs that were closer together (i.e., 16 and 23.5 Hz, 32.5 and 40 Hz) and this combination did not produce any involuntary attention switches.

Experimental procedure
An attention switch paradigm was used to direct attention to the stimulus presented in the designated ear for the dichotic stimuli, (see Fig. 1). The trial started with a fixation cross presented at the center of the screen for 500 ms. Then, a cue in the form of the words 'RIGHT' or 'LEFT' appeared on the screen indicating the participants which ear to attend to and after 1 second the set of paired stimuli (16 or 23.5 Hz; 32.5 or 40 Hz) were presented for 30 seconds. The cue remained on the screen for the duration of the stimuli. The participants were instructed to attend to the ear cued and press the response button as fast as they can whenever they heard a change in modulation frequency of the stimuli ('target'). A total of 72 trials were presented in one experimental session. Out of these 72 trials, 48 were standard trials that contained no targets and 24 trials had targets in them. In 12 target trials, the location of the targets and attention cue were same, i.e.,

if the cue was 'RIGHT', the target also appeared during right ear stimulation; these trials represent the 'congruent' condition. The 'incongruent' condition consisted of the remaining 12 target trials in which the cue and the stimulation ear were at opposite locations. The reaction times for detecting the targets were recorded and slower reaction times were expected in the incongruent condition compared to the congruent one (assuming that attention manipulation had been successful).

Electrophysiological recording

The participants were seated on a comfortable chair while the electrode cap was fitted. Prior to the fitting of the electrode cap, the scalp of each participant was combed to reduce the time taken to achieve the optimal scalp electrode impedance [21]. The raw electroencephalograph (EEG) was recorded with a BioSemi Active-Two amplifier system (BioSemi, Amsterdam, Netherlands). The 64 Ag-AgCl electrodes were mounted on a nylon electrode cap according to the international standard 10-10 system [22]. There were two electrodes on the electrode cap (CMS & DRL) which served as online references. Six additional electrodes were also placed on the participants. Four of them were bipolar electrodes placed above and below the left eye and outer canthi of both the eyes to monitor vertical and horizontal eye movements (EOG channels) respectively and two electrodes were placed on two mastoids. The raw EEG recording was sampled at 512 Hz with online band-pass filtering of .05–200 Hz. This raw EEG data was stored for every participant for later offline analysis.

EEG data analysis

The pre-processing and analysis of the stored raw EEG data was carried out using EEGLAB version 10 [23] and custom written functions in MATLAB (The Mathworks, Natick, MA). Initially, any obvious artifact was removed after visually inspecting the data. Then the EEG data was re-referenced to the average of both the mastoids. The resultant EEG activity was band-pass filtered (1 Hz high pass and 70 Hz low pass; 12 dB per octave roll-off). The filtered data then was epoched into a pre-stimulus period of 200 ms and post stimulus period of 30 seconds. Only the standard trials were included in the EEG analysis. The epoched data then was subjected to *runica*, an ICA (Independent component analysis) algorithm incorporated in EEGLAB to detect and remove eye blinks, horizontal eye movements and other artifacts (muscle, line noise artifacts). The ICA algorithm resulted in 64 components and based on the scalp topography, activity power spectrum and activity over trials, the artifactual components were identified and removed from the EEG data. To remove the effect of onset and offset ERP responses, the epochs were averaged from 1 s to 29.5 s in the ICA corrected epochs to form ASSR responses. The averaged ASSR responses were calculated for each modulation frequency in four conditions namely, 'right attended', 'right unattended', 'left attended' and 'left unattended'.

These time domain ASSR responses were then subjected to a Fourier transformation using a custom written MATLAB script to convert them into frequency domain (FFTs). The FFTs were used to calculate the absolute ASSR power for each condition for every

modulation frequency at the two most lateral electrodes (T7 and T8) on the scalp depicting left and right hemispheric activity respectively. These two electrodes were selected as the greater distance between the locations of T7 and T8 makes them the best electrodes to compare neural activity between the two hemispheres, as opposed to using two fronto-central electrodes. To determine if the ASSR at the modulation frequencies of interest evoked at T7 and T8 was significant across participants, the mean absolute power at the two neighboring frequencies on the either side of the modulation frequency were computed and compared with the power at the modulation frequency of interest using a t-test in the resultant FFTs. Results revealed that across all the conditions the power of the ASSR at the frequency of interest was a significant response.

Data analysis

To determine how attention modulates the ASSR as a function of modulation frequency and hemisphere by ear of stimulation (ipsilateral and contralateral), the data on the absolute power of the ASSR obtained through FFT was subjected to a 4 ('modulation frequency'; 16 Hz, 23.5 Hz, 32.5 Hz & 40 Hz)×2 ('stimulation ear'; left vs. right)×2 ('attention'; attended vs. unattended)×2 ('hemisphere by stimulation' (ipsilateral vs. contralateral)) within participant factorial ANOVA. The reaction times obtained in the target detection task were also analyzed with a 4×2×2 repeated measures ANOVA, with 'Frequency' (four modulation frequencies), 'congruency' (congruent vs. incongruent) and 'stimulation ear' (left vs. right) as within participant factors. This analysis provided an index of the differential attention paid to the experimental stimuli. For both above mentioned ANOVA analyses, wherever the assumption of sphericity was violated the Greenhouse-Geisser correction was applied. The significant results obtained are reported in the section below.

Results

Reaction times

Table 2 shows the reaction times obtained for four modulation frequencies across congruent and incongruent conditions. The ANOVA results indicated that congruency significantly altered the reaction times $(F(1,17) = 24.77, \ p<.001, \ \eta_p^2 = .56)$ and the modulation frequencies and the ear of stimulation had no significant main effect on reaction times. As evident from Table 2, reaction times were slower when participants attended to targets in the incongruent conditions across the different modulation frequencies. Similar reaction times between right and left ears and slower response times to targets in incongruent conditions across modulation frequencies when considered together, suggest that participants paid and sustained attention to the appropriate ear as instructed at the beginning of each trial.

ASSR

Fig. 2 and Fig. 3 show the grand mean FFTs of the ipsilateral and contralateral activation patterns for the 16 Hz/23.5 Hz and 32.5 Hz/40 Hz modulation frequencies respectively as a function

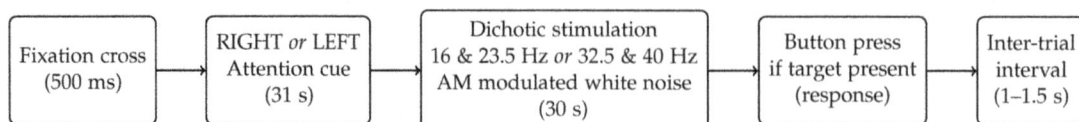

| Fixation cross (500 ms) | → | RIGHT *or* LEFT Attention cue (31 s) | → | Dichotic stimulation 16 & 23.5 Hz *or* 32.5 & 40 Hz AM modulated white noise (30 s) | → | Button press if target present (response) | → | Inter-trial interval (1–1.5 s) |

Figure 1. A depiction of the trial sequence.

Table 2. Mean reaction times for targets across modulation frequencies for the congruent and incongruent condition. Standard deviations are given in parentheses.

Frequency	Congruent		Incongruent	
	Left	Right	Left	Right
16 Hz	493 (134.27)	489 (116.85)	531 (138.71)	574 (168.75)
23.5 Hz	492 (122.04)	535 (144.49)	559 (139.36)	584 (152.18)
32.5 Hz	532 (152.54)	532 (133.57)	572 (127.33)	596 (117.65)
40 Hz	510 (153.30)	501 (149.97)	587 (141.44)	545 (142.54)

of attention (i.e., presented to the attended and unattended ear). The presence of clear and robust peaks in the FFTs indicates that the multiple frequencies presented had the desired effect of driving auditory responses at those frequencies. The results of repeated measures ANOVA revealed that there was a significant three-way interaction between frequency, attention and activation pattern, $F(3,66) = 5.76$, $p = .005$, $\eta_p^2 = .20$ (there was no significant main effect of modulation frequency, attention, ear of stimulation or hemisphere by stimulation). To understand this complex three way interaction, first the ipsilateral and contralateral activations were combined from the two ears for each attended and unattended condition across the four modulation frequencies. Then, a follow up two-way ANOVA was computed with factors 'attention' (attended & unattended) and 'hemisphere by stimulation' (ipsilateral & contralateral) for each modulation frequency (16 Hz, 23.5 Hz, 32.5 Hz & 40 Hz).

The results of this ANOVA revealed that there was no significant main effect of attention and hemisphere by stimulation across all the modulation frequencies. There was a significant interaction between these factors for the 16 Hz $(F(1,22) = 14.40$, $p = .001$, $\eta_p^2 = .39)$ and 23.5 Hz $(F(1,22) = 10.47$, $p = .004$, $\eta_p^2 = .32)$ modulation frequencies. To investigate this interaction, subsequent one-way ANOVAs were conducted on each 16 Hz and 23.5 Hz modulation frequency. For the 16 Hz modulation, the power of the ASSR for attended compared to the unattended stimuli was significantly suppressed for ipsilateral activation $(F(1,22) = 9.17$, $p = .005)$ and significantly enhanced for contralateral activation $(F(1,22) = 9.93$, $p = .006)$. A similar significant suppression on attended ipsilateral stimulation was found for 23.5 Hz, $(F(1,22) = 8.46$, $p = .008)$, but attention did not affect contralateral stimulation $(F(1,22) = .21$, $p = .64)$. For 32.5 Hz and 40 Hz AM frequencies, attention did not alter the power of the ASSR, although the change in power was in the enhancement direction for 32.5 Hz and suppression for 40 Hz for both ipsilateral and contralateral stimulation, respectively. These results are illustrated in Fig. 4. The complete statistical analysis has been summarized in supplementary Table S1.

Discussion

The aim of the present research was to determine the extent to which auditory sustained selective attention modulates the strength of ASSR for ipsilateral and contralateral stimulation across different modulation frequencies. The results from the behavioral task demonstrated an effect of selective attention: responses were slower to incongruent (target presented on the unattended side) versus congruent targets depicting successful manipulation of attention. Below we consider the effects of this allocation of attention on the ASSR as a function of the various experimental manipulations.

Attentional modulation of ASSR

To our knowledge, this is the first study that has used a frequency tagging paradigm with more than two modulation frequencies to test the effect of attention on ASSR. This design allows for the direct comparison of the effect of attention on ASSR by multiple modulation frequencies. Our results indicated that attention significantly modulated the power of ASSR and, except for two studies [13,14] listed in Table 1, our results are in general agreement with other studies. The inconsistencies with the results of the studies in Table 1 may be explained by the differences in the experimental tasks used to manipulate the attention. The participants in the current study (and in [15,24]) attended to a change in the modulation frequency or the temporal envelope of stimuli which revealed modulation of ASSR. In the two studies that failed to show any significant modulation of ASSR power [13,14], the participants' task was to attend to changes in carrier frequency (or to spectral change). This difference in task raises the possibility that the attentional modulation of the ASSR requires that attention be directed to modulation frequency change rather than a change in the carrier frequency. In other words, it appears that attending to the stimulus parameter that drive the ASSR (modulation frequency) is essential for its modulation whereas attending to any other stimulus change (carrier frequency) is not. Further, we found that the attentional modulation of ASSR depended on the modulation frequencies and pattern of activation, which are discussed below.

Attentional modulation of ASSR across modulation frequencies and hemispheric dominance

The results indicated that selective attention influenced the power of ASSR for the 16 and 23.5 Hz modulation frequencies whereas this was not the case for the two other modulation frequencies used. These results are in general agreement with two studies (see Table 1), that also reported significant modulation by attention for 20–29 Hz ASSR [15,24]. It has been reported that white noise when amplitude modulated using a range of modulation frequencies (4–256 Hz) tends to preferentially stimulate different parts of central auditory pathway [9]. That is, the primary auditory cortex and the neural structures closer to the cortex like the medial geniculate body and a portion of lower brainstem appear to be more sensitive to 16–32 Hz AM frequencies, whereas the lower brainstem structures are more responsive to >40 Hz AM frequencies. Based on this selective responsiveness of neural structures within the auditory system, we suggest that assemblies more proximal to the cortex are likely to be more susceptible to attentional effects than those more distal from the cortex. Such a differential sensitivity would result in lower modulation frequencies being the ones most likely to show an attention effect. This claim that the activity of neural structures

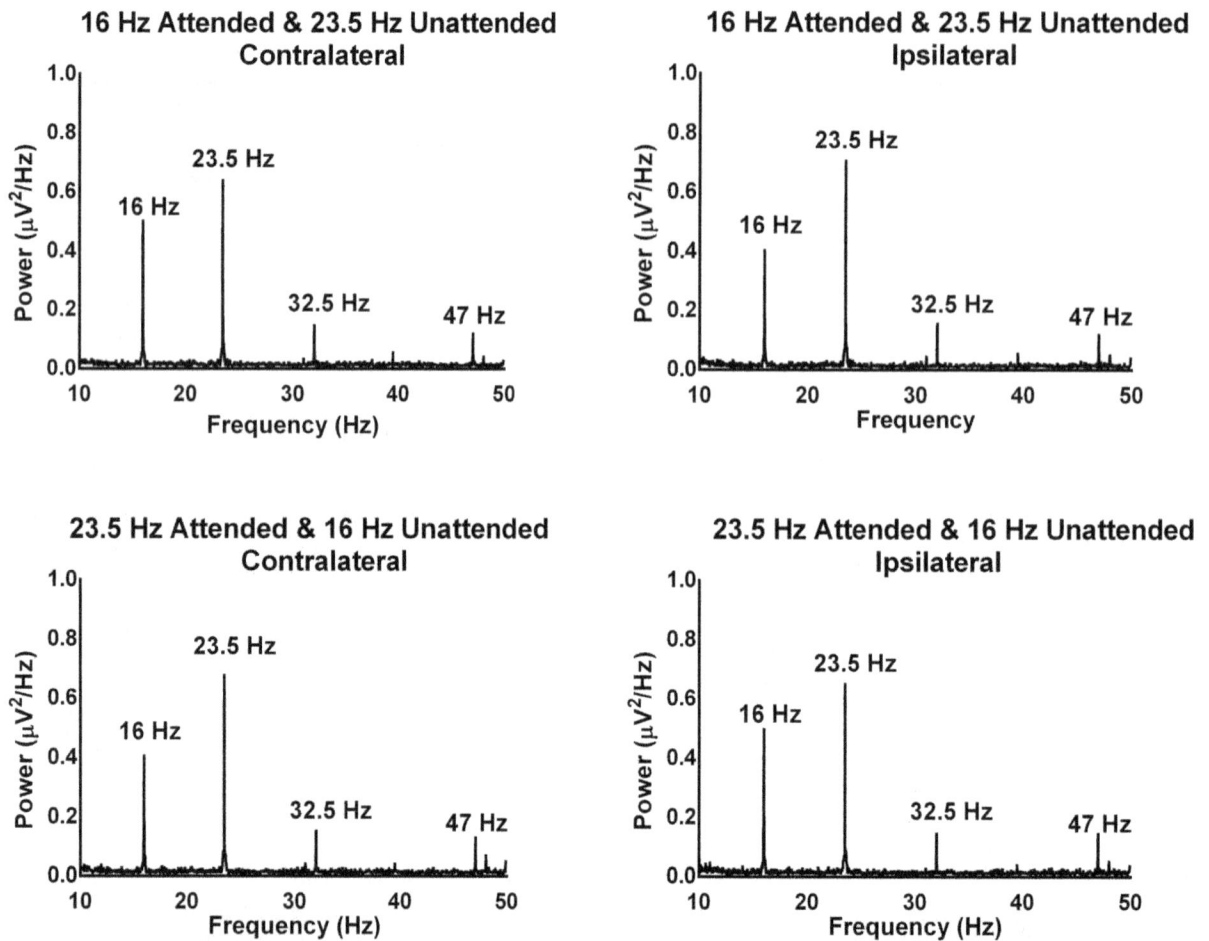

Figure 2. The grand mean FFTs for 16 and 23.5 Hz modulation frequencies during attended and unattended conditions across ipsilateral and contralateral activations combined from the two electrodes (T7 & T8). The power in the FFTs is an absolute value expressed in terms of squared microvolts per every 1 Hz of frequency (μV^2/Hz). The first harmonics for both 16 and 23.5 Hz are also shown.

higher in auditory system will be more open to attention modulation than those located down the auditory hierarchy is supported by a series of studies that have reported no effects of attention on auditory brainstem responses [1].

The results of the present study are inconsistent with the results of a number of previous studies that have found significant modulation of ASSR by attention for modulation rates between 35–45 Hz [16,17,19]. In line with the explanation proposed by Müller et al to clarify the lack of attentional modulation of 45 Hz ASSR in their study, this discrepancy might have stemmed from methodological differences between the studies. For example, Skosnik et al. found attention effects only for 45 Hz ASSR and not 20 Hz ASSR (they also used binaural stimulation of these frequencies with clicks as carrier signals in an oddball paradigm). Ross et al. used only monaural stimulation in their target detection task for 40 Hz ASSR (change in modulation frequency) and used a concurrent visual control task for unattended condition, thus involving two modalities in contrast to the present study that investigated effect of attention with in a single modality. Lastly, in a MEG study, Bharadwaj et al used rapid presentation of vowels (A, E, I, O and U) at 35 and 45 Hz spatially to the participants two ears based on his/her head related transfer functions. The task was to attend to one spatial stream and count a particular vowel in that stream and like Ross et al a visual control task was used as an unattended condition.

In the current study, there was no separate unattended control condition as we considered the modulation frequency presented opposite to the attended ear to be unattended. Furthermore, we suggest that in examining the effects of auditory selective attention on ASSR, it is important that the unattended or control condition should only involve the auditory modality. That is, a visual attention control task in an auditory selective paradigm may stimulate additional cortical areas and pathways apart from auditory ones; hence the results will not be specific to auditory stimulation alone. The differences in the stimulation pattern (binaural vs. monaural vs. dichotic), unattended conditions (visual control vs. attention switch) between previous studies [16,17,19] and the present study might indicate that the current results are specific to the experimental manipulations we used and as such do not conflict with previous results per se. In support of the idea that modulation effects might be influenced by the precise paradigm used, our paradigm was based on Müller et al's paradigm in terms of having an attention switching task between the ears and to detect a change in modulation frequencies. They also reported attention effects only for 20 Hz and not 45 Hz modulation frequencies.

As shown in Table 1, previous research found significant attentional modulation of ASSR either in left hemisphere and right ear [15,17,24] or in the right hemisphere [14]. Since the task in the current study was to detect a change in the modulation

32.5 Hz Attended & 40 Hz Unattended Contralateral

32.5 Hz Attended & 40 Hz Unattended Ipsilateral

40 Hz Attended & 32.5 Hz Unattended Contralateral

40 Hz Attended & 32.5 Hz Unattended Ipsilateral

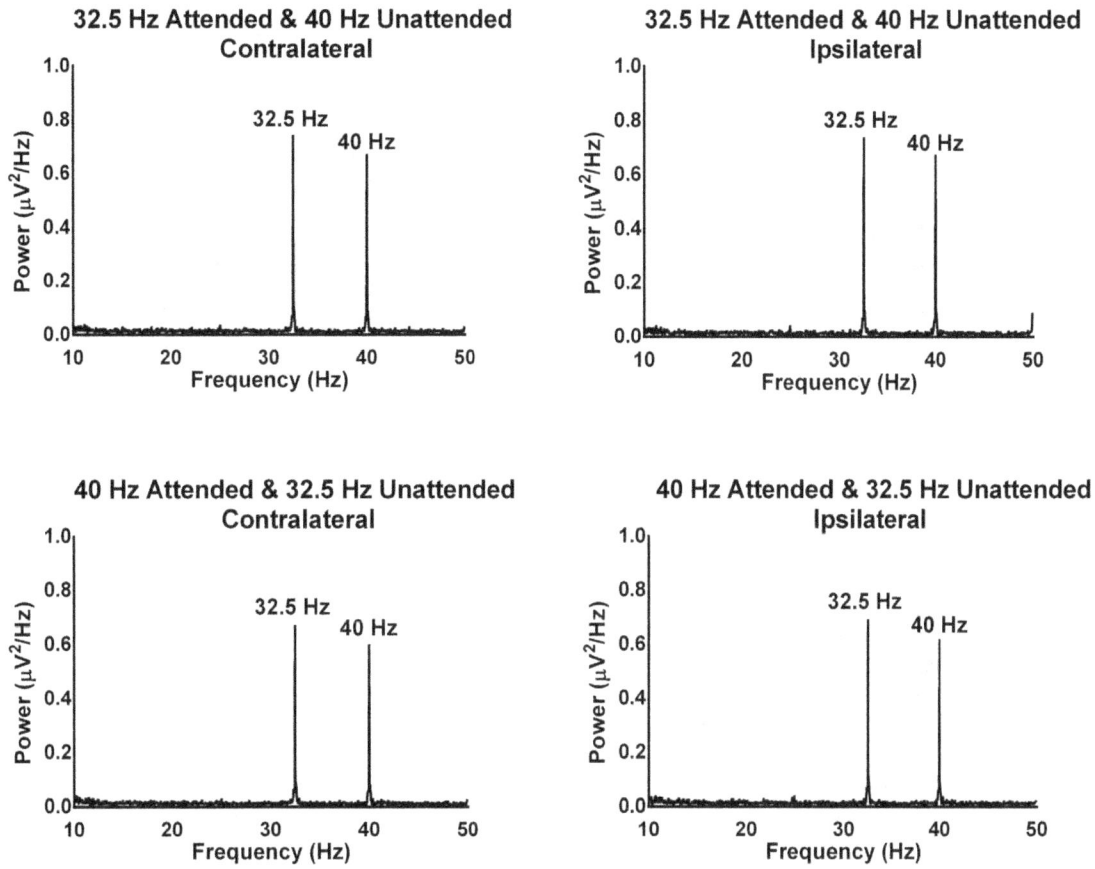

Figure 3. The grand mean FFTs for 32.5 and 40 Hz modulation frequencies during attended and unattended conditions across ipsilateral and contralateral activations combined from the two electrodes (T7 & T8). The power in the FFTs is an absolute value expressed in terms of squared microvolts per every 1 Hz of frequency (μV^2/Hz).

frequency, i.e., a change in the temporal envelope, left hemisphere laterality was expected for the attentional modulation as opposed to right hemisphere when a change in carrier frequency was to be detected (spectral change; [14]). However, the results revealed neither an ear effect nor any hemispheric laterality effect. The reason for the lack of an influence of hemispheric laterality is not clear. A notable difference between our study and previous ones is that we used white noise as a carrier signal, whereas previous studies used pure tones of different frequencies (see Table 1). We employed white noise as a carrier signal to evoke reliable, robust and larger ASSR responses since the white noise activates a larger region of the basilar membrane, which in turn provides more sensory input to higher cortical structures [25]. Except for one study [16] that used vowels as stimuli to evoke ASSR, other studies used pure tones as carrier signals and have reported attentional modulation of ASSR in either left or right hemisphere. The type of carrier signal (broadband or pure tone) or the band width of the carrier signal (large for white noise and small for pure tone) might determine the laterality of the ASSR when modulated by the attention. In line with the findings of previous studies that have showed hemispheric laterality of ASSR, it is plausible that that narrow band carrier signal when used to evoke ASSR is more likely to elicit clear hemisphere laterality during attentional modulation as compared to a broadband signal as in present study. Support to this proposal comes from a recent experiment [26] on hemispheric laterality of various auditory processing tasks such as gap detection, frequency discrimination and intensity

discrimination. The results showed that no hemispheric lateralization was found for psychoacoustic thresholds obtained from these tasks with broad band stimuli whereas clear left hemisphere laterality was found for pure tones.

Additionally, it has been reported that in conventional central masking scenarios, the power of the ASSR reduces in both the hemispheres when evoked monaurally in the presence of contralaterally presented continuous white noise [27]. Applying similar principles to the results of the present study, it is possible that the continuous white noise stimulation from each ear might have reduced the power of ASSR in both hemispheres and in effect eliminated any hemispheric differences that might have been evident during attentional modulation. Though, it must be noted that this account is speculative and further systematic investigations would be needed to confirm this.

Attentional modulation of ASSR across ipsilateral and contralateral activations

It was found that attention differentially affected ASSR power as a function of ipsilateral versus contralateral stimulation. When attended, the ASSR was suppressed for ipsilateral stimulation at modulation frequencies of 16 and 23.5 Hz and enhanced for contralateral stimulation at 16 Hz (the effect for 23.5 Hz was in the enhancement direction but was not significant). In general, these results agree with those of Müller et al who also reported similar suppression and enhancement effects for 20 Hz frequency

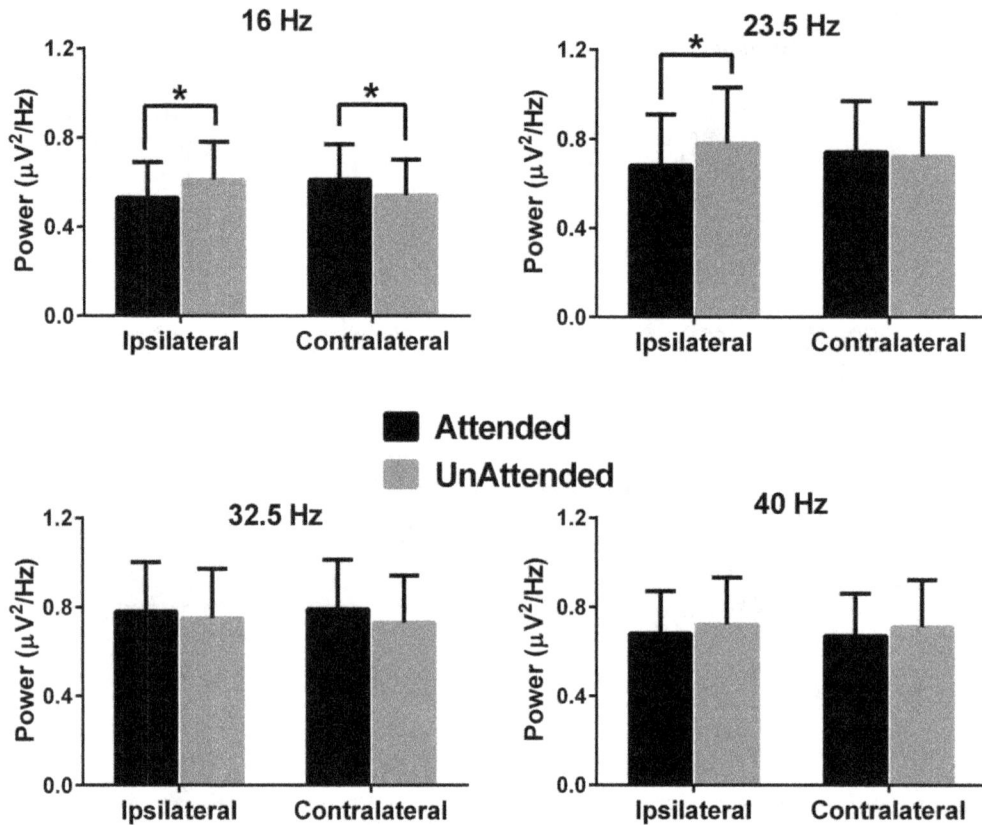

Figure 4. The bar graphs represent the absolute power measured from FFTs, when white noise was modulated with a particular modulation frequency and was attended or unattended. The bars represent neural activity from the ipsilateral and contralateral activations combined from T7 and T8 sites. An asterisk above the bar graphs indicates significant differences at $p<.05$.

for ipsilateral and contralateral stimulation, respectively and did not find any significant effects for the 45 Hz ASSR.

Müller et al. explained these findings based on an experiment by Staines et al. [28] that examined the somatosensory system and where an enhancement for contralateral and suppression for ipsilateral stimulation was found. In the study by Staines et al it was found that task relevant stimulation increased the BOLD response in the somatosensory cortex contralateral to stimulation and decreased it in the ipsilateral one. Staines et al. pointed out that this was unexpected since the suppression in the ipsilateral cortex occurred in response to task-relevant somatosensory stimulation (the task was to detect a change in frequency of vibrotactile stimulation, no matter on what side it occurred). The explanation that was given for this inhibitory effect was that, making the ipsilateral cortex less responsive would mitigate the effects that potentially conflicting inputs would have on a behaviorally relevant task. Müller et al. explained their ASSR modulation assuming that information is likely to be more relevant when processed by the contralateral mechanisms than when processed by ipsilateral ones. That is, relevant contralateral activity gets enhanced by attention whereas ipsilateral activity gets suppressed. A problem with this account is that the basis of the assumption that relevant and irrelevant stimulation map to contralateral and ipsilateral mechanisms has not been made clear. Also, the ipsilateral effect has not been found across stimulation frequencies. For example, Bhardwaj et al. found an enhancement effect for contralateral ASSR for 35 Hz and 45 Hz modulations but no ipsilateral effect for these modulation frequencies.

There are several other approaches for explaining the finding that attention leads to contralateral enhancement and ipsilateral suppression. One approach builds on two proposals that have been made about findings using dichotic listening. First, it has been reported that the dichotic listening leads to a cortical level competition between the two auditory inputs from the two ears [8,12]. This competition may lead to either summation or suppression of neural responses. Fujiki et al. [8] and Kaneko et al. [12] found suppression of ipsilateral activity in both the hemispheres during dichotic listening when compared with monaural stimulation. While there was no task associated with Fujiki et al's and Kaneko et al's frequency tagging paradigms, the listeners were attending to the stimuli. The present study which employed a task-relevant dichotic listening frequency tagging paradigm would have produced similar ipsilateral suppressive effects on ASSR power. The binaural rivalry from the two ears in response to dichotic stimulation led to the suppression of ipsilateral activity during attention. Secondly, it is well-known that during dichotic listening, there is a shift of hemispheric balance towards the hemisphere contralateral to the stimulation owing to the relatively large number of contralateral neural connections [29]. This property might have led to enhanced and larger ASSR on attention for the contralateral side during dichotic stimulation in the present study. It should be pointed out that the suppression and summation of ASSR reported for dichotic listening in Fujiki et a. [8] and Kaneko et al. [12] was with higher modulation frequencies (26, 39 & 41 Hz) than those used in present study. Given this, and the lack of ipsilateral suppression by Bhardawaj et al. [16] and that the differential effects of attention in the present study were present only for two of the four tested modulation frequencies, it would appear that attentional effects on the ASSR are complex and likely depend on the experimental procedures used to manipulate attention. We therefore suggest that our interpretation of attentional effects on ASSR based on dichotic listening should be viewed with some caution.

A slightly different explanation suggests that the pattern of enhancement and inhibition as a function of neural connectivity may be ultimately due to the anatomical arrangement and function of the inferior colliculus (IC). The IC contains EI cells (excitatory-inhibitory cells) that enhance contralateral input and suppresses the ipsilateral input [30,31]. This arrangement may influence processing at cortical regions and result in relative inhibition of ipsilateral activity and enhancement of contralateral activity. It is known that, selective attention enhances the underlying neuronal output and increases the synchronization of the local neuronal output [32]. Accordingly, during selective attention the overall neural firing of the EI cells at the level of ICs will also increase; with EI cells being excitatory and inhibitory in nature, the increased output will be inhibited at ipsilateral cortex and enhanced on the contralateral cortex. Indeed, bilateral activation at the level of ICs in an auditory selective attention task, where the participants had to selectively attend to an increasing or decreasing pitch in one ear and ignore the stimulus in the other, has been reported [33]. Rinne et al. [33] observed increased activations at the level of ICs, while attending the stimuli contralaterally than ipsilaterally. These findings suggests that on attention, the selective auditory processing at cortical level is mediated both by the increased neuronal output at the level of ICs and by the excitatory-inhibitory properties of the EI cells which alter the contralateral and ipsilateral activations at cortical level.

Conclusions

The results of the present study indicate that modulation of ASSR by selective attention: 1) depends upon the modulation frequencies used in the paradigm (with 16 and 23.5 Hz being modulated by attention). 2) Also depends upon the pattern of activation at the cortical level, with contralateral activations from either ear enhanced the ASSR and ipsilateral activations suppressed the ASSR. 3) Can be probed efficiently using a frequency tagging paradigm in which participants monitor a change in the temporal envelope.

The results of the present study contribute to the limited but emerging body of research on auditory selective attention using an ecologically valid frequency tagging scenario and also stress the importance of replication of research. Future studies may usefully look into the attentional modulation of low frequencies (3–8 Hz) to which primary and secondary auditory cortices are highly responsive. Based on current findings we would predict a significant modulation of low frequency ASSR as well. Also an experimental comparison between different carrier stimuli is required to examine the relationship between ipsilateral/contralateral activations and attention.

Author Contributions

Conceived and designed the experiments: YM CD JK. Performed the experiments: YM CD. Analyzed the data: YM. Contributed reagents/materials/analysis tools: YM. Wrote the paper: YM CD JK.

References

1. Giard M-H, Fort A, Mouchetant-Rostaing Y, Pernier J (2000) Neurophysiological mechanisms of auditory selective attention in humans. Front Biosci 5: d84.
2. Choi I, Rajaram S, Varghese LA, Shin-Cunningham BG (2013) Quantifying attentional modulation of auditory-evoked responses from single trial electroencephalography. Front Hum Neurosci 7: 115.
3. Hillyard SA, Hink RF, Schwent VL, Picton TW (1973) Electrical signs of selective attention in the human brain. Science 182: 177–180.
4. Woldorff MG, Gallen CC, Hampson SA, Hillyard SA, Pantev C, et al. (1993) Modulation of early sensory processing in human auditory cortex during auditory selective attention. Proc Natl Acad Sci 90: 8722–8726.
5. Michie PT, Solowij N, Crawford JM, Glue LC (1993) The effects of between-source discriminability on attended and unattended auditory ERPs. Psychophysiology 30: 205–220.
6. Reagan D (1989) Human brain electrophysiology: Evoked potentials and evoked magnetic fields in science and medicine. New York: Elsevier. 546 p.
7. Picton TW, John MS, Dimitrijevic A, Purcell D (2003) Human auditory steady-state responses. Int J Audiol 42: 177–219.
8. Fujiki N, Jousmaki V, Hari R (2002) Neuromagnetic responses to frequency-tagged sounds: a new method to follow inputs from each ear to the human auditory cortex during binaural hearing. J Neuroscience 22: RC205.
9. Giraud A-L, Lorenzi C, Ashburner J, Wable J, Johnsrude I, et al. (2000) Representation of the temporal envelope of sounds in the human brain. J Neurophysiol 84: 1588–1598.
10. Liégeois-Chauvel C, Lorenzi C, Trébuchon A, Régis J, Chauvel P (2004) Temporal envelope processing in the human left and right auditory cortices. Cereb Cortex 14: 731–740.
11. Miller LM, Escabi MA, Read HL, Schreiner CE (2002) Spectrotemporal receptive fields in the lemniscal auditory thalamus and cortex. J Neurophysiol 87: 516–527.
12. Kaneko K, Fujiki N, Hari R (2003) Binaural interaction in the human auditory cortex revealed by neuromagnetic frequency tagging: no effect of stimulus intensity. Hear Res 183: 1–6.
13. Linden DR, Picton TW, Gilles H, Kenneth BC (1987) Human auditory steady-state evoked potentials during selective attention. Electroenceph Clin Neurophysiol 66: 145–159.
14. Lazzouni L, Ross B, Voss P, Lepore F (2010) Neuromagnetic auditory steady-state responses to amplitude modulated sounds following dichotic or monaural presentation. Clin Neurophysiol 121: 200–207.

15. Müller N, Schlee W, Hartmann T, Lorenz I, Weisz N (2009) Top-down modulation of the auditory steady-state response in a task-switch paradigm. Front Hum Neurosci 3:1.
16. Bharadwaj HM, Lee AKC, Shin-Cunningham BG (2014) Measuring auditory selective attention using frequency tagging. Front Integr Neurosci 8: 1.
17. Ross B, Picton T, Herdman A, Pantev C (2004) The effect of attention on the auditory steady-state response. Neurol Clin Neurophysiol 22–22.
18. Evans E (1982) Functions of the auditory system. In: Barlow HB, Mollon, JD, editors. The senses. Cambridge: Cambridge University Press. p.239.
19. Skosnik PD, Krishnan GP, O'Donnell BF (2007) The effect of selective attention on the gamma-band auditory steady-state response. Neuroscie Lett 420: 223–228.
20. John MS, Dimitrijevic A, Picton TW (2003) Efficient stimuloi for evoking auditory steady-state responses. Ear Hear 24: 406–423.
21. Mahajan Y, McArthur G (2010) Does combing the scalp reduce scalp electrode impedances? J Neurosci Meth 188: 287–289.
22. Oostenveld R, Praamstra P (2001) The five percent electrode system for high-resolution EEG and ERP measurements. Clin Neurophysiol 112: 713–719.
23. Delorme A, Makeig S (2004) EEGLAB: an open source toolbox for analysis of single-trial EEG dynamics including independent component analysis. J Neurosci Meth 134: 9–21.
24. Bidet-Caulet A, Fischer C, Besle J, Aguera PE, Giard MH, et al. (2007) Effects of selective attention on the electrophysiological representation of concurrent sounds in the human auditory cortex. J Neurosci 27: 9252–9261.
25. Ross B (2014) Steady-state auditory evoked responses. In: Celesia GG, editor. Handbook of clinical neurophysiology: Disorders of peripheral and central auditory processing. Amsterdam: Elsevier. 10: pp. 137–154.
26. Sininger YS, Bhatara A (2012). Laterality of basic auditory perception. Laterality 17: 129–149.
27. Kawase T, Maki A, Kanno A, Nakasato N, Sato M, et al. (2012) Contralateral white noise attenuates 40-Hz auditory steady-state fields but not N100m in auditory evoked fields. Neuroimage 59: 1037–1042.
28. Staines WR, Graham SJ, Black SE, McIlroy WE (2002) Task-relevant modulation of contralateral and ipsilateral primary somatosensory cortex and the role of a prefrontal-cortical sensory gating system. Neuroimage 15: 190–199.
29. Hugdalh K, Westerhausen R, Alho K, Medvedev S, Laine M, Hämäläinen H (2009) Attention and cognitive control: unfolding the dichotic listening story. Scand J Psychol 50: 11–22.

30. Sanes DH, Malone BJ, Semple MN (1998) Role of synaptic inhibition in processing of dynamic binaural level stimuli. J Neurosci 18: 794–803.

31. Xiong XR, Liang F, Li H, Mesik L, Zhang KK, et al. (2013) Interaural level difference-dependent gain control and synaptic scaling underlying binaural computation. Neuron 79: 738–753.

32. Womelsdorf T, Fries P (2007) The role of neuronal synchronization in selective attention. Curr Opin Neurobiol 17: 154–160.

33. Rinne T, Balk MH, Koistinen S, Autti T, Alho K, Sams M (2008) Auditory selective attention modulates activation of human inferior colliculus. J Neurophysiol 100: 3323–3327.

10

The Relationship between Brain Morphology and Polysomnography in Healthy Good Sleepers

Matthias A. Reinhard[1], Wolfram Regen[1], Chiara Baglioni[1], Christoph Nissen[1], Bernd Feige[1], Jürgen Hennig[2], Dieter Riemann[1], Kai Spiegelhalder[1]*

1 Department of Psychiatry and Psychotherapy, University Medical Center Freiburg, Freiburg, Germany, 2 Department of Diagnostic Radiology, University Medical Center Freiburg, Freiburg, Germany

Abstract

Background: Normal sleep continuity and architecture show remarkable inter-individual variability. Previous studies suggest that brain morphology may explain inter-individual differences in sleep variables.

Method: Thirty-eight healthy subjects spent two consecutive nights at the sleep laboratory with polysomnographic monitoring. Furthermore, high-resolution T1-weighted MRI datasets were acquired in all participants. EEG sleep recordings were analyzed using standard sleep staging criteria and power spectral analysis. Using the FreeSurfer software for automated segmentation, 174 variables were determined representing the volume and thickness of cortical segments and the volume of subcortical brain areas. Regression analyses were performed to examine the relationship with polysomnographic and spectral EEG power variables.

Results: The analysis did not provide any support for the a-priori formulated hypotheses of an association between brain morphology and polysomnographic variables. Exploratory analyses revealed that the thickness of the left caudal anterior cingulate cortex was positively associated with EEG beta2 power (24–32 Hz) during REM sleep. The volume of the left postcentral gyrus was positively associated with periodic leg movements during sleep (PLMS).

Conclusions: The function of the anterior cingulate cortex as well as EEG beta power during REM sleep have been related to dreaming and sleep-related memory consolidation, which may explain the observed correlation. Increased volumes of the postcentral gyrus may be the result of increased sensory input associated with PLMS. However, due to the exploratory nature of the corresponding analyses, these results have to be replicated before drawing firm conclusions.

Editor: Bogdan Draganski, Centre Hospitalier Universitaire Vaudois Lausanne - CHUV, UNIL, Switzerland

Funding: KS and DR have received funding by the Else Kroener-Fresenius-Stiftung (2011_A208; http://www.ekfs.de/). CB and DR have received funding from the European Community's Seventh Framework Programme (People, Marie Curie Actions, Intra-European Fellowship, FP7-PEOPLE-IEF-2008; http://cordis.europa.eu/fp7/home_en.html) under grant agreement n. 235321. The funders had no role in study design, data collection and analysis, decision to publish, or preparation of the manuscript.

Competing Interests: The authors have declared that no competing interests exist.

* Email: Kai.Spiegelhalder@uniklinik-freiburg.de

Introduction

Normal sleep shows remarkable variability among individuals. This variability applies to polysomnographically determined sleep variables like sleep duration and sleep efficiency [1], sleep spindles [2], EEG sigma activity [3] and total EEG spectral power [4]. In contrast, when analyzing night-to-night variability within an individual, some sleep variables are remarkably stable [5]. This stability was found in standard polysomnographic variables [1], and especially in EEG spectral power values during different sleep stages [1,4] as well as in the frequency and topography of sleep spindles [2]. De Gennaro et al. used the term "fingerprint" to describe this high intra-individual stability in sleep EEG parameters [3]. It is plausible to assume that this high intra-individual stability results from stable neurobiological factors, as for example

the morphology of the brain which is closely linked to brain function [6].

Recently, some research has focused on elucidating the association between brain morphology and inter-individual differences in sleep parameters [5,7]. Up to now, these studies focused on EEG spectral power variables because of their particularly high intra-individual stability. Buchmann et al. found a significant correlation between the size of the anterior corpus callosum and the maximal spectral power of slow wave activity (SWA) [7]. Saletin et al., instead, reported that the slow wave amplitude correlated positively with the gray matter volume of the orbitofrontal cortex and the cingulate cortex [5]. Only one study to date has investigated the correlation between subjectively reported sleep continuity variables and specific brain structures in healthy individuals [8]. The authors found a positive correlation between hippocampal volumes in children and self-reported sleep duration.

In summary, no clear picture has emerged from previous investigations and none of the reported findings has been replicated. Furthermore, the association between standard polysomnographic parameters and brain morphology have not been investigated up to now. Therefore, the aim of the current study was to further contribute to our understanding of the relationship between brain morphology and polysomnographic variables by investigating a well-defined sample of healthy good sleepers. The analyses were carried out in two steps. First, the following a-priori hypotheses were tested based on the results of previous work: (1) SWA is significantly correlated with the morphology of the orbitofrontal cortex, the cingulate cortex and the anterior corpus callosum; (2) There is a significant positive correlation between the hippocampal volume and total sleep time. Second, an explorative approach was chosen in order to further explore the associations between polysomnographic variables and other variables of brain morphology.

Materials and Methods

Participants

Forty healthy subjects, who were recruited through local advertisements, were included in the current study. Two participants were excluded from the analysis because of pathologic MRI scans. Thus, the final sample consisted of 38 healthy good sleepers. The data stems from the control group of a project on insomnia morphometry [9,10]. A semistandardized psychiatric and sleep-related interview was conducted by an experienced psychiatrist to rule out any history of psychiatric disorder, shift work, or sleep disorder. Furthermore, all participants underwent a standard physical examination, including electrocardiogram, electroencephalogram (EEG), and routine laboratory investigation (blood cell count; liver, renal and thyroid function) to exclude those with serious medical conditions. All participants were right-handed, as assessed with the Edinburgh Handedness Inventory [11], and free of any psychoactive medication. Participants with a periodic leg movements (PLMS) during sleep arousal index per total sleep time (TST) of more than 5.0/h or a sleep apnea index per TST of more than 5.0/h were not included in the current study. The study was conducted in accordance with the Declaration of Helsinki. The study protocol was approved by the Institutional Review Board of the University Medical Center Freiburg. All participants gave their informed written consent prior to inclusion in the study.

Polysomnography

All participants underwent 2 consecutive nights of polysomnography. The first night served as an adaptation and screening night to rule out sleep apnea, periodic leg movements in sleep, and occult sleep disorder pathology. Sleep was recorded on 24-channel Sagura EEG-polysomnographs for 8 h from "lights out" (22:00 to 23:00) until "lights on" (06:00 to 07:00). All recordings included EEG (F4-M1; C4-M1; O2-M1), electrooculogram (horizontal and vertical) and electromyogram (submental), and were scored visually by experienced raters according to the American Academy of Sleep Medicine criteria [12]. In the first night, all participants were screened for apneas and periodic leg movements by monitoring abdominal and thoracic effort, nasal airflow, oxymetry, and bilateral tibialis anterior EMG. Sleep recordings were evaluated for the following parameters of sleep continuity: TST; sleep efficiency (ratio of TST to time in bed×100%); sleep onset latency defined as time from lights out until sleep onset

(defined as first epoch of stage 2); wake after sleep onset (WASO) defined as difference between sleep period time (SPT; time from sleep onset until final awakening) and TST; number of awakenings; and arousal index. Sleep architecture parameters were amounts of stages 1 and 2, slow wave sleep (SWS) and rapid eye movement sleep (REM) as percentage of SPT. Leg movements and sleep apnea were evaluated according to standard criteria. All participants had to refrain from alcohol, caffeine, and daytime naps during the recording days.

Spectral analysis

A standard procedure was used for EEG spectral analysis (see e.g. [13]). During the night, continuous EEG (C3 referenced to the right ear) was amplified with a time constant of 0.3 s and a low pass at 70 Hz (12 dB/octave), digitized at 200 Hz and stored for off-line analysis. An all-night spectral analysis was performed on the same 30-s epochs for which sleep stages had been determined. Within each epoch, spectral power was calculated using the fast Fourier transform (FFT) algorithm from 22 windows (512-points each) overlapping by half, resulting in a spectral resolution of 0.39 Hz. Within each FFT window, the EEG was demeaned and detrended by subtracting the linear least-squares regression line before applying a Welch window and calculating the FFT. The 22 spectral power estimates were averaged to increase the stability of the estimate. The goal of the further analysis was to minimize the effects of confounding variables on the spectra averaged across epochs, such as the number of movements or arousals and other sleep parameters that can be analyzed separately. This was done by two techniques: (a) arousals and myoclonias were visually marked during staging and epochs including any such events were excluded from the analysis; (b) a fully automatic exclusion of 'deviant' epochs from the average was performed. Deviant epochs were those containing movements or arousals as determined during staging; furthermore, the total (0.8–48 Hz) and gamma-band (32–48 Hz) log power of each epoch were related to the corresponding median-filtered value (the median of values in the 5 min preceding and 5 min following the epoch) and an epoch was excluded if the deviation was larger than the difference between the median and the first quartile of all median-filtered values across the night. In this way, artifacts mainly restricted to low frequencies (such as EOG events) as well as those occurring mainly in higher frequencies (such as EMG contamination) were eliminated in a data-driven way. All-night spectral power averages were obtained across all artifact-free epochs of sleep stage 2 and REM sleep separately. The analysis of NREM sleep was restricted to stage 2 sleep in order to eliminate the influence of different NREM sleep stage distributions across subjects.

The logarithmic (base e) spectra for artifact-free sleep epochs were averaged across each night separately for NREM stage 2 and REM sleep. Logarithmic spectral band power was calculated after adding the spectral power values of FFT bins with center frequency within the following frequency bands: delta1 (0.1–1.0 Hz), delta2 (1.0–3.5 Hz), theta (3.5–8 Hz), alpha (8–12 Hz), sigma1 (12–14 Hz), sigma2 (14–16 Hz), beta1 (16–24 Hz), beta2 (24–32 Hz), and gamma (32–48 Hz). Additionally, the total band (0.1–48 Hz) was calculated.

MRI acquisition and analysis

High-resolution T1-weighted MRI datasets were acquired on a 3-Tesla scanner (Magnetom TIM-Trio, Siemens, Erlangen, Germany) using an MPRAGE sequence (repetition time (TR) 2.2 sec; echo time (TE) 2.6 msec; 160 sagittal slices of 256×256 voxels, $1.0 \times 1.0 \times 1.0$ mm^3 [14]). The MRI investigations were carried out between 7 days and 3 months after the PSG

Table 1. Polysomnographic data of the first and second night (means ± standard deviations).

	Night 1	Night 2
Total sleep time (min)	379.1±56.2	416.3±24.0
Sleep efficiency (%)	80.2±10.0	86.7±5.0
Sleep onset latency (min)	20.7±19.0	17.8±16.5
Sleep period time (min)	446.0±46.7	457.9±22.5
Number of awakenings	38.0±15.8	35.4±13.7
Wake after sleep onset (min)	66.8±40.2	41.6±16.8
Arousal index (h^{-1})	16.9±6.1	14.2±5.7
Stage 1 (% SPT)	11.3±5.2	8.7±4.5
Stage 2 (% SPT)	49.9±8.7	53.8±5.9
SWS (% SPT)	6.8±6.6	8.9±7.2
REM (% SPT)	17.1±5.1	19.5±3.8
Leg movements (during TST)	39.1±34.6	-
Leg movements with arousal (during TST)	4.9±7.7	-
PLMS (during TST)	14.4±21.9	-
PLMS with arousal (during TST)	2.3±4.8	-
PLMS index (h^{-1} TST)	2.4±3.7	-
PLMS index with arousal (h^{-1} TST)	0.4±0.8	-
Apnea hypopnea index (h^{-1} TST)	3.6±4.0	-
Sleep apnea index (h^{-1} TST)	0.4±0.7	-

SPT: sleep period time; SWS: slow wave sleep; REM: rapid eye movement sleep; PLMS: periodic leg movements during sleep; TST: total sleep time.

recordings. All scans were inspected for motion artefacts and for the absence of pathologic findings by a neurologist under the supervision of a board-certified neuroradiologist.

FreeSurfer-based morphometry

Cortical surface reconstruction and volumetric segmentation was performed using the FreeSurfer software, version 5.1.0 (Athinoula A. Martinos Center for Biomedical Imaging; http://surfer.nmr.mgh.harvard.edu/). The technical details of this procedure have been described in previous publications [15,16,17].

For quality control, segmentations were visually inspected for each participant by two independent raters (K.S. and W.R.) on a slice-by-slice basis. However, no manual corrections were necessary for the automatic segmentation results. 38 subcortical volumes ("aseg.stats" files) as well as cortical volume and thickness values of 68 structures ("aparc.stats" files) based on the Killiany/Desikan cortical parcellation [18] were extracted from FreeSurfer, resulting in a total of 174 measures per participant. Additionally, intracranial volume (ICV) was extracted.

Statistical analysis

The data analysis was conducted with the software IBM SPSS Statistics 20.0 (SPSS Inc., Chicago, IL, USA). For descriptive purposes, age and sex effects were investigated. Pearson's correlation was used to determine the association between ICV and age. A t-test for independent groups was performed to test for ICV differences between sexes. Furthermore, a multivariate ANOVA with the 174 morphometric variables as dependent variables was calculated to explore possible sex differences. Mean correlations were calculated using Fisher's Z transformation to describe the association of age with morphometric volumes and thicknesses, respectively.

In order to investigate the relationship between polysomnographic parameters and brain morphometry, univariate linear regression analyses were carried out. In each of these analyses, one polysomnographic parameter was used as dependent variable and one of the 174 morphometric variable was used as independent variable. Intracranial volume (ICV), age and sex were included as covariates in all of these analyses. Non-standardized b-values as well as T-and p-values of the analyses are reported.

For testing hypothesis 1, NREM delta1 and delta2 power of the second night were used as dependent variables and the following variables as independent variables: left medial orbitofrontal volume, right medial orbitofrontal volume, left posterior cingulate volume, right posterior cingulate volume, volume of the anterior corpus callosum. Of note, the posterior cingulate is the region defined by FreeSurfer that most closely approximates the middle cingulate cortex described by Saletin et al. [5]. To obtain a better comparison with the results of Buchmann et al. [7], the regression analyses concerning the anterior corpus callosum were recalculated without correction for ICV and after limiting the study sample to those with an age <40 years. Hypothesis 2 was tested with TST of the second night as dependent variable and the hippocampal volume of the left and right hemisphere as independent variables. Overall, 14 hypothesis-based analyses were carried out. For each of these, the level of significance was set at p<.05 (two-tailed).

The explorative data analysis was also conducted using the above described ICV-, age- and sex-adjusted regression analyses. For each of 39 polysomnographic parameter (11 sleep continuity and sleep architecture variables of the second night [see Table 1], 8 leg movement and respiratory parameters of the first night [see Table 1], and 20 power spectral analysis parameters of the second night [see Table 2]), 174 regression analyses were calculated (in sum, 6786 regression analyses). P-values were corrected using the false discovery rate (FDR [19]) separately for each dependent

Table 2. Power of EEG frequency spectra in REM sleep and NREM stage 2 (means and standard deviations).

		REM		NREM stage 2	
		Night 1	**Night 2**	**Night 1**	**Night 2**
Total	(0.1–48 Hz)	4.34±0.35	4.38±0.31	5.49±0.30	5.45±0.26
Delta1	(0.1–1.0 Hz)	3.15±0.51	3.17±0.41	4.68±0.40	4.61±0.33
Delta2	(1.0–3.5 Hz)	3.08±0.34	3.14±0.35	4.24±0.25	4.24±0.25
Theta	(3.5–8.0 Hz)	2.77±0.30	2.84±0.33	3.50±0.33	3.53±0.35
Alpha	(8–12 Hz)	1.89±0.36	1.93±0.39	2.73±0.41	2.75±0.45
Sigma1	(12–14 Hz)	0.43±0.39	0.43±0.43	1.59±0.50	1.56±0.55
Sigma2	(14–16 Hz)	0.17±0.38	0.16±0.41	0.67±0.50	0.63±0.54
Beta1	(16–24 Hz)	1.02±0.36	1.02±0.39	0.83±0.34	0.79±0.38
Beta2	(24–32 Hz)	0.00±0.54	-0.02±0.60	-0.34±0.35	-0.38±0.44
Gamma	(32–48 Hz)	-1.59±0.58	-1.62±0.62	-1.69±0.47	-1.75±0.51

REM = rapid eye movement sleep; NREM = non rapid eye movement sleep.

variable. The FDR-corrected level of significance was set at p<.05 (two-tailed) for these analyses.

Results

Sample characteristics

The group consisted of 17 men and 21 women with a mean age of 39.6±8.9 years (range: 27–57 years). The mean intracranial volume (ICV) was 1087.7±100.9 cm^3. ICV was not correlated with age ($r = -.11$, $p = .52$), and men had a higher ICV than women ($t[36] = 5.62$, $p<.001$).

The mean correlations of age with morphometric volumes and thicknesses were $r = -.32$, ($t[105] = -13.46$, $p<.001$) and $r = -.26$ ($t[67] = -10.52$, $p<.001$), respectively. A multivariate ANOVA with all 174 morphometric variables as dependent variables missed overall significance ($F[36;1] = 5.01$, $p = .34$) for the independent variable sex.

Polysomnographic data of the sample are presented in Table 1. Data for power of EEG frequency spectra are presented in Table 2.

Testing a-priori hypotheses

Hypothesis 1: Regression analyses did not reveal any significant association between NREM delta1 or delta2 power and the medial orbitofrontal volume (NREM delta1 and left medial orbitofrontal volume: $b = 8.1*10^{-5}$, $t[33] = 0.70$, $p = .49$; NREM delta2 and left medial orbitofrontal volume: $b = 1.3*10^{-4}$, $t[33] = 1.70$, $p = .10$; NREM delta1 and right medial orbitofrontal volume: $b = 8.2*10^{-5}$, $t[33] = 0.80$, $p = .43$; NREM delta2 and right medial orbitofrontal volume: $b = 8.0*10^{-5}$, $t[33] = 1.18$, $p = .25$), posterior cingulate volume (NREM delta1 and left posterior cingulate cortex: $b = -5.1*10^{-5}$, $t[33] = -0.42$, $p = .68$; NREM delta2 and left posterior cingulate cortex: $b = 1.2*10^{-4}$, $t[33] = 1.61$, $p = .12$; NREM delta1 and right posterior cingulate cortex: $b = 7.4*10^{-5}$, $t[33] = 0.68$, $p = .50$; NREM delta2 and right posterior cingulate cortex: $b = 6.1*10^{-5}$, $t[33] = 0.85$, $p = .40$), and the volume of the anterior corpus callosum (NREM delta1: $b = 1.2*10^{-4}$, $t[33] = 0.28$, $p = .78$; NREM delta2: $b = 4.1*10^{-4}$, $t[33] = 1.47$, $p = .15$). After limiting the study sample to those with an age <40 years (11 men, 9 women; age: 32.3±3.4 years) and eliminating ICV from the list of covariates (to obtain a better comparison with the results of Buchmann et al. [7]), regression analyses revealed no

significant relationship between the volume of the anterior corpus callosum and NREM delta1 or delta2 (NREM delta1: $b = -3.6*10^{-4}$, $t[33] = -0.63$, $p = .54$; NREM delta2: $b = 2.2*10^{-4}$, $t[33] = 0.64$, $p = .53$).

Hypothesis 2: Hippocampal volumes were not significantly correlated with TST (left hippocampus: $b = 4.7*10^{-3}$, $t[33] = 0.38$, $p = .71$; right hippocampus: $b = 1.9*10^{-3}$, $t[33] = 0.19$, $p = .85$).

Explorative analyses

Table 3 lists the results of the explorative data analyses that survived FDR correction.

3.3.1 Standard polysomnographic variables. The volume of the left postcentral gyrus was positively correlated with the number of leg movements, the number of PLMS, and the PLMS index (Table 3). Figure 1 shows the corresponding scatter plots. Of note, the associations between the right-hemispheric postcentral volume and the leg movement-related variables pointed in the same direction as the ones for the left-hemispheric postcentral volume. However, these results did not survive FDR correction (number of leg movements: $b = 0.020$, $t[33] = 3.03$, $p = .004$, uncorrected, $p = 0.38$, corrected; number of PLMS: $b = 0.013$, $t[33] = 3.30$, $p = .002$, uncorrected, $p = 0.20$, corrected; PLMS index: $b = 2.1*10^{-3}$, $t[33] = 3.02$, $p = .005$, uncorrected, $p = 0.17$, corrected). The correlations between the left postcentral volume and arousal-associated leg movement variables did also not survive FDR correction (leg movement with arousal: $b = 4.1*10^{-3}$, $t[33] = 3.26$, $p = .003$, uncorrected, $p = 0.45$, corrected; PLMS with arousal: $b = 2.4*10^{-3}$, $t[33] = 3.14$, $p = .004$, uncorrected, $p = 0.62$, corrected; PLMS arousal index: $b = 3.9*10^{-3}$, $t[33] = 3.24$, $p = .003$, uncorrected, $p = 0.47$, corrected).

3.3.2 Spectral analysis. There was a significant relationship between the thickness of the left caudal anterior cingulate cortex (ACC) and beta2 power in REM sleep (see Table 3). Figure 1 shows the corresponding scatter plot. One participant showed a remarkably increased thickness of the left caudal ACC and remarkably high beta2 values during REM sleep (thickness: 3.5 standard deviation [SD] above of the sample's mean; beta2: 4.5 SD above the sample's mean). This participant showed increased beta activity in both nights and selectively during REM sleep. However, with regard to other EEG or sociodemographic variables, no explanation for this deviation could be found. Brain segmentation of this participant was rechecked and, again, rated as

Table 3. Significant relationships between brain structures and polysomnographic variables after FDR correction (adjusted p-values are reported).

				b	t(33)	p
Gyrus postcentralis	L	V	leg movements	0.022	4.57	.01
Gyrus postcentralis	L	V	PLMS	0.015	5.36	.001
Gyrus postcentralis	L	V	PLMS index	$2.6*10^{-3}$	5.13	.002
Caudal ACC	L	T	REM beta2	2.109	4.66	.01

L = left hemisphere; V = volume; PLMS: periodic leg movements during sleep; ACC: anterior cingulate cortex; T = thickness; REM = rapid eye movement sleep.

adequate. The scatter plots show that this participant strongly affects the regression analyses. As a consequence, these results should be interpreted with caution.

Discussion

Testing a-priori hypotheses

The presented data did not provide any support for the a-priori formulated hypotheses of an association between brain morphology and polysomnographic variables. Several potential reasons for this have to be discussed.

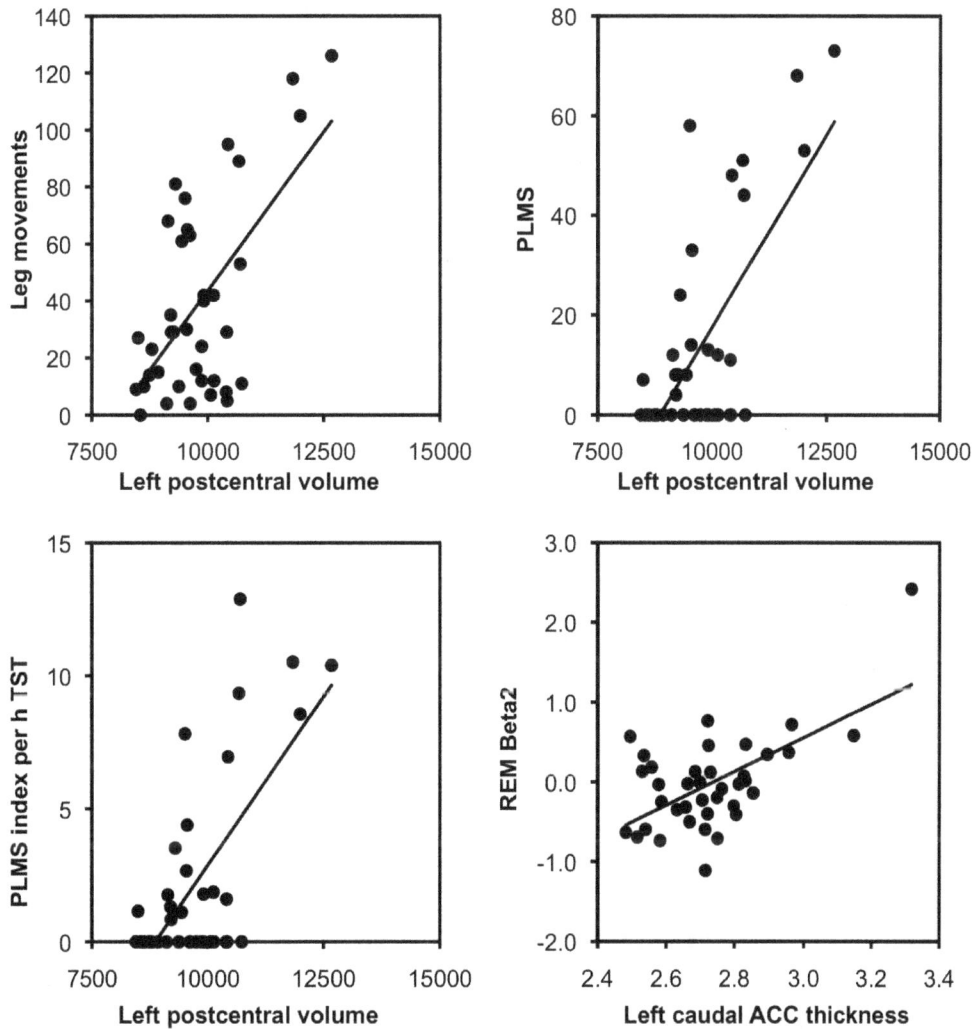

Figure 1. Scatter plots of relationships between brain structures and polysomnographic parameters. Presented volumes are age-, sex- and ICV-adjusted by using the residual method. Solid lines represent regression lines. ACC = anterior cingulate cortex; ICV = intracranial brain volume; PLMS = periodic leg movements during sleep; REM = rapid eye movement sleep; TST = total sleep time.

First, the current study used an automated segmentation technique based on the FreeSurfer tool. While Buchmann et al. [7] used the same software for their analyses, Saletin et al. [5] investigated their sample by using voxel based morphometry, which may detect more subtle differences in localized areas of the brain and may be better suited for subcortical structures with small surface areas (see [18]). Furthermore, in contrast to Buchmann et al. [7], the analyses of the current study were corrected for the influence of ICV, which is a standard technique in brain morphometry studies to reduce the impact of different brain sizes.

Second, the EEG data was processed differently. Saletin et al. [5] calculated SWA amplitude for selected NREM sleep episodes (including stage 2 and SWS) in the frequency range 0.5–4 Hz. Buchmann et al. [7], in comparison, used a rather unique parameter, the maximal SWA (0.5–4.5 Hz) during NREM sleep. The current study instead used all-night power spectral analysis within defined frequency bands, a common method in this field [20].

Last, with respect to the non-replication of the association between total sleep time and hippocampus volumes, the current study investigated adults in contrast to the investigation by Taki et al. [8] who investigated children aged 5 through 18 years. It has also to be noted that Taki et al. had a considerably larger power due to a larger sample size ($N = 290$). Finally, the results are difficult to compare because Taki et al. investigated the association between brain morphology and subjective sleep (measured with a self-assessment questionnaire) without including polysomnographic measurements.

Despite these differences between this study and previous investigations, the current results suggest that other variables than brain morphology contribute substantially to the explanation of variance in PSG parameters.

Explorative analyses

The results of the current study suggest a positive correlation between the volume of the left postcentral gyrus and leg movements during sleep. The association between the volume of the right postcentral gyrus and leg movements during sleep pointed in the same direction. Up to now, the association between brain morphology and leg movements during sleep has not been studied. However, PLMS are a frequent symptom of the restless legs syndrome (RLS) [21], a condition that has been suggested to be associated with morphometric postcentral gyrus alterations before (see [22] for an overview). Furthermore, Margariti et al. [23] showed an increased activation of the left postcentral gyrus during nocturnal leg movements in RLS patients using fMRI. As morphometric studies suggest a positive impact of the activity of a structure on its size [6], an increased postcentral gyrus volume may be the consequence of an increased activity of the postcentral gyrus, an observation that fits well with the uncomfortable and unpleasant sensations of RLS patients. The current study suggests that even PLMS without RLS are associated with an increased postcentral volume, maybe due to a similar mechanistic pathway.

A further important observation of the current study was the positive association between the thickness of the left caudal ACC and EEG beta2 power during REM sleep. In general, beta power is assumed to be a marker of local neuronal processing [24]. However, the underlying causes and/or consequences of beta power during REM sleep remain unclear. High-frequency activity during REM sleep may represent dreaming [25], memory consolidation [26,27] or, more broadly, a chronic increase of arousal levels [28]. Interestingly, the ACC, as an important interface for the regulation and integration of cognitive and emotional processes [29] has also been linked to dreaming and memory processes [30,31]. With respect to the link between both ACC and EEG beta power to arousal levels, it should be noted that a recent morphometric investigation found increased ACC volumes in primary insomnia patients [32], a disorder which is characterized by increased arousal levels [33], which are, in turn, assumed to be reflected in increased levels of nocturnal spectral beta power [28]. This is in line with the results of the current investigation and suggests that the ACC may be involved in the modulation of arousal levels during sleep. However, it has to be noted that the causal pathways between ACC thickness, spectral beta power during REM sleep and the above-mentioned sleep-related processes (dreaming, sleep-related memory consolidation, arousal) remain unclear due to the cross-sectional design of the current investigation.

Limitations

Several limitations have to be discussed with respect to the current results and interpretations. First, although the current sample is well characterized, it is a convenience sample possibly reducing external validity. In particular, the sample had a comparably low sleep efficiency and high number of awakenings [34]. However, in comparison with previous studies the present sample appears to be representative of other healthy participants of the sleep laboratory in Freiburg [35]. Second, it should be noted that, in the current study, PLMS was measured only during the first night. As Hornyak et al. reported a large variability in the occurrence of PLMS [36] future studies may investigate the association between brain morphology and PLMS measured across multiple nights. Third, subcortical structures with smaller surface areas are probably less reliably segmented by FreeSurfer than cortical structures [18], and, thus, voxel-based morphometry may be a better option for subcortical structures. Last, the current study used a cross-sectional design. A longitudinal approach would reveal maturation processes and neural plasticity. In this context, a study of a sample of children and adolescents would be of particular interest.

Conclusions

The presented data did not provide any support for the a-priori formulated hypotheses regarding the association between brain morphology and polysomnographic variables. However, exploratory data analysis revealed a significant relationship between the postcentral volume and the occurrence of PLMS which may be the result of an increased sensory input associated with PLMS. Additionally, the ACC thickness was positively associated with beta2 power during REM sleep. This may be explained by an involvement of both ACC and beta power in dreaming, sleep-related memory consolidation and arousal levels.

Author Contributions

Conceived and designed the experiments: KS CN JH DR. Performed the experiments: KS CB. Analyzed the data: MAR WR BF KS. Contributed to the writing of the manuscript: MAR WR CB CN BF JH DR KS. Drafting the manuscript: MAR KS. Revising the manuscript critically for important intellectual content: WR CB CN BF JH DR. Final approval of the manuscript and agreement to be accountable for all aspects of the work: MAR WR CB CN BF JH DR KS.

References

1. Tucker AM, Dinges DF, Van Dongen HPA (2007) Trait interindividual differences in the sleep physiology of healthy young adults. J Sleep Res 16: 170–180. Available: http://dx.doi.org/10.1111/j.1365-2869.2007.00594.x.
2. Werth E, Achermann P, Dijk DJ, Borbély AA (1997) Spindle frequency activity in the sleep EEG: individual differences and topographical distribution. Electroencephalogr Clin Neurophysiol 103: 535–542. Available: http://dx.doi.org/10.1016/S0013-4694(97)00070-9.
3. De Gennaro L, Ferrara M, Vecchio F, Curcio G, Bertini M (2005) An electroencephalographic fingerprint of human sleep. Neuroimage 26: 114–122. Available: http://dx.doi.org/10.1016/j.neuroimage.2005.01.020.
4. Lewandowski A, Rosipal R, Dorffner G (2013) On the individuality of sleep EEG spectra. J Psychophysiol 27: 105–112. Available: http://dx.doi.org/10.1027/0269-8803/a000092.
5. Saletin JM, van der Helm E, Walker MP (2013) Structural brain correlates of human sleep oscillations. Neuroimage 83: 658–668. Available: http://dx.doi.org/10.1016/j.neuroimage.2013.06.021.
6. May A, Gaser C (2006) Magnetic resonance-based morphometry: a window into structural plasticity of the brain. Curr Opin Neurol 19: 407–411.
7. Buchmann A, Kurth S, Ringli M, Geiger A, Jenni OG, et al. (2011) Anatomical markers of sleep slow wave activity derived from structural magnetic resonance images. J Sleep Res 20: 506–513. Available: http://dx.doi.org/10.1111/j.1365-2869.2011.00916.x.
8. Taki Y, Hashizume H, Thyreau B, Sassa Y, Takeuchi H, et al. (2012) Sleep duration during weekdays affects hippocampal gray matter volume in healthy children. Neuroimage 60: 471–475. Available: http://dx.doi.org/10.1016/j.neuroimage.2011.11.072.
9. Spiegelhalder K, Regen W, Baglioni C, Klöppel S, Abdulkadir A, et al. (2013) Insomnia does not appear to be associated with substantial structural brain changes. Sleep 36: 731–737. Available: http://dx.doi.org/10.5665/sleep.2638.
10. Spiegelhalder K, Regen W, Prem M, Baglioni C, Nissen C, et al. (2014) Reduced anterior internal capsule white matter integrity in primary insomnias. Hum Brain Mapp 35: 3431–3438. Available: http://dx.doi.org/10.1002/hbm.22412.
11. Oldfield RC (1971) The assessment and analysis of handedness: the Edinburgh inventory. Neuropsychologia 9: 97–113. Available: http://dx.doi.org/10.1016/0028-3932(71)90067-4.
12. American Academy of Sleep Medicine (2007) The AASM Manual for the Scoring of Sleep and Associated Events: Rules, Terminology and Technical Specifications. Westchester: American Academy of Sleep Medicine.
13. Spiegelhalder K, Regen W, Feige B, Holz J, Piosczyk H, et al. (2012) Increased EEG sigma and beta power during NREM sleep in primary insomnia. Biol Psychol 91: 329–333. Available: http://dx.doi.org/10.1016/j.biopsycho.2012.08.009.
14. Mugler JP, Brookeman JR (1990) Three-dimensional magnetization-prepared rapid gradient-echo imaging (3D MP RAGE). Magn Reson Med 15: 152–157.
15. Fischl B, Dale AM (2000) Measuring the thickness of the human cerebral cortex from magnetic resonance images. Proc Natl Acad Sci 97: 11050–11055. Available: http://dx.doi.org/10.1073/pnas.200033797.
16. Fischl B (2012) FreeSurfer. Neuroimage 62: 774–781. Available: http://dx.doi.org/10.1016/j.neuroimage.2012.01.021.
17. Fischl B, Salat DH, Busa E, Albert M, Dieterich M, et al. (2002) Whole brain segmentation: automated labeling of neuroanatomical structures in the human brain. Neuron 33: 341–355. Available: http://dx.doi.org/10.1016/S0896-6273(02)00569-X.
18. Desikan RS, Ségonne F, Fischl B, Quinn BT, Dickerson BC, et al. (2006) An automated labeling system for subdividing the human cerebral cortex on MRI scans into gyral based regions of interest. Neuroimage 31: 968–980. Available: http://dx.doi.org/10.1016/j.neuroimage.2006.01.021.
19. Benjamini Y, Hochberg Y (1995) Controlling the false discovery rate: a practical and powerful approach to multiple testing. J R Statist Soc Ser B (Methodological), 57: 289–300.
20. Achermann P, Dijk DJ, Brunner DP, Borbély AA (1993) A model of human sleep homeostasis based on EEG slow-wave activity: quantitative comparison of data and simulations. Brain Res Bull 31: 97–113. Available: http://dx.doi.org/10.1016/0361-9230(93)90016-5.
21. Hening W (2004) The clinical neurophysiology of the restless legs syndrome and periodic limb movements. Part I: diagnosis, assessment, and characterization. Clin Neurophysiol 115: 1965–1974. Available: http://dx.doi.org/10.1016/j.clinph.2004.03.032.
22. Rizzo G, Manners D, Vetrugno R, Tonon C, Malucelli E, et al. (2012) Combined brain voxel-based morphometry and diffusion tensor imaging study in idiopathic restless legs syndrome patients. Eur J Neurol 19: 1045–1049. Available: http://dx.doi.org/10.1111/j.1468-1331.2011.03604.x.
23. Margariti PN, Astrakas LG, Tsouli SG, Hadjigeorgiou GM, Konitsiotis S, et al. (2012) Investigation of unmedicated early onset restless legs syndrome by voxel-based morphometry, T2 relaxometry, and functional MR imaging during the night-time hours. Am J Neuroradiol 33: 667–672. Available: http://dx.doi.org/10.3174/ajnr.A2829.
24. Engel AK, Fries P (2010) Beta-band oscillations – signalling the status quo? Curr Opin Neurobiol 20: 156–165. Available: http://dx.doi.org/10.1016/j.conb.2010.02.015.
25. Llinas R, Ribary U (1993) Coherent 40-Hz oscillation characterizes dream state in humans. Proc Natl Acad Sci 90: 2078–2081. Available: http://dx.doi.org/10.1073/pnas.90.5.2078.
26. Quyen MLV, Staba R, Bragin A, Dickson C, Valderrama M, et al. (2010) Large-scale microelectrode recordings of high-frequency gamma oscillations in human cortex during sleep. J Neurosci 30: 7770–7782. Available: http://dx.doi.org/10.1523/jneurosci.5049-09.2010.
27. Rasch B, Born J (2013) About sleep's role in memory. Physiol Rev 93: 681–766. Available: http://dx.doi.org/10.1152/physrev.00032.2012.
28. Perlis ML, Merica H, Smith MT, Giles DE (2001) Beta EEG activity and insomnia. Sleep Med Rev 5: 365–376. Available: http://dx.doi.org/10.1053/smrv.2001.0151.
29. Rushworth MFS, Behrens TEJ, Rudebeck PH, Walton ME (2007) Contrasting roles for cingulate and orbitofrontal cortex in decisions and social behaviour. Trends Cogn Sci 11: 168–176. Available: http://dx.doi.org/10.1016/j.tics.2007.01.004.
30. Hobson JA (2009) REM sleep and dreaming: towards a theory of proto-consciousness. Nat Rev Neurosci 10: 803–813. Available: http://dx.doi.org/10.1038/nrn2716.
31. Maquet P, Laureys S, Peigneux P, Fuchs S, Petiau C, et al. (2000) Experience-dependent changes in cerebral activation during human REM sleep. Nat Neurosci 3: 831–836. Available: http://dx.doi.org/10.1038/77744.
32. Winkelman JW, Plante DT, Schoerning L, Benson K, Buxton OM, et al. (2013) Increased rostral anterior cingulate cortex volume in chronic primary insomnia. Sleep 36: 991–998. Available: http://dx.doi.org/10.5665/sleep.2794.
33. Riemann D, Spiegelhalder K, Feige B, Voderholzer U, Berger M, et al. (2010) The hyperarousal model of insomnia: A review of the concept and its evidence. Sleep Med Rev 14: 19–31. Available: http://dx.doi.org/10.1016/j.smrv.2009.04.002.
34. Ohayon MM, Carskadon MA, Guilleminault C, Vitiello MV (2004) Meta-analysis of quantitative sleep parameters from childhood to old age in healthy individuals: developing normative sleep values across the human lifespan. Sleep 27: 1255–1274.
35. Feige B, Al-Shajlawi A, Nissen C, Voderholzer U, Hornyak M, et al. (2008) Does REM sleep contribute to subjective wake time in primary insomnia? A comparison of polysomnographic and subjective sleep in 100 patients. J Sleep Res 17: 180–190. Available: http://dx.doi.org/10.1111/j.1365-2869.2008.00651.x.
36. Hornyak M, Kopasz M, Feige B, Riemann D, Voderholzer U (2005) Variability of periodic leg movements in various sleep disorders: implications for clinical and pathophysiologic studies. Sleep 28: 331–335.

11

Early Postnatal EEG Features of Perinatal Arterial Ischaemic Stroke with Seizures

Evonne Low[1], Sean R. Mathieson[2], Nathan J. Stevenson[1], Vicki Livingstone[1], C. Anthony Ryan[1], Conor O. Bogue[1], Janet M. Rennie[2], Geraldine B. Boylan[1]*

1 Neonatal Brain Research Group, Irish Centre for Fetal and Neonatal Translational Research, Department of Paediatrics and Child Health, University College Cork, Cork, Ireland, 2 Elizabeth Garrett Anderson Institute for Women's Health, University College London Hospital, London, United Kingdom

Abstract

Background: Stroke is the second most common cause of seizures in term neonates and is associated with abnormal long-term neurodevelopmental outcome in some cases.

Objective: To aid diagnosis earlier in the postnatal period, our aim was to describe the characteristic EEG patterns in term neonates with perinatal arterial ischaemic stroke (PAIS) seizures.

Design: Retrospective observational study.

Patients: Neonates >37 weeks born between 2003 and 2011 in two hospitals.

Method: Continuous multichannel video-EEG was used to analyze the background patterns and characteristics of seizures. Each EEG was assessed for continuity, symmetry, characteristic features and sleep cycling; morphology of electrographic seizures was also examined. Each seizure was categorized as electrographic-only or electroclinical; the percentage of seizure events for each seizure type was also summarized.

Results: Nine neonates with PAIS seizures and EEG monitoring were identified. While EEG continuity was present in all cases, the background pattern showed suppression over the infarcted side; this was quite marked (>50% amplitude reduction) when the lesion was large. Characteristic unilateral bursts of theta activity with sharp or spike waves intermixed were seen in all cases. Sleep cycling was generally present but was more disturbed over the infarcted side. Seizures demonstrated a characteristic pattern; focal sharp waves/spike-polyspikes were seen at frequency of 1–2 Hz and phase reversal over the central region was common. Electrographic-only seizure events were more frequent compared to electroclinical seizure events (78 *vs* 22%).

Conclusions: Focal electrographic and electroclinical seizures with ipsilateral suppression of the background activity and focal sharp waves are strong indicators of PAIS. Approximately 80% of seizure events were the result of clinically unsuspected seizures in neonates with PAIS. Prolonged and continuous multichannel video-EEG monitoring is advocated for adequate seizure surveillance.

Editor: Natasha M. Maurits, University Medical Center Groningen UMCG, Netherlands

Funding: E.L. was funded by a Wellcome Trust Translational Award UK (85249/z/08/z) and N.J.S. received funding from Science Foundation Ireland Principal Investigator Award (10/IN.1/B3036). This work was also partly undertaken at University London Hospitals/University College London, which received a proportion of funding from the Department of National Institute for Health Research and Biomedical Research Centers funding scheme. The funders had no role in study design, data collection and analysis, decision to publish, or preparation of the manuscript.

Competing Interests: The authors have declared that no competing interests exist.

* Email: G.Boylan@ucc.ie

Introduction

Perinatal arterial ischaemic stroke (PAIS) occurs approximately 1 in 2500 livebirths and is recognized as a common cause of early onset neonatal seizures. [1] Approximately 20% of neonatal seizures are due to PAIS, [2] and neonatal seizures have been noted in up to 26% of neonates with PAIS. [3] Generally, neonates with PAIS are non-encephalopathic but those with significant seizure burden can be neurologically abnormal, making the distinction from seizures due to other causes such as hypoxia-ischaemia difficult in the acute neonatal period. [4] The diagnosis of PAIS should be suspected when seizures are observed in non-encephalopathic neonates within the first 48 hours of birth. [5] While cranial ultrasound scans have been shown to have good diagnostic capabilities when performed after day 4, [6] confirmation of diagnosis is only reliably achieved with magnetic resonance imaging (MRI); however this facility is not readily available in many institutions.

Electroencephalogram (EEG) or amplitude integrated-EEG (aEEG) is now one of the first diagnostic tools available at the cotside in the neonatal intensive care unit for the assessment of cerebral function. Most studies in PAIS have described EEG changes in the first week after birth, but typical changes observed in the first 48 hours after birth have not been described. Early EEG may distinguish neonates with PAIS from those with hypoxic-ischaemic encephalopathy (HIE) [3] and other aetiologies, providing invaluable support for clinical decision-making and counselling. The aEEG has been used to obtain additional information in neonates with PAIS by van Rooij et al. [7] and Mercuri et al. [8]; however these studies have not given details on the characteristics of electrographic seizures. Early accurate recognition of PAIS would be helpful in distinguishing neonates with seizures who do not fulfil the current criteria for therapeutic hypothermia, but who require thrombophilic screening and high quality MRI for diagnosis and prognosis. The aim of our study was to characterize the early postnatal EEG findings in term neonates with PAIS who had seizures.

Methods

Ethics statement

This study was approved by the Clinical Research Ethics Committees of the Cork Teaching hospitals, Ireland and the National Health Service in the United Kingdom (UK), via the Integrated Research Application Service. Written, informed consent was obtained from at least one parent of each neonate who participated in this study.

Patients

Neonates were enrolled from Cork University Maternity Hospital (CUMH), Ireland between June 2003 and October 2011 and University College London Hospital (UCLH), UK from January 2009 to October 2011 as part of an ongoing study of neonatal seizures. Neonates >37 weeks gestation were enrolled for EEG monitoring if they fulfilled at least one of the following criteria: Apgar score <6 at five minutes; a continued need for resuscitation after birth; any clinical evidence of encephalopathy or seizures within 72 hours of age. The diagnosis of PAIS was based on neuroimaging evidence of focal infarction affecting at most two arterial territories. Study analysis included only neonates with PAIS who had electrographic seizures. Neonates with HIE, infections, inborn errors of metabolism, blood disorders, venous or multiple infarctions were excluded due to differing pathogeneses and clinical manifestations when compared to those with focal arterial infarction.

Clinical features

All clinical seizures were treated as well as seizures recognized by the clinical team interpreting the aEEG. The aEEG used to confirm suspected seizures was also used as an aid in clinical decision-making at the cotside. Concern regarding any abnormal behaviour or aEEG pattern prompted a review of the multichannel EEG from the neurophysiologist in each hospital. Immediate reporting of the multichannel EEG was not always available; the aEEG and clinical suspicion were the mainstays of seizure diagnosis. Phenobarbitone was the first-line anticonvulsant administered to a maximum dose of 40 mg/kg intravenously. Second-line anticonvulsants were administered if clinical and/or electrographic seizures recurred following phenobarbitone administration. In both hospitals, second-line anticonvulsant was either intravenous phenytoin or midazolam. Although standardized protocols for the use of anticonvulsants were similar in both hospitals, the choice of second-line anticonvulsant administration was at the discretion of the attending neonatologist. The timing and dose of each anticonvulsant as well as morphine administered were recorded in all neonates.

EEG features

Clinical details of all neonates were obtained at the time of monitoring. Throughout the study, EEG recording methods were identical at both hospitals. A Nicolet monitor (Carefusion NeuroCare, Wisconsin, USA) was used to record multichannel video-EEG, using the 10–20 system of electrode placement modified for neonates. [9] EEG monitoring was commenced when recruitment criteria were met and continued for at least 20 hours. Scalp electrodes were placed at F3, F4, C3, C4, T3, T4, O1, O2 and Cz locations to record EEG activity from the frontal, central, temporal and occipital areas. Parietal electrodes (P3–P4) were also used where possible. Impedances below five kΩ were maintained. Simultaneous bilateral aEEG trends, electrocardiogram and respiration traces were also displayed on the monitor.

All EEG recordings from each neonate were independently reviewed by an experienced neonatal electroencephalographer (GBB). The entire background EEG pattern was graded and assessed for continuity, symmetry, synchrony and other specific features. Sleep cycling was assessed as being present, absent or disturbed in each neonate; a disturbed sleep cycling signified an interruption to the expected sleep cycle architecture of healthy term neonates. [10] Significant EEG suppression was defined as EEG activity below five μV in all EEG channels for at least 10 seconds respectively. The morphology of seizures was also assessed. An electrographic seizure was defined as a sudden and evolving repetitive stereotyped waveform with a definite start, middle and end, lasting for at least 10 seconds [11] on at least one EEG channel. Status epilepticus was defined as continuous or accumulative electrographic seizure activity lasting ≥50% of a one-hour period. [12]

Any associated clinical correlates with all electrographic seizures annotated were analyzed using the simultaneous video recording. Electrographic-only seizures were defined as clear electrographic seizures without any clinical correlates. [13] Electroclinical seizures were defined as electrographic seizures accompanied with behavioural correlates. Clinical seizures were defined as paroxysmal alterations in neurological function (behaviour, motor or autonomic); the description was based on those categorized by Volpe. [2] Subtle seizures were defined as paroxysmal behaviours (including changes in autonomic parameters) which were not clearly clonic, tonic or myoclonic seizures [2] and included behaviours such as eye blinking, pedalling or cycling movements of the limbs, hiccups, sucking or chewing movements and apnoeic spells.

Radiographic features

MRI studies were performed in a Siemens Avanto 1.5 Tesla unit (Siemens Ag, Erlangen, Germany) and CT scanning was performed using a Toshiba Aquilion 4-detector row CT (Toshiba, Tochigi-ken, Japan). All imaging studies were performed without sedation. Neonates were transferred to the MRI scanner in an MRI-compatible incubator with integrated neonatal array coils (MR Diagnostics Incubator, Lammers Medical Technology GmbH, Luebeck, Germany). The arterial territory and estimated size of cerebral infarction based on methods described by Marks et al., [14] were reported by an experienced paediatric radiologist (COB).

Statistical analysis

The total seizure burden was defined as the total duration of recorded electrographic seizures in minutes. Electrographic seizure window was defined as the timepoint between the first and last recorded electrographic seizure in hours. Seizure burden was also expressed in terms of seizure per hour and was calculated using a formula:

Seizure burden = total seizure burden (minutes)/ electrographic seizure window (hours).

In each neonate, the mean seizure duration is calculated as the proportion of the total seizure burden in seconds relative to the number of seizures.

Mean seizure duration = total seizure burden (in seconds) / total number of seizures.

To avoid neonates with many seizures having much influence on the results, summary measures were calculated for each neonate. These summary measures were percentages of the number of seizure events and the seizure burden (seizure duration in minutes) associated with electrographic-only, electroclinical seizures and the duration when viewing of the video was obscured (for example during a medical procedure); they were calculated relative to the total number of electrographic seizures and the total seizure burden (seizure duration in minutes). For example:

% number of electrographic-only seizures = (the number of electrographic-only seizures/ the total number of seizures) * 100

% seizure burden of electrographic-only seizures = (the seizure burden of electrographic-only seizures/ the total seizure burden) * 100

% number of electroclinical seizures = (the number of electroclinical seizures/ the total number of seizures) * 100

% seizure burden of electroclinical seizures = (the seizure burden of electroclinical seizures/ the total seizure burden) * 100.

These summary measures were then described across all neonates using medians and interquartile ranges (IQR). For paired comparisons, the Wilcoxon signed-rank test was used. All statistical analyses were performed using SPSS Statistics 20.0 (IBM SPSS Statistics, Illinois, USA). All tests were two-sided; p-value <0.05 was considered to be statistically significant.

Results

During the study, nine neonates with PAIS who had continuous early EEG monitoring had electrographic seizures. Five neonates had coagulation testing and none had thrombophilic disorders. Table 1 lists the clinical demographics and outlines the MRI findings in eight of the nine neonates with various degrees of middle cerebral artery (MCA) infarction; one neonate had CT imaging. Cranial imaging was undertaken at a median (IQR) of 5 (3–12) days after birth.

Table 2 summarizes the background EEG and seizure characteristics for each neonate. In all neonates, a continuous background pattern was present but voltage suppression and intermittent sharp theta discharges were seen over the infarcted side (figure 1). Background EEG suppression was greatest in cases where the estimated size of infarction was larger than 66% of one hemisphere. Sleep cycling was present in all cases but disturbed in 5 of the 9 neonates. The morphology of seizures in neonates with PAIS showed a characteristic pattern in all cases (figure 2). Spike and polyspike waves at a frequency of 1–2 Hz were seen over the infarcted side and phase reversal of these spikes over the central region was evident as the seizure evolved. Higher frequency temporal discharges were seen during apnoea in a neonate who presented with dusky episodes.

Of 536 electrographic seizures identified from multichannel EEG in this cohort of neonates with PAIS; 519 were classified (table 2). Accumulatively, there were more electrographic-only seizure events (n = 405; 78%) than electroclinical seizure events

(n = 114; 22%). Summary measures of each neonate showed that the median (IQR) electrographic-only seizure events was higher than electroclinical seizure events [66 (52–90) *vs* 29 (8–40)%; p = 0.051]. Subtle seizures were noted in six of nine neonates and manifested activities such as pedalling or cycling movements of the limbs, sucking or chewing movements. Other occasional subtle seizures noted were hiccups and eye blinking episodes. When electroclinical seizures were subdivided, there were more subtle (n = 61; 12%) than clonic seizures (n = 53; 10%) [median (IQR) of subtle *vs* clonic seizures = 12 (0–22) *vs* 7 (2–24)%; p = 0.553]. The median percentage of seizure burden of electrographic-only was higher than electroclinical seizures [49 (31–88) *vs* 44 (12–51)%; p = 0.515]. This is despite the significantly shorter median duration of electrographic-only when compared to electroclinical seizures [100 (55–173) *vs* 181 (95–359) seconds; p<0.001].

The temporal distribution of electrographic-only and electroclinical seizures with anticonvulsant administration superimposed for each neonate are shown in figure 3. In four of nine neonates (cases 1, 2, 3 and 6), anticonvulsants were administered prior to prolonged multichannel EEG monitoring, hence before the first electrographic seizure. All nine neonates with PAIS received first-line anticonvulsants at 34 (20–46) hours while seven neonates received second-line anticonvulsants at 48 (29–66) hours.

Discussion

The background EEG generally showed suppression over the affected side; this was quite marked (>50% amplitude reduction) if the infarction was large. Characteristic unilateral theta bursts with intermixed sharp or spike waves were seen in all cases over the infarcted side. Sleep cycling was generally present but was more disturbed over the infarcted side. Seizures in neonates with PAIS appear to have a characteristic pattern and in all cases, focal sharp waves/spike-polyspike seizure discharges were seen at a frequency of 1–2 Hz over the area of infarction. In our experience, the morphology of these seizures is quite characteristic and markedly different from seizures due to HIE. [15] All neonates in our series had MCA involvement; seizures were generally seen over the central region and phase reversal of spike and polyspike discharges were a common finding. This is the first study to describe these characteristic EEG findings in a series of neonates with PAIS in the early postnatal period; these findings may prove very useful for early diagnosis of neonates with seizures.

Indeed PAIS tends to be a clinical diagnosis when three important findings are present: no clear history of HIE, seizure onset beyond 12 hours after birth and focal seizures. In many instances when the affected cases are discussed retrospectively, subtle details are often missed; they usually revealed a slightly complicated antenatal history such as mild changes on the cardiotocogram or meconium stained delivery. [16] Apgar scores and clinical history may be subjective. We advocate the use of the EEG as an adjunct to suggest the early diagnosis of PAIS during the neonatal period when clinical suspicions are aroused.

Comparing one-channel with the two-channel aEEG recordings in 34 neonates who had seizures due to unilateral brain injury, van Rooij et al. showed more varied seizures patterns, asymmetry in the background activity and a difference in sleep cycling on the ipsilateral side, [7] however this study gave no specific analysis on a subgroup of neonates who had PAIS (n = 5) or specifically those who had MCA involvement (n = 3). Using a four-channel aEEG in 19 neonates with PAIS (6 neonates with asymmetrical and 2 with bilateral sharp waves/ spikes, 8 no seizures, 3 not recorded), Mercuri et al. showed that the presence of seizures accompanied by a normal background EEG was not related to abnormal

Table 1. Demographics and neuroimaging features of neonates in the order of increasing seizure burden.

Neonate	1	2	3	4	5	6	7	8	9
Birthweight (grams)	3700	3740	3750	3410	2830	3420	3160	3670	3480
Gestation (weeks)	40	35	41	41	39	41	39	41	41
Gender	Male	Male	Male	Female	Female	Female	Male	Male	Male
Perinatal events	None	Polyhydramnios, PROM (36 h)	NRCTG	None	NRCTG, PROM (>13 h)	None	NRTCG	FTP	FTP
Mode of delivery	VV	VV	EMCS	Forceps	EMCS	Ventouse	EMCS	EMCS	EMCS
First pH	7.42	7.04	7.13	7.29	7.00	7.34	7.30	7.41	7.27
5 min Apgar	10	9	9	10	6	7	10	10	10
Age at first clinical seizure (hours)	36	54	20	6	47	33	15	18	33
First clinical seizure	RUL	Dusky episodes	LS	RS	LLL	RS	RUL	RUL	LUL
Age at EEG (hours)	54	55	26	9	53	3	18	19	36
Age at first recorded EEG seizure (hours)	54	60	26	9	53	39	19	19	36
EEG duration (hours)	25	70	49	39	44	46	49	63	229
Cerebral infarction	LMCA	LMCA	RMCA	LMCA, RMCA	RMCA	LMCA	LMCA	LMCA, LPCA	RMCA
Age at cranial imaging (days)	5	8	29	3	10	3	2	3	14
Estimated size of infarction (%)	<33	>66	<33	<33	33–66	33–66	<33	>66	33–66

EMCS, emergency Caesarean section; FTP, failure to progress; LLL, left lower limb clonic; LMCA, left middle cerebral artery; LPCA, left posterior cerebral artery; LS, left-sided clonic; LUL, left upper limb clonic movements; NRCTG, non-reassuring cardiotocogram; PROM, premature rupture of membranes; RMCA, right middle cerebral artery; RS, right-sided clonic; RUL, right upper limb clonic; VV, vertex vaginal.

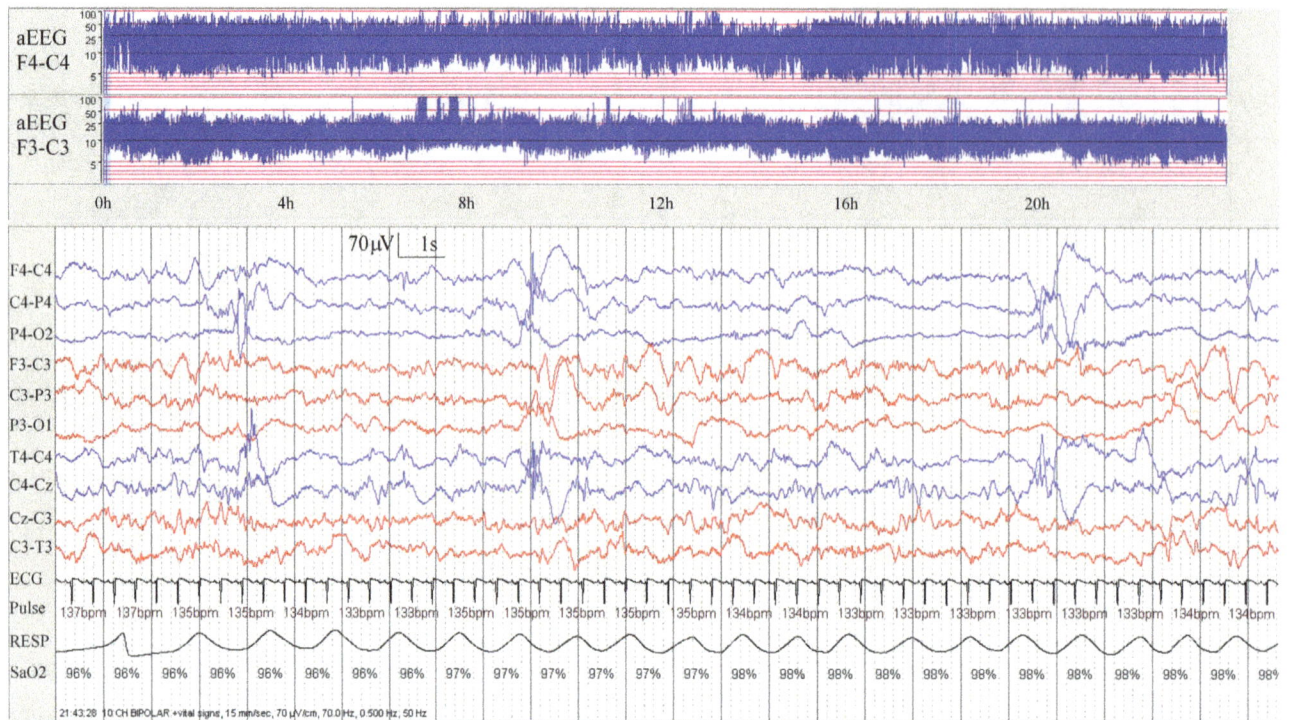

Figure 1. Background EEG pattern in a neonate (case 9) with a right middle cerebral artery infarction. Note the mild voltage reduction over the right hemisphere on EEG (blue channels) which is also evident on the aEEG with a wider band on the right in comparison to the left side. In addition, intermittent right-sided bursts of higher voltage sharpened theta activity are also evident. Some sleep cycling is also present over the left albeit disturbed but this is absent over the right side.

outcome; [8] this indicates that both factors are poor predictors of outcome. Although our study was not aimed to assess outcome, we believe that an abnormal background and the presences of seizures have a much higher prognostic value. Also, the study by Mercuri *et al.* had not assessed seizures as an independent factor in determining outcome. [8] Multichannel EEG has been shown to be more accurate than the aEEG in detecting seizures. Our EEG findings based on multichannel EEG recordings are similar to studies by van Rooij *et al.* [7] and Mercuri *et al.* [8] which used the aEEG, however we have provided more details on the characteristics of seizures early in the neonatal period in terms of seizure morphology and more detailed seizure characteristics in a cohort of neonates with PAIS.

Several studies have reported the electrographic seizure burden in neonates with HIE, [17], [18] but none has quantified seizure burden in neonates with PAIS using continuous multichannel EEG. A study by Rafay *et al.* compared the EEG characteristics between neonates with PAIS and HIE; [3] they showed that there was no significant difference in the number of neonates who had electrographic seizures (PAIS *vs* HIE: 7/27 *vs* 13/35; p = 0.350]. Although their study contributed further to our understanding of neonatal seizures, the results were limited because EEG findings were described exclusively from EEG reports generated by a neurophysiology service. In our study, we have explored further on the multichannel EEG recordings. The overall seizure burden was high in our study; prolonged multichannel video-EEG monitoring showed that the number of seizures is higher than clinically apparent. In our study, anticonvulsants were administered when there was a clinical concern of seizures. The use of anticonvulsants may have resulted in more electrographic-only seizures [19]; and in our study we have shown that 80% of seizure events were

electrographic-only seizures. The high number of seizures which we uncovered in this group of neonates was surprising but reinforces the need for early and continuous EEG monitoring in this group of neonates. In comparison, electroclinical dissociation has been reported to occur up to 28% of neonates with HIE; however this figure was based on aEEG findings in neonates above 32 weeks gestation and its association with anticonvulsant administration was not described. [20] The studies by van Rooij *et al.* [7] and Mercuri *et al.* [8] did not provide information on the dissociation of seizures. Many of the previous studies reported the clinical response to anticonvulsants without any EEG monitoring. [21–23] It is known that anticonvulsants can be a sedative agent and lead to electroclinical uncoupling or dissociation. [24] Clinical seizures are therefore a poor indicator when it comes to assessing the response to anticonvulsants; hence the true response of anticonvulsants in seizure control in neonates with PAIS remains unknown. Our study highlights that despite the use of anticonvulsants, under tight EEG monitoring, there are still ongoing electrographic seizures in neonates with PAIS. Neonatologists should be aware of this when treating neonates with PAIS who are already treated with initial anticonvulsants, particularly in the absence of EEG monitoring. This also explains why several neonates in our study had many hours of repetitive seizures and were not treated with anticonvulsants. We believe that this study is the first to demonstrate the high seizure burden in PAIS using continuous multichannel EEG monitoring and is thus of significant and practical clinical importance.

The MCA is the most commonly involved artery for ischaemic infarction in term neonates (the posterior branch irrigates the occipital, temporal and posterior parietal areas, while the anterior branch irrigates the prefrontal, precentral, central and anterior

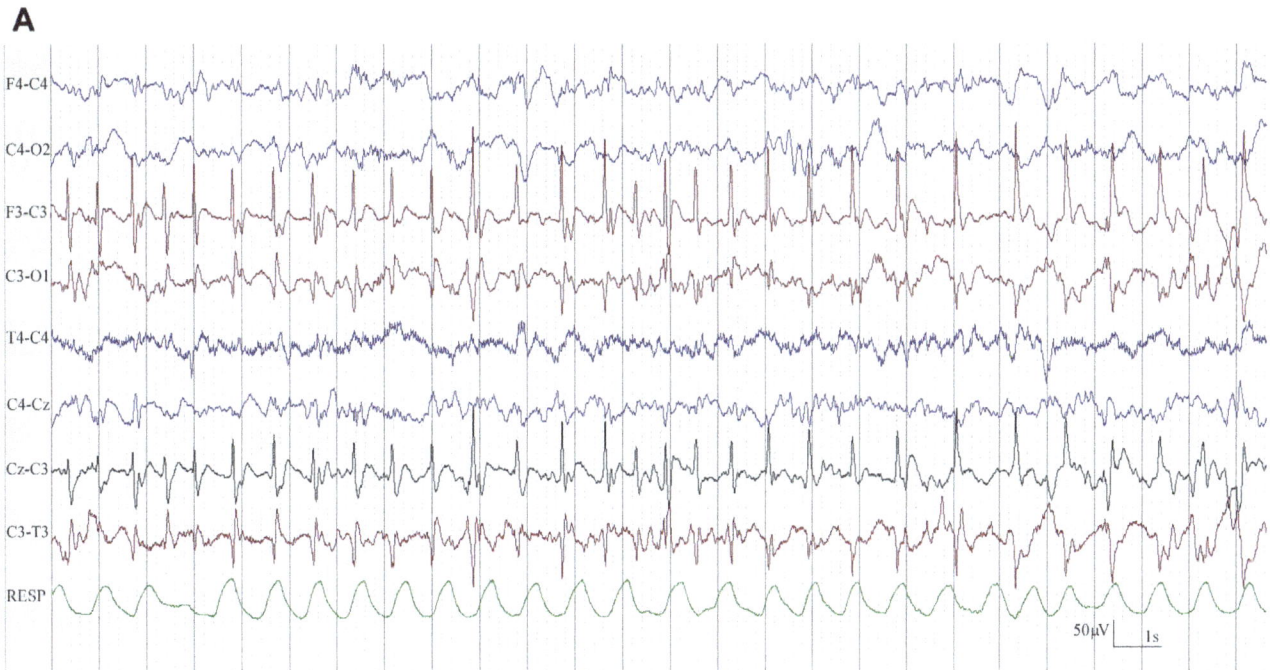

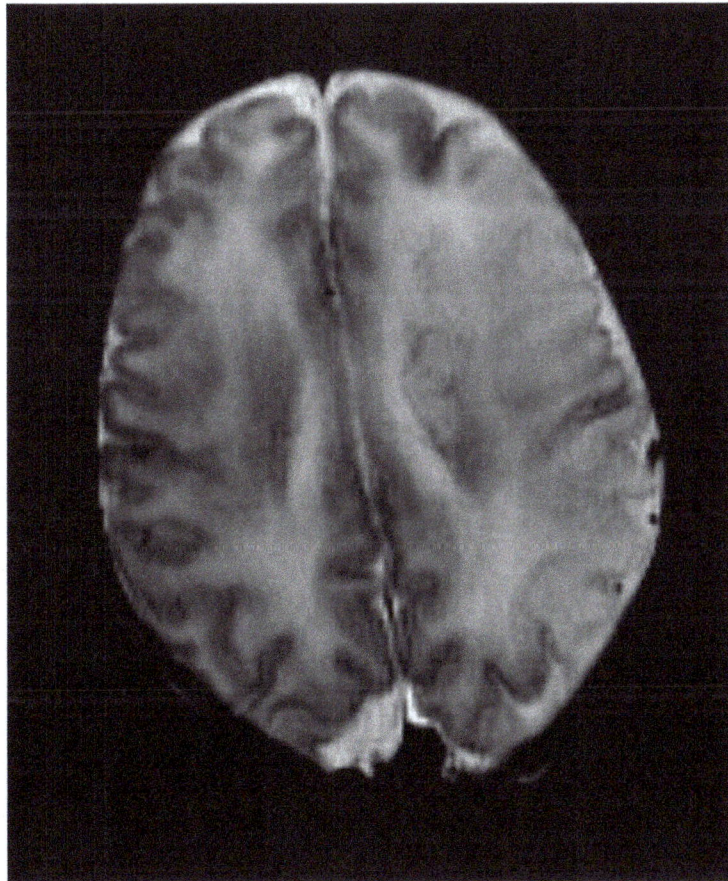

Figure 2. A. EEG in a neonate (case 6). Seizures arising from the left hemisphere corresponding with a left middle cerebral artery infarction on cranial MRI. **B. Cranial MRI in a neonate (case 6).** The sequence is an axial T2 turbo spin echo performed on day 7 of life. Note the characteristic focal spike and wave discharges over the left hemisphere with phase reversal over the left central region.

Table 2. Characteristics of EEG and seizures.

Neonate	1	2	3	4	5	6	7	8	9
Summary of background EEG feature									
Continuous activity	Yes	Yes	Yes	Yes	Yes	Yes	Yes	Yes	Yes
Symmetry	Left mild suppression	Left significant suppression	Right mild suppression	Good	Right mild suppression	Good	Good	Left significant suppression	Right mild suppression
Intermittent features	Left-sided sharp sharp bursts	Left-sided theta sharp waves	Right focal sharp waves	Left-sided sharp waves in quiet sleep	Right-sided theta sharp waves	Left-sided theta sharp waves	Left-sided focal sharp theta waves	Left-sided theta sharp waves	Right-sided sharp waves
Sleep cycling	Normal bilaterally	Disturbed unilaterally	Disturbed bilaterally	Disturbed bilaterally	Normal bilaterally	Normal bilaterally	Disturbed unilaterally	Disturbed unilaterally	Normal bilaterally
Seizure morphology	Focal spikes over left central with phase reversal	Focal spikes over left central with phase reversal	Focal spikes over right central with phase reversal	Focal spikes & polyspikes over left central with phase reversal	Focal spikes & polyspikes over right central with phase reversal	Focal spikes over left central with phase reversal	Focal spikes over left central with phase reversal	Focal spikes & polyspikes over left central with phase reversal	Focal spikes & polyspikes over right central with phase reversal
Summary of seizure burden									
Total seizure burden (minutes)	19	67	101	133	162	201	266	327	332
Seizure burden (minutes/hour)	2.70	7.28	27.60	5.53	10.27	18.15	12.77	9.25	6.18
Mean seizure duration (seconds)	370	98	356	362	120	523	143	195	146
Seizure window (hours)	7	9	4	24	16	11	21	35	54
Status epilepticus	None	None	Yes	None	None	Yes	Yes	Yes	Yes
Number of seizures (n)	3	41	17	22	81	23	112	101	136
Seizure classification									
Electrographic-only seizures: n (%)	0 (0)	27 (66)	8 (47)	20 (91)	77 (95)	13 (57)	77 (69)	62 (61)	121 (89)
Electrographic-only seizure burden: minutes (%)	0 (0)	28 (42)	26 (25)	129 (97)	146 (90)	74 (37)	129 (49)	244 (74)	282 (85)
Electroclinical seizures: n (%)	2 (66)	10 (24)	7 (41)	1 (4.5)	3 (3.7)	9 (39)	32 (29)	35 (35)	15 (11)
Electroclinical seizure burden: minutes (%)	18 (95)	30 (44)	48 (48)	3 (2)	15 (9)	108 (54)	126 (47)	80 (24)	50 (15)
Clonic/subtle seizures: n	2/0	0/10D	5/2C	1/0	3/0	0/9S	17/15S	16/19Y	9/6M
Video obscured: n (%)	1 (33)	4 (10)	2 (12)	1 (4.5)	1 (1.3)	1 (4)	3 (2)	4 (4)	0 (0)

Subtle seizures: C, cycling movements of the limbs; D, desaturations; M, mouthing and smacking; S, sucking; Y, yawning.

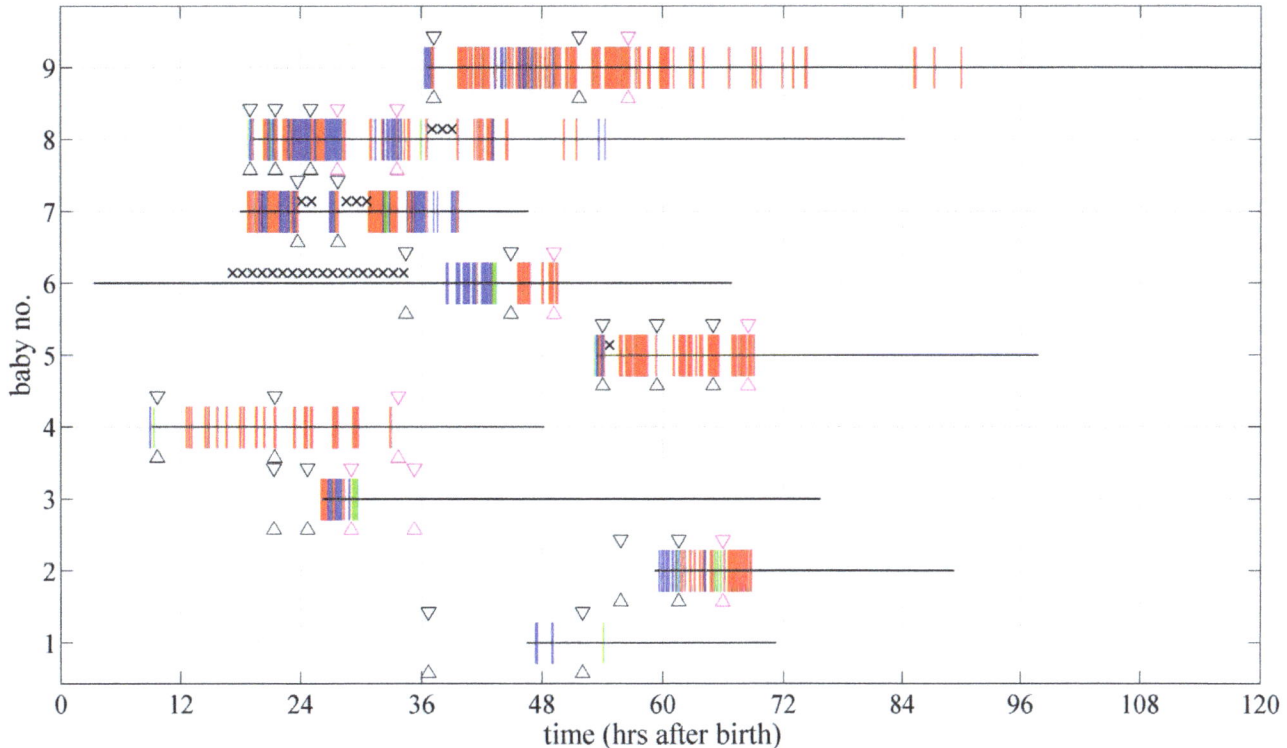

Figure 3. Characteristics of seizures and anticonvulsant administration in each neonate. Vertical red lines denote the presence of electrographic-only seizures, vertical blue lines denote electroclinical seizures and vertical green lines denote obscured seizures. Horizontal black line denotes the period of EEG monitoring. Black crosses denote missing data. Timepoints bounded by black arrows denote the first-line anticonvulsant administration while the magenta arrows denote the second-line anticonvulsant administration.

parietal areas). [25] Clinical signs may not manifest if the motor cortical strip is not involved. [25] All neonates in our study had some degree of MCA involvement; at some timepoint a clinical correlate (often very subtle) was evident. Although typically neonates with PAIS are non-encephalopathic, [26] hypotonia, poor sucking reflex and irritability have been described. [27] Subtle seizures in our cohort involved mainly oral-buccal-lingual movements (four of six neonates); this is in line with other studies. [2], [28] In PAIS, autonomic dysfunction such as apnoeic spells [29], [30] has been reported in up to 36% of neonates; [31] only one neonate in our study presented with apnoea before any anticonvulsant administration. Other subtle seizures which have been previously described included eye blinking, vertical nystagmus and thumb adduction, [29] but multichannel EEG monitoring was not applied, thus the accuracy of these clinical signs is unknown. Our results support the suggestion for low threshold in initiating EEG monitoring when there is any suspicion of unusual movements which may be seizures.

To date, reported incidences of seizures in neonates with PAIS are mainly based on observation of neonatal behaviours, [22], [32] rather than on multichannel EEG which is the gold standard for accurate detection of neonatal seizures. [18], [33–35] Approximately 20% of neonatal seizures in term neonates are due to PAIS. [2] Conversely, while neonatal seizures have been noted in 26% of neonates with PAIS, [3] we believe these numbers could be much higher if detection of seizures is based on prolonged multichannel EEG monitoring. A limitation of our study is the small number of neonates with PAIS. In our cohort of neonates, all accept one neonate (case 2) was captured when they presented with

hemiconvulsions before discharge shortly after birth in our 2 neonatal units. We only included neonates that presented with clear PAIS involving at most 2 arterial territories and who had continuous multichannel EEG monitoring as soon as possible after their presentation with seizures. While being monitored, these neonates with seizures showed asymmetrical characteristics on the EEG. In this period, other neonates would have presented but did not have continuous EEG monitoring undertaken. It is difficult to diagnose all neonates with PAIS in the neonatal period as the majority of term neonates affected by PAIS are asymptomatic; [1] appearing clinically well enough to be sent to the postnatal ward shortly after birth. In our 2 units, there is a policy of early maternal and neonatal discharge. Any neonate presenting with seizures after they were discharged would have been readmitted to regional paediatric hospitals, not the neonatal units. Even though our number of neonates with PAIS is small, we believe that the novelty here is having captured a number of neonates who had early and long duration of multichannel EEG monitoring.

In our study, EEG monitoring was initiated only after clinical seizures were observed in the first 3 days of life; we have shown that the age of first clinical seizure and first recorded EEG seizure [33 (17–42) and 36 (19–54) hours] were within 72 hours of age. This is current practice in most neonatal units as there are no existing early indicators to identify neonates with PAIS, hence it is possible that neonates with PAIS and electrographic-only seizures may have been missed during our recording period. Early EEG monitoring may have a role in providing an early indicator of PAIS, as early EEG from three hours after delivery has been shown to demonstrate occasional focal sharp waves over the infarcted region which became more frequent, complex and of higher amplitude in quiet sleep. [36]

In conclusion, EEG in neonates with PAIS demonstrated distinctive features in the background EEG and morphology of seizures. These features were present from very early after birth. Given the ease with which EEG monitoring can now be performed at the cotside, careful EEG analysis may prove very useful for early diagnosis of PAIS. For the first time, we have also quantified the seizure burden in neonates with PAIS using multichannel video-EEG. The majority of seizures in neonates with PAIS will escape detection without prolonged multichannel EEG monitoring.

Acknowledgments

Special thanks to the medical and nursing staff from the neonatal intensive care units in CUMH, UCLH and the parents who gave permission for their babies to be studied.

The views expressed in this publication are those of the authors and not necessarily those of the Department of Health in the United Kingdom.

Author Contributions

Conceived and designed the experiments: GBB JMR. Performed the experiments: EL GBB SRM. Analyzed the data: EL GBB SRM NJS. Contributed reagents/materials/analysis tools: EL GBB SRM NJS VL. Wrote the paper: EL SRM NJS VL CAR COB JMR GBB. Provided reports and measurements on the cranial imaging scans: COB.

References

1. Lynch JK, Nelson KB (2001) Epidemiology of perinatal stroke. Curr Opin Pediatr 13: 499–505.
2. Volpe JJ (2008) Neonatal Seizures. In: Neurology of the Newborn. Philadelphia, PA: WB Saunders Company. pp. 203–244.
3. Rafay MF, Cortez MA, de Veber GA, Tan-Dy C, Al-Futaisi A, et al. (2009) Predictive value of clinical and EEG features in the diagnosis of stroke and hypoxic ischemic encephalopathy in neonates with seizures. Stroke 40: 2402–2407.
4. Ramaswamy V, Miller SP, Barkovich AJ, Partridge JC, Ferriero DM (2004) Perinatal stroke in term infants with neonatal encephalopathy. Neurology 62: 2088–2091.
5. Rutherford MA, Ramenghi LA, Cowan FM (2012) Neonatal stroke. Arch Dis Child Fetal Neonatal Ed 97:F377–F384.
6. Cowan F, Mercuri E, Groenendaal F, Bassi L, Ricci D, et al. (2005) Does cranial ultrasound imaging identify arterial cerebral infarction in term neonates? Arch Dis Child Fetal Neonatal Ed 90:F252–F256.
7. van Rooij LG, de Vries LS, van Huffelen AC, Toet MC (2010) Additional value of two-channel amplitude integrated EEG recording in full-term infants with unilateral brain injury. Arch Dis Child Fetal Neonatal Ed 95:F160–F168.
8. Mercuri E, Rutherford M, Cowan F, Pennock J, Counsell S, et al. (1999) Early prognostic indicators of outcome in infants with neonatal cerebral infarction: a clinical, electroencephalogram, and magnetic resonance imaging study. Pediatrics 103: 39–46.
9. Klem GH, Luders HO, Jasper HH, Elger C (1999) The ten-twenty electrode system of the International Federation. The International Federation of Clinical Neurophysiology. Electroencephalogr Clin Neurophysiol Suppl 52: 3–6.
10. Lamblin MD, Walls EE, Andre M (2013). The electroencephalogram of the full-term newborn: review of normal features and hypoxic-ischemic encephalopathy patterns. Neurophysiol Clin 43: 267–287.
11. Clancy RR (2006) Prolonged electroencephalogram monitoring for seizures and their treatment. Clin Perinatol 33: 649–665.
12. Ortibus EL, Sum JM, Hahn JS (1996) Predictive value of EEG for outcome and epilepsy following neonatal seizures. Electroencephalogr Clin Neurophysiol 98: 175–185.
13. Weiner SP, Painter MJ, Geva D, Guthrie RD, Scher MS (1991) Neonatal seizures: electroclinical dissociation. Pediatr Neurol 7: 363–368.
14. Marks MP, Holmgren EB, Fox AJ, Patel S, von Kummer R, et al. (1999) Evaluation of early computed tomographic findings in acute ischemic stroke. Stroke 30: 389–392.
15. Lynch N, Low E, Rennie JM, Boylan GB (2011). Comparison of seizure characteristics in full term neonates with stroke and hypoxic-ischemic encephalopathy. Arch Dis Child 96:A39.
16. Mercuri E (2001) Early diagnostic and prognostic indicators in full term infants with neonatal cerebral infarction: an integrated clinical, neuroradiological and EEG approach. Minerva Pediatr 53: 305–311.
17. Clancy RR, Legido A (1987) The exact ictal and interictal duration of electroencephalographic neonatal seizures. Epilepsia 28: 537–541.
18. Murray DM, Boylan GB, Ali I, Ryan CA, Murphy BP, et al. (2008) Defining the gap between electrographic seizure burden, clinical expression and staff recognition of neonatal seizures. Arch Dis Child Fetal Neonatal Ed 93:F187–F191.
19. Glykys J, Dzhala VI, Kuchibhotla KV, Feng G, Kuner T, et al. (2009) Differences in cortical versus subcortical GABAergic signaling: a candidate mechanism of electroclinical uncoupling of neonatal seizures. Neuron 63: 657–672.
20. Vasiljevic B, Maglajlic-Djukic S, Gojnic M (2012) The prognostic value of amplitude-integrated electroencephalography in neonates with hypoxic-ischemic encephalopathy. Vojnosanit Pregl 69: 492–499.
21. Estan J, Hope P (1997) Unilateral neonatal cerebral infarction in full term infants. Arch Dis Child Fetal Neonatal Ed 76:F88–F93.
22. Golomb MR, Garg BP, Carvalho KS, Johnson CS, Williams LS (2007) Perinatal stroke and the risk of developing childhood epilepsy. J Pediatr 151: 409–413.
23. Rando T, Ricci D, Mercuri E, Frisone MF, Luciano R, et al. (2000) Periodic lateralized epileptiform discharges (PLEDs) as early indicator of stroke in full-term newborns. Neuropediatrics 31: 202–205.
24. Boylan GB, Rennie JM, Pressler RM, Wilson G, Morton M, et al. (2002) Phenobarbitone, neonatal seizures, and video-EEG. Arch Dis Child Fetal Neonatal Ed 86:F165–F170.
25. Govaert P, Matthys E, Zecic A, Roelens F, Oostra A, et al. (2000) Perinatal cortical infarction within middle cerebral artery trunks. Arch Dis Child Fetal Neonatal Ed 82:F59–F63.
26. Cowan F, Rutherford M, Groenendaal F, Eken P, Mercuri E, et al. (2003) Origin and timing of brain lesions in term infants with neonatal encephalopathy. Lancet 361: 736–742.
27. Miller V (2000) Neonatal cerebral infarction. Semin Pediatr Neurol 7: 278–288.
28. Pinto LC, Giliberti P (2001) Neonatal seizures: background EEG activity and the electroclinical correlation in full-term neonates with hypoxic-ischemic encephalopathy. Analysis by computer-synchronized long-term polygraphic video-EEG monitoring. Epileptic Disord 3: 125–132.
29. Fujimoto S, Yokochi K, Togari H, Nishimura Y, Inukai K, et al. (1992) Neonatal cerebral infarction: symptoms, CT findings and prognosis. Brain Dev 14: 48–52.
30. Hoogstraate SR, Lequin MH, Huysman MA, Ahmed S, Govaert PP (2009) Apnoea in relation to neonatal temporal lobe haemorrhage. Eur J Paediatr Neurol 13: 356–361.
31. Sreenan C, Bhargava R, Robertson CM (2000) Cerebral infarction in the term newborn: clinical presentation and long-term outcome. J Pediatr 137: 351–355.
32. Kirton A, Armstrong-Wells J, Chang T, Deveber G, Rivkin MJ, et al. (2011) Symptomatic neonatal arterial ischemic stroke: the International Pediatric Stroke Study. Pediatrics 128:e1402–e1410.
33. Glass HC, Wirrell E (2009) Controversies in neonatal seizure management. J Child Neurol 24: 591–599.
34. Low E, Boylan GB, Mathieson SR, Murray DM, Korotchikova I, et al. (2012) Cooling and seizure burden in term neonates: an observational study. Arch Dis Child Fetal Neonatal Ed 97:F267–F272.
35. Wusthoff CJ, Dlugos DJ, Gutierrez-Colina A, Wang A, Cook N, et al. (2011) Electrographic seizures during therapeutic hypothermia for neonatal hypoxic-ischemic encephalopathy. J Child Neurol 26: 724–728.
36. Walsh BH, Low E, Bogue CO, Murray DM, Boylan GB (2011) Early continuous video electroencephalography in neonatal stroke. Dev Med Child Neurol 53: 89–92.

12

Exploring Combinations of Auditory and Visual Stimuli for Gaze-Independent Brain-Computer Interfaces

Xingwei An[1,2]*, **Johannes Höhne**[2,3], **Dong Ming**[1]*, **Benjamin Blankertz**[2]

1 Department of Biomedical Engineering, Tianjin University, Tianjin, China, **2** Neurotechnology Group, Berlin Institute of Technology, Berlin, Germany, **3** Machine Learning Group, Berlin Institute of Technology, Berlin, Germany

Abstract

For Brain-Computer Interface (BCI) systems that are designed for users with severe impairments of the oculomotor system, an appropriate mode of presenting stimuli to the user is crucial. To investigate whether multi-sensory integration can be exploited in the gaze-independent event-related potentials (ERP) speller and to enhance BCI performance, we designed a visual-auditory speller. We investigate the possibility to enhance stimulus presentation by combining visual and auditory stimuli within gaze-independent spellers. In this study with N = 15 healthy users, two different ways of combining the two sensory modalities are proposed: simultaneous redundant streams (Combined-Speller) and interleaved independent streams (Parallel-Speller). Unimodal stimuli were applied as control conditions. The workload, ERP components, classification accuracy and resulting spelling speed were analyzed for each condition. The Combined-speller showed a lower workload than uni-modal paradigms, without the sacrifice of spelling performance. Besides, shorter latencies, lower amplitudes, as well as a shift of the temporal and spatial distribution of discriminative information were observed for Combined-speller. These results are important and are inspirations for future studies to search the reason for these differences. For the more innovative and demanding Parallel-Speller, where the auditory and visual domains are independent from each other, a proof of concept was obtained: fifteen users could spell online with a mean accuracy of 87.7% (chance level <3%) showing a competitive average speed of 1.65 symbols per minute. The fact that it requires only one selection period per symbol makes it a good candidate for a fast communication channel. It brings a new insight into the true multisensory stimuli paradigms. Novel approaches for combining two sensory modalities were designed here, which are valuable for the development of ERP-based BCI paradigms.

Editor: Virginie van Wassenhove, CEA.DSV.I2BM.NeuroSpin, France

Funding: This work was supported by the China Scholarship Council and National Natural Science Foundation of China (Grant No. 81222021). Furthermore, the authors acknowledge financial support by the BMBF Grant Nos. 16SV5839 and 01GQ0850, by the European ICT Programme Project FP7-224631. This paper only reflects the authors' views and funding agencies are not liable for any use that may be made of the information contained herein. The funders had no role in study design, data collection and analysis, decision to publish, or preparation of the manuscript.

Competing Interests: The authors have declared that no competing interests exist.

* Email: xing-wei.an@hotmail.com (XA); richardming@tju.edu.cn (DM)

Introduction

Brain-computer interfaces (BCIs) can provide direct communication by non-muscular methods for people with severe motor impairments [1,2]. Most BCI systems either are based on modulations of local brain oscillations (mostly sensorimotor rhythms (SMRs)) that are induced by certain voluntary control strategies such as Motor Imagery based techniques [3,4], or they exploit event-related potentials (ERPs) that are modulated according to the allocation of attention to selected stimuli. While SMR-based BCIs have the advantage of providing a continuous control signal (in time and magnitude), ERP-based BCIs are commonly considered to be more stable [5] and more efficient for selection tasks, such as mental typewriting. In ERP-based spellers, users can select symbols by directing their attention to stimuli, from the visual, auditory or tactile domain.

The Matrix Speller designed by Farwell and Donchin [6] was the first approach to provide communication to users with severe motor disabilities based on ERPs. It is remarkable that this early approach is still popular, and many novel variants have been devised that still follow the original idea quite closely. Some of these approaches have optimized the exploitation of visual evoked potentials (VEPs) that are elicited by stimuli within the foveal field [7,8]. Also, it is the Matrix Speller that is employed in one of the rare cases of 'home use' BCIs by a paralyzed user [9]. However, it was shown in [10,11] that the performance of the Matrix Speller depends critically on the user's ability to fixate the target character which limits its applicability to users with a certain degree of oculomotor control. To also accommodate users with impaired ocular motor control, recent studies proposed alternative paradigms to implement gaze-independent visual BCI spellers, see [12,13,14,15,16]. For an overview of gaze-independent spellers see [17].

As an alternative paradigm for users with limited or even no vision several research groups investigate spellers based on tactile or somatosensory [18,19] and auditory [20,21,22] stimuli. Paradigms with somatosensory stimuli were considered as a suitable alternative for vision and/or hearing impaired BCI users. Studies about auditory stimuli [20,21,22] examined approaches similar to the visual matrix speller, mapping different sounds to rows and/or columns of the symbol matrix, such as the words from 1 to 10 (for a 5*5 matrix), and 6 environmental sounds (for 6*6 matrix). A novel approach that allowed considerably higher transmission rates was proposed by Schreuder and colleagues [23,24]. The key idea was to employ spatially distributed auditory stimuli, which allowed a fast presentation speed and an easier allocation of attention. Höhne et al. [25,26] introduced a variant of that approach that uses less spatial directions but adds pitch or just the sound of the letters as independent features. More recently, it was shown that the use of syllables as natural stimuli not only improved the users' ergonomic ratings but also increased the classification accuracy [27]. Klobassa et al. [21] used a multimodal audio-visual speller paradigm to provide a better 'training' in initial sessions to finally use mono-auditory speller.

Instead of uni-modal stimuli paradigms, researchers started to focus on using bimodal stimuli [18,28,29,30,31]. Talsma and colleagues [32] reviewed the developments in the understanding of the interaction between attention and multi-sensory processing, focusing on studies using audio-visual stimulus material. Their review also identified several important directions and challenges for future research in this field. Teder-Sälejärvi et al. [28] used randomized sequences of unimodal (auditory (**A**) or visual (**V**)) and simultaneous bimodal (**AV**) stimuli presented to right- or left-field locations. The results in that study showed overlapping but distinctive patterns of multisensory integration for spatially congruent and incongruent **AV** stimuli. Belitski and his colleagues [30] presented an extension of the matrix speller using a so-called 'visual+auditory' paradigm as a transient process for best performance and moved smoothly to purely auditory. Results demonstrated the effectiveness of this approach with this transient process. It was also found that the 'visual + auditory' stimuli increased the average strength of the stimulus response in matrix-speller style BCIs, when compared to unimodal stimuli. However, this study refers only to gaze-dependent visual spellers. Though it was not designed for ERP spelling, Thurlings and her team [31] investigated the effect of bimodal visual-tactile stimulus presentation on the ERP components, BCI performance and participants' task performance. Results of this study showed enhanced early components (N1), which may enhance the BCI performance, while also showed reduced late ERP components (P300).

We live in a multisensory world in which we are continuously deluged with stimulus input through multiple sensory pathways [32]. Therefore it is important to address the following questions: (1) Can multi-sensory integration be exploited in a gaze-independent ERP speller in order to enhance BCI performance? (2) Is there any difference of brain response between single and multi-sensory stimuli? (3) Is it possible to use a BCI paradigm with two independent channels, coding different information?

To answer these questions, we designed a visual-auditory speller (called Combined-Speller, denoted as **AV**) by simultaneous presentation of visual stimuli and auditory stimuli. To enable a comparison with the uni-modal speller paradigms, the mono-visual (denoted as **V**) and mono-auditory (denoted as **A**) spellers are also studied in addition. For answering the third question, we propose a new and truly multi-modal BCI approach (called Parallel-Speller, denoted as **V*A**). In the Parallel-Speller, the visual and auditory stimuli are coded independently.

Material and Methods

Participants

Fifteen healthy subjects (8 female) aged 24-34 (mean 26.9 ± 2.63 years) participated in this study. Two of the participants had already participated in earlier BCI experiments. Each participant did not suffer from a neurological disease and had normal hearing. They also provided written informed consent confirming the notification of the experimental process, the using of the data and the personal right of themselves. Subjects were paid for their participation with 8€/hour, and the entire experiment lasted 3 to 4 hours. The study was approved by the Ethics Committee of the Charité University Hospital (number EA4/110/09).

Stimuli

This study compares four different conditions related to sensory modalities that can be used to drive a BCI speller. Two conditions use stimuli in one sensory modality only, labeled **V** for visual speller and **A** for auditory speller. These experimental settings are similar to existing speller paradigms and have been used for comparison with the novel multimodal spellers. The speller of the **AV** condition (Combined-Speller) uses simultaneous auditory and visual stimuli as redundant information, while the Parallel-Speller (**V*A** condition) exploits alternating auditory and visual cues as independent streams. Figure 1 and Figure 2 show the course of the experiment. The three conditions **V**, **A**, and **AV** used a vocabulary of thirty symbols and a two periods selection procedure as explained below (Figure 1), while condition **V*A** allows to select one out of thirty six symbols within a single selection period (Figure 2). The thirty-symbol alphabet comprised the standard Latin alphabet, punctuation marks '.' and ',', a space symbol '_' and a backspace symbol '<' that could be used to erase the previous symbol. The thirty six-symbol alphabet extended the thirty-symbol alphabet by additional control keys (lower cases 's' for 'Shift', 'c' for 'Ctrl', 'A' for 'Alt', 'p' for 'Space') and punctuation marks ('-' and '?').

In all conditions, the selection of one symbol is coded by two selection steps of one out of six targets each. In the first selection step, a group of symbols (e.g., 'ABCDE') is selected, while in the second selection step one symbol of that group is selected. In the condition **V*A** both steps are performed at the same time (one by each modality), while in the other speller they are performed subsequently. For the serial selection, each group contains five characters (or symbols) and one symbol ('^') that serves as a backdoor to return to the group selection step that can be used in case of an erroneous group selection. In the concurrent selection of group and symbol in condition A*V, the backdoor functionality makes no sense. Therefore, additional symbols were used as replacement. (A different option would have been to have only five symbols per group such that the symbol stage would only be a five class selection. This would have been an advantage with respect to the accuracy of the Parallel-Speller. However, as the focus of this study was the comparison of the multimodal speller with the unimodal spellers, the preference was given to keep the complexity of the selections constant.).

It is important to note that before each selection period, a countdown was launched. It included the intensification of the visual and (or) auditory target stimuli for three times. This was followed by the pre-flashing of the last 3 digits (3, 2, 1) synchronized with the subsequent stimulus sequence. The design of the countdown part did not only provide a cue for the targets but also helped the participant to get used to the flashing frequency.

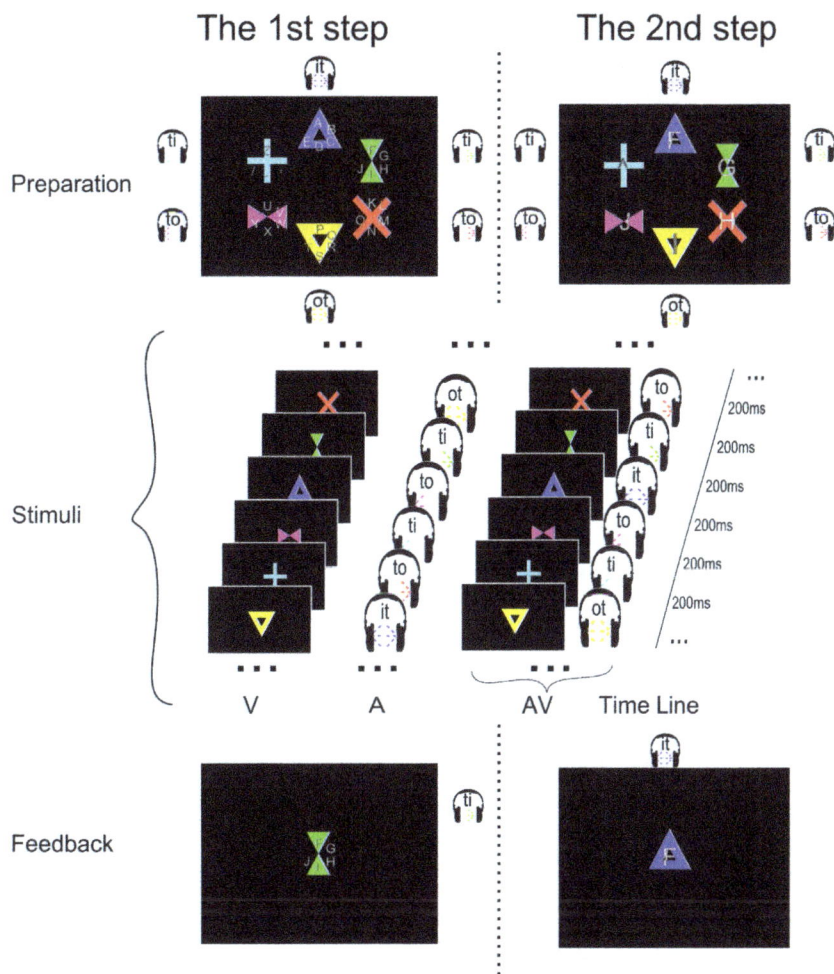

Figure 1. Visualization of the experimental design of the experiment for unimodal speller (Visual: V and Auditory: A) and Combined-Speller (AV). The left column shows the first selection period for group selection. The right column shows the second selection period for symbol selection. The upper channel shows the 'target cue' part before stimuli start, including the cue for showing the position (or voice) of the target and the countdown part for hint of the start. The middle panel shows the time sequence of each stimuli paradigm. The lower panel shows the feedback after each selection period. For the first selection period, the group of the target symbol was chosen, and the symbols in that group will re-distributed into these six visual shapes (the last shape, light blue cross, was left blank as the 'backdoor' symbol) according to their position in the chosen group.

In condition **V**, visual stimuli were presented as in the Center Speller [12]. The Center Speller is a gaze-independent speller, where participants attend to the center of the screen at which the 6 stimuli are presented in a pseudo-random sequence. Six different stimuli were designed such that they had a unique geometrical shape and color (Figure 1), providing two distinct features for visual discrimination. During the presentation of the stimuli, the geometrical shapes were presented centrally in a sequential fashion. The duration of each stimulus was 130 ms and the stimulus onset asynchrony (SOA) was kept at 200 ms. The reason for choosing 130 ms as the duration of the visual stimuli was to match the duration of the auditory stimuli (see below).

In condition **A**, auditory stimuli were presented in a similar fashion as in [25]. We used only 6 stimuli in this study (Figure 1). Short spoken syllables (left 'ti', left 'to', middle 'it', middle 'ot', right 'ti', right 'to') were sung with different pitches by three speakers (bass, tenor and soprano human voices) as stimuli. Every speaker was presented only from one fixed direction (bass: from the left, tenor: from the middle, soprano: from the right). For each direction we recorded 2 stimuli (stimuli with vowel 'i' and stimuli

with vowel 'o'). The stimuli with the vowel 'i' (left 'ti', middle 'it' and right 'ti') were recorded with high pitch (A#) and the stimuli with vowel 'o' (left 'to', middle 'ot' and right 'to') were recorded with comparatively low pitch (C#). All of the auditory stimuli were kept within 130 ms as the duration of the visual stimuli. The SOA was also chosen to be 200 ms, such that conditions **V** and **A** were the analog in most aspects but used different sensory modalities.

In condition **AV**, corresponding visual and auditory stimuli were presented simultaneously, while those two concurrent streams coded the same information, see Figure 1. Therefore, targets in the visual sequence always appear at the very same time as targets in the auditory sequence. Senkowski et al. reported the timing of multimodal stimuli to be a crucial aspect [33]. Thus, we investigated the optimal delay in a pilot experiment and finally set the timing that auditory stimuli were presented about 17 ms (1 fame of a 60 Hz monitor) earlier than the corresponding visual stimuli. Participants were instructed to concentrate on the combined visual and auditory stimuli at the same time.

During conditions **V**, **A**, and **AV**, the order of stimuli was randomized within each repetition with the constraint that the

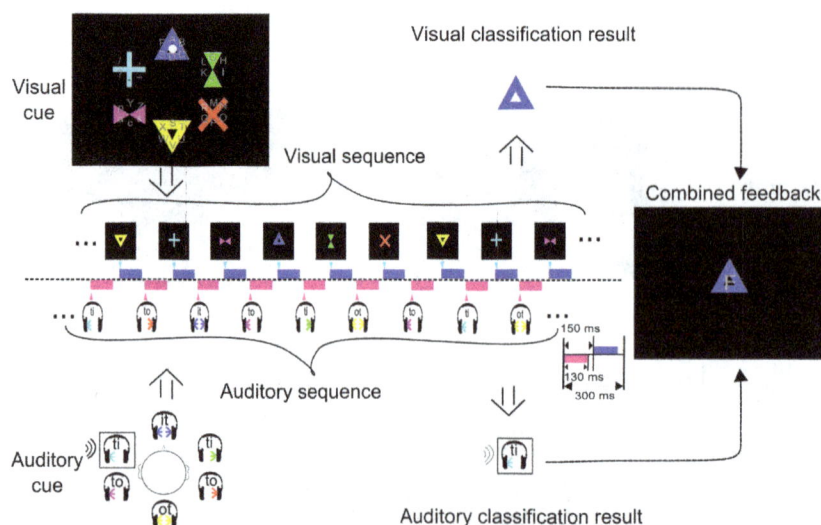

Figure 2. Visualization of the experimental design of the experiment for Parallel-Speller (V*A). Six symbols locate in each group, making a total of thirty-six symbols. The presentation of the visual stimuli was used to choose the group the symbol was in. The position of the symbol in the group was selected through the auditory domain. The upper panel shows the sequence of visual target selection, and the lower panel shows that of the auditory target selection.

same stimulus could not appear with less than two different stimuli in between. Participants were instructed to count the number of target occurrences to help them focus on the stimuli.

In condition **V*A**, the same visual and auditory stimuli have been used, but they were presented as independent sequences. The SOA in each sequence was 300 ms and the onset between auditory and visual cues was 150 ms, with 130 ms duration of each stimuli, see Figure 2. To spell a letter, the group was selected through visual stream, while the within-group selection was done via the auditory domain. That way, two independent decisions are made parallel. For example, to select the symbol 'F', which is the sixth symbol in the first group (cf. Figure 2 visual cue), the target in the visual sequence is the blue triangle and in the auditory sequence the base 'ti' (cf. Figure 2 auditory cue). As it was described above selections of visual and auditory targets were made simultaneously and independently. However those two channels stimuli were alternatively presented in a rapid sequence (see Figure 2 visual and auditory sequences). After several presentations of each stimulus (10 repetitions were used in this experiment), the binary classification and multiclass selection was performed independently for each stimulus domain – resulting in a visual and an auditory output. Combining the visual and auditory output, the final symbol was spelled (see Figure 2).

Note that due to the independence of the two streams, targets in the visual and in the auditory sequence occur at different times in both sequences. The minimum inter-target distance within each modality (visual target to visual target or auditory target to auditory target, cf. Figure 2) is three stimuli and equivalently 900 ms. However, it may happen that two target presentations are only 150 ms apart (e.g. the time between a visual target and auditory target). This cannot be circumvented, as any combination of group and symbol-with-group can be the pair of targets.

Procedure

Visual stimuli were presented on a 19' TFT screen with a refresh rate of 60 Hz and a resolution of 1280*1024 px². Auditory stimuli were presented through a light neckband headphone (Sennheiser PMX 200) that was positioned comfortably. Partici-

pants were seated in a comfortable chair at a distance of about 1 m from the screen. During the preparation of the EEG, the written and verbal instructions were provided. Thereafter, subjects were instructed to sit still, relax and try to minimize eye movements (try not to blink, though it is inevitable) during the course of a trial.

There were 2 offline calibration runs for each the conditions **V**, **A**, and **AV**. In each calibration run, participants are provided with a sequence of 6 symbols for which they have to perform the 'selections' by allocating attention to the corresponding target stimuli. In total, there were 12 symbols (6 symbols * 2 calibration runs) for each condition in the calibration phase. The sequence of symbols to spell was randomly selected from all available symbols, and this differed between subjects. The 6 runs of the 3 conditions (**V**, **A**, **AV**) were conducted in pseudo-randomly order.

After the calibration phase, offline analysis was conducted to train a classifier (see [34] and Section 2.4) on the collected data of condition **AV**. After a short pause, participants were instructed to complete one self-conceived word (without telling the experimenter) in free spelling mode comprising 6–10 symbols with condition **AV**. During free spelling, participants could use the backdoor symbol '^' (which is contained in every group) to cancel the selection of the group and use the backspace symbol ('<') to erase the previous symbol, if a wrong group or symbol was selected. Free-spelling was conducted as motivation and for getting familiar with online spelling. Thereafter, participants were asked to spell twenty predefined symbols in the so-called copy-spelling mode (again condition **AV**). In contrast to free-spelling, erroneously selected symbols needed not to be deleted as in the free spelling part. As a two-period spelling paradigm, the spelling in condition **AV** faces the problem that the first period (group selection) could be wrong, which will definitely lead to wrong symbol selection. In this study, the default visual and auditory targets in the second period were the same as the correct target should be, no matter the correct group was selected or not. From the symbols the participants selected, it is easy to analyze the accuracy in each period.

Condition **V*A** was conducted after a short break. The reason for having this condition always at the end was that participants should have experienced the simpler conditions first in order to be able to cope with this more demanding condition. This training effect was conjectured to outweigh the possible detrimental effect of fatigue that may occur at the end of the experiment. Participants underwent a calibration of 4 runs (6 symbols in each run), a free spelling phase where self-chosen words could be spelled, and finally the copy spelling of a predefined sentence.

In the calibration phase, there were similar countdown and feedback parts for each trial to select the target symbol. The intensification of the target in the countdown part was a flashing circle in the center of the target visual shape with the target auditory stimuli presented through the earphone (both for three times), followed by the pre-flashing of the last 3 digits (3, 2, 1) synchronized with the subsequent stimulus sequence. Only one selection period was needed to choose the target symbol. The visual stimuli and auditory stimuli were presented independently and alternatively as described in Section 2.2. Considering the complexity of the task, it is difficult to quickly count the number of targets occurrences. There were 20 target occurrences in 18 s. It is possible that visual target and auditory target may occur consequently. In this circumstance, participants need to count two numbers in 600 ms. Thus participants were not asked to count the number target occurrences, but just to pay attention to the target stimuli in the auditory as well as in the visual stream. After the presentation of 10 repetitions of the stimuli (since the task is difficult than other paradigms, more repetitions were used here), the outputs of the visual and auditory classification were made according to these two stimuli streams.

The offline analysis for condition **V*A** were conducted after the calibration phase, followed by free spelling and copy spelling runs. During free spelling, the participants could spell any word without telling the experimenter, and could use the backspace symbol ('/') to erase the previous symbol, if a wrong symbol was selected. Thereafter, twenty predefined symbols (the same as in condition **AV**) in the so-called copy-spelling mode without erasing the wrong symbols selected.

For this whole experiment, we have ten calibration runs in total. Each calibration run lasts for less than 3 minutes, while 6 symbols are spelled. For conditions **V**, **A** and **AV**, there are 2 selection periods for choosing a symbol, compared to only one selection period for per symbol in condition **V*A**. Besides the calibration runs, for condition **AV** and **V*A**, free spelling and copy spelling runs were also conducted after their calibration runs. Neither copy spelling nor free spelling was done with unimodal stimuli (condition **V** and **A**). Between each run, participants could rest for 2–5 min. There is no break within runs.

Data acquisition and analysis

Electroencephalogram (EEG) signals were acquired using a Fast'n Easy Cap (EasyCap GmbH, Munich, Germany) with 63 Ag/AgCl electrodes placed at the standard positions of the international 10–20 system. Channels were referenced to the nose, with the Ground electrode located at the front (at position AFz). Electrooculogram (EOG) signals were recorded additionally. Signals were amplified using two 32-channel amplifiers (Brain Amp by Brain Products, Munich, Germany), sampled at 1 kHz. Further online and offline analysis was performed in Matlab. Statistical analysis was performed with both IBM SPSS statistics 20 and MATLAB. The visual and auditory feedback was implemented using the open source framework PyFF (Venthur et al., 2010).

To evaluate the workload of each condition, participants were asked to fill in the NASA TLX questionnaire (NASA Human Performance Research Group, 1987) after the calibration phase of each condition. It was introduced as a measure of usability in BCI by Pasqualotto et al. [35] and Riccio et al. [36], and it has been used to compare the workload for a visual and an auditory speller by Käthner et al. [37]. It was used here as a multidimensional rating procedure to derive an overall workload score based on a weighted average of ratings on six sub-scales (Mental workload, Physical workload, Temporal workload, Performance, Effort needed and Frustration) for each condition. There were fifteen pair-wise comparisons of each two of the six subscales (Mental vs. Physical, Mental vs. Temporal, and Physical vs. Temporal, et al.) for the participants to choose the subscale in the comparison which weighs more for the whole workload. The subscale wins in each pair-wise comparison will count 1. So the sum score of the weightings is fifteen. A high score reveals an increased importance for workload.

Generally, EEG is prone to various sources of noise arising from factors such as 50 Hz power noise or ECG artifacts. Moreover, the discriminative components of the ERP are mainly found below 40 Hz. A Chebychev filter was therefore applied for offline analysis, using a passband up to 40 Hz and a stopband starting at 49 Hz and then down sampled to 100 Hz. It removes particularly well the line noise and other high-frequency noise [12,23]. For online classification, signals were subsampled to 100 Hz without prior filtering. The continuous signals were then segmented into epochs between -150ms and 800 ms relative to each stimulus onset, using the first 150ms as a baseline.

Classification was based on spatio-temporal features [34] and preceded as in [12] and [16]. For each condition, the sample-wise r^2 coefficients (augmented with the sign of the difference) were calculated for *targets* vs. *nontargets*. Five time intervals in which those coefficients indicated highly discriminative information were generally determined heuristically [34] but sometimes manually adjusted by the experimenter (for example when the time intervals were chosen before the onset of the stimuli, the experimenter should choose one after the onset instead). Spatio-temporal features were determined from single-trials by averaging all samples within those intervals for each channel. This provides feature-vectors with dimensionality 63 (number of EEG channels) times 5 (number of time intervals), i.e. 315. For classification, regularized Linear Discriminant Analysis (LDA) with shrinkage regularization of the covariance matrix was used, see [34] for details. Classification was done for each stimulus, as a binary task to distinguish the *target* sub-trials from the *non-target* sub-trials. For online classification, in each selection period, one out of six stimuli had to be chosen (the one that was attended by the participant with highest probability). To that end, real-valued classifier outputs (distance to the separating hyperplane) were averaged for each of the six stimuli across all available repetitions and the stimulus with the highest scores was selected. In this study the number of repetitions was six for condition **AV** and ten for condition **V*A**.

In an offline analysis, the temporal distribution as well as the spatial distribution class discriminative information was investigated for each participant and condition. Therefore, the accuracy of a classifier was estimated which was trained either on all channels and sliding time intervals (window size = 20 ms, step size = 5 ms) or only one channel and heuristically determined time intervals.

As Schreuder et al. [38] has shown that the number of repetitions can significantly impact BCI performance, the BCI performance when using smaller numbers of repetitions was also estimated in offline analysis. Cross-validation was used to evaluate the classification performance based on the calibration data, also for the unimodal conditions with which no online spelling has been performed.

Though in general context the Information Transfer Rate (ITR) is a reasonable performance measure text, we consider the actual symbols per minute (SPM) for spelling applications is more straightforward and realistic [38]. For single level interfaces, a correct selection counts as +1 symbol. An erroneous selection counts as -1 symbol, to account for the added effort of performing a backspace. We used the formula described in [38] to investigate the SPM for each speller:

$$\text{symbols per minute} = 60/\text{time per symbol} \qquad (1)$$

$$E = \text{Percent correct-Percent erroneous} \qquad (2)$$

$$\text{SPM} = \text{symbols per minute} * E \qquad (3)$$

Need to notice that the *time per symbol* includes all the necessary overhead including countdown part, classification and feedback time.

Results

In this study, we investigate and compare workload, ERP components, classification accuracy and spelling speed in each speller. We compare all of these features among condition **V**, **A**, and **AV** to investigate whether multi-sensory stimuli enhance BCI performance in the gaze-independent speller and to find the difference among brain response. We also present those results for condition V*A to study the possibility to use a BCI paradigm with two independent channels coding different information.

Behavioral data

The subjective workload that was imposed in each spelling condition was estimated based on the NASA TLX questionnaire. The left column of Figure 3 shows the mean rating with SD (standard deviation, stands for the standard deviation of the sampling distribution of the rating score) for each subscale and the overall weighted workload with SEM (standard error of the mean) for each condition. Also the grand averaged weights of the subscales were plotted on the right of the figure.

Results show that condition **AV** has the lowest, while condition **V*A** has the highest subjective workload for each sub-scale and overall. The data of workload has an approximate Gaussian distribution (K-S test, p>0.05), and they have equal sample variances (Levene tests, p> 0.05). Univariate ANOVA of the workload with factor *condition* and *subscale* was conducted. The results show significant effects of factors *condition* (p <.001) and *subscale* (p <.001), but no significant effects on *condition*subscale* (p = .967). Pairwise comparison was also conducted on *conditions*. Significant differences were found for each comparison of conditions **A**, **AV**, and **V*A** (p <.050). Condition V and V*A also have significant difference (p <.001). The overall workload of all 4 conditions follow an approximate Gaussian distribution (K-S test, p = .980).The results do not show significant difference among conditions **V**, **A**, and **AV** (p>.01), but significant difference (p <.01) between condition A*V and the other three conditions (**V, A, AV**). Moreover, the pie chart plot of weightings for the subscales reveals the subscale *Mental* (*30.3*%) to be the most important factor of workload, followed by *Effort* (*17.0*%).

Event-related potentials

Figure 4 depicts the grand-average (N = 15 participants) of the event-related potentials (ERPs) and spatial-temporal diversities of the class-discriminative information of the first 3 conditions (left: **V**, middle: **A**, right: **AV**). FC5 electrode was used in [27] for the early negative auditory ERP components. In visual P3-speller literatures, PO7, P7 and (or) P8 were used to check the early negative ERP components. Also concerning the ERP scalp maps in Figure 4, we choose the three channels (Cz, FC5 and P7) to analysis. These three channels of grand averaged ERPs are plotted on the top of the figure. The matrix plots under the ERPs show the spatial-temporal discriminative information (signed r^2) of *targets* vs. *non-targets* in each condition. To compare each component across different conditions, scalp maps of the class-discriminative information (r^2) are shown for 4 fixed time intervals, which are marked in the ERP plots. The components shown in this 4 time intervals are denoted as 'N1', 'N2', 'P3' and 'P4', according to the polarity and the order of the components.

In condition **V**, there is a prominent negative component 250-350 ms after stimulus onset located at lateral parieto-occipital electrodes (P7, P9) with higher amplitudes on the left hemisphere. This component is referred to as N2. The ERPs at P7 in Figure 4.1a depicts the difference of grand average ERPs between *targets* and *nontargets*. As expected, a positive component is observed approximately 350-560 ms (channel Cz) after the stimulus onset (referred to as P3 components). As seen from the spatial-temporal distribution matrix plot (Figure 4.1b), the positive component starts from the centro-parietal area and extends to the surrounding electrodes. The decay of the discriminative information of this component progresses from occipital to frontal electrodes, see Figure 4.1b.

In condition **A**, all components have lower amplitudes compared to the corresponding components in condition **V**, which is in agreement with existing literature. An early negative component observed at approximately 150-230 ms (referred as N1 component) occurs at fronto-central areas. As already observed by Höhne et al. [27], this component is stronger on the left hemisphere than on the right hemisphere. The P3 component starts at around 360 ms with a focus in the central area.

Figure 4.3 depicts the ERPs and topographies of the class-discriminative information in condition **AV**. The N1 component in condition **AV** occurs around the frontal area with a higher amplitude on the left hemisphere, which is similar to condition **A**. The N2 component observed at parieto-occipital electrodes shows a similar but weaker response compared with that in condition **V**. The P3 component starts from the fronto-central area between 350 ms and 500 ms, showing an earlier discriminative response than that in condition **V** similar as in condition **A**. Surprisingly, the decay of the P3 component progresses from the front to the occipital area (Figure 4.3b) vary much in contract to the condition **V**.

Figure 5 shows the ANOVA (using Matlab) results of ERP response for conditions **V**, **A**, and **AV** (Left: Targets, right: Non-Targets). The ERP response has significant differences of 3 conditions were marked light blue (p <.05). Light pink marked time-zones show the significant difference between condition **V** and **AV** (p <.05). The early components of the ERP response after stimulus onset show significant differences both for Targets and Non-Targets, which might indicate that those difference was influenced by the stimuli properties of different stimuli. Light pinked zones could indicate the influence of auditory stimuli to visual stimuli response. No obvious significant difference was found for P300 components during 250–450 ms. Thus, the characteristics of the individual auditory stimuli influence rather

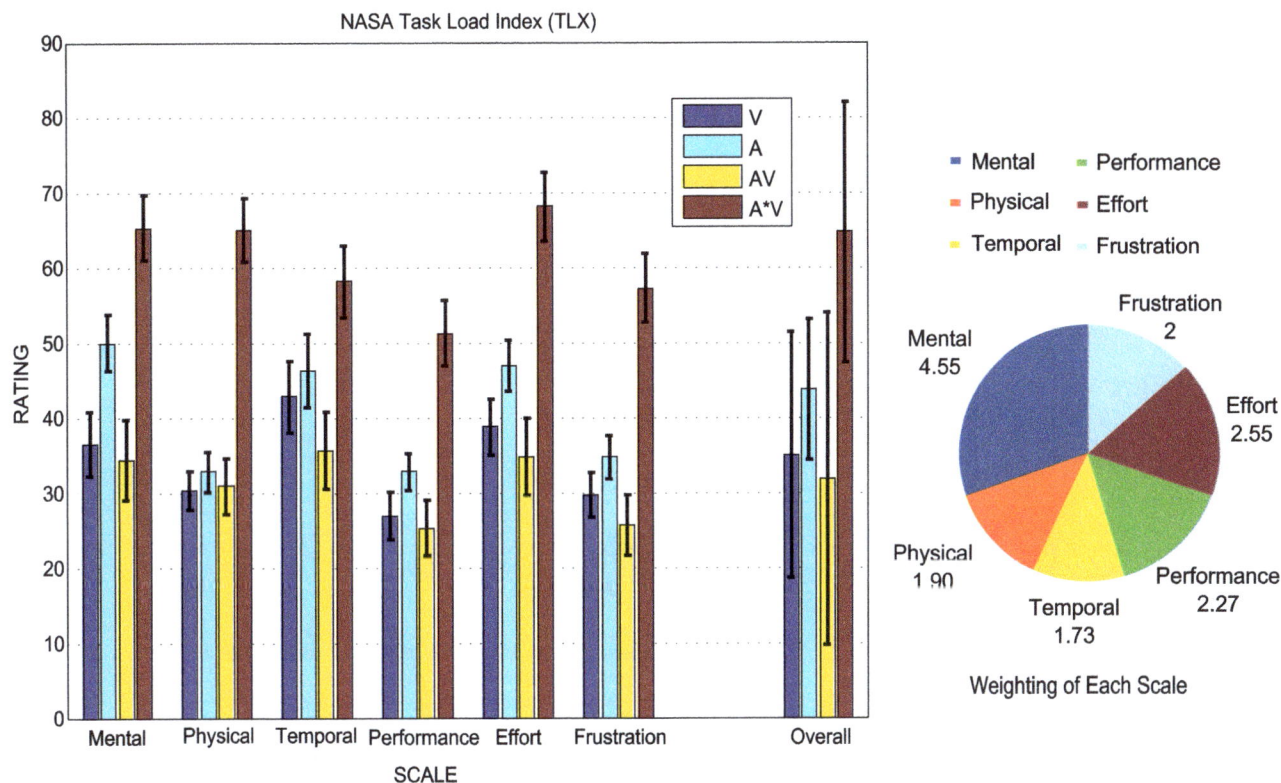

Figure 3. The NASA TLX workload and the overall weighted score of different conditions. The left column shows the mean rating with the standard deviation (SD) for each subscale and the overall weighted workload for each condition. The pie chart shows the grand-averaged weighting for each subscale. The total weighting is 15, due to 15 pair-wise comparisons of the sub-scales (see section 2.4).

the early ERP components, while later components are not affected.

Figure 6 show the ERPs (as well as the ANOVA results) and class-discriminative information (signed r^2) separately for visual and auditory stimuli in condition **V*A** (left: visual; right: auditory). The upper two subfigures show the ANOVA results of Targets versus Non-Targets for visual and auditory stimuli independently. Significant differences are found at large time zones for Target versus Non-Target ERP response. For the grand averaged visual response, the negative component at occipital area is observed at 250–380 ms after the visual stimulus onset, and the positive component at the central area occurs at 450 ms. The auditory negative component is observed at frontal areas from 100 to 250 ms and the positive response appears at the central area between 400 and 500 ms.

Offline binary accuracy

The single trial classification accuracies for each condition, which have an approximate Gaussian distribution (K-S test, p> 0.05) and equal sample variances (Levene tests, p = .875), were estimated and depicted in Figure 7. ANOVA of the accuracies with the factor condition was conducted. As expected, the classification accuracies in condition **V** and **AV** are significantly better than that in condition **A** ($p < .001$). However, there is no significant difference between condition **V** and condition **AV** ($p = 1$). No significant differences were found between V and V|A*V as well as between A and A|A*V (p>.05).

Figure 8.a depicts the grand average temporal distribution of discriminative information. To investigate which time intervals contribute most to classification success, a time window of 20 ms

and time step of 5 ms were used to calculate the temporal distribution of the classifications. Cross-validation results of those features for each time point provide a temporal distribution of the multivariate discriminative information. The curve for condition **A** shows lower classification accuracy compared to condition **V** for the whole time period except for the early interval 200–260 ms. Condition **AV** effectively exploits the early components of both modalities with accuracies above both unimodal conditions between 200 and 300 ms. However, starting from about 380 ms the results of **AV** are inferior to those of **V**, which is in line with the observation of the earlier decay of the P3 component in the bimodal condition (see Figure 4).

Analogously to Figure 8.a, Figure 8.b shows the temporal evolution of the discriminative information for condition **V*A**. It is quite similar to the results for the unimodal conditions in Figure 8.a. However, surprisingly, for the auditory stimuli in the Parallel-Speller (**V*A**), the discriminative information starts earlier than in the unimodal condition **A**, which may be due to an increased level of attention.

Complementary to Figures 8, the spatial distribution of the discriminative information is displayed in Figure 9. The top row shows the results of the first 3 conditions (**V, A, AV**). In condition **V**, higher accuracies of the occipital electrodes suggest that visual and visual-attentional components are essential ingredients for classification. Discriminative information from cognitive processes as reflected in the P3 is spatially more wide spread and therefore not so prominent is this display of single channel analysis. Classification accuracies for condition **A** show the importance of fronto-central electrodes in particular on the left hemisphere,

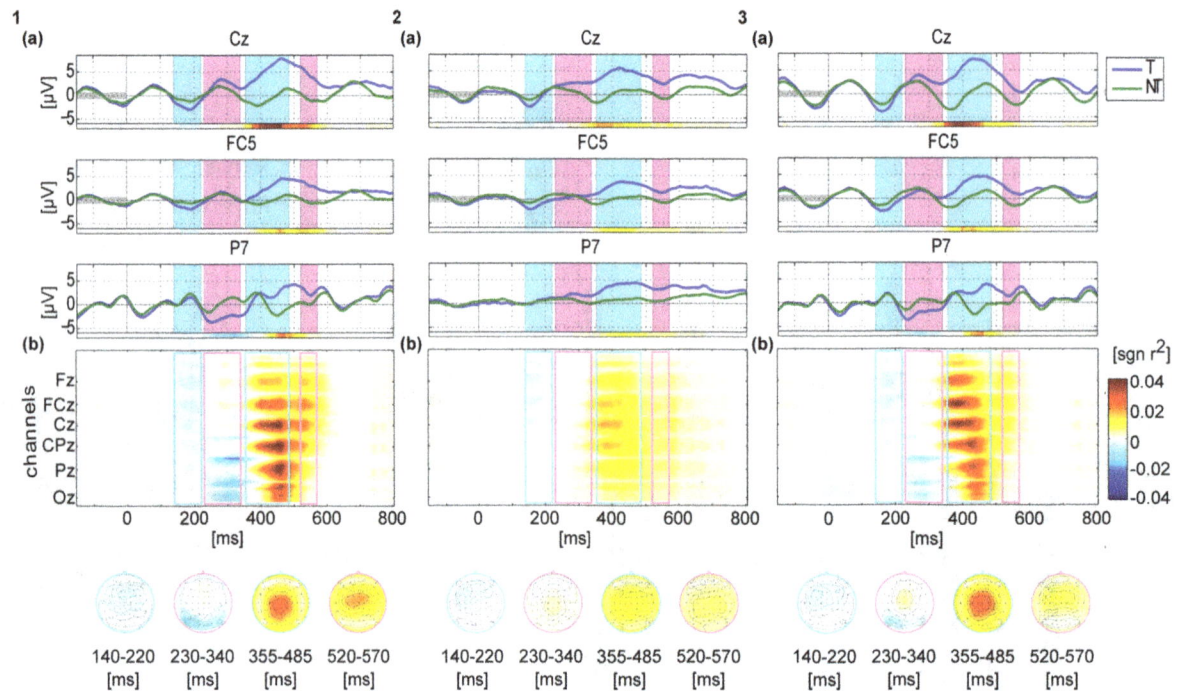

Figure 4. Grand averaged ERP and spatio-temporal diversity of the class-discriminative information for the first 3 conditions. Conditions are arranged in columns (left: **V**, middle: **A**, right: **AV**). All plots share the same color scale. The top row shows the ERPs for targets and non-targets of three selected electrodes Cz, FC5 and P7. The pink and green shade areas in each plot marked the time intervals, for which the scalp maps are shown at the bottom also colored accordingly. The colored bar underneath of each plot gives the signed correlation coefficient (sign r^2). It indicated the difference between target and non-target classes for the chosen channel. In the middle, the spatio-temporal distribution of class-discriminative information was shown as a matrix plot, under which also the scalp maps of the chosen intervals were shown depicting the averaged r^2 values within the time intervals. The matrix plot shows the signed r^2 values for each EEG channel and for each time point. The light-blue and light-magenta rectangles depicted the chosen time interval as the shaded area in the top rows.

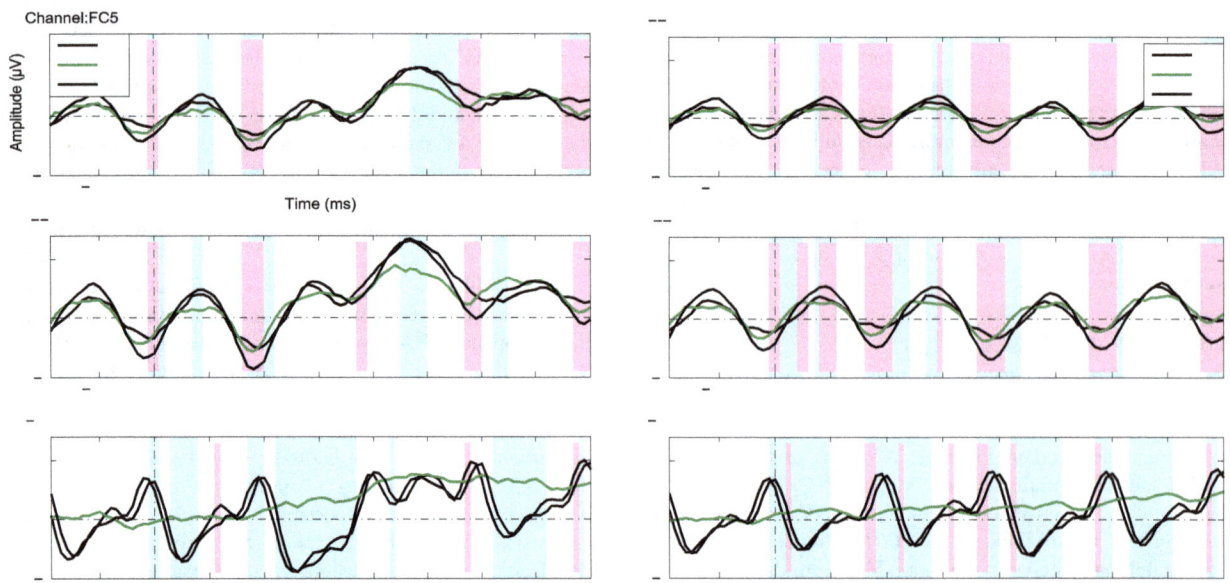

Figure 5. The ANOVA results of ERP response with factor *condition* **(conditions V, A, and AV; left: Targets, right: Non-Targets).** The time intervals with significant difference of ERP response for conditions **V**, **A**, and **AV** was marked light blue (p <.05). The pink-marked time-zones show the time intervals that have significant difference of conditions **V** and **AV** (p <.05).

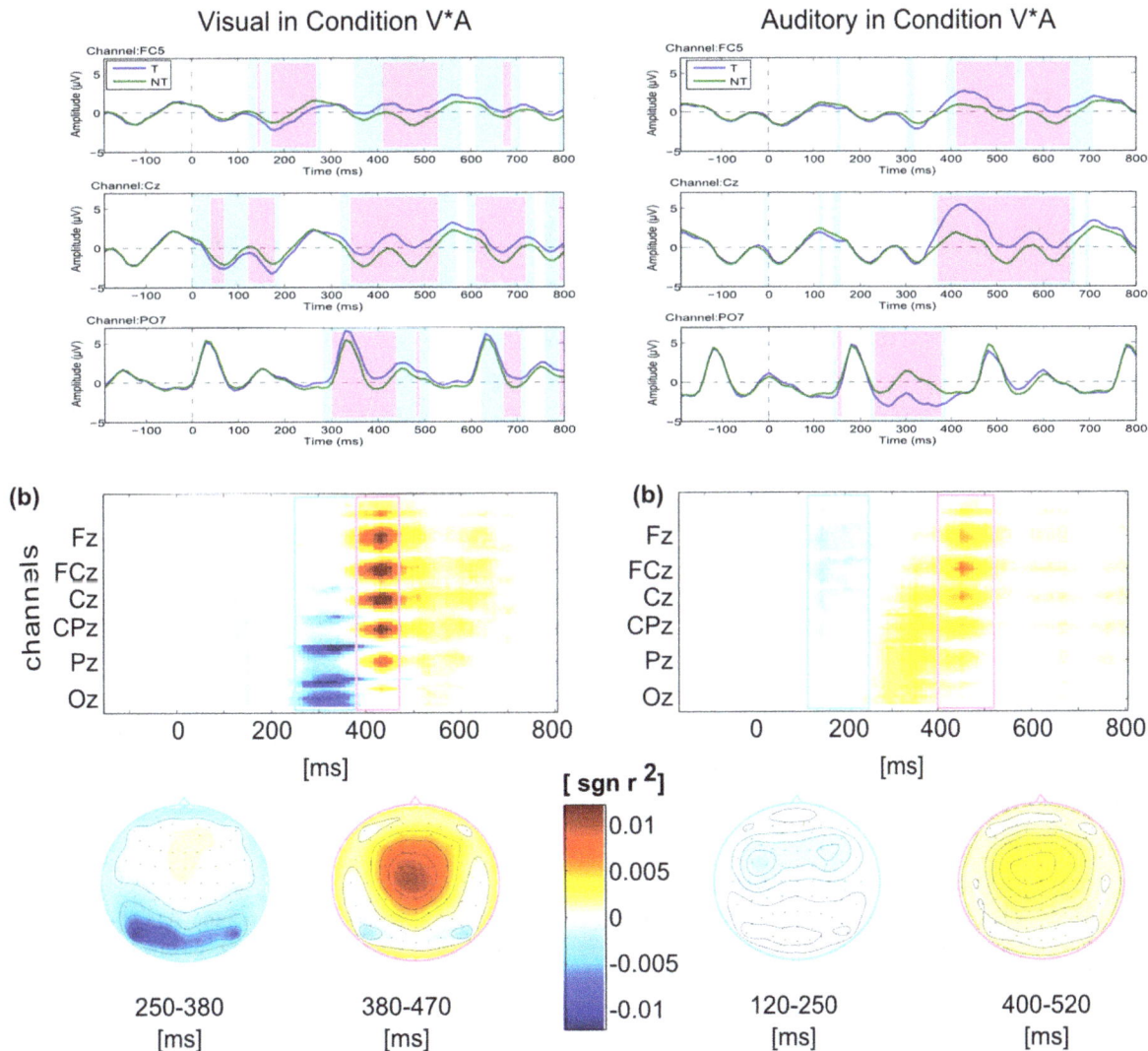

Figure 6. The ANOVA results of ERP response and class-discriminance (signed r^2) maps of Targets versus Non-Targets in condition V*A. The two columns show the ERP responses for visual (left) and auditory (right) stimuli independently in condition **V*A**. The first row shows the ERP responses for the three selected electrodes FC5, Cz and PO7. The time intervals with significant difference of ERP response for Targets and Non-Targets was marked light blue ($p < .05$). The pink-marked time-zones show the time intervals that have more significant difference with $p < .01$. Spatio-temporal diversities of the class-discriminative information are shown in the second row. All plots share the same color scale (different scale in the colorbar compared to Figure 4). The spatial distribution of class-discriminant information is depicted with scalpmaps for two time intervals.

which is in line with the ERP results shown in Figure 4. The asymmetry also exists in condition **AV**.

The classification accuracies in condition **V*A** are lower than in the other conditions. Therefore, in the second row a different scale for the colormap is used for better display. Apart from the lower absolute value, the maps of classification accuracy look similar to the maps for the corresponding uni-modal conditions in the row above. The occipital area of the map for V|V*A seems to show a stronger lateralization to the left side than the maps of the visual-only condition.

Online Spelling Results

Figure 10 depicts the results of conditions **AV** and **V*A** in the online copy-spelling mode of this study. Each participant had to spell 20 symbols ('AUDIO_VISUAL_SPELLER') in both paradigms.

For condition **AV** (Combined-Speller), 6 repetitions of the stimuli were used for each selection, and two selection periods (group selection and symbol selection) have been conducted for each symbol. The blue bar in Figure 10 shows the symbol accuracies in condition **AV**. More than *73.3%* participants (11 in 15 participants) could get accuracy over *90%*. Only 2 of all the participants got accuracy under *80%*. The mean accuracy is *92.0%* (chance level *<3%*) with a speed of more than 2 symbols per minute.

In the Parallel-Speller (condition **V*A**) 10 repetitions of the stimuli have been used. The visual stimuli coded the group and the auditory stimuli coded the position of the symbol in the visual group. Since there is no pause or the need for correcting selection errors during copy-spelling, all of the participants finished this part within 10 min. The red and green bars in Figure 10 shows the visual (**V**) and auditory (**A**) selection accuracies separately. The visual selections for thirteen participants are over 90.0%, while

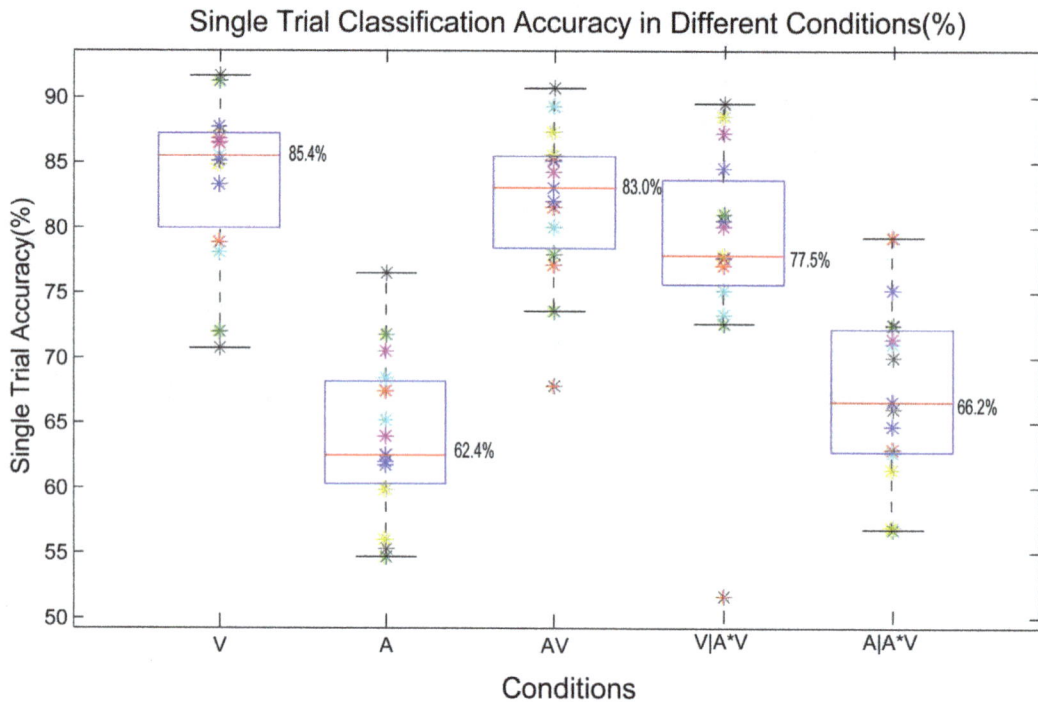

Figure 7. Single trial classification accuracies in different conditions for the binary *target* vs *non-target* discrimination. Accuracies are estimated by cross-validation on the calibration data using class-wise normalized loss function (chance level = 0.5). Each colored '*' represents the accuracy for each participant in giving conditions. The edges of the blue box in each column reveal the 25% and 75% data range. The central red mark is the median accuracy overall the participants in the giving condition.

only six participants could get accuracies over 90.0% for the auditory condition. Thus, the selection errors of the symbols are mostly due to an error of the auditory-based selection. Eleven of the participants achieved at least *80.0%* accuracy. Four participants spelled less than 16 correct symbols, thus displaying a selection accuracy of below 80%. All users could spell online with a mean accuracy of 87.7% (chance level <3%) showing a competitive average speed of 1.65 symbols per minute.

We also performed offline simulations where we determined the spelling speed (symbols/minute) as a function of the number of the sequences using the calibration data. Figure 11 shows the results for different conditions. ANOVA measures with factors *condition* and *number of repetitions* was conducted to investigate the significance of each factor for the first 3 conditions. The results show significant effects of factors *condition* ($p < .001$), *number of repetitions* ($p < .001$) but no significant effect of the factor

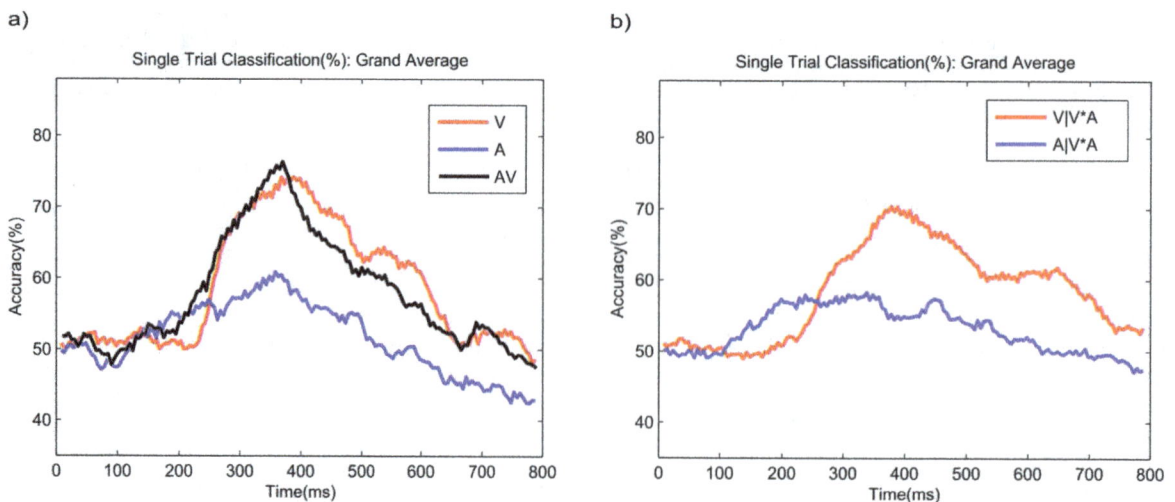

a)

b)

Figure 8. The grand averaged temporal distribution of discriminative information for each condition. a) The single trial classification for the unimodal spellers and Combined Speller (red: condition **V**; blue: condition **A**; black: condition **AV**). b) The temporal distribution of the single trial classification accuracy for condition **V*A** (red: visual classification; blue: auditory classification). The time window used in this study is 20 ms with a time step of 5 ms.

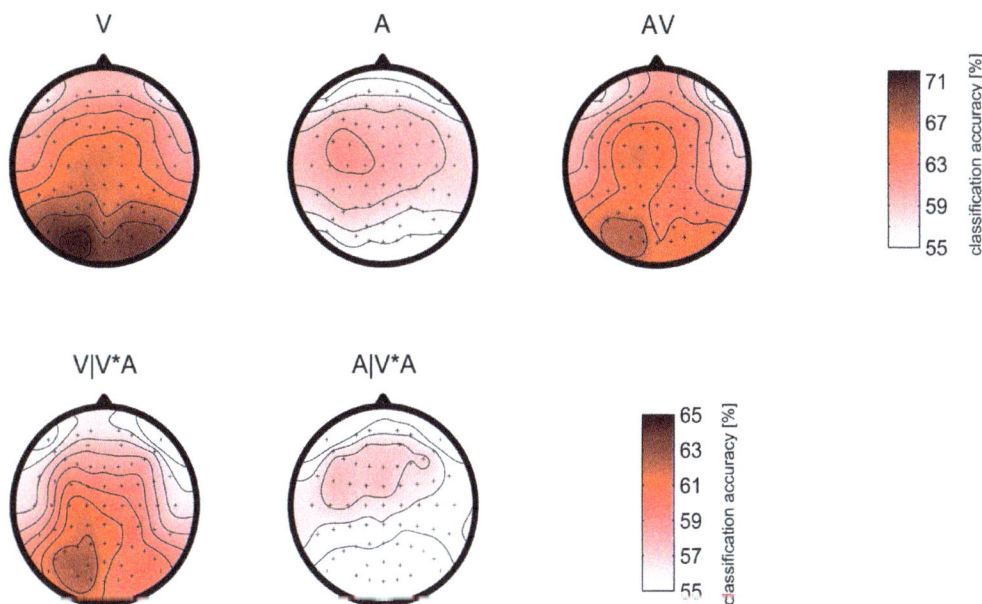

Figure 9. Spatial distribution of classification performance. Classification was made for each electrode individually. The time intervals were chosen by a heuristic between [0 800] after the stimulus onset. The grand average for each of the condition is shown and the binary classification accuracies are indicated by color gradients. The plots in the first row use the same color scale as shown on the right of that row. The figures in the second row use a different color bar as shown on the right of the second row.

condition * repetition ($p = .210$). However, concerning only the offline stimulation results of the spelling speed for conditions **V** and **AV**, there were significant effects of the *repetition* ($F = 21.996$, p $= 0$) factor, but no significant effect of the *condition* ($F = 3.125$, $p = 0.079$) and the *condition * repetition* ($F = .067$, $p = .997$) factors.

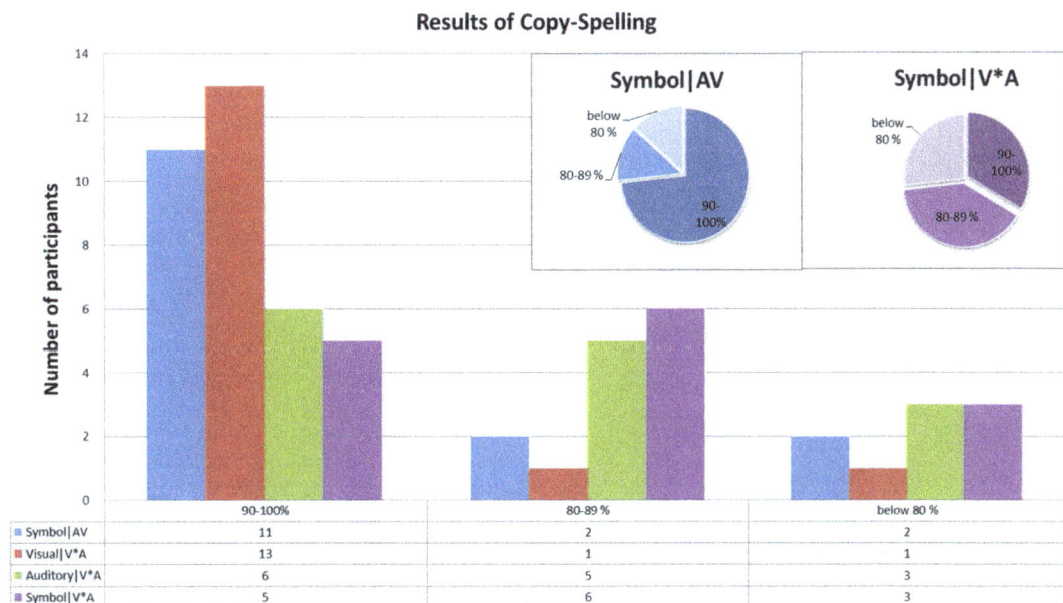

Figure 10. The distribution results of online copy spelling. The histogram shows the number of participants, whose classification accuracies were located in each accuracy scale. The accuracies were separated into 7 scales. 'Symble|AV' stands for the symbol selection accuracies in condition **AV**, and 'Symbol|V*A' stands for the symbol selection accuracies in condition **V*A**. The red bar, which is noted as 'Visual|V*A', represents the visual selection accuracies in condition **V*A**. The green bar, denoted as 'Auditory|V*A', shows the auditory selection accuracies distribution. The blue-dominant pie chart shows the proportion of each accuracy scale for the symbol selection accuracies in condition AV. The purple-dominant pie chart shows the proportion in condition **V*A**.

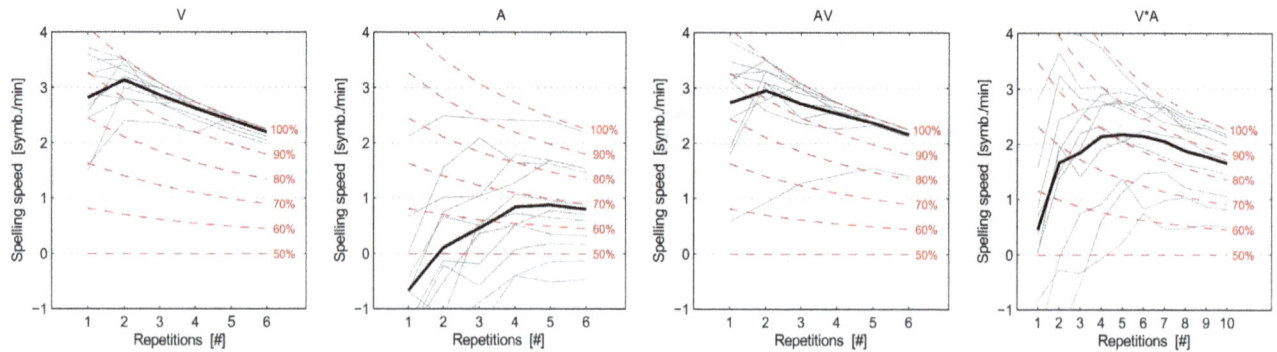

Figure 11. Spelling speed for each of the 4 conditions plotted against the number of repetitions. Thin gray lines depict results for single participants and the solid black line depicts the mean. Red dashed lines represent the spelling speed for fixed levels of symbol selection accuracy. Spelling accuracy for the empirical data (solid black line) can be deduced by comparing the black solid line to the red dashed lines. The accuracy is based on the calibration data for each condition.

Discussion

To answer the questions mentioned in section 1, two ways of combining visual and auditory stimuli were investigated: the first one employed simultaneous visual and auditory stimuli which represent the same information (called Combined-Speller, denoted as AV). The second one used two independent streams of visual and auditory stimuli which allow integrating two selection periods into a single one (called Parallel-Speller, denoted as V*A). There were two central goals in this study: first, to evaluate the advantages and disadvantages of the Combined-Speller and to compare it with the uni-modal paradigms (comparing workload, ERP response and discrimination information); second, to demonstrate the feasibility and usability of the Parallel-Speller (discussing the ERP response, spelling speed and so on), in which two independent decisions are made parallel.

Comparing the Combined-Speller with uni-modal paradigms

Workload. In our study, workload was used as a measure of usability of a system. Mental demand is the major factor for the weighted overall workload. Thus it is important to reduce the mental workload when operating a BCI system. It was reported in [36] that the workload for an auditory speller was significant higher than that for a (gaze-dependent) visual speller. Similar result but not significant difference was obtained here for an auditory compared with a gaze-independent visual paradigm. In particular, participants mentioned the difficulty of ignoring the non-targets, which had the same syllables or came from the same speakers as the target stimuli. However, when being asked after the whole experiment, some participants felt it was easier to attend uni-modal auditory speller compared with uni-modal visual speller, especially after having to focus on the center of the screen for such long time. The workload for the Combined-Speller (condition AV) was insignificantly lower than that for the mono-visual and mono-auditory paradigms. However, Participants (except one) mentioned that they were more relaxed during the Combined-Speller without always intensively focusing to either the visual stimuli or the auditory stimuli. Some participants regarded the target auditory stimuli as cues for the coming visual target, while others regarded the visual stimuli as cues instead. Thus, one can get to the conclusion that with an increasing runtime of the experiment, the Combined-Speller is the best choice with respect to workload, not only because the low workload it needs during

spelling, but also the changing of modality to release the mental workload.

The ERP and class-discrimination information. Belitski et al. [30] reported that multi-modal (audio+visual) stimulation increased the average strength of the stimulus response in matrix speller style BCIs, when compared to either visual or auditory stimulation in isolation. Thurling et al. [31], however, reported an enhanced N1 and reduced P300 in bimodal visual-tactile paradigm.

Detailed results were derived in our study. From Figure 4, we could find that the peak of the visual N1 component of Combined-Speller is shifted to the left hemisphere. This might be due to the evoked responses of the auditory stimulation. The discriminability of the N2 component is reduced compared to the uni-modal visual speller, with a possible explanation that the positive response caused by the auditory stimuli affected the negative response for visual stimuli at the same time. Focusing on the following positive components, we find that the P3 component in the Combined-Speller had a shorter latency than in the mono-visual paradigm. While the P3 component in the unimodal visual speller featured a second component with more frontal focus, this sub-component was absent in the bimodal condition. However, the exact mechanism of the response in the Combined-Speller remains to be investigated in further studies.

From the statistical analysis of the ERPs (Figure 5) for 3 channels, we could find that the early ERP components show significant improvements (i.e. increased discriminability) in the Combined-Speller compared to the uni-modal visual and auditory spellers. The time intervals marked in light blue and pink show the significant difference amongst the three conditions. Thus, the bimodal stimulation in condition **AV** mainly impacts the early ERP components such as P1 and N1. No obvious significant difference were found during P300 component from 250 – 450 ms between conditions **V** and **AV**. However, both conditions yield to significantly higher P300 amplitude than condition A. Since channel PO7 reflects mostly on the visual processing, conditions **V** and **AV** don't show significant differences at that channel.

The spatial information of the discriminant information shown in Figure 9 reveals two important findings: the visual response area was affected by the auditory stimuli, with the central higher classification area shifting left as the auditory stimuli; the occipital electrodes featured less classification accuracies in Combined-Speller than that in the uni-modal visual speller. As possible reason, it can be speculated that less attention was allocated to the visual stimuli due to the concurrent auditory stimulation.

Thus, visual stimuli with concurrent auditory stimuli have significant difference between single modal visual and auditory stimuli. ERP difference was mostly on early exogenous components during 0 – 200 ms after stimuli onset and in frontal and central electrodes.

Parallel-Speller

In previous studies [21,30,31], multi-modal spelling paradigms all used visual and auditory stimuli to convey the same information. Our study used for the first time visual and auditory stimuli to convey different information in parallel. The workload of the parallel speller is considerably higher than for the other three spellers.

Figure 6 provides an overview over the class-discriminative information for the Parallel-Speller. The negative and positive components occurred at specific area were clearly found for visual and auditory stimuli respectively in Parallel-Speller. It shows that the visual and auditory stimuli could work independently, though having a higher workload used (according to Figure 3).

Besides, the temporal and spatial distribution of single trial classification accuracy also showed a possible classifier for visual and auditory stimuli respectively, similar though lower accuracies and tightened response area as uni-modal visual and auditory stimuli.

Performances of Combined-Speller and Parallel-Speller

Riccio et al. [17] provides a comparison of most BCI spellers with visual and (or) auditory stimuli. The comparison was discussed and depicted in a table (Table 1 in [17]) through the accuracy, bits per symbol, symbols per minute and bits per minute of the BCIs. Most spellers using auditory or visual + auditory stimuli have accuracies less than 70% and ITR less than 1.9 bits per minute if the total number of selections is more than twenty. Concerning the visual stimuli, only one (out of thirteen) speller has an ITR up to 10 bits per minute. We describe the Combined-Speller and the Parallel-Speller. Compared to the gaze-independent spellers reviewed by Riccio et al. [17], our paradigms featured competitive selection accuracies (94.9% for Combined-Speller and 85.9% for Parallel-Speller) and overall BCI performances (ITR of 10.01 and 8.85 bits per minute respectively).

The spelling speed (symbols per minute), which is one of the evaluation of the feasibility of spelling system, shows that for the Parallel-Speller most participants could spell 2 symbols per minute when 5 repetitions were used. Two participants could even spell about 3.5 symbols per minute when 2 repetitions were used, which is comparable even better than other paradigms. All of the above results prove the feasibility and usability of the Parallel-Speller.

Furthermore, slower spelling speeds have been obtained with the parallel speller. Apart from the slower spelling speed, several participants indicated a preference for the Parallel-Speller, due to the fact that there is only one period to select a symbol. Several measures to be taken in future developments can be expected to give improvement in this respect: (a) Due to the more difficult task, some training might be required. (b) Given the difference in detectability in the sensory domains, an uneven distribution of the auditory and visual stimuli might be beneficial. For example, if

symbols are distributed in eight groups of four each, double the number of repetitions for auditory stimuli can be collected. (c) The current study used a considerable 'overhead' for the selection procedure in the Parallel-Speller. The 'overhead' contains the countdown part (hint for the target stimuli or a blank period for remember the targets, and the pre-flashing of the last digits), the classification time (to compute the result selections) and feedback (to show the selected group or symbols on the screen), more information was described in section 2.3. In this study, the stimulation time for each symbol in Parallel-Speller was about 18 s, while the 'overhead' (the countdown, classification and feedback) occupied about 10 s. For Combined-Speller, the stimulation time for each symbol was 2*7.2 s, while the 'overhead' was about 2*6.1 s. We assume that after practicing with the Parallel-Speller, the assistant time could reduce to 6.1 s as in Combined-Speller. (d) An optimal stopping method (Schreuder et al, 2013) could be employed to enhance the performance for the Parallel-Speller.

The Parallel-Speller is a novel approach for an ERP speller, which provides new insight into multisensory processing. Moreover, it represents a way to practice these two human sensory channels.

Conclusions

In a multisensory world, it might be advisable to also use multisensory stimulation for BCI applications. We approached this topic by comparing unimodal stimuli (from either visual or auditory domain), with multisensory stimuli from both domains. We studies two kinds of multisensory integration in an ERP-based BCI speller: the Combined-Speller and the Parallel-Speller.

For the Combined-Speller, most participants pointed out the positive aspect that it is not necessary to continuously locate attention to a fixed modality. The ERP response as well as the distribution of discriminative information was observed to be different for combined-speller compared to unimodal stimuli. It remains an area of future research to exploit such differences. Comparing the Combined-Speller to uni-modal paradigms we found shorter latencies, lower amplitudes, as well as a shift of the temporal and spatial distribution of discriminative information. As it was already suggested in this study, the Combined-Speller is a good choice for BCI speller with a low workload.

Moreover, a novel multimodal stimulus paradigm, called 'Parallel-Speller', was introduced. The Parallel-Speller combines two independent streams of stimuli, enabling a 1-out-of-36 decision with a single step. However, the workload is increased compared to all other conditions. The results for its classification and brain response showed that it is possible to apply such a truly multimodal paradigm. We hope that the new way of combining sensory modalities could stimulate further discussions and novel applications.

Author Contributions

Conceived and designed the experiments: XWA JH BB DM. Performed the experiments: XWA JH. Analyzed the data: XWA JH. Contributed reagents/materials/analysis tools: BB. Wrote the paper: XWA JH BB DM.

References

1. Wolpaw JR, Wolpaw EW (2012) Brain-Computer Interfaces: Principles and Practice. Oxford University Press.
2. Dornhege G (2007) Toward Brain-Computer Interfacing. MIT Press.
3. Wolpaw JR, McFarland DJ (2004) Control of a two-dimensional movement signal by a noninvasive brain-computer interface in humans. Proc Natl Acad Sci USA 101: 17849–54.
4. Blankertz B, Dornhege G, Krauledat M, Müller KR, Curio G (2007) The non-invasive Berlin brain-computer interface: fast acquisition of effective performance in untrained subjects. Neuroimage 37: 539–50.
5. Mak JN, Wolpaw JR (2009) Clinical applications of brain-computer interface: current state and future prospects. IEEE Rev Biomed Eng 2: 187–99.

6. Farwell LA, Donchin E (1988) Talking off the top of your head: toward a mental prosthesis utilizing event-related brain potentials. Electroencephalogr Clin Neurophysiol 70: 510–23.

7. Zhang D, Song H, Xu H, Wu W, Gao S, et al. (2012) An N200 speller integration the spatial profile for the detection of the non-control state. J.Neural Eng 9: 026016.

8. Bin G, Gao X, Wang Y, Li Y, Hong B, et al. (2011) A high-speed BCI based on code modulation VEP. J Neural Eng 8: 025015.

9. Sellers EW, Vauqhan TM, Wolpaw JR (2010) A brain-computer interface for long-term independent home use. Amyotroph Lateral Scler 11 (5): 449–55.

10. Brunner P, Joshi S, Briskin S, Wolpaw JR, Bischof H, et al. (2010) Does the 'P300' speller depend on eye gaze?. J Neural Eng7: 056013.

11. Treder MS, Blankertz B (2010) (C)overt attention and visual speller design in an ERP-based brain-computer interface. Behavioral and Brain Function 6: 28.

12. Treder MS, Schmidt NM, Blankertz B (2011) Gaze-independent brain–computer interfaces based on covert attention and feature attention. J Neural Eng 8: 066003.

13. Schaeff S, Treder MS, Venthur B, Blankertz B (2012) Exploring motion VEPs for gaze-independent communication. J Neural Eng 9: 045006.

14. Liu Y, Zhou Z, Hu D (2011) Gaze-independent brain-computer speller with covert visual search tasks. Clin Neurophysiol 122(6): 1127–36.

15. Aloise F, Aricò P, Schettini F, Riccio A, Salinari S, et al. (2012) A covert attention P300-based brain-computer interface: Geospell. Ergonomics 55(5): 538–551.

16. Acqualaqna L, Blankertz B (2013) Gaze-independent BCI-spelling using rapid serial visual presentation (RSVP). Clin Neurophysiol 124(5): 901–8.

17. Riccio A, Mattia D, Simione L, Olivetti M, Cincotti F (2012) Eye-gaze independent EEG-based brain-computer interfaces for communication. J Neural Eng 9(4): 045001.

18. Brouwer A-M, van Erp JBF, Aloise F, Cincotti F (2010) Tactile, Visual, and Bimodal P300s: Could Bimodal P300s Boost BCI Performance? SRX Neuroscience 2010: 1–9.

19. Van der Waal M, Severens M, Geuze J, Desain P (2012) Introducing the tactile speller: an ERP-based brain–computer interface for communication. Journal of Neural Engineering 9: 045002.

20. Kübler A, Furdea A, Halder S, Hammer EM, Nijboer F, et al. (2009) A brain-computer interface controlled auditory event-related potential (p300) spelling system for locked-in patients. Annals of the New York Academy of Sciences 1157: 90–100.

21. Klobassa DS, Vaughan TM, Brunner P, Schwartz NE, Wolpaw JR, et al. (2009) Toward a high-through put auditory P300-based brain-computer interface. Clin Neurophysiol 120(7): 1252–61.

22. Halder S, Hammer EM, Kleih SC, Bogdan M, Rosenstiel W, et al. (2013) Prediction of auditory and visual p300 brain-computer interface aptitude. PloS one 8: e53513.

23. Schreuder M, Blankertz B, Tangermann M (2010) A New Auditory Multi-Class Brain-Computer Interface Paradigm: Spatial Hearing as an Informative Cue. PloS One 5: e9813.

24. Schreuder M, Rost T, Tangermann M (2011) Listen, you are writing! Speeding up online spelling with a dynamic auditory BCI. Front Neuroscience 5: 112.

25. Höhne J, Schreuder M, Blankertz B, Tangermann M (2011) A Novel 9-Class Auditory ERP Paradigm Driving a Predictive Text Entry System. Front Neurosci 5: 99.

26. Höhne J, Tangermann M (2014) Towards user-friendly spelling with an auditory brain-computer interface: the CharStreamer paradigm. PloS One 9: e98322.

27. Höhne J, Krenzlin K, Dähne S, Tangermann M (2012) Natural stimuli improve auditory BCIs with respect to ergonomics and performance. J Neural Eng 9: 045003.

28. Teder-Sälejärvi WA, Di Russo F, McDonald JJ, Hillyard SA (2005) Effects of spatial congruity on audio-visual multimodal integration. Journal of Cognitive Neuroscience 17: 1396–409. doi:10.1162/0898929054985383.

29. Campanella S, Bruyer R, Froidbise S, Rossignol M, Joassin F, et al. (2010) Is two better than one? A cross-modal oddball paradigm reveals greater sensitivity of the P300 to emotional face-voice associations. Clincal Neurophysiology 121: 1855–1862.

30. Belitski A, Farquhar J, Desain P (2011) P300 audio-visual speller. J Neural Eng 8: 025022.

31. Thurling ME, Brouwer Am, Van Erp JBF, Blankertz B, Werkhoven PJ (2012) Does bimodal stimulus presentation increase ERP components usable in BCIs? J Neural Eng 9: 045005.

32. Talsma D, Senkowski D, Soto-Faraco S, Woldorff MG (2010) The multifaceted interplay between attention and multisensory integration. Trends Cogn Sci 14: 400–10.

33. Senkowski D, Talsma D, Grigutsch M (2007) Good times for multisensory integration: effects of the precision of temporal synchrony as revealed by gamma-band oscillations. Neuropsychologia 45: 561–571.

34. Blankertz B, Lemm S, Treder MS, Haufe S, Müller KR (2011) Single-trial analysis and classification of ERP components-a tutorial. Neuroimage 56: 814–825.

35. Pasqualotto E, Simonetta A, Gnisci V, Federici S, Olivetti M (2011) BelardinelliToward a usability evaluation of BCIs. Int J Bioelectromagn 13: 121–22.

36. Riccio A, Leotta F, Bianchi L, Aloise F, Zickler C, et al. (2011) Workload measurement in a communication application operated through a P300-based brain-computer interface. J Neural Eng 8: 025028.

37. Käthner I, Ruf CA, Pasqualotto E, Braun C, Birbaumer N, et al. (2013) A po auditory P300 brain-computer interface with directional cues. Clin Neurophyisol 124: 327–38.

38. Schreuder M, Höhne J, Blankertz B, Haufe S, Dickhaus T, et al. (2013) Optimizing event-related potentail based brain-computer interface: a systematic evaluation of dynamic stopping methods. J Neural Eng 10: 036025.

13

Remembering the Object You Fear: Brain Potentials during Recognition of Spiders in Spider-Fearful Individuals

Jaroslaw M. Michalowski[2*], **Mathias Weymar**[1], **Alfons O. Hamm**[1]

1 Department of Biological and Clinical Psychology, University of Greifswald, Greifswald, Germany, **2** Faculty of Psychology, University of Warsaw, Warszawa, Poland

Abstract

In the present study we investigated long-term memory for unpleasant, neutral and spider pictures in 15 spider-fearful and 15 non-fearful control individuals using behavioral and electrophysiological measures. During the initial (incidental) encoding, pictures were passively viewed in three separate blocks and were subsequently rated for valence and arousal. A recognition memory task was performed one week later in which old and new unpleasant, neutral and spider pictures were presented. Replicating previous results, we found enhanced memory performance and higher confidence ratings for unpleasant when compared to neutral materials in both animal fearful individuals and controls. When compared to controls high animal fearful individuals also showed a tendency towards better memory accuracy and significantly higher confidence during recognition of spider pictures, suggesting that memory of objects prompting specific fear is also facilitated in fearful individuals. In line, spider-fearful but not control participants responded with larger ERP positivity for correctly recognized old when compared to correctly rejected new spider pictures, thus showing the same effects in the neural signature of emotional memory for feared objects that were already discovered for other emotional materials. The increased fear memory for phobic materials observed in the present study in spider-fearful individuals might result in an enhanced fear response and reinforce negative beliefs aggravating anxiety symptomatology and hindering recovery.

Editor: Allan Siegel, University of Medicine & Dentistry of NJ - New Jersey Medical School, United States of America

Funding: The research was supported in part by a grant from the University of Warsaw to the first author, BST 164600/2015 and in part by a grant from the National Science Centre to the first author, 2013/11/N/HS6/01401. The funders had no role in study design, data collection and analysis, decision to publish, or preparation of the manuscript.

Competing Interests: The authors have declared that no competing interests exist.

* Email: jmichalowski@psych.uw.edu.pl

Introduction

Individuals suffering from specific phobias exhibit an excessive and unreasonable fear of their phobia-relevant objects or feared situations. Moreover, phobic individuals detect even minor signals of upcoming threat at a very early processing stage [1–2]. When the threat cue does not disappear or even approaches, this increased attention is followed by defensive response mobilization, as indexed by cardiac acceleration and startle potentiation [3] to prepare the organism for effective escape if possible.

It is well established that our survival depends not only on the ability to activate such functional behavioral adjustments to threatening situations but also to increase the chance that survival-relevant information is available in the future [4]. In fact, multiple evidence suggest that emotionally arousing events are better remembered than affectively neutral events (for review see [5–6]) as demonstrated in studies using free recall [7] and recognition memory procedures [8–10]. The question arises whether mnemonic processing of feared objects also varies with inter-individual fear status? One might expect that individuals with specific phobia show better memory of their feared objects due to stronger emotional arousal elicited by these events. Previous studies, however, have found mixed results. One Positron Emission Tomography (PET) study [11] found better memory discrimina-

tion for phobic pictures compared to non-phobic pictures in participants with animal phobia. Moreover, in this study the memory performance covaried with amygdala activation and electrodermal activity during encoding, supporting the arousal hypothesis [5–6]. In contrast, studies using words as stimuli did not find memory enhancing effects for phobia-relevant words in explicit memory tests such as recognition or recall [12–14]. For instance, memory recall for a spider word presented in a continuous stream of neutral pictures did not differ between spider phobics and non-phobic controls [12]. In another study, spider phobic participants recalled fewer spider related words (e.g., cobweb, fangs) compared to neutral words, in the presence of a live spider [14] Similarly, Thorpe and Salkovskis [13] observed that individuals with spider phobia did not differ from non-fearful controls in their recognition memory (hits and false alarms) for live spiders presented in video clips. Moreover, even poorer recognition memory for big dead spiders was observed for individuals with animal phobia compared to non-phobic participants in the study by Watts, Trezise, and Sharrock [15].

Several methodological issues might have contributed to these inconsistent findings: First, phobic stimulation might engage an avoidance tendency, as postulated in the attention-avoidance hypothesis [16], and/or overload the encoding capacities interfering with subsequent detailed processing of phobia-relevant information. In fact, previous eye movement data showed that individuals with specific phobia tend to avoid a detailed perceptual analysis of their feared objects after an increased initial orienting [17–18]. Second, the poorer quality of cognitive representations and reduced memory performance for phobic stimuli might result from short intervals between initial stimulus presentation and the memory test. A number of studies revealed that the storage of emotional material benefits from longer consolidation intervals [6], [19–21]. Using longer time intervals resulted in a higher memory accuracy and recollective experience for emotionally arousing relative to neutral events when compared to short (immediate) time lags. Third, arousal levels of the spider material could vary across the different experiments. For instance, arousal levels are lower for words than for affective pictures in general [22–23], thus pictorial materials of spiders may be more effective in prompting emotional arousal [11] than spider-related words leading to better memory performance for pictures than for words.

Thus, in the present study, we used pictorial scenes, a longer memory consolidation interval (1-week), and increased the number of repetitions during encoding to counteract shallow encoding due to possible avoidance tendencies engaged by phobic stimulation. In addition, we investigated recognition memory using Event-Related Potentials (ERPs), which provides a more direct insight into memory processing mechanisms [24]. Numerous studies reported differences in the ERP waveform between items presented for the first time and repeated items (for review see [25]). Specifically, during recognition, correctly recognized old stimuli reliably elicited a more positive-going ERP deflection than correctly classified new stimuli. An early frontal old/new difference between 300 and 500 ms has been linked to familiarity-based recognition [26] and a later occurring (~400–800 ms) centro-parietal old/new effect was suggested to index successful recollection of information [27–29]. Importantly, previous ERP studies found that this later centro-parietal old/new effect is more pronounced for emotional, relative to neutral words [30], [31], facial expressions [32] and natural scenes [23], indicating that better recognition of emotional events is related to explicit recollection [6].

In the present study we presented unpleasant, neutral and spider pictures to spider-fearful and control individuals and tested recognition memory for these materials. Considering previous evidence suggesting that the storage of emotional material benefit from longer consolidation intervals [6], [19–21], we used a delay of 7 days between encoding and memory test. Moreover, given the high homogeneity of phobia-relevant spider pictures these materials are more difficult to memorize when compared to images depicting neutral and unpleasant scenes. In order to overcome this problem and to ensure that there is an appropriate amount of trials for analyzing EPRs we included photographs depicting different exemplars of spiders and increased initial picture presentation time and frequency. Accordingly, during encoding session, each picture was presented three times to ensure deeper encoding. We expected to replicate previous findings of better recognition memory and larger ERP old/new difference for emotional (unpleasant and spider pictures) pictures, compared to neutral pictures. Moreover, if spiders induce more emotional arousal in spider-fearful individuals than in controls, memory for spider pictures should be better in the high fearful relative to the control group. Previous ERP studies [1], [33–35] observed facilitated perceptual processing of spider pictures in spider-fearful relative to control individuals presumably in the P1, Early Posterior Negativity (EPN), and Late Positive Potentials (LPP).

We also tested whether such ERP differences occur during recognition when old and pictures are presented.

Materials and Methods

Participants

31 students from the University of Greifswald participated in two study sessions (encoding and recognition). Participants were selected from a pool of 532 students from the University of Greifswald who were screened with the German version of the 31-item spider phobia questionnaire (SPQ; German version, [36]). 16 participants (15 females) scoring above the 85th percentile of the distribution on the SPQ were included in the spider-fearful group (M = 19.7, SD = 3.1) and 15 female participants scoring below the 33th percentile of the distribution were included in the non-fearful control group (M = 3.5, SD = 1.4). The groups did not differ in general anxiety as measured by the State-Trait Anxiety Inventory (STAI-T, [37]), t (28)<1, ns. Participants received either course credit or 24 Euros for participation. The study protocol was approved by the Research Ethics Committee of the Faculty of Psychology University of Warsaw. All subjects gave their written informed consent. Data from one female spider-fearful participant were excluded from further analyses because of excessive EEG artifacts.

Stimulus Materials and procedure

Overall, 256 color photographs were selected from the International Affective Picture System (IAPS; [38]) and from our own picture pool (see [39–42]). The pictures included 128 neutral (e.g., landscapes, buildings and neutral people), 64 unpleasant (e.g., mutilation, human and animal attack), and 64 fear-relevant pictures of spiders.

During the encoding session, participants viewed a set of 160 pictures presented within three separate blocks: 32 neutral pictures (block 1), 32 neutral intermixed with 32 spider pictures (block 2), and 32 neutral intermixed with 32 unpleasant pictures (block 3, see Figure 1). The block order was counterbalanced across participants. In each block pictures were presented twice in a pseudo-random order with the restriction that the same picture could not occur on two consecutive trials. Each picture was presented for 1500 ms, preceded by a fixation cross (1000 ms) and followed by an intertrial interval (ITI) of 750, 1000, or 1250 ms (in random order). The color of the fixation cross (blue or green or dark yellow equated in brightness) signaled the category of the upcoming picture. Assignment of colors to the specific picture category (neutral, unpleasant, spider) was counterbalanced across subjects. A cue signaling neutral pictures remained the same across all three experimental blocks. At the end of the session each participant was asked to view each picture as long as desired and to press a button to terminate picture presentation. After each picture offset valence and arousal ratings were collected using a computerized version of the Self-Assessment Manikin [43]. During the encoding session, no mention of a memory test was made (incidental encoding). These first session ERP data are reported elsewhere.

One week after the encoding session, 96 old and 96 new pictures (32 neutral, 32 unpleasant, and 32 spider pictures, respectively) were presented for 2500 ms and participants were instructed to decide for each picture whether it has been presented before in the study by pressing a button marked "yes" or "no" after picture offset. Following the recognition decision, participants rated the recognition confidence (see [10], [44]) on an 11-point Likert scale (0 – not confident, 10 – absolutely confident). At the end of the recognition session the EEG sensors were removed and valence and arousal ratings for all new pictures were obtained from the

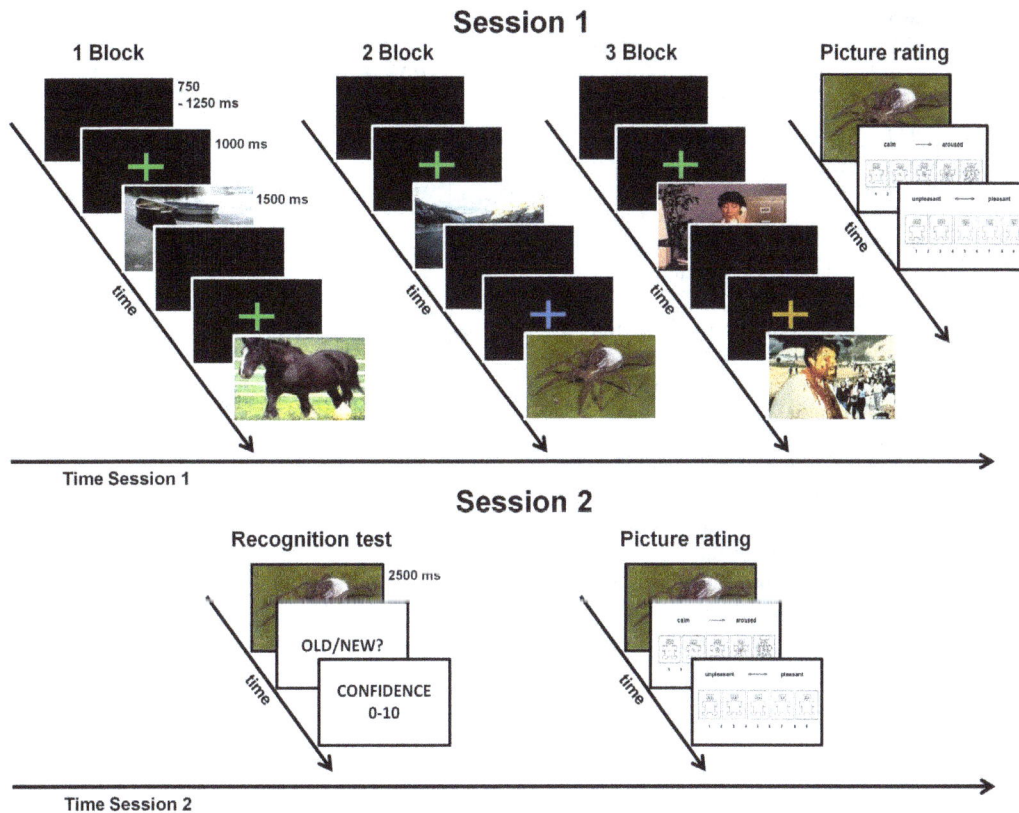

Figure 1. Illustration of the experimental procedure. In the first session (top) 3 separate picture blocks (neutral, spider and neutral, unpleasant and neutral) were presented in a randomized order. Within each block pictures were preceded by a fixation cross in one of three different colors that signaled the category of an upcoming picture. At the end of this session pictures were rated for valence and arousal. In the second session (bottom) old and new pictures were presented and participants were asked to decide for each picture whether it has been presented before in the study or not (OLD/NEW?) and to rate their confidence (0–10). Finally, new pictures were rated for valence and arousal.

participants using the Self-Assessment Manikin [43]. During both sessions participants were seated in a recliner in a dimly lit and sound-attenuated room in front of a 20-inch (50.8 cm) computer monitor located approximately 1.5 m from their eyes (11° of visual angle).

Data acquisition, recording and reduction

Electrophysiological data were collected from the scalp using a 256-sensor net (Electrical Geodesics, Inc., Eugene, OR). Electrode impedance was kept below 30 kΩ as recommended by the manufacturer. EEG data were continuously recorded with the vertex sensor as a reference electrode, in the 0.1–100 Hz frequency range with a sampling rate of 250 Hz. Continuous electroencephalography (EEG) data were low pass filtered at 40 Hz using digital filtering before stimulus synchronized epochs lasting from -120 ms to 1000 ms relative to the picture onset were extracted. Data editing and artifact rejection were based on a method for statistical control of artifacts [45]. Artifact rejection was based upon boundary values of three parameters: maximal absolute value over time, standard deviation over time, and maximal temporal gradient over time. First, the data with common (vertex) reference were used to detect and reject channels with artifacts. Eye movement and blink artifacts were reduced using a regression-based procedure as implemented in BioSig [46]. Second, the data were transformed to averaged reference and global artifacts were detected and contaminated trials excluded from further analysis. Overall, approximately 25% of the trials

were rejected because of artifacts. The rejected trials were equally distributed across picture categories and groups. For the remaining trials, rejected single channels were estimated by a spherical spline interpolation on the basis of all remaining sensors on a trial-by-trial base. Data reported are baseline-corrected and converted to an average reference.

Statistical data analysis

Behavioral Data. Hit rate (H), false alarm (FA), recognition accuracy (Pr (p (hit)$-$p (false alarms)) and response bias Br (p (false alarms)/p $(1-Pr)$) were analyzed in the recognition task. According to Snodgrass and Corwin [47] greater Pr values indicate better discrimination between old and new items. Br values higher than 0.5 indicate liberal response criteria (bias to respond "old") and lower than 0.5 suggest conservative response criteria (bias to respond "new"). These behavioral performance measures were analyzed with repeated measures analysis of variance (ANOVA) including Picture Category (neutral vs., unpleasant vs., phobia-relevant) as a within-subject factor and Group (spider fear vs., control) as a between-subject factor.

Confidence ratings were analyzed with repeated measures ANOVAs including Memory (old vs. new) and Picture Category as within-subject factors as well as Group as a between-subject factor. Valence and arousal ratings as well as the viewing time were analyzed separately using an ANOVA involving Group as a between-subject factors and Picture Category as a within-subject factor.

Event-Related Potentials. As in previous studies [10], [48], visual inspection of the ERP waveforms as well as single-sensor waveform analyses were used in concert to identify the temporal and spatial characteristics of the old/new ERP effects. For the single-sensor waveform analyses, repeated measures ANOVAs including the within-factors Picture Category (neutral vs., unpleasant vs., phobia-relevant) and Memory (old vs., new) as well as the between-factor Group (spider fear vs., control) were carried out for each time point after picture onset and each individual sensor (cf. [48]). To avoid false positives and to ensure a more stringent alpha-level adjustment, significant effects were only considered meaningful when observed for at least eight continuous data points (32 ms) and two neighboring sensors. These analyses revealed differences in the ERP waveforms for correctly recognized old and new pictures as well as the effects of emotional ERP modulation. For detailed analyses of these effects, mean amplitudes averaged within time windows and sensor clusters identified by both visual inspection and single-sensor waveform analyses were included in further statistical analyses. The ERP old/new effect and the emotional LPP modulation were analyzed within the time window from 400 to 800 ms after picture onset in two central sensor clusters comprising the following sensors: 9, 44, 45, 52, 53, 59, 60, 66, 78, 79, 80, 88, 89 in the left hemisphere and 130, 131, 132, 142, 143, 144, 154, 155, 164, 183, 184, 185, 186 in the right hemisphere (see inlet in Figure 2). The P1 was scored in the time window 124–172 ms in two posterior sensor clusters including 96, 97, 98, 106, 107, 108, 115, 116, 117, 124, 125 in the left hemisphere and 138, 139, 149, 150, 151, 152, 159, 160, 161, 169, 170 in the right hemisphere. The EPN was scored in the time window 200–300 ms for two posterior sensor clusters: 114, 115, 116, 121, 122, 123, 124, 133, 134, 135, 136 in the left hemisphere and 148, 149, 150, 157, 158, 159, 166, 167, 168, 174, 175 in the right hemisphere. Further analyses were carried out by calculating repeated measures ANOVAs including Picture Category, Memory, and Laterality (right vs. left) as within factors and Group as a between factor. Follow-up ANOVAs were calculated for each picture category including Memory (old vs., new) and Laterality (right vs., left) as within factors and Group as a between factor. In order to analyze the emotional ERP modulation, we further compared emotional (spider or unpleasant pictures) with neutral picture contents. For effects involving repeated measures, the Greenhouse-Geisser correction of degrees of freedom was applied.

Results

Behavioral Data

Ratings and viewing times. Hedonic valence and arousal ratings corresponded with the IAPS norms [38]. When compared to neutral images pictures depicting unpleasant scenes and spiders were rated as more unpleasant, Picture Category, F (1.691, 56) = 262.37, $p < .001$, $\eta 2 = .90$, and more arousing, Picture Category, F (1.867, 56) = 196.20, $p < .001$, $\eta 2 = .87$. These differences were modulated by group, Picture Category × Group, $Fs > 31$, $ps < .001$. As expected, individuals with spider fear rated pictures of spiders as more arousing and more unpleasant than control subjects, ts (28) > 6, $ps < .001$. The two experimental groups did not differ in the arousal and valence ratings for neutral pictures, ts (28) < 1.3, ns, and in the arousal ratings for unpleasant pictures, ts (28) < 1.3, ns. The latter picture category was rated as more unpleasant in the spider fear when compared to the control group, t (28) = 2.2, $p < .05$. Similar viewing times were found for the three picture categories, Picture Category, F (1.538, 56) = 2.88, $p = .080$, $\eta 2 = .09$, Picture Category × Group, F (1.538, 56) = .97, $p = .367$, $\eta 2 = .03$. Follow-up tests revealed shorter viewing

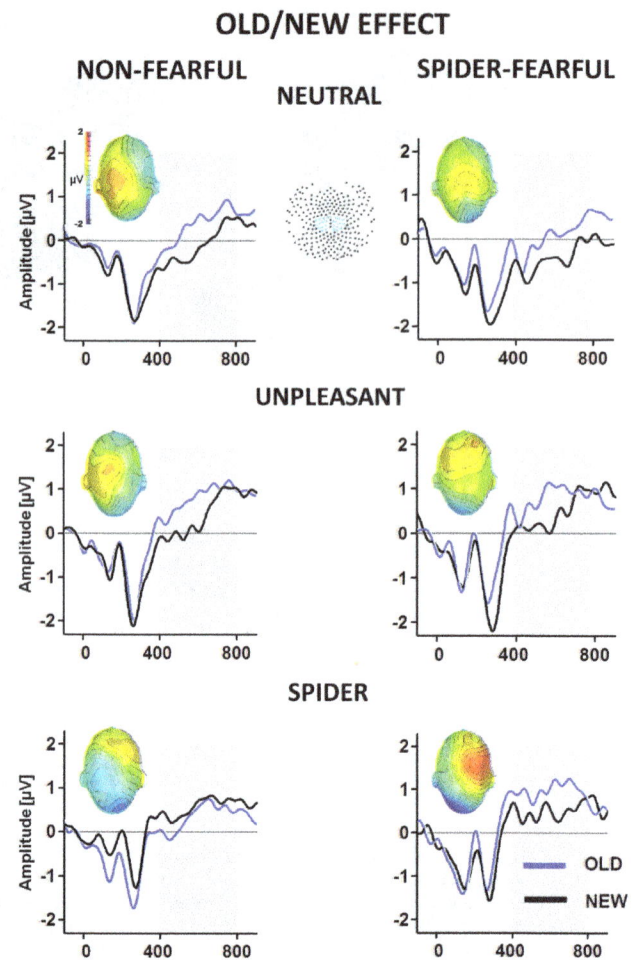

Figure 2. ERP old/new effect in non-fearful and spider-fearful individuals exposed to pictures of naturalistic scenes. The Figure highlights ERP waveforms averaged across centro-parietal channel cluster (see inlet) elicited by correctly classified old and new neutral, unpleasant and spider pictures as well as topographical difference maps (old minus new) displayed for non-fearful control (left) and spider-fearful individuals (right). Shaded areas mark the time interval 400–800 ms selected for the analysis of the ERP old/new effect.

durations of spider pictures in spider-fearful than control individuals, t (28) = 2.2, $p < .05$, and no group differences in the viewing time for the two other picture categories, ts (28) < 1.3, ns.

Memory performance. Table 1 shows the memory performance data (hits, false alarms, discrimination index, response bias and mean confidence ratings) as a function of picture category and group. As expected, hit rates varied as a function of Picture Category, F (1.274, 56) = 49.03, $p < .001$, $\eta 2 = .64$. Replicating previous findings, unpleasant pictures were better remembered than neutral pictures, F (1, 28) = 8.35, $p < .01$, $\eta 2 = .23$. Unpleasant, F (1, 28) = 66.98, $p < .001$, $\eta 2 = .71$, but also neutral pictures, F (1, 28) = 40.66, $p < .001$, $\eta 2 = .59$, were better recognized than pictures depicting spiders. Hit rates did not differ between groups, Picture Category × Group, F (1.274, 56) < 1, ns. Statistical analyses calculated for false alarms rates resulted in significant effect of Picture Category, F (1.539, 56) = 34.70, $p < .001$, $\eta 2 = .55$, and the interaction Group × Picture Category showed a trend towards significance, F (1.539, 56) = 3.29, $p = .059$, $\eta 2 = .11$. False alarms rates were lower for unpleasant when compared to neutral pictures, F (1, 28) = 39.26, $p < .001$, $\eta 2 = .58$, an effect that did not differ between both groups, Picture Category×Group, F (1, 28)< 1, ns. Moreover, there were significantly higher false alarms rates for spider than for unpleasant pictures, F (1, 28) = 54.02, p<.001, $\eta 2$ = .66, and neutral pictures, F (1, 28) = 13.40, p<.01, $\eta 2$ = .32. The <u>discrimination index</u> also differed as a function of Picture Category, F (1.363, 56) = 116.46, p<.001, $\eta 2$ = .81. Better discrimination was observed for unpleasant than neutral and spider pictures, F (1, 28) = 60.77, p<.001, $\eta 2$ = .68, and F (1, 28) = 172.04, p<.001, $\eta 2$ = .86, respectively. Moreover, the discriminability was significantly poorer for spider when compared to neutral pictures, F (1, 28) = 78.17, p<.001, $\eta 2$ = .74. Overall ANOVAs did not show differences in the <u>response bias</u> between the three different picture categories, F (1.795, 56) = 1.73, <u>ns</u>. Although discrimination index Pr was higher and response bias Br was more conservative for spiders in spider-fearful participants (see Table 1), Pr and Br did not differ as a function of Group, Fs (1, 28)<1.3, <u>ns</u>, or Picture Category×Group, F (1.363, 28) = 1.07, <u>ns</u> and F (1.795, 28) = .62, <u>ns</u> for Pr and Br, respectively.

Confidence ratings

Overall, the analyses of confidence ratings calculated for correctly remembered old and correctly rejected new pictures demonstrated significant effects of Picture Category, F (2, 56) = 70.74, p<.001, $\eta 2$ = .72, and Picture Category×Group, F (2, 56) = 7.74, p<.01, $\eta 2$ = .22. Unpleasant pictures received higher confidence ratings than neutral and spider pictures, Picture Category, Fs (1, 28) = 83.31, p<001, $\eta 2$ = .75. and F (1, 28) = 90.53, p<.001, $\eta 2$ = .76, respectively. Moreover, neutral pictures were also remembered with higher confidence than spider pictures, Picture Category, F (1, 28) = 42.25, p<.001, $\eta 2$ = .60. Importantly, confidence ratings were higher for correctly recognized spider pictures in the spider fear than the control group, Group, F (1, 28) = 5.20, p<.05, $\eta 2$ = .16, see Table 1. No group effects were found for the other stimulus materials Fs (1, 28)<1, <u>ns</u>.

Event Related Potentials

The ERP waveforms are displayed in Figure 2. Replicating previous studies, correctly recognized old pictures elicited overall more positive ERP amplitudes over centro-parietal scalp areas than correctly rejected new pictures, Memory, F (1, 28) = 22.29, p<.001, $\eta 2$ = .44, Memory×Picture Category, F (1.634, 56) = 1.50, p = .23, $\eta 2$ = .05, Memory×Picture Category×Group, F (1.634, 56) = 2.18, p = .13, $\eta 2$ = .07. For unpleasant and neutral

pictures this significant old/new difference, Memory, Fs (1, 28)≥ 5.5, ps<.05 did not differ between both groups, Memory×Group, Fs (1, 28)<1, <u>ns</u>. In contrast, analyses performed for spider pictures revealed significant differences in the ERP old/new effect between the spider fear and the control group, Memory×Group, F (1, 28) = 7.0, p<.05, $\eta 2$ = .20. Post-hoc tests showed that old spider pictures prompted an enhanced positivity compared to new pictures in spider-fearful participants, F (1, 14) = 5.01, p<.05, $\eta 2$ = .26, but not in controls, F (1, 14) = 1.99, p = .18, $\eta 2$ = .12 (see also bottom panel in Figure 2). Although number of hits and correct rejections were lowest for spider pictures, there were enough trials (average: 16) for this picture category that could be included in waveform analysis. Based on previous studies we also tested for early frontal ERP old/new differences [26] in a 300 to 500 ms time window. We found a significant difference between correctly classified old when compared to new pictures, Memory, F (1, 28) = 11.2, p<.01. However, this early frontally located old/ new difference was not modulated by picture content and did not differ between both experimental groups.

Replicating previous ERP studies [1], [49], the P1 was overall more pronounced in spider-fearful than control individuals, Group, F (1, 28) = 4.0, p = 0.5, $\eta 2$ = .13, Picture Category×Group F (1.848, 56)<1, ns. Moreover, as in earlier studies [1], [33], [35], an increased EPN and LPP was found when viewing unpleasant and spider pictures, compared to neutral material, Picture Category, F (1.408, 56) = 14.50, p<.001, $\eta 2$ = .34 and Picture Category F (1.634, 56) = 22.76, p<.001, $\eta 2$ = .45, for the EPN and LPP, respectively. The effects of an enhanced EPN and LPP for spider when compared to neutral pictures were significantly more pronounced in spider fearful when compared to control participants, Picture Category×Group, F (1, 28) = 23.35, p<.001, $\eta 2$ = 0.44 and Picture Category×Group, F (1, 28) = 6.65, p<.05, $\eta 2$ = 19, for the EPN and LPP, respectively. Unpleasant and neutral picture comparisons did not reveal any significant group differences, Fs (1, 28)<1, <u>ns</u>. When calculated for each single picture category the EPN and LPP did not differ as a function of group, Fs (1, 28)<1, ns.

Discussion

In the present study we used behavioral and electrophysiological measures to investigate long-term recognition memory for unpleasant, neutral and spider pictures in individuals with spider

Table 1. Behavioral data.

	H	FA	Pr	Br	Confidence (Old)	Confidence (New)
Unpleasant						
Control	.93 (.07)	.05 (.06)	.88 (.09)	.45 (.41)	9.4 (.57)	8.8 (.73)
Spider Fear	.94 (.07)	.06 (.08)	.88 (.09)	.54 (.38)	9.4 (.65)	8.9 (.72)
Neutral						
Control	.89 (.10)	.13 (.08)	.76 (.11)	.57 (.32)	9.0 (.77)	7.5 (1.10)
Spider Fear	.90 (.08)	.14 (.12)	.76 (.13)	.60 (.30)	9.1 (.84)	7.9 (1.45)
Spider						
Control	.69 (.16)	.26 (.14)	.43 (.17)	.46 (.22)	7.2 (1.33)	6.0 (2.10)
Spider Fear	.68 (.20)	.18 (.07)	.50 (.16)	.40 (.20)	8.1 (1.19)	7.6 (1.49)

<u>Note</u>: Mean hit rates (H), false alarm rates (FA), discrimination index (Pr) and response bias (Br) in percentages and confidence ratings (0 – not confident, 10 – absolutely confident) for each picture category and experimental group. Numbers in parentheses represent SD.

fear and non-fearful controls. Replicating previous findings, we found enhanced recognition memory performance accompanied with better confidence ratings for unpleasant when compared to neutral pictures [8], [9], [10], [50]. Memory performance for these materials did not differ between both groups. In the ERPs, enhanced positivity was found for remembered "old" when compared to correctly classified "new" pictures [23], [26]. This ERP old/new effect was observed over centro-parietal scalp areas during the 400–800 ms time interval, indicating recollection-based recognition. Contrary to our expectations, the ERP old-new difference did not differ between neutral and unpleasant pictures as in earlier studies using long retention intervals (e.g., [10], [44], [51]). This lack of interaction was due to the strong old/new effect observed for neutral pictures and not due to a weak old/new effect for unpleasant pictures, both effects are strong and statistically significant. Methodological reasons might account for this deviant pattern of results. In contrast to earlier studies [10], [44], [51], in which pictures were only presented once during encoding, pictures were shown for multiple times in the present study, probably facilitating ERP old-new differences [52], particularly for neutral stimuli. Moreover, a number of neutral pictures were presented in blocks that did not include unpleasant (or spider) pictures. Recent studies found that memory for neutral pictures is better when presented in pure blocks than mixed with emotional stimuli (e.g., [53–56]), indicating that neutral pictures in pure blocks may allocate more attentional resources for a detailed analysis than in mixed blocks, resulting in elaborate internal representations and a more pronounced ERP old/new effect for these cues.

One major aim of the current study was to investigate whether we would find different behavioral and/or electrophysiological memory effects for the phobia-relevant material in low and high fear volunteers. In general, our findings indicate that spider pictures were recognized with lower accuracy and confidence in memory than pictures depicting unpleasant and neutral scenes. This seems to be surprising because pictures of spiders are generally more emotional (more arousing and unpleasant) than neutral pictures as indicated by stimulus ratings and electrocortical responses (e.g., [1]) and thus should be better remembered than neutral pictures. On the other hand, given that different spider pictures comprise a very homogenous category where individual exemplars of the category share very similar features, item-similarity between old and new stimuli might have impaired memory performance because spider photographs were perceptually harder to differentiate, even though they included different kinds of spiders displayed with different positions and backgrounds. The poorer discrimination index and the lower confidence ratings for this picture category are in line with this interpretation. Memory accuracy for spider pictures, however, tended to be higher and false alarms were significantly lower in individuals with high spider fear compared to the non-fearful control groups, suggesting that memory performance for these stimuli was better in spider-fearful individuals than in controls. Moreover, participants with spider fear were significantly more confident in their memory decisions for spider pictures than controls indicating a fear-related memory bias. Mirroring this behavioral pattern, significant centro-parietal ERP old-new differences in response to spider pictures were only observed in spider-fearful, but not in control individuals. Because the centro-parietal old-new effect is assumed to reflect recognition memory based on recollection of rich contextual details of the learned event [26], [44], our ERP finding indicates that fear-relevant material was better recollected in spider fearful participants than controls.

Enhanced recollection for fear-relevant material observed in individuals with spider fear when compared to the control group is probably initiated already during the encoding and storage. In fact, the extraction of meaning during the elaborated stimulus processing is supposed to lead to the formation of inter-item associations and enhanced memory consolidation [57–59]. Indeed, multiple studies found [1], [33], [34], [35], [60], [61] facilitated processing of fear-related stimuli in individuals with elevated specific fears, as revealed by early and late ERP differences, an effect that was suggested to reflect a state of enhanced attention to feared stimulus materials Such prioritized stimulus processing was also evident during picture viewing at recognition in our study. Enhanced perceptual processing of phobia-related stimuli was also reported in several functional neuroimaging studies showing increased activations in the lateral occipital, posterior parietal, and inferior temporal cortex in specific phobic volunteers during processing of their feared pictures relative to neutral materials [62–65]. Confirming the assumption that the facilitated perceptual stimulus processing may be regulated by limbic structures, individuals with small animal phobia also exhibited increased amygdala and insula activations during their feared picture encoding [42], [62], [65], [66–69]. A recent PET study performed by Ahs and collaborators [11] demonstrated that these phobic stimuli that prompted stronger amygdala and parahippocampal activations were correlated with better memory for feared stimuli.

In sum, our results indicate that fear-relevant stimuli may be deeply encoded and easily recollected in spider-fearful individuals. Previous studies indicate that the exposure to a phobic stimulus is associated with increased retrieval of fear memories and unpleasant post-event recollection, which results in an enhanced fear response [70]. Unfortunately, these processes might strengthen the phobic response maintaining or even aggravating anxiety symptomatology. Moreover, resulting in an increased avoidance and reinforcing negative beliefs these processes might hinder recovery and interfere with exposure during treatment [16]. Reducing stimulus associated memory retrieval might have potentially beneficial effects on extinction-based psychotherapy. In this context, recent studies focused on promising retrieval-impairing effects of stress and glucocorticoids [71–72]. In addition, acute stress induced shortly before extinction was demonstrated to reduce expectancy ratings during the retrieval test that was performed on a subsequent day [73]. This suggests that glucocorticoids might facilitate the consolidation of extinction memory, which may also enhance extinction-based treatment programs [71], [74], [75].

Taken together, the present data indicate enhanced memory processing for phobia-relevant materials in spider-fearful participants. Moreover, we also found that spider-fearful individuals allocate more attentional resources for evaluative processing of phobia-relevant pictures than non-anxious controls. Future research may consider focusing on the relationship between fear memory retrieval, extinction memory and symptom reduction in the course of treatment as well as in the post-treatment phase.

Acknowledgments

We are grateful to Max Hübner for his help with data collection and to Christiane A. Pané-Farré for her personal support.

Author Contributions

Conceived and designed the experiments: JMM MW AOH. Performed the experiments: JMM. Analyzed the data: JMM MW. Contributed reagents/ materials/analysis tools: JMM MW AOH. Wrote the paper: JMM MW AOH.

References

1. Michalowski JM, Melzig CA, Weike AI, Stockburger J, Schupp HT, et al. (2009) Brain dynamics in spider-phobic individuals exposed to phobia-relevant and other emotional stimuli. Emotion 9(3): 306–315.

2. Weymar M, Gerdes ABM, Löw A, Alpers GW, Hamm AO (2013) Early enhanced attention, selection and inhibition in specific fear. Psychophysiology 50: 139–148.

3. Hamm A, Cuthbert BN, Globisch J, Vaitl D (1997) Fear and the startle reflex: Blink modulation and autonomic response patterns in animal and mutilation fearful subjects. Psychophysiology 34: 97–107.

4. Dolan RJ (2002) Emotion, cognition, and behavior. Science 298: 1191–1194.

5. McGaugh JL (2004) The amygdale modulates the consolidation of memories of emotionally arousing experiences. Ann Rev Neurosci 27: 1–28.

6. LaBar KS, Cabeza R (2006) Cognitive neuroscience of emotional memory. Nature Neurosci Rev 7: 54–64.

7. Bradley MM, Greenwald MK, Petry MC, Lang PJ (1992) Remembering pictures: Pleasure and arousal in memory. J Exp Psychol [Learn Mem Cogn] 18: 379–390.

8. Dolcos F, LaBar KS, Cabeza R (2005) Remembering one year later: Role of the amygdala and medial temporal lobe memory system in retrieving emotional memories. P Natl Acad Sci USA 102: 2626–2631.

9. Ochsner KN (2000) Are affective events richly recollected or simply familiar? The experience and process of recognizing feelings past. J Exp Psychol [General] 129(2): 242–261.

10. Weymar M, Löw A, Melzig CA, Hamm AO (2009) Enhanced long-term recollection for emotional pictures: Evidence from high-density ERPs. Psychophysiology 46: 1200–1207.

11. Ahs F, Palmquist AM, Pissiota A, Appel L, Franz O, et al. (2011) Arousal modulation of memory and amygdala-parahippocampal connectivity: a PET-psychophysiology study in specific phobia. Psychophysiology 48(11): 1463–1469.

12. Kulas JF, Conger JC, Smolin JM (2003) The effects of emotion on memory: An investigation of attentional bias. J Anxiety Disord 17: 103–113.

13. Thorpe SJ, Salkovskis PM (2000) Recall and Recognition Memory for Spider Information. J Anxiety Disord 14 (4): 359–375.

14. Watts FN, Dalgleish T (1991) Memory for phobia-related words in spider phobics. Cognition Emotion 5: 313–329.

15. Watts FN, Trezise L, Sharrock R (1986) Processing of phobic stimuli. British Journal of Clin Psychol 25: 253–259.

16. Williams JMG, Watts FN, MacLeod C, Mathews A (1997) Cognitive psychology and emotional disorders. Chichester, UK: Wiley.

17. Pflugshaupt T, Mosimann UP, Schmitt WJ, von Wartburg R, Wurtz P, et al. (2007) To look or not to look at threat? Scanpath differences within a group of spider phobics. J Anxiety Disord 21: 353–366.

18. Tolin DF, Lohr JM, Lee TC Sawchuk CN (1999) Visual avoidance in specific phobia. Behav Rest Ther 37: 63–70.

19. Quevedo J, Sant'Anna MK, Madruga M, Lovato I, de Paris F, et al. (2003) Differential effects of emotional arousal in short- and long-term memory in healthy adults. Neurobiol Learn Mem 79(2): 132–135.

20. Sharot T, Phelps EA (2004) How arousal modulates memory: Dientangling the effects of attention and retention. CABN 3: 294–306.

21. Sharot T, Yonelinas AP (2008) Differential time-dependent effects of emotion on recollective experience and memory for contextual information. Cognition 106: 538–547.

22. Keil A (2006) Macroscopic brain dynamics during verbal and pictorial processing of affective stimuli. Prog Brain Res 156: 217–232.

23. Weymar M, Hamm AO (2013) Electrophysiological signature of emotional memories. In: Linden M, Rutkowski K, editors. Hunting memories and beneficial forgetting. Elsevier Insights. pp. 21–35.

24. Voss JL, Paller KA (2008) Brain substrates of implicit and explicit memory: The importance of concurrently acquired neural signals of both memory types. Neuropsychologia 16: 3021–3029.

25. Rugg MD, Allan K (2000) Event-related potential studies of memory. In: Tulving GE, Craik FIM, editors. The Oxford Handbook of Memory. Oxford, UK: Oxford University Press. pp. 521–537.

26. Rugg MD, Curran T (2007) Event-related potentials and recognition memory. Trends Cogn Sci 11(6): 251–257.

27. Curran T (2000) Brain potentials of recollection and familiarity. Mem Cognition 28: 923–938.

28. Friedman D, Johnson RJ (2000) Event-related potential (ERP) studies of memory encoding and retrieval: A selective review. Microsc Res Tech 51: 6–28.

29. Mecklinger A (2000) Interfacing mind and brain: A neurocognitive model of recognition memory. Psychophysiology 37: 565–582.

30. Dietrich DE, Waller C, Johannes S, Wieringa B, Emrich HM, et al. (2001) Differential effects of emotional content on: event-related potentials in word recognition memory. Neuropsychobiology 43: 96–101.

31. Inaba M, Nomura M, Ohira H (2005) Neural evidence of effects of emotional valence on word recognition. Int J Psychophys 57: 165–173.

32. Johansson M, Mecklinger A, Treese AC (2004) Recognition memory for emotional and neutral faces: An event-related potential study. J Cogn Neurosci 16: 1840–1853.

33. Kolassa IT, Musial F, Mohr A, Trippe RH, Miltner WHR (2005) Electrophysiological correlates of threat processing in spider phobics. Psychophysiology 42: 520–530.

34. Leutgeb V, Schäfer A, Schienle A (2009) An event-related potential study on exposure therapy for patients suffering from spider phobia. Biol Psychol 82: 293–300.

35. Miltner WHR, Trippe RH, Krieschel S, Gutberlet I, Hecht H, et al. (2005) Event-related brain potentials and affective responses to threat in spider/snake-phobic and non-phobic subjects. Internat J Psychophysiol 57: 43–52.

36. Hamm AO (2006). Spezifische Phobien. Göttingen: Hogrefe.

37. Spielberger CD, Gorssuch RL, Lushene PR, Vagg PR, Jacobs GA (1983) Manual for the Trait-State Anxiety Inventory. Consulting Psychologists Press, Inc.

38. Lang PJ, Bradley MM, Cuthbert BN (2008) International Affective Picture System (IAPS):Affective ratings of pictures and instruction manual. (Tech. Rep. No. A-8). Gainesville, FL: University of Florida.

39. Hamm A, Cuthbert BN, Globisch J, Vaitl D (1997) Fear and the startle reflex: Blink modulation and autonomic response patterns in animal and mutilation fearful subjects. Psychophysiology 34: 97–107.

40. Globisch J, Hamm A, Esteves F, Öhman A (1999) Fear appears fast: Temporal course of startle reflex potentiation in animal fearful subjects. Psychophysiology 36: 66–75.

41. Michalowski JM, Pané-Farré CA, Löw A, Hamm AO (2012) Modulation of the ERP repetition effects during exposure to phobia-relevant and other affective pictures in spider phobia. Internat J Psychophysiol 85: 55–61.

42. Wendt J, Lotze M, Weike AI, Hosten N, Hamm AO (2008) Brain activation and defensive response mobilization during sustained exposure to phobia-related and other affective pictures in spider phobia. Psychophysiology 45: 205–215.

43. Bradley MM, Lang PJ (1994) Measuring emotion: The Self-Assessment Manikin and the semantic differential. J Behav Ther Exp Psychiatry 25: 49–59.

44. Weymar M, Löw A, Hamm AO (2011) Emotional Memories are Resilient to Time: Evidence from the Parietal ERP Old/New Effect. Hum Brain Mapp 32(4): 632–640.

45. Junghöfer M, Elbert T, Tucker D, Rockstroh B (2000) Statistical control of artifacts in dense array EEG/MEG studies. Psychophysiology 37: 523–532.

46. Schloegl A, Keinrath C, Zimmermann D, Scherer R, Leeb R, et al. (2007) A fully automated correction method of EOG artifacts in EEG recordings. Clin Neurophysiol 118(1): 98–104.

47. Snodgrass JG, Corwin J (1988) Pragmatics of measuring recognition memory: applications to dementia and amnesia. J Exp Psychol [General] 117(1): 34–50.

48. Schupp HT, Junghöfer M, Weike AI, Hamm AO (2003) Attention and emotion: An ERP analysis of facilitated emotional stimulus processing. Neuroreport 14: 1107–1110.

49. Kolassa IT, Musial F, Kolassa S, Miltner WHR (2006) Event-related potentials when identifying or color-naming threatening schematic stimuli in spider phobic and non-phobic individuals. BMC Psychiatry 6: 38.

50. Sharot T, Delgado MR, Phelps EA, (2004) How emotion enhances the feeling of remembering. Neuroscience 7(12): 1376–1380.

51. Schaefer A, Pottage CL, Rickart AJ (2011) Electrophysiological memories of remembering emotional pictures. Neuroimage 54: 714–724.

52. Ferrari V, Bradley MM, Codispoti M, Karlsson M, Lang PJ (2012) Repetition and brain potentials when recognizing neutral scenes: task and emotion differences. Soc Cogn Affect Neurosci 8(8): 847–854. doi:10.1093/scan/nss081.

53. Dewhurst SA, Parry LA (2000) Emotionality, distinctiveness, and recollective experience. Eur J Cogn Psychol 12: 541–551.

54. Grühn D, Scheibe S, Baltes PB (2007) Reduced negativity effect in older adults' memory for emotional pictures: The heterogeneity-homogeneity list paradigm. Psychol Aging 22(3): 644–649.

55. Hadley CB, MacKay DG (2006) Does emotion help or hinder immediate memory? Arousal versus priority-binding mechanisms. J Exp Psychol [Learn Mem Cogn] 32(1): 79–88.

56. Watts S, Buratto LG, Brotherhood EV, Barnacle GE, Schaefer A (2014) The neural fate of neutral information in emotion-enhanced memory. Psychophysiology 51(7): 673–84.

57. Cowan N (1995) Attention and memory: An integrated framework. New York, NY: Oxford University Press.

58. Craik FIM, Lockhart R (1972) Levels of processing: A framework for memory research. J Verb Learn Verb Beh 11: 671–684.

59. Craik FIM, Tulving E (1975) Depth of processing and the retention of words in episodic memory. J Mem Lang 27: 23–39.

60. Mühlberger A, Wiedemann G, Hermann MJ, Pauli P (2006) Phylo- and ontogenetic fears and the expectation of danger: differences between spider- and flight-phobic-students in cognitive and physiological responses to disorder specific stimuli. J of Abnorm Psychol 115: 580–589.

61. Weymar M, Keil A, Hamm AO (2013) Timing the fearful brain: Hypervigilance and spatial attention in early visual perception. Soc Cogn Affect Neurosci 9(5): 723–729.

62. Dilger S, Straube T, Mentzel HJ, Fitzek C, Reichenbach HR, et al. (2003) Brain activation to phobia-related pictures in spider phobic humans: an event-related functional magnetic resonance imaging study. Neurosci Lett 348: 29–32.

63. Fredrikson M, Wik G, Annas P, Ericson K, Stone-Erlander S (1995) Functional neuroanatomy of visually elicited simple phobic fear: Additional data and theoretical analysis. Psychophysiology 32: 43–48.

64. Paquette V, Lévesque J, Mensour B, Leroux JM, Beaudoin G, et al. (2003) Change the mind and you change the brain: Effects of cognitive-behavioral therapy on the neural correlates of spider phobia. NeuroImage 18: 401–409.

65. Sabatinelli D, Bradley MM, Fitzsimmons JR, Lang PJ (2005) Parallel amygdala and inferotemporal activation reflect emotional intensity and fear relevance. NeuroImage 24: 1265–1270.

66. Carlsson K, Petersson KM, Lundquist D, Karlsson A, Ingvar M, et al. (2004) Fear and the amygdala: Manipulation of awarness generates differential cerebral responses to phobic and fear-relevant (but nonfeared) stimuli. Emotion 4: 340–353.

67. Fredrikson M, Furmark T (2003) Amygdaloid regional cerebral blood flow and subjective fear during symptom provocation in anxiety disorders. Ann NY Acad Sci 985: 341–347.

68. Schienle A, Schäfer A, Walter B, Stark R, Vaitl D (2005) Elevated disgust sensitivity in blood phobia. Cognition Emotion 19: 1229–1241.

69. Straube T, Mentzel HJ, Miltner WHR (2006) Neural mechanisms of automatic and direct processing of phobogenic stimuli in specific phobia. Biol Psychiat 59: 162–170.

70. Cuthbert BN, Lang PJ, Strauss C, Drobes D, Patrick CJ, et al. (2003) The physiology of anxiety disorder: fear memory imagery. Psychophysiology 40(3): 407–422.

71. de Quervain DJ, Bentz D, Michael T, Bolt OC, Wiederhold BK, et al. (2011) Glucocorticoids enhance extinction-based psychotherapy. P Natl Acad Sci USA 108: 6621–6625. doi: 10.1073/pnas.10118214108.

72. Kuhlmann S, Piel M, Wolf OT (2005) Impaired memory retrieval after psychosocial stress in healthy young men. J Neurosci 25: 2977–2982. doi:10.1523/JNEUROSCI.5139-04.2005.

73. Bentz D, Michael T, Wilhelm FH, Hartmann FR, Kunz S, et al. (2013) Influence of stress on fear memory processin an aversive differential conditioning paradigm in humans. Psychoneuroendocrino 38: 1186–1197. doi: 10.1016/j.psyneuen.2012.12.018.

74. Bentz D, Michael T, de Quervain DJ, Wilhelm FH (2010) Enhancing exposure therapy for anxiety disorders with glucocorticoids: from basic mechanisms of emotional learning to clinical applications. J Anxiety Disord 24: 223–230. doi: 10.1016/j.janxdis.2009.10.011.

75. Soravia LM, Heinrichs M, Aerni A, Maroni C, Schielling G, et al. (2006) Glucocorticoids reduce phobic fear in humans. P Natl Acad Sci USA 103: 5585–5590. doi: 10.1073/pnas.0509184103.

14

Like or Dislike? Affective Preference Modulates Neural Response to Others' Gains and Losses

Yang Wang[1,2,9], **Chen Qu**[2,9], **Qiuling Luo**[1], **Lulu Qu**[1], **Xuebing Li**[3*]

1 School of Psychology, Center for the Study of Applied Psychology, South China Normal University, Guangzhou, China, **2** Department of Psychology, The Chinese University of Hong Kong, Hong Kong, S.A.R., China, **3** Key Laboratory of Mental Health, Institute of Psychology, Chinese Academy of Sciences, Beijing, China

Abstract

Previous studies have demonstrated that the brain responds differentially to others' gains and losses relative to one's own, moderated by social context factors such as competition and interpersonal relationships. In the current study, we tested the hypothesis that the neural response to others' outcomes could be modulated by a short-term induced affective preference. We engaged 17 men and 18 women in a social-exchange game, in which two confederates played fairly or unfairly. Both men and women rated the fair player as likable and the unfair players as unlikable. Afterwards, ERPs were recorded while participants observed each confederate playing a gambling game individually. This study examines feedback related negativity (FRN), an ERP component sensitive to negative feedback. ANOVA showed a significant interaction in which females but not males displayed stronger FRNs when observing likable players' outcomes compared to unlikable ones'. However, males did not respond differently under either circumstance. These findings suggest that, at least in females, the neural response is influenced by a short-term induced affective preference.

Editor: Marin Pavlova, University of Tuebingen Medical School, Germany

Funding: This work was supported by: the National Nature Science Foundation of China (Grant No. 31000504, 30930031, 30900441: http://www.nsfc.gov.cn/publish/portal0/default.htm); Humanities and Social Sciences project, Ministry of Education of China (Grant No. 09YJXLX008); Humanities and Social Sciences project, Ministry of Education of China (Grant No. 09YJXLX008: http://xm.sinoss.net/indexAction!to_index.action); Guangdong Philosophy social science planning youth project (Grant No. 09SXLQ002: http://www.gdpplgopss.gov.cn/); and the Key Laboratory of Mental Health of Institute of Psychology of Chinese Academy of Sciences. The funders had no role in study design, data collection and analysis, decision to publish, or preparation of the manuscript.

Competing Interests: The authors have declared that no competing interests exist.

* Email: lixb@psych.ac.cn

⑨ These authors contributed equally to this work.

Introduction

Although committing an error or receiving a negative feedback is generally considered to be an unpleasant event, it is crucial for learning and for adjusting future behavior. Converging evidence implies that FRN (feedback-related negativity), an ERP component generated from the anterior cingulate cortex (ACC), is generally more pronounced for negative outcomes of our own performances. The FRN peaks approximately 200-300 ms after feedback onset, and is related to the learning of information that can guide subsequent behaviors [1–4]. As social creatures, humans learn not only from their own experiences but also by observing others' behaviors during social interactions [5]. A growing number of studies have demonstrated that observing another's monetary loss elicits an FRN effect that is similar, both in morphology and scalp distribution, to a loss that is directly experienced, a pattern commonly referred to as oFRN (observational-FRN)[5–7]. This phenomenon implies that the neural process underlying "learning by observation" resembles the process underlying "learning by doing". This similarity allows us to avoid negative results that are potentially dangerous without having to experience them directly.

By manipulating the relationship between an observer and another person, previous studies suggested that the oFRN might be driven by two processes. First, one may evaluate the observer's outcome from an egocentric perspective when one's own benefit is involved. For example, the research in which an observer and a performer were in competition so that the observer lost when the performer won and vice versa, showed that the oFRN in response to wins of the performer was similar to that in response to losses of the observer[8,9]. Even participating in one's own separate gambling game alongside the observational task could affect feelings about others. Leng and Zhou (2010) explored the differing neural responses to friends and strangers when the observer was engaged in the same gambling game, and failed to find a differentiation of FRN responses between friend and stranger observations. This finding was interpreted as shown that participation itself might draw their attention from other's performance to their own benefit, potentially diminishing the expected differences in neural response toward friends versus strangers[10].

Second, an observer may evaluate a performer's outcome empathically and emotionally when it has no consequence for the self. Modulation of the oFRN occurs when the observer's outcomes are unrelated to the performer's, and the existence of a long-term relationship has been found to modulate the magnitude of oFRN when self-involvement is not a factor in the experiment. Ma and colleagues removed the observer's own gambling from the experimental design, so that participants only observed and evaluated the outcomes of friends versus strangers. Once the observers' egocentric focus on their own results was no longer a factor, there was a larger oFRN effect associated with friends' outcomes than with strangers' [11]. It seems like that the greater the self-benefit is involved, the more that egocentrism and cognitive evaluation reduce the emotional response toward others' results. The less self-benefit is involved, the more emotion influences the oFRN.

However, the design that does not include participation in the same gambling game cannot exclude personal involvement as an influence on oFRN. It also could be argued that it is the potential benefits gained from the success of the other person in a long-term relationship that results in the differentiation seen in the oFRN phase. For example, a friend might pay for drinks after winning a game. Therefore,it is unclear whether the stronger response to friends' losses and gains is due to the social context or to this potential personal benefits.

Another possible interpretation of the larger oFRN in response to friends' outcomes is that one may generally attend more to friends than to strangers because of higher familiarity. The purpose of the present study was to investigate the degree to which the oFRN is moderated by affective preference when controlling for potential benefit and familiarity. A variation on the trust game was used to establish a short-term affective preference for two strangers [12]. In the game, one confederate was fair and generous, while the other was unfair and selfish, leading to varying affective preferences on the part of the participant. Then, the two confederates played a gambling game individually while the participant observed. Event-related potentials (ERPs) were recorded during the observation phase. This paradigm allowed us to explore how a learned affective preference influences neural responses toward liked and disliked strangers. It was expected that the learned affective preference would result in a larger oFRN toward the likable player than toward the unlikable one.

Gender differences were also examined in the current study. Although females are better at recognizing emotions and at expressing themselves emotionally, males show greater responses when presented with threatening emotions such as fear, anger and dominance (see a review, [13]). For example, females tend to be sensitive to both positive (happy) and negative (angry) emotions, but males are primarily sensitive to the negative one (i.e., angry) [14]. This pattern might be due to sex differences in hormones, chromosomes, and brain structures [13]. Besides gender differences in the emotion expression and recognition, females often have a stronger empathic responses than males and score higher on self-reported empathy [15]. When accessing others' emotions females showed increased activation in the right inferior frontal cortex while there is no differential activations in males. Females also recruit areas of the human mirror system, which has been claimed to be related to the capacity for empathy, to a higher degree than males during both self assessing and other assessing tasks [16]. Furthermore, from an evolutionary perspective, males might benefit more than females from competition. For example, the copulation frequency of male elephant seals during breeding seasons is related directly to success in male-male competition. Low competitive males that reached maturity are prevented from mating by the highest ranking males[17]. There is also evidence that in humans, an intergroup conflict has profound effects on males in particular compared with females [18,19].

Considering the fact that females showed stronger emotion sensitivity and empathy responses compared to males, it might be easier for them to distinguish the results of fair players and unfair players, whereas males might be especially more sensitive to unfair players only, and might even use an egocentric evaluation path to process unfair players' results, and present a reversed oFRN pattern. This hypothesis is further supported by Singer and colleges' findings that women showed more empathy toward fair versus unfair players' pain, whereas men's reward region was activated even when they faced unfair players' losses[12]. Thus, we predict that compared to women, men would show stronger sensitivity to unfair players' results.

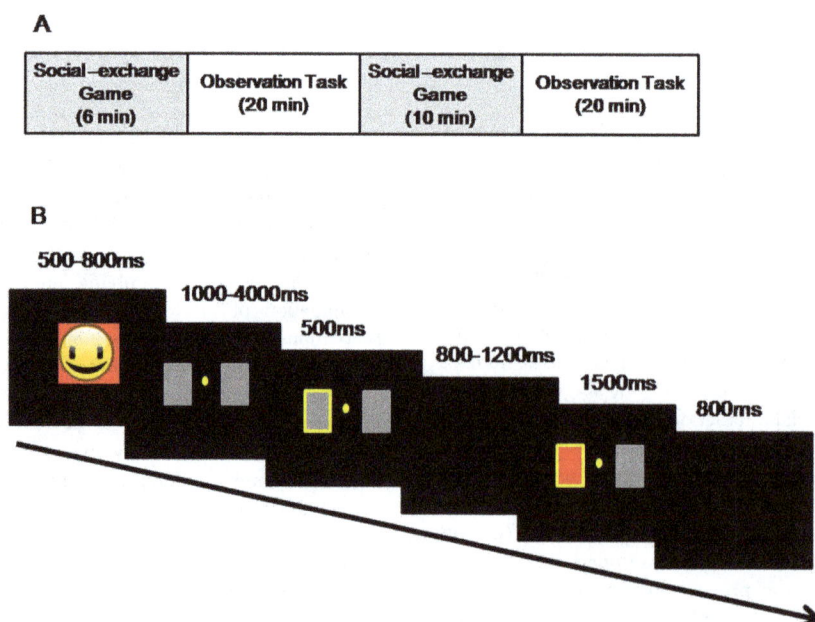

Figure 1. (A) Schematic representation of the experimental procedure. The study included two independent experiments. One experiment was a social exchange game and the other one was an observation task. Each experiment consisted of two blocks which were alternated, and the study ended with a behavioral assessment. (B) Observation task: overview. (The vectogram for the human face used here is provided for illustration, photographs of human faces were used in the study.)

Methods

The study was approved by the Ethics Committee of the department of Psychology at South China Normal University. Written informed consents were obtained from participants, and they had the right to discontinue participation at any time.

Forty participants (20 male and 20 female) aged 19–25 years (Mean = 22 years, SD = 2.1 years) were recruited from South China Normal University, China. Five participants (three male and two female) were excluded from ERP data analysis, one because one fell asleep during the experiment and the other four because they correctly identified the other two "participants" as confederates. All participants had normal or corrected-to-normal vision and no history of neurobiological or psychiatric disorders. Participants were paid 30 yuan (about $4.50) for their participation.

Procedure

Participants sat in an electrically shielded room about 1 m away from and in front of a 17-inch CRT while their EEG was recorded simultaneously. They were told that two other students were sitting in different rooms and would play games with them. There would be three separate games: one was related to "social exchange", one was an "observational-learning task", and one was related to "grouping-social exchange" in which participants would be able to invite one co-player to form a team to compete against the other team. Participants did not actually play the third game which was mentioned only to assure participants that they were playing with real people rather than a computer program.

Each of the two games was divided into two sections. The experiment started with one section of the social exchange game, followed by two sections of the observational learning task which was interspersed by a second section of the social exchange game. At the end of the experiment, participants completed a behavioral assessment, see Fig. 1(A). They were then fully debriefed about the aims and methods of the study. Participation in the entire study took around one hour and thirty minutes.

Social-exchange game

We used a revised trust game, which has also been adopted in previous studies to induce participants' feeling of like and dislike towards strangers[12,20]. In the traditional trust game, subject A could choose any amount of money from zero to ten dollars, to send to subject B. The amount of money would be tripled by the time it reached subject B. Subject B would then decide how much of the tripled money to keep and how much to send back to the sender [20]. In the current study, each experimental group was composed of one participant and two same-gender strangers. The participant always had the first move and was given the choice of "trusting" the confederate by sending 10 starting points or "mistrusting" by keeping the points. According to the game rules, points sent would be tripled. A confederate who received these 30 points reciprocated by sending between 0 and 10 points back, which were also tripled. The fair player reciprocated with large amounts, whereas the unfair player reciprocated with small amounts.

Photos of the two confederates and the participant, taken before the experiment, were used in a computer program to remind participants whose turn it was and to make the setup more convincing. The photos had backgrounds with different colors: blue for participants, red for one confederate, and green for the other (counterbalanced across participants). The same colors were displayed on playing cards in the observation task so that participants could easily distinguish between likable and unlikable confederates easily.

Observational-learning task

Following the exchange game, participants were informed that the two participants they played with would then play a gambling game individually in which they would win money or lose money from their original payment. To maintain their attention, participants were asked to count the number of losses or gains in each block.

The observation task consisted of 240 trials: 120 games played by the unfair confederate and 120 by the fair confederate. The 240 trials were split into 12 blocks of 20 trials, each performed by one confederate. The gambling task was adapted from Gehring and Willoughby's (2002) classic task, illustrated in Fig. 1(B). In the original task, the participant was asked to choose from two squares, each of which contained the number 5 or 25. After the choice, each square turned red or green indicating whether the participant lost or won such amount of money[21]. In the current study, each trial began with the participant's photo ($3.5° \times 5°$) against a black background for 500–800 ms. Two gray squares then appeared, laid out horizontally, for 1000–4000 ms. Each subtended $1.6° \times 1.6°$, and the visual angle between the centers of the two squares was 3 degrees. The player whose turn it was selected one card with a key press, pressing the 'F' key for the left card or 'J' for the right card. The chosen card was then highlighted with a yellow border for 500 ms. After another 800–1200 ms interval, the background of the performer's chosen card turned the color displayed in his/her social-exchange game, with a '+' or '−' on it to show whether he/she gained or lost on that trial. The inter-stimulus interval was 800 ms.

Electrophysiological recordings

EEGs were recorded from 32 scalp sites using tin electrodes mounted in an elastic cap (Brainproducts, Munich, Germany) with the reference on the left mastoid. Eye blinks were monitored with electrodes located in four places: above and below the right eye and 1.5 cm lateral to the left and right external canthi. All electrode recordings were referenced to an electrode placed on the left mastoid, and electrode impedances were kept below 5 k Ohm for all recordings. Off-line analysis was performed using Brain Vision Analyzer software (Brainproducts). The electrophysiological signals were filtered with a bandpass of 0.01–100 Hz and digitized at a rate of 500 Hz. Trials with amplitudes of more than $\pm$ 100 uV in EEG voltages were excluded from further analysis. EEG data were digitally filtered below 30 Hz (24 dB/Octave) and re-referenced offline to linked mastoid electrodes. ERPs time locked to feedback (gains and losses) were averaged for epochs of 1000 ms, using a 200 ms pre-feedback baseline.

The ERP components analyzed in this study include the FRN and P300. For the purpose of statistical analysis, we selected two electrodes, Fz and FCz, in the anterior frontal midline area for FRN, because the FRN effect was largest at these electrodes, and they had been commonly found to produce large FRN effects in previous studies[22–25].

A 2 (gain vs. loss) by 2 (likable vs. unlikable) by 2 (female vs. male) repeated-measures ANOVA on the peak latencies of FRN found only a significant gender difference, $F(1, 33) = 9.099$, $p = .005$, $\eta 2 = .216$, in which males displayed a shorter peak FRN latency (266.89 ± 7.70 ms) than did females (299.28 ± 7.49 ms). Other main and interaction effects were all non-significant ($p > .05$). Based on this, we chose a different time window for FRN in analyses on females and males. FRN was defined as the mean

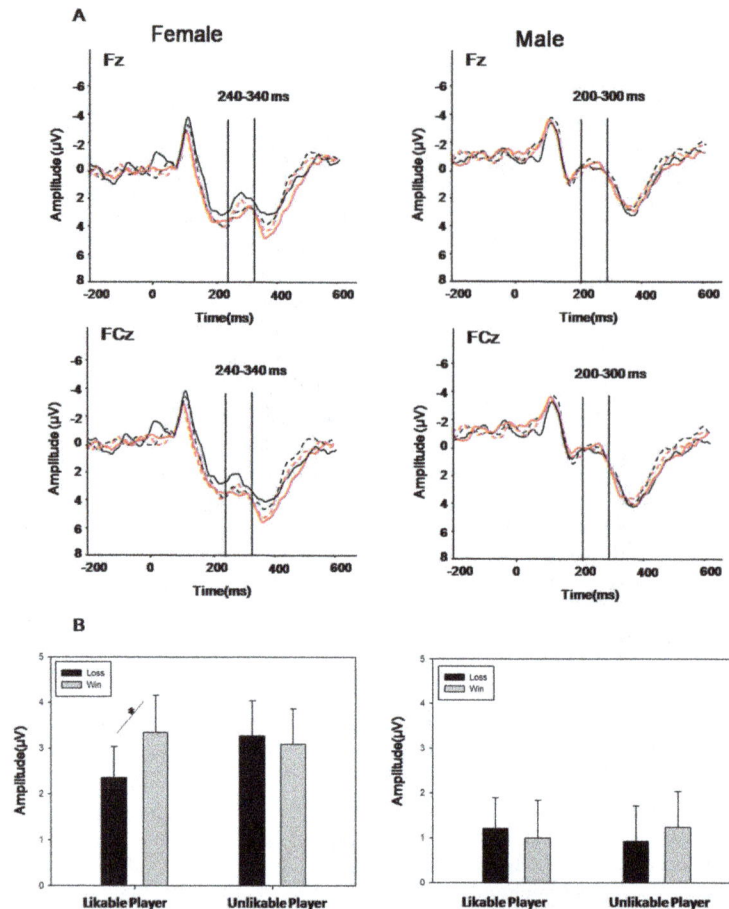

Figure 2. The ERP grand-average waveforms and the amplitudes of the FRN. (A) The grand-averaged ERP waveforms aligned at the onset of feedback stimuli for likable and unlikable players' performance (recorded for Fz and FCz sites). The left panel shows data from females, and the right panel shows data for males. (B) FRN response to win and loss outcomes of likable and unlikable players based on gender.

amplitude of the outcome distributed on the anterior scalp at 240–340 ms for females and at 200–300 ms for males.

Results

Rating-task results

To check whether the affective-preference manipulation worked, participants performed a likeability trait rating task at the end of the experiment using a 7-point Likert scale ranging from -3 (unlikable) to 3 (ikable). There was a significant difference between perceptions of the two strangers ($F(1, 33) = 194.15, p < .01$, $\eta^2 = .885$), indicating a preference for the fair player (Mean = 2.51, $SD = 0.13$) over the unfair one (Mean $= -1.14$, $SD = 1.22$). No significant gender difference was found ($F < 1$).

ERP results

Fig. 2(A) shows the event-related potentials for gains and losses at Fz, based on likeability and gender. The analysis of mean FRN amplitudes with four factors (agency, valence, gender, electrode) revealed only one significant interaction effect a three-way interaction among agency, valence and gender ($F(1, 33) = 4.60$, $p = 0.039$, $\eta^2 = .12$), indicating that the FRN was influenced by both affective preference and gender. No other significant main effect or interaction effects were found. Follow-up simple-effects analysis showed that, for women, the main effect of valence was

significant when observing likable players' outcomes ($F(1, 33) = 4.42$, $p = .043$, $\eta^2 = .535$), whereas the comparison between unlikable players' loses and gains was not significant ($F(1, 33) = 0.37$, $p = .574$). Mean ERP amplitudes were significantly more negative in response to the likable players' losses ($2.354 \pm 0.677 \mu V$) than to their wins ($3.27 \pm 0.768 \mu V$) in females ($F(1,33) = 4.42$, $p = 0.043$). Female participants also showed more negative mean ERP amplitudes in response to the likable players' losses ($2.354 \pm 0.677 \mu V$) than to those of the unlikable player ($3.343 \pm 0.813 \mu V$) ($F(1, 33) = 5.92$, $p = 0.021$, $\eta^2 = .551$, See Fig. 2(B). However, for men, the main effect of valence was not significant when neither observing likable players' performance (p = .538) nor unlikable players' performance (p = .592).

Discussion

Previous researches on the FRN effect under observation conditions have focused on manipulating the relationship between self and others by taking advantage of long-term friendships or by using a benefit-related competition situation. The present study, using trust game and gambling game, extends this work by examining the gender difference in how the short-term social interaction induces affective preference modulation in oFRN. The results suggest a gender-based difference in rapidly processing others' losses and gains. For females, the likable performers' losses elicited larger oFRN than did those of unlikable performers.

Although males rated the fair player as more likable, they did not display significantly different responses toward the two performers. The results imply an existence of emotional and empathic explanation of oFRN.

The female having generally sensitive neural response for distinguishing likable from unlikable strangers is concordant with previous studies and implies an empathetic and emotional account of oFRN. It has been reported that female participants categorized a friend's loss as equivalently negative to their own even in a competitive situation[26]. The dual-processes hypothesis suggests that the other person's status as a personal acquaintance might have enhanced females' empathic responses, overriding the egocentric evaluative component for female participants[9]. In addition, empathy might be the cause of observational FRN[9-11,26]. In the previous studies, the size of the FRN effect varied as a function of whether an action was performed by a friend or by a stranger[11]. In another study, females showed a smaller empathic response toward unfair players' pain[12]. In the present study, the greater FRN responses for the likable player in the observation condition, similar to responses induced by feedback information concerning the observer's own results, under the observation condition may be related to a stronger empathic response toward the likable player. When observing the unlikable players' results, the observer's reduced empathic response might result in a non-significant FRN effect. These results might also be supported by Wilson's selection theory in which the units of evolution is group instead of individual, and highly cooperative groups have an evolutionary advantage over poorly cooperative groups [27]. People tend to cooperate with in-group members whereas they compete with out-group members to benefit themselves. From this perspective, the human tribal inclination has evolved to help humans categorize individuals based on their group membership, and treat in-group members benevolently and out-group members malevolently[19]. The likable player in our study might be considered as an in-group member while the unlikable player might be treated as an out group member. Thus, we observed a disassociation between the responses to these two members.

Crucially, the current study revealed a gender effect in which females responded differently toward likable versus unlikable performers, whereas males did not. This inconsistent response toward two strangers suggests that, in females, not only long-term relationships but also the affective link established through short-term social interaction can affect early neural responses to the consequences of actions unrelated to one's own interests. We suggest that this phenomenan is caused by different empathic responses in females from that in males. The gender-based differences in empathy have been widely reported. Using self-report questionnaires, females showed superiority in empathy in the general population and even among persons with Asperger Syndrome(AS)/high-functioning autism(HFA) [15]. Using voxel-based morphometry analysis, concurrent with the dispositional empathy measures, researchers also found that young adult females had significantly larger gray matter volume locatged in the mirror-neuron system, which is highly related in empathy

ability[28]. Females showed earlier and stronger brain processing of the action's purpose in the females brain compared with males in an ERP study[29]. Females were also more accurate when their feelings of the target[30].

Gender-based differences in emotion sensitivity and interpersonal sensitivity might also be a reason for the gender differences were found in the current study. Females often perform better in various emotional tasks than males. Studies focused on sex differences in facial expression processing found that female advantage in decoding of emotional cues both in adults and children[31].Consistently, females displayed superior performance in affective arousal and expression of emotion over males. For instance, increased corrugator activity for angry faces and increased zygomatic activity for happy faces were more pronounced for females compared to males[32]. Unpleasant and high arousing stimuli also evoked stronger N100 and N200 in females compared to males[33].

In addition, Singer and her coworkers found that males expressed a desire for revenge when observing players who had just betrayed them by administering pain[12]. However, males' hypothesized reversed responses toward unfair player did not occur in our study. It is possible that males did not process the information. This explanation might be supported by the shorter latency of oFRN in males compared with that in females. Females' automatic response toward others may lead to a longer latency in which to make sure that they could separate the likable player and unlikable one, whereas the males, who finished the evaluation phrase in a shorter time, could not finish an precise evaluation. Males' weaker empathic/emotional response and lower level of social sensitivity might not allow them to separate their representations of the two strangers within a few hundred million seconds. Finally, from an evolutionary perspective, males should show stronger sensitivity to unfair players' results, but our results were not completely in line with the evolutionary hypothesis. However, the rapid evaluation failure does not mean it will not work in the long run. Using more extreme targets (people one hates), the revenge effect on oFRN might be possible.

By manipulating observers' affective preferences toward different performers through trust games and by removing the effect of self-benefit, the present study found that females displayed a stronger FRN effect when observing likable players' outcomes compared to unlikable players' and a stronger P300 response toward unlikable ones; males did not display any difference in their responses toward the two strangers. These findings suggest that, at least in females, outcome evaluation can be affected by short-term affective preference even when the person being observed is a total stranger.

Author Contributions

Conceived and designed the experiments: YW CQ XbL. Performed the experiments: YW QL LQ. Analyzed the data: YW. Wrote the paper: YW CQ XbL.

References

1. Falkenstein M, Hohnsbein J, Hoormann J, Blanke L (1991) Effects of crossmodal divided attention on late ERP components. II. Error processing in choice reaction tasks. Electroencephalogr Clin Neurophysiol 78(6): 447–455.
2. Gehring WJ, Willoughby AR (2002) The medial frontal cortex and the rapid processing of monetary gains and losses. Science 295(5563): 2279–2282.
3. Nieuwenhuis S, Holroyd CB, Mol N, Coles MG (2004) Reinforcement-related brain potentials from medial frontal cortex: origins and functional significance. Neurosci Biobehav Rev 28(4): 441–448.
4. Nieuwenhuis S, Yeung N, Holroyd CB, Schurger A (2004) Sensitivity of electrophysiological activity from medial frontal cortex to utilitarian and performance feedback. Cereb Cortex 14(7): 741–747.
5. Frey SH, Gerry VE (2006) Modulation of neural activity during observational learning of actions and their sequential orders. J Neurosci 26(51): 13194–13201.
6. Fukushima H, Hiraki K (2009) Whose loss is it? Human electrophysiological correlates of non-self reward processing. Soc Neurosci 4(3): 261–275.
7. Yu RJ, Zhou XL (2006) Brain responses to outcomes of one's own and other's performance in a gambling task. Neuroreport 17(16): 1747–1751.

8. Itagaki S, Katayama J (2008) Self-relevant criteria determine the evaluation of outcomes induced by others. Neuroreport 19(3): 383–387.

9. Marco-Pallares J, Kramer UM, Strehl S, Schroder A, Munte TF (2010) When decisions of others matter to me: an electrophysiological analysis. Bmc Neuroscience 11: 86

10. Leng Y, Zhou XL (2010) Modulation of the brain activity in outcome evaluation by interpersonal relationship: An ERP study. Neuropsychologia 48(2): 448–455.

11. Ma QG, Shen QA, Xu Q, Li DD, Shu LC, et al. (2011) Empathic responses to others' gains and losses: An electrophysiological investigation. Neuroimage 54(3): 2472–2480.

12. Singer T, Seymour B, O'Doherty JP, Stephan KE, Dolan RJ, et al. (2006) Empathic neural responses are modulated by the perceived fairness of others. Nature 439(7075): 466–469.

13. Kret ME, De Gelder B (2012) A review on sex differences in processing emotional signals. Neuropsychologia 50(7): 1211–21.

14. Biele C, Grabowska A (2006) Sex differences in perception of emotion intensity in dynamic and static facial expressions. Exp Brain Res 171(1): 1–6.

15. Baron-Cohen S, Wheelwright S (2004) The empathy quotient: An investigation of adults with Asperger syndrome or high functioning autism, and normal sex differences. J Autism Dev Disord 34(2): 163–175.

16. Schulte-Ruther M, Markowitsch HJ, Shah NJ, Fink GR, Piefke M (2008) Gender differences in brain networks supporting empathy. Neuroimage: 42(1): 393–403.

17. Leboeuf BJ (1974) Male-Male Competition and Reproductive Success in Elephant Seals. Amer Zool 14(1): 163–176.

18. Van Vugt MD, De Cremer, Janssen DP (2007) Gender differences in cooperation and competition - The male-warrior hypothesis. Psychol Sci 18(1): 19–23.

19. Van Vugt M (2009) Sex Differences in Intergroup Competition, Aggression, and Warfare The Male Warrior Hypothesis. Values, Empathy, and Fairness across Social Barriers 1167: 124–134.

20. Berg J, Dickhaut J, Mccabe K (1995) Trust, Reciprocity, and Social-History. Games and Economic Behavior 10(1): 122–142.

21. Gehring WJ, Willoughby AR (2002) The medial frontal cortex and the rapid processing of monetary gains and losses. Science 295(5563): 2279–2282.

22. Cohen MX, Ranganath C (2007) Reinforcement learning signals predict future decisions. Journal Neurosci 27(2): 371–378.

23. Zhou Z, Yu R, Zhou X (2010) To do or not to do? Action enlarges the FRN and P300 effects in outcome evaluation. Neuropsychologia 48(12): 3606–3613.

24. Hajcak G, Moser JS, Holroyd CB, Simons RF (2006) The feedback-related negativity reflects the binary evaluation of good versus bad outcomes. Biol Psychol 71(2): 148–154.

25. Holroyd CB, Hajcak G, Larsen JT (2006) The good, the bad and the neutral: electrophysiological responses to feedback stimuli. Brain Res 1105(1): 93–101.

26. Fukushima H, Hiraki K (2006) Perceiving an opponent's loss: gender-related differences in the medial-frontal negativity. Social Cognitive & Affective Neurosci 1(2): 149–157.

27. Nowak MA, Tarnita CE, Wilson EO (2010) The evolution of eusociality. Nature 466(7310): 1057–1062.

28. Cheng Y, Chou KH, Decety J, Chen IY, Hung D (2009) Sex differences in the neuroanatomy of human mirror-neuron system: a voxel-based morphometric investigation. Neuroscience 158(2): 713–720.

29. Proverbio AM, Riva F, Zani A (2010) When neurons do not mirror the agent's intentions: Sex differences in neural coding of goal-directed actions. Neuropsychologia 48(5) 1454–1463.

30. Klein KJ, Hodges SD (2001) Gender differences, motivation, and empathic accuracy: When it pays to understand. Personality and Social Psychology Bulletin 27(6): 720–730.

31. McClure EB (2000) A meta-analytic review of sex differences in facial expression processing and their development in infants, children, and adolescents. Psychol Bull 126(3): 424–453.

32. Dimberg U, Lundquist LO (1990) Gender differences in facial reactions to facial expressions. Biol Psychol 30(2): 151–159.

33. Lithari C, Frantzidis CA, Papadelis C, Vivas AB, Klados MA (2010) Are females more responsive to emotional stimuli? A neurophysiological study across arousal and valence dimensions. Brain Topogr 23(1): 27–40.

15

Revealing a Brain Network Endophenotype in Families with Idiopathic Generalised Epilepsy

Fahmida A. Chowdhury[1,2$\P$], **Wessel Woldman**[3$\P$], **Thomas H. B. FitzGerald**[1,4], **Robert D. C. Elwes**[2], **Lina Nashef**[2], **John R. Terry**[3‡], **Mark P. Richardson**[1,2*‡]

1 Institute of Psychiatry, Psychology and Neuroscience, King's College London, London, United Kingdom, **2** Centre for Epilepsy, King's College Hospital, London, United Kingdom, **3** College of Engineering, Mathematics and Physical Sciences, University of Exeter, Exeter, United Kingdom, **4** Wellcome Trust Centre for Neuroimaging, UCL, London, United Kingdom

Abstract

Idiopathic generalised epilepsy (IGE) has a genetic basis. The mechanism of seizure expression is not fully known, but is assumed to involve large-scale brain networks. We hypothesised that abnormal brain network properties would be detected using EEG in patients with IGE, and would be manifest as a familial endophenotype in their unaffected first-degree relatives. We studied 117 participants: 35 patients with IGE, 42 unaffected first-degree relatives, and 40 normal controls, using scalp EEG. Graph theory was used to describe brain network topology in five frequency bands for each subject. Frequency bands were chosen based on a published Spectral Factor Analysis study which demonstrated these bands to be optimally robust and independent. Groups were compared, using Bonferroni correction to account for nonindependent measures and multiple groups. Degree distribution variance was greater in patients and relatives than controls in the 6–9 Hz band ($p = 0.0005$, $p = 0.0009$ respectively). Mean degree was greater in patients than healthy controls in the 6–9 Hz band ($p = 0.0064$). Clustering coefficient was higher in patients and relatives than controls in the 6–9 Hz band ($p = 0.0025$, $p = 0.0013$). Characteristic path length did not differ between groups. No differences were found between patients and unaffected relatives. These findings suggest brain network topology differs between patients with IGE and normal controls, and that some of these network measures show similar deviations in patients and in unaffected relatives who do not have epilepsy. This suggests brain network topology may be an inherited endophenotype of IGE, present in unaffected relatives who do not have epilepsy, as well as in affected patients. We propose that abnormal brain network topology may be an endophenotype of IGE, though not in itself sufficient to cause epilepsy.

Editor: Satoru Hayasaka, Wake Forest School of Medicine, United States of America

Funding: FAC was funded by a Clinical Research Training Fellowship from the Medical Research Council UK (G0701310, www.mrc.ac.uk). MPR was supported in part by the National Institute for Health Research Biomedical Research Centre at the South London and Maudsley NHS Foundation Trust (http://www.nihr.ac.uk/infrastructure/Pages/infrastructure_biomedical_research_centres.aspx). MPR and JRT are supported by a Medical Research Council UK Programme Grant (MR/K013998/1, www.mrc.ac.uk). The funders had no role in study design, data collection and analysis, decision to publish, or preparation of the manuscript.

Competing Interests: The authors have declared that no competing interests exist.

* Email: mark.richardson@kcl.ac.uk

$\P$ These authors contributed equally to this work.

¶ FAC and WW are first authors on this work.

‡ JRT and MPR also contributed equally to this work and are last authors on this work.

Introduction

Idiopathic generalised epilepsy (IGE) comprises a group of clinical syndromes which account for 15–20% of all epilepsies [1]. Although the classification scheme for the epilepsies is evolving, the concept of IGE remains robust, consisting of a set of epilepsy disorders characterised by specific well-recognised generalised seizure types. Although IGE may very rarely be a monogenic disorder in a few families [2], typically it has a complex inheritance suggesting susceptibility is associated with multiple genes [3].

Generalised spike-wave (GSW) seen in EEG is a hallmark of IGE, and reflects abnormal hypersynchronous electrical activity within brain networks. There is at present much interest concerning the structural and functional nature of brain networks in which seizures arise [4] and how these factors give rise to specific seizure types or epilepsy syndromes. The complexity of the brain makes it challenging to study, but a well-developed approach to characterising complex networks, graph theory, has recently had a substantial impact on the investigation of data relating to brain networks [5]. Graph theory enables local and global characteristics of network connectivity to be computed and compared between subjects. Brain networks can be inferred from EEG by examining the patterns of association between EEG signals (correlation, synchronisation etc), based on the ability of EEG to capture information about multiple brain sources of activity. It is assumed that neuronal activity in distributed brain networks is reflected in multiple sources of independent activity detectable in scalp EEG, and that examining interactions between the signals obtained by different EEG electrodes is a reasonable proxy for examining interactions between the underlying sources which constitute the brain network. Graph theory can be used to summarize structural topological features of brain networks; these structural properties may have a key influence on the dynamics which the network can generate [4]. Abnormality of brain dynamics is evident in epilepsy as the paroxysmal occurrence of seizures, therefore it is logical to propose that these abnormal dynamics may be dependent on abnormal network topology. The aim of this study is to use graph theory applied to EEG to explore the hypothesis that abnormal properties of brain networks are a component of the inherited phenotype in IGE.

Investigations of the complex genetics of brain disorder have in some instances made important progress through investigating endophenotypes, heritable traits with a simpler genetic basis than the full disorder, which may be present in family members who do not have the disease [6]. Measures of network topology have been suggested as potential endophenotypes [5]. It is noteworthy that some basic EEG-derived network metrics obtained using graph theory, particularly clustering coefficient and average path length, show high heritability in healthy subjects, especially in the alpha frequency band [7,8]. Studies of the maturation of brain networks in children [9] suggest that normal development is characterised by a gradual alteration of the balance between the strength of local connectivity, presumably reflecting cortical localisation of function, and the strength of long-range connections which presumably reflects the functional integration between localised regions required for normal brain function. From a graph theoretic perspective, this balance is reflected in the small-world index. Given that IGE may often have onset in childhood and remit with maturation, we specifically hypothesise that brain networks in people with IGE and their relatives will show altered network properties compared to healthy controls, and that this may have a basis in aberrant development.

Interpretation of EEG in a clinical setting typically uses five broad frequency bands defined according to prominent features visible to an expert observer. A recent literature has sought to establish the frequency bands in which EEG oscillatory activity is maximally independent, hypothesising that such maximally-independent bands may represent different neurobiological generators, and may be optimally sensitive to differences between subjects or experimental manipulations. Although the conventional clinical EEG frequency bands relate to qualitative features seen in the EEG, it is not necessarily the case that these conventional bands optimally reflect the underlying generators. Furthermore, given that brain network features in the alpha band may show evidence of heritability [7,8], and that antiepileptic drug treatment my alter peak alpha frequency [10], we particularly focus on the alpha range through dividing into sub-bands. Here, we adopt the frequency bands defined by Spectral Factor Analysis (SFA) in two independent datasets of resting EEG activity [11], in which these bands were shown to be extremely robust to a range of methods used to determine the bands, artefact rejection schemes and scalp electrode positions.

Materials and Methods

Recruitment and selection of participants

Subjects with IGE were identified from five hospitals in London and outlying regions, and were a consecutive series that met the inclusion and exclusion criteria and were able to participate. Inclusion criteria for patients were age>18 years old, a diagnosis of IGE, and ≥2 family members with epilepsy according to self-

report. Twenty-eight families were recruited; in 16 families the reported presence of epilepsy in more than one family member was confirmed by us from history and investigation; in the other 12 families, the reportedly affected family members were not available for assessment. In addition to the affected probands, clinically unaffected first degree relatives were recruited from the 28 families. These unaffected relatives were interviewed in detail by a neurologist (FAC) and had no evidence of symptomatic seizures from detailed history. Furthermore, in addition to the EEG study carried out as part of this investigation, all unaffected relatives underwent diagnostic MRI which was in all cases normal. Healthy participants with no personal or family history of neurological or psychiatric diseases were recruited via a local research participant database. Participants were excluded if they had any other neuropsychiatric condition or a full scale IQ (FSIQ) <70. Ethical approval was obtained from King's College Hospital Research Ethics Committee (08/H0808/157). Written informed consent was obtained from all participants. We recently reported the neuropsychometric findings in this cohort of patients, relatives and controls [12].

EEG acquisition

Conventional 10–20 scalp EEG was collected using a NicoletOne system (Viasys Healthcare, San Diego, California, USA), 19 channels, sampling rate 256 Hz, bandpass filtered 0.3–70 Hz. EEG was carried out using the same system in the same recording room, undertaken by the same EEG technologist using conventional measurement techniques to determine electrode positions. Collection of subjects from the different groups was interleaved over the duration of the study. Ten minutes of awake EEG in all participants and 40 minutes of sleep was obtained where possible. Where specific consent was obtained, hyperventilation and photic stimulation were carried out. Here we examined only the awake EEG.

Conventional expert EEG analysis

The EEGs were reviewed independently by two reviewers (FC and RE). The following features were noted: presence of GSW; focal abnormalities including spikes, sharp waves and slow waves; response to photic stimulation; and normal variants.

Quantitative EEG analysis

EEG data was referenced to the channel average. A single 20 s epoch was selected which included continuous dominant background rhythm with eyes closed, without any artefacts, epileptiform abnormalities or patterns indicating drowsiness or arousal. Epoch selection for analysis was carried out by one investigator (TF) who was blinded to subject group. These EEG epochs were used for all the subsequent analysis methods described below. Our analyses used 5 frequency bands defined from previous literature applying SFA to resting EEG: 1–5 Hz, 6–9 Hz, 10–11 Hz, 12–19 Hz and 21–70 Hz. Although different from the conventional clinical EEG frequency bands, the bands we used here were shown to be extremely robust to a range of methods used to identify the maximally independent bands, artefact rejection schemes and scalp electrode positions [11].

Analyses were performed using a combination of EEGlab toolbox [13], the Brain Connectivity Toolbox [14], in addition to our own custom Matlab (Mathworks, Natick, Massachusetts, USA) scripts for band-pass filtering the EEG data to optimise the rectangular drop-off at the boundary between frequency bands.

Construction of weighted undirected graphs

The Hilbert transform was applied to the band-pass filtered EEG to generate instantaneous phase and amplitude estimates. For each electrode pair and each frequency band, we calculated the phase-locking factor (PLF) [15], a value between 0 and 1 reflecting the strength of synchronous activity between each pair. We assumed that each electrode is represented by a vertex in a graph with edge strength between vertices determined by the relevant PLF. All PLF analyses were carried out using custom scripts implemented in Matlab (available from authors on request). Note that we therefore construct weighted graphs, with each edge taking the value of the corresponding PLF.

Degree distribution, clustering coefficient, characteristic path length

For each individual, we characterise the degree distribution by establishing the strength of each vertex through summing the PLF values associated with the edges connected to that vertex and then using the mean and variance of these vertex strengths, denoted by K and D respectively. The clustering coefficient C indexes the tendency of a network to form local clusters; the path length L is a measure of how well the nodes of the network are interconnected [16]. C and L are sensitive to changes in network degree distribution [16,17]. To control for this, we calculated normalised metrics $\hat{C} = \frac{C}{C^{surr}}$ and $\hat{L} = \frac{L}{L^{surr}}$ where C^{surr} and L^{surr} are the mean clustering coefficient and characteristic path length of a distribution of 500 surrogate random networks [16,17]. We calculated $\hat{C}$ and $\hat{L}$ for each subject for each frequency band network. All network topology analyses were carried out using the Brain Connectivity Toolbox [14].

Statistical testing

To explore differences in the proportions of each group showing qualitative EEG abnormalities we used a Chi-squared test with significance threshold of p = 0.05 two-tailed, Bonferroni-corrected for three between-group comparisons.

Prior to testing, all quantitative measures were tested for normality and a non-normal distribution was observed. Thus a non-parametric Kruskal-Wallis test was used to examine for effects in each measure across the three groups and five frequency bands; results were declared significant at p<0.05 two-tailed, Bonferroni corrected for five frequency bands. Where the Kruskall-Wallis test was significant, we investigated further using Mann-Whitney tests to compare between pairs of groups for each frequency band. Results were declared significant when p<0.05 after Bonferroni correction for three between-group comparisons.

Results

We studied 117 participants: 40 normal controls (20 female, mean age 30.7 yrs), 35 patients with IGE (21 female, mean age 34.4 yrs), and 42 unaffected first-degree relatives of patients with IGE (19 female, mean age 36.0 yrs). The age and gender distributions of the groups were not significantly different (all p> 0.05 uncorrected). Clinical details of the patients who participated in the study are presented in Table 1. Thirteen patients and 8 relatives refused photic stimulation because of the risk of provoking a seizure.

Qualitative Analysis

Patients were more likely to have generalised epileptiform discharges compared with relatives and controls (17/35 patients, 2/42 relatives, 0/40 controls; chi-squared with Fisher's exact test,

one-sided p<0.0001 Bonferroni corrected in both instances), but there was no significant difference in the proportion of relatives with generalised epileptiform discharges compared with normal controls (p = 0.27 uncorrected). There were no significant differences between any pair of groups in the proportions of subjects with focal discharges, positive photoparoxysmal response or normal variants.

Graph theoretic metrics (Figure 1, Table 2)

Mean degree (K) differed between the groups only in the 6–9 Hz band (Kruskall-Wallis p = 0.0064, Bonferroni corrected for five frequency bands). Subsequent comparison of group pairs revealed that K was higher in the patients than normal controls (Mann-Whitney p = 0.0008, Bonferroni corrected for three between-group comparisons); in relatives, K was higher than healthy controls and lower than patients but did not differ significantly from either group. Degree distribution variance (D) showed a difference between the three groups only in the 6–9 Hz band (p = 0.0005, Bonferroni corrected for five frequency bands). Examining paired comparisons between groups, D was higher in patients and relatives than in normals in this band (p = 0.0005 and p = 0.0009 respectively, Bonferroni corrected). Clustering coefficient ($\hat{C}$) differed between the three groups only in the 6–9 Hz band (p = 0.0018, Bonferroni corrected). $\hat{C}$ was greater in the patients and relatives than in normal controls (p = 0.0025 and p = 0.0013 respectively, both Bonferroni corrected). There were no differences between groups for $\hat{L}$. There were no other significant differences or trends between groups in any other frequency band, comparing controls, patients and relatives. In particular, there were no differences between patient and relative groups in any frequency band for any measure.

Discussion

In this study we show that brain network topology, as inferred from scalp EEG, differs between normal subjects and patients with IGE. Moreover, we show that brain network topology differs between normal subjects and unaffected first-degree relatives of people with IGE – and that unaffected relatives and patients have similar networks. Although it is conceivable that EEG network features in the patients may differ from normal subjects as a result of antiepileptic drug treatment, the unaffected relatives were not taking medication. We conclude that brain network topology may be a component of an inherited endophenotype of IGE, and not dependent on medication effects.

We have previously reviewed in detail the literature describing brain networks in epilepsy using a wide range of approaches, not only graph theory [18]. We are not aware of prior literature examining brain network data from unaffected relatives of patients with IGE; however there is a small published literature examining brain networks of patients with IGE, using graph theory methods, in comparison with normal controls. A small study examined interictal MEG in five adults with absence epilepsy and five matched controls [19]. Using coherence as the measure of interaction between channels, the authors found that average node strength, clustering coefficient, and global efficiency were all greater in patients than normal controls; these findings would be in keeping with ours. A group of 26 adults with IGE characterised by generalized tonic-clonic seizures was compared with 26 normal controls using fMRI and DTI [20]. The brain was parcellated into a large number of nodes, and connectivity between all pairs of nodes estimated from both datasets. The results were somewhat inconsistent between methods, but a decrease in small worldness and a decrease in clustering coefficient were found comparing

Table 1. Clinical characteristics of the patients.

Gender	Age	Syndrome	Age of onset (years)	Seizures and frequency	Time since last seizure	Medications (total daily dose mg)	EEG	MRI
M	26	GTCS	5	GTCS 1/month	2 weeks	Sodium Valproate 1600, Topiramate 200, Lamotrigine 100	GSW	Normal
M	25	GTCS	11	GTCS 3/month	3 weeks	Sodium Valproate 300	GSW	Normal
F	45	GTCS	2	SF	36 years	(none)	Normal	N/A
M	31	GTCS	8	GTCS 6/year	1 month	Sodium Valproate 2000, Zonisamide 250, Levetiracetam 500, Lamotrigine 100	GSW, Ph+	N/A
F	18	JAE	7	GTCS 1/month, Abs SF	1 week	Ethosuximide 250, Lamotrigine 600	GSW	Normal
F	20	GTCS	0.5	SF	9 years	(none)	Normal	N/A
M	49	GTCS	26	SF	1 year	(none)	GSW	Normal
F	21	JAE	10	SF	4 years	Lamotrigine 400, Ethosuximide 500	GSW	Normal
F	20	JME	13	MJ weekly, GTCS SF	1 week	Sodium Valproate 1000	GSW	Normal
M	59	JME	14	SF	10 years	(none)	GSW	N/A
F	19	GTCS	15	GTCS 4/year	3 months	Levetiracetam 2000	GSW	Normal
F	28	Unclassified	20	SF	7 years	Carbamazepine 200	Normal	Normal
F	23	CAE	8	SF	6 years	Sodium Valproate 800, Lamotrigine 25	GSW	Normal
M	48	JME	17	SF	5 years	Sodium Valproate 1500, Topiramate 200, Carbamazepine 600	GSW, PSW	N/A
F	32	CAE	4	GTCS SF, Abs weekly	1 weeks	(none)	GSW	N/A
M	30	Unclassified	11	SF	3 years	(none)	Normal	N/A
F	28	JME	15	SF	13 years	Sodium Valproate 1400	PSW	N/A
F	41	JME	11	GTCS rare, MJ weekly	1 week	Levetiracetam 1000, Lamotrigine 500, Zonisamide 200	GSW, PSW	N/A
M	45	CAE	3	SF	2 years	Sodium Valproate 1400, Levetiracetam 2000	GSW	N/A
M	31	Unclassified	8	SF	10 years	Sodium Valproate 400	Normal	Normal
M	27	Unclassified	16	SF	10 years	Carbamazepine 1200	Normal	N/A
F	39	GTCS	22	SF	10 years	Carbamazepine 200	GSW	Normal
M	28	CAE	4	SF	5 years	Sodium Valproate 600, Levetiracetam 750, Lamotrigine 250	GSW	N/A
F	18	JME	15	MJ SF, GTCS 1/month	4 months	Levetiracetam 1000	GSW	N/A
F	36	GTCS	21	GTCS 2/year	2 months	Levetiracetam 1750	GSW, Ph+	Normal
F	43	CAE	7	SF	10 years	(none)	GSW	N/A
M	28	GTCS	8	SF	1 year	Sodium Valproate 400	GSW	N/A
F	53	GTCS	3	GTCS SF, Abs daily	1 day	(none)	GSW, Ph+	Normal
F	33	JAE	12	GTCS 3/year	4 months	Topiramate 400	GSW, Ph+	Normal
F	55	GTCS	16	SF	25 years	(none)	Normal	N/A
M	26	CAE	5	SF	8 years	(none)	GSW	N/A
F	47	JAE	11	Abs daily, GTCS SF	1 day	Levetiracetam 2000	PSW	Normal
M	25	JME	14	GTCS 5/year, MJ weekly	1 week	Valproate	GSW	Normal
F	20	JME	15	MJ 2/month	2 weeks	Lamotrigine 400, Levetiracetam 1500	GSW	Normal
F	21	Absences with eyelid myoclonia	6	Abs daily, MJ weekly	1 day	Lamotrigine 500	PSW	N/A

CAE childhood absence epilepsy, GTCS generalised tonic clonic seizures only, JAE juvenile absence epilepsy, JME juvenile myoclonic epilepsy, MJ myoclonic jerks, Abs absences, Ph + Photosensitivity; GSW generalised spike and wave, PSW polyspike and wave; SF Seizure Free; N/a not available.

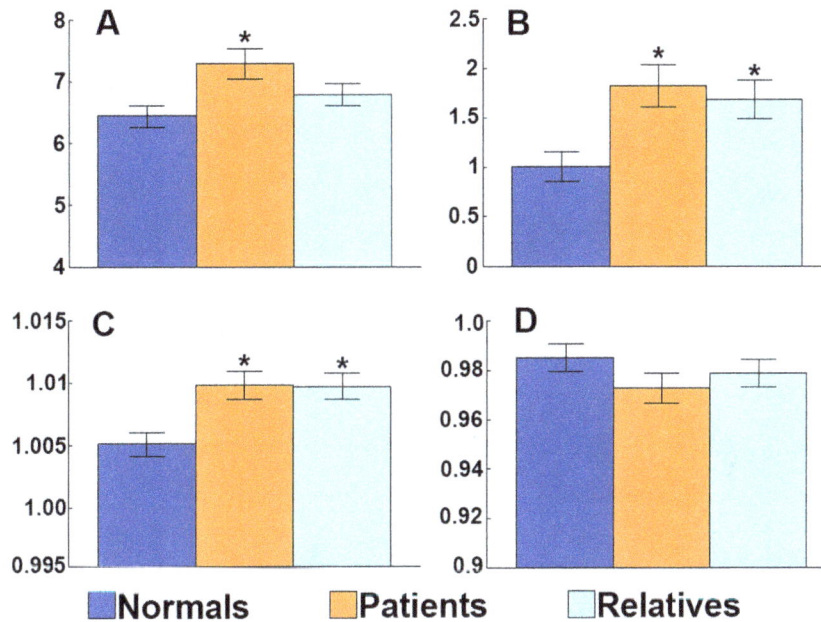

Figure 1. An abnormal EEG network topology is an endophenotype of IGE, present in patients and first-degree relatives. Group means +/− standard error of the mean are shown for: (A) mean degree K, (B) mean degree variance D, (C) clustering coefficient $\hat{C}$, and (D) normalised path length $\hat{L}$, in the 6–9 Hz band. Normal controls (dark blue), patients with IGE (orange), and first-degree relatives of patients with IGE (light blue). * = $p<0.05$ Bonferroni corrected compared with normal controls.

patients with normals. A further study also used DTI to compare brain networks in 18 children with childhood absence epilepsy with 18 matched normal controls [21]. This study found that the network connection strength, clustering coefficient, local efficiency and global efficiency were decreased in the patients, and the characteristic path length increased. Although some of these findings are contradictory to our findings and those of [19], at the current time, it is extremely difficult to reconcile results found with MRI methods with those found using EEG/MEG.

Animal models of childhood absence epilepsy (CAE) show abnormalities in a complex brain network comprising a combination of a focal cortical region which drives the onset of generalised seizure discharges in thalamocortical networks, and an abnormality of anterior transcallosal pathways [22,23]; this transcallosal abnormality has also been found in human juvenile myoclonic epilepsy (JME) [24], hence there is a justification to propose that large-scale brain network abnormalities are a feature of IGE. A large study of recent-onset IGE demonstrated 34–49% failed to achieve 12-month remission with first-line antiepileptic drugs [25], indicating an urgent need for better treatment based on improved mechanistic understanding of IGE. This improved understanding is likely to emerge from detailed phenotyping, genotyping, and the development of explanatory models. It seems likely that seizures emerge in large-scale brain networks through the interaction between brain network structure and the dynamics of the brain regions which constitute the network nodes [26]. We introduce the term "brain network ictogenicity" to describe the likelihood seizures will emerge from a brain network. In this study, we show that one contributor to brain network ictogenicity – network structure – is abnormal in IGE patients compared with healthy controls, and that a similar abnormality is observed in the unaffected relatives of the patients. We propose that our findings in the current study contribute to a more detailed phenotype of IGE and have implications for future genetic studies.

Fundamental to our approach is to identify a brain network endophenotype of IGE. An endophenotype is a heritable trait which is a component of a disorder or associated with high liability to develop the disorder. An endophenotype may be present in family members who do not have the disease, hence increasing the power of genetic studies, and its inheritance is likely to be simpler than the full disorder [6]. This concept has been extensively exploited in other common brain disorders with complex inheritance, such as schizophrenia [27]. Given the universal availability of EEG, and that GSW is a cardinal feature of IGE, EEG is an obvious place to look for an IGE endophenotype. It has been shown that 0.5% of unaffected adults and 1.8% of unaffected children under 16 yrs may show GSW [28,29]. Unaffected first-degree relatives of patients with IGE show a much higher prevalence of GSW: 8–40% of unaffected siblings under 16 yrs had GSW when awake and up to 72% when asleep [30,31]; but only 6–9% of unaffected siblings over 16 yrs had GSW [31,32]. Therefore GSW may be an endophenotype of limited usefulness in adults, since, if IGE is explained by complex inheritance, at least 50% of first-degree relatives of patients with IGE should share one or more genes contributing to the IGE phenotype.

Conventional expert EEG review of our subjects revealed GSW in 49% of patients, 5% of relatives and zero controls; these findings are expected, and suggest that our cohort is unexceptional. Finding GSW in some "unaffected" relatives might suggest the possibility that some relatives in fact have unsuspected epilepsy. Although we concede this is possible, our detailed assessment of the relatives did not reveal any evidence of symptomatic seizures in any of the unaffected relatives group; post hoc exclusion of the two relatives with GSW does not alter the effects found.

Measures of EEG network topology differed between groups, revealing strong similarities between brain networks of patients and first degree relatives. For networks inferred from EEG band-pass filtered in the 6–9 Hz band, both the mean degree and mean degree variance was lower in normals than either patients or

Table 2. Summary of effects found comparing three groups (normal controls, patients, relatives).

Measure	Comparison	1–5 Hz		6–9 Hz		10–11 Hz		12–19 Hz		21–70 Hz	
		Uncorr.	Bonferroni corrected	Uncorr.	Bonferroni corrected	Uncorr.	Bonferroni corrected	Uncorr.	Bonferroni corrected	Uncorr.	Bonferroni corrected
Mean degree	difference between groups	0.9513		0.0013	0.0064	0.9321		0.5501		0.5435	
Mean degree	normals vs patients			0.0003	0.0008						
Mean degree	normals vs relatives			0.0514							
Mean degree	relatives vs patients			0.0718							
Mean degree variance	difference between groups	0.8795		0.0001	0.0005	0.8533		0.6280		0.0441	0.2206.
Mean degree variance	normals vs patients			0.0002	0.0005						
Mean degree variance	normals vs relatives			0.0003	0.0009						
Mean degree variance	relatives vs patients			0.5947							
Clustering coefficient	difference between groups	0.9003		0.0004	0.0018	0.7291		0.5370		0.1315	
Clustering coefficient	normals vs patients			0.0008	0.0025						
Clustering coefficient	normals vs relatives			0.0004	0.0013						
Clustering coefficient	relatives vs patients			0.8780							
Characteristic path length	difference between groups	0.5920		0.0814		0.4343		0.3798		0.8177	
Characteristic path length	normals vs patients										
Characteristic path length	normals vs relatives										
Characteristic path length	relatives vs patients										

For details of Bonferroni correction see Methods. Uncorr = uncorrected.

relatives. This indicates that the variability in the number of connections per network node is greater in patients and relatives, revealing the existence of a brain network endophenotype characterised by both unusually overconnected brain regions (hubs) and underconnected brain regions.

Comparison of epilepsy patients taking antiepileptic drugs with unmedicated normal controls introduces the potential confound that effects found may be due to the drugs and not due to the disease. We cannot exclude this possibility in our study. However, the relatives were unmedicated, therefore the comparison of relatives with controls does not suffer this confound.

Our network analyses were carried out in "sensor space" – that is, networks were constructed which described the interactions between activities at the EEG electrodes, rather than the interactions between the brain sources which generated these activities. The limited spatial sampling of routine clinical EEG would not readily permit source reconstruction, but future studies should attempt to identify the origins of these network properties in the brain.

We chose to examine weighted graphs, in contrast to some studies (eg. [33]) which have examined unweighted graphs. An unweighted graph is produced by choosing a threshold for edge weight, and assigning the value of an edge as either zero or one according to this threshold. As has been discussed in detail elsewhere [34], there are limitations to either approach. One practical limitation in our data is that our networks have only 19 nodes, therefore the range of possible network degree is limited; the consequence of this is that defining an unweighted network using a high threshold (or low network degree) would have the consequence that many networks will fall apart into disconnected components and therefore could not be validly compared; whereas using a low threshold (or high network degree) would have the outcome that the networks would tend to be fully connected (ie. every possible edge is present) therefore there would be very limited possibility to identify any difference between networks. Given these limitations, we argue that using a weighted unthresholded approach is preferable. Furthermore, some studies have compared between groups the weights of individual edges; we chose here to examine global properties, but have also examined for differences in individual edge strength finding no differences that survived Bonferroni correction.

There is an inherent problem in work of this kind, which may be described as the problem of reducing bias due to common sources of EEG activity seen at more than one scalp electrode, and which encompasses both the selection of reference electrode and consideration of the effect of volume conduction in selection of the method to determine interaction between EEG timeseries. The problem of common sources is well-known and does not have a single optimal solution [35] [36] [37]. We chose here to use an average reference, and to use a measure of interaction between EEG timeseries, PLF, which detects synchronization at zero phase lag. Note that previous work shows this combination of measure and reference is able to detect real differences in synchronization [37]; we are currently examining alternative measures of synchronization which may be less sensitive to volume conduction.

An important consideration in any experimental work is whether results are reliable and can be reproduced. An important strength of our study is the sample size: we have 117 subjects, and detected very large effect sizes, which is a strong defence against error. However, an important question is whether results are stable if a different epoch of EEG data were chosen from each subject. The difficulty of identifying artefact-free EEG data epochs of 20 s from every subject should not be underestimated – EEG is highly prone to movement, blink and other artefacts – and we chose to identify artefact-free epochs rather than clean the data using artefact removal tools. Hence, we were not able to find more than one suitable epoch for every subject. Nonetheless, post hoc, we sought to examine the stability of our findings by dividing the single epoch from each subject into two equal non-overlapping epochs of half the length (which we labelled epoch 1 and epoch 2). We repeated an identical analysis for both epochs from all subjects: in the analysis of the full 20 s epoch, we report five pairwise comparisons that reached significance using Bonferroni correction; using epoch 1 for every subject, the same 5 comparisons remained significant; using the epoch 2, three of the five comparisons remained significant and two were at the level of strong trend (and were significant without Bonferroni correction). Furthermore, the comparison between patients and relatives of mean degree, degree distribution variance, and clustering coefficient revealed no differences using the full 20 s epoch, and also revealed no differences using either epoch 1 or epoch 2. Therefore, our findings are reproducible within two non-overlapping epochs of EEG data. Nonetheless, we recognise that the reliability of our findings needs to be established in an independent dataset.

It is not yet established whether individual syndromes of IGE are entirely unrelated, with no shared aetiologic, genetic or mechanistic factors, or represent a continuum or set of overlapping disorders with important shared pathophysiology. We recognise in this context a divergence of views between those who seek to identify individual syndromes on the basis of highly detailed phenotyping, and those who seek common aetiological and mechanistic factors across the range of common IGE syndromes, as we do here. In this study, we specifically seek shared factors between families and between different IGE syndromes, hypothesising that there are likely to be shared genetic and mechanistic factors between different IGE syndromes [38] [39,40]. We note this approach has been highly successful in recent genetic studies, which have identified recurrent chromosomal microdeletions as the most frequent identifiable genetic factor associated with all the common IGE syndromes studied here [41–43]. For example, the most frequently identified microdeletions each accounted for patients with at least three of the four common IGE syndromes included in our study here [42]: Microdeletions at 15q11.2 were identified in patients with JME, JAE, CAE and GTCS; microdeletions at16p13.11 were found in JME, CAE and GTCS; and microdeletions at 15q13.3 were found in JAE, JME and CAE. We argue that these genetic findings strongly support our argument that a similar brain network endophenotype might be found across the range of common IGE syndromes.

In summary, we show here for the first time the existence of a brain network endophenotype of IGE, present in relatives and patients. We propose that our findings have significant implications for the current mechanistic understanding of IGE, and for future phenotyping and genetics studies.

Acknowledgments

We are grateful for the expert assistance of Mrs Devyani Amin (Chief EEG Technician) and her team.

Author Contributions

Conceived and designed the experiments: FAC WW THBF RDCE LN JRT MPR. Performed the experiments: FAC. Analyzed the data: FAC WW THBF RDCE JRT. Contributed reagents/materials/analysis tools: RDCE LN JRT. Wrote the paper: FAC WW THBF RDCE LN JRT MPR.

References

1. Jallon P, Latour P (2005) Epidemiology of idiopathic generalized epilepsies. Epilepsia 46 Suppl 9: 10–14.
2. Helbig I, Scheffer IE, Mulley JC, Berkovic SF (2008) Navigating the channels and beyond: unravelling the genetics of the epilepsies. Lancet Neurol 7: 231–245.
3. Pal DK, Strug LJ, Greenberg DA (2008) Evaluating candidate genes in common epilepsies and the nature of evidence. Epilepsia 49: 386–392.
4. Richardson M (2010) Current themes in neuroimaging of epilepsy: brain networks, dynamic phenomena, and clinical relevance. Clin Neurophysiol 121: 1153–1175.
5. Bullmore E, Sporns O (2009) Complex brain networks: graph theoretical analysis of structural and functional systems. Nat Rev Neurosci 10: 186–198.
6. Gottesman II, Gould TD (2003) The endophenotype concept in psychiatry: etymology and strategic intentions. Am J Psychiatry 160: 636–645.
7. Smit DJ, Stam CJ, Posthuma D, Boomsma DI, de Geus EJ (2008) Heritability of "small-world" networks in the brain: a graph theoretical analysis of resting-state EEG functional connectivity. Hum Brain Mapp 29: 1368–1378.
8. Smit DJ, Boersma M, van Beijsterveldt CE, Posthuma D, Boomsma DI, et al. (2010) Endophenotypes in a dynamically connected brain. Behav Genet 40: 167–177.
9. Power JD, Fair DA, Schlaggar BL, Petersen SE (2010) The development of human functional brain networks. Neuron 67: 735–748.
10. Tuunainen A, Nousiainen U, Pilke A, Mervaala E, Partanen J, et al. (1995) Spectral EEG during short-term discontinuation of antiepileptic medication in partial epilepsy. Epilepsia 36: 817–823.
11. Shackman AJ, McMenamin BW, Maxwell JS, Greischar LL, Davidson RJ (2010) Identifying robust and sensitive frequency bands for interrogating neural oscillations. Neuroimage 51: 1319–1333.
12. Chowdhury FA, Elwes RDC, Koutroumanidis M, Morris RG, Nashef L, et al. (in press) Impaired cognitive function in IGE and unaffected family members: an epilepsy endophenotype. Epilepsia.
13. Delorme A, Makeig S (2004) EEGLAB: an open source toolbox for analysis of single-trial EEG dynamics including independent component analysis. J Neurosci Methods 134: 9–21.
14. Rubinov M, Sporns O (2010) Complex network measures of brain connectivity: uses and interpretations. Neuroimage 52: 1059–1069.
15. Tass P, Rosenblum MG, Weule J, Kurths J, Pikovsky A, et al. (1998) Detection of n:m phase locking from noisy data: application to magnetoencephalography. Phys Rev Lett 81: 3291–3294.
16. Stam CJ, de Haan W, Daffertshofer A, Jones BF, Manshanden I, et al. (2009) Graph theoretical analysis of magnetoencephalographic functional connectivity in Alzheimer's disease. Brain 132: 213–224.
17. Stam CJ, Jones BF, Nolte G, Breakspear M, Scheltens P (2007) Small-world networks and functional connectivity in Alzheimer's disease. Cereb Cortex 17: 92–99.
18. Richardson MP (2012) Large scale brain models of epilepsy: dynamics meets connectomics. J Neurol Neurosurg Psychiatry 83: 1238–1248.
19. Chavez M, Valencia M, Navarro V, Latora V, Martinerie J (2010) Functional modularity of background activities in normal and epileptic brain networks. Phys Rev Lett 104: 118701.
20. Zhang Z, Liao W, Chen H, Mantini D, Ding JR, et al. (2011) Altered functional-structural coupling of large-scale brain networks in idiopathic generalized epilepsy. Brain 134: 2912–2928.
21. Xue K, Luo C, Zhang D, Yang T, Li J, et al. (2014) Diffusion tensor tractography reveals disrupted structural connectivity in childhood absence epilepsy. Epilepsy Res 108: 125–138.
22. Meeren H, van Luijtelaar G, Lopes da Silva F, Coenen A (2005) Evolving concepts on the pathophysiology of absence seizures: the cortical focus theory. Arch Neurol 62: 371–376.
23. Chahboune H, Mishra AM, DeSalvo MN, Staib LH, Purcaro M, et al. (2009) DTI abnormalities in anterior corpus callosum of rats with spike-wave epilepsy. Neuroimage 47: 459–466.
24. O'Muircheartaigh J, Vollmar C, Barker GJ, Kumari V, Symms MR, et al. (2011) Focal structural changes and cognitive dysfunction in juvenile myoclonic epilepsy. Neurology 76: 34–40.
25. Marson A, Jacoby A, Johnson A, Kim L, Gamble C, et al. (2005) Immediate versus deferred antiepileptic drug treatment for early epilepsy and single seizures: a randomised controlled trial. Lancet 365: 2007–2013.
26. Terry JR, Benjamin O, Richardson MP (2012) Seizure generation: The role of nodes and networks. Epilepsia 53: e166–169.
27. Allen AJ, Griss ME, Folley BS, Hawkins KA, Pearlson GD (2009) Endophenotypes in schizophrenia: a selective review. Schizophr Res 109: 24–37.
28. Gregory RP, Oates T, Merry RT (1993) Electroencephalogram epileptiform abnormalities in candidates for aircrew training. Electroencephalogr Clin Neurophysiol 86: 75–77.
29. Gerken H, Doose H (1973) On the genetics of EEG-anomalies in childhood 3. Spikes and waves. Neuropadiatrie 4: 88–97.
30. Degen R, Degen HE, Roth C (1990) Some genetic aspects of idiopathic and symptomatic absence seizures: waking and sleep EEGs in siblings. Epilepsia 31: 784–794.
31. Doose H, Baier WK (1987) Genetic factors in epilepsies with primarily generalised minor seizures. Neuropaediatrics 18 (Suppl 1): 1–64.
32. Jayalakshmi SS, Mohandas S, Sailaja S, Borgohain R (2006) Clinical and electroencephalographic study of first-degree relatives and probands with juvenile myoclonic epilepsy. Seizure 15: 177–183.
33. Quraan MA, McCormick C, Cohn M, Valiante TA, McAndrews MP (2013) Altered resting state brain dynamics in temporal lobe epilepsy can be observed in spectral power, functional connectivity and graph theory metrics. PLoS One 8: e68609.
34. van Wijk BC, Stam CJ, Daffertshofer A (2010) Comparing brain networks of different size and connectivity density using graph theory. PLoS One 5: e13701.
35. Guevara R, Velazquez JL, Nenadovic V, Wennberg R, Senjanovic G, et al. (2005) Phase synchronization measurements using electroencephalographic recordings: what can we really say about neuronal synchrony? Neuroinformatics 3: 301–314.
36. Peraza LR, Asghar AU, Green G, Halliday DM (2012) Volume conduction effects in brain network inference from electroencephalographic recordings using phase lag index. J Neurosci Methods 207: 189–199.
37. Stam CJ, Nolte G, Daffertshofer A (2007) Phase lag index: assessment of functional connectivity from multi channel EEG and MEG with diminished bias from common sources. Hum Brain Mapp 28: 1178–1193.
38. Andermann F, Berkovic SF (2001) Idiopathic generalized epilepsy with generalized and other seizures in adolescence. Epilepsia 42: 317–320.
39. Blumenfeld H (2005) Cellular and network mechanisms of spike-wave seizures. Epilepsia 46 Suppl 9: 21–33.
40. Motelow JE, Blumenfeld H (2009) Functional neuroimaging of spike-wave seizures. Methods Mol Biol 489: 189–209.
41. Helbig I, Mefford HC, Sharp AJ, Guipponi M, Fichera M, et al. (2009) 15q13.3 microdeletions increase risk of idiopathic generalized epilepsy. Nat Genet 41: 160–162.
42. de Kovel CG, Trucks H, Helbig I, Mefford HC, Baker C, et al. (2010) Recurrent microdeletions at 15q11.2 and 16p13.11 predispose to idiopathic generalized epilepsies. Brain 133: 23–32.
43. Dibbens LM, Mullen S, Helbig I, Mefford HC, Bayly MA, et al. (2009) Familial and sporadic 15q13.3 microdeletions in idiopathic generalized epilepsy: precedent for disorders with complex inheritance. Hum Mol Genet 18: 3626–3631.

16

Effect of Familiarity on Reward Anticipation in Children with and without Autism Spectrum Disorders

Katherine K. M. Stavropoulos*, Leslie J. Carver

Psychology Department, University of California San Diego, La Jolla, California, United States of America

Abstract

Background: Previous research on the reward system in autism spectrum disorders (ASD) suggests that children with ASD anticipate and process social rewards differently than typically developing (TD) children—but has focused on the reward value of unfamiliar face stimuli. Children with ASD process faces differently than their TD peers. Previous research has focused on face processing of unfamiliar faces, but less is known about how children with ASD process familiar faces. The current study investigated how children with ASD anticipate rewards accompanied by familiar versus unfamiliar faces.

Methods: The stimulus preceding negativity (SPN) of the event-related potential (ERP) was utilized to measure reward anticipation. Participants were 6- to 10-year-olds with ($N = 14$) and without ($N = 14$) ASD. Children were presented with rewards accompanied by incidental face or non-face stimuli that were either familiar (caregivers) or unfamiliar. All non-face stimuli were composed of scrambled face elements in the shape of arrows, controlling for visual properties.

Results: No significant differences between familiar versus unfamiliar faces were found for either group. When collapsing across familiarity, TD children showed larger reward anticipation to face versus non-face stimuli, whereas children with ASD did not show differential responses to these stimulus types. Magnitude of reward anticipation to faces was significantly correlated with behavioral measures of social impairment in the ASD group.

Conclusions: The findings do not provide evidence for differential reward anticipation for familiar versus unfamiliar face stimuli in children with or without ASD. These findings replicate previous work suggesting that TD children anticipate rewards accompanied by social stimuli more than rewards accompanied by non-social stimuli. The results do not support the idea that familiarity normalizes reward anticipation in children with ASD. Our findings also suggest that magnitude of reward anticipation to faces is correlated with levels of social impairment for children with ASD.

Editor: Gabriel S. Dichter, UNC Chapel Hill, United States of America

Funding: This work was supported by an Autism Speaks Dennis Weatherstone Predoctoral Fellowship awarded to KKMS (grant 7844). The funders had no rule in study design, data collection and analysis, decision to publish, or preparation of the manuscript.

Competing Interests: The authors have declared that no competing interests exist.

* Email: kmeltzoff@gmail.com

Introduction

Autism spectrum disorder (ASD) is a disorder defined by social-communicative deficits and repetitive and restricted behaviors. ASD is estimated to effect up to 1 in 68 children in the US (Centers for Disease Control and Prevention [CDC], 2014). Children with ASD have well documented difficulties in multiple aspects of social communication, including eye contact [1,2], language [3], and joint attention [1], in addition to having repetitive behaviors and restricted interests.

Several theories have emerged concerning why individuals with ASD are impaired relative to their neurotypical peers in social abilities. One is the social motivation hypothesis [4–9]. According to this idea, children with ASD are less intrinsically motivated to attend to and engage with others, which leads to downstream social deficits. The social motivation hypothesis might predict, then, that children with ASD need to be more motivated than TD children in order to find faces rewarding. In the current study, we

tested the hypothesis that, although unfamiliar faces may not be rewarding for children with ASD, a socially important familiar face, such a caregiver's face, may have greater reward value than an unfamiliar face.

There is reason to believe that children with autism might respond differently to a caregiver's face than to other, unfamiliar faces. Previous literature has investigated how children with and without ASD react to their caregivers, and whether attachment relationships differ between the two groups. The attachment literature suggests that children with ASD show somewhat typical and secure attachment relationships to their caregivers [10,11], although a recent meta-analysis suggested that children with ASD are less likely to be securely attached compared to TD children and those with other developmental disorders [12]. Given the suggestion that children with ASD may react to their parents similarly to TD children despite their social impairments, it is possible that familiar faces may be particularly salient to children with ASD, and may "normalize" the neural responses of people with ASD [13]. While this is an intriguing possibility, no prior study has directly investigated the effect of face familiarity on the brain's reward system in ASD. The current study was designed to investigate whether familiar faces would increase reward anticipation in children with ASD compared to their TD peers.

Previous literature has documented different neural responses in individuals with ASD compared to their TD peers when viewing unfamiliar faces [14–16]. The relatively small literature on the effect of familiarity in ASD has been limited to the effect of familiarity on face processing [13,17–25]. The studies on familiarity have varied results, likely due to inter-study differences in participants' age, methodologies, and stimuli. Previous literature on the reward system in ASD has also had mixed results, with some studies finding reward deficits in social rewards only, and others finding global reward deficits. One recent study has integrated these two lines of research and investigated familiar versus unfamiliar faces, as well as monetary rewards in a behavioral paradigm and found that both face and monetary rewards improved behavioral performance for individuals with and without ASD in a go/no-go task [26]. In order to setup and motivate the current study, we next briefly review the research on the reward system in ASD individuals using electrophysiology, functional neuroimaging, and combined methodologies, and then review previous research on the effect of familiar faces in ASD.

Reward System in ASD

Electrophysiological studies. Event-related potentials (ERP) are brain potentials recorded at the surface of the scalp. These recordings reflect synchronous firing of groups of synapses, and have been used to measure the time course of brain activity related to the anticipation or processing of specific discrete events.

ERPs have been used to study the reward system in ASD. Three studies have compared reward anticipation between TD individuals and those with ASD [27–29]. One study used a probabilistic learning task with monetary rewards and found that children with ASD and ADHD demonstrated larger neural responses than TD children when anticipating positive outcomes, but equivalent responses when anticipating negative outcomes [27]. A second study measured attentional ERP components in response to cues triggering trials with social vs. nonsocial rewards and found that TD children exhibited larger attentional components during reward versus non-reward conditions, but children with autism did not. In addition, children with autism exhibited smaller attentional components after cues initiating social reward anticipation trials [28]. A third study measured neural correlates of reward anticipation in a guessing game task with social and nonsocial rewards and found group differences such that children with ASD showed reduced brain activity when anticipating rewards accompanied by intact versus scrambled faces [29]. Taken together, ERP studies of social reward anticipation provide evidence that individuals with ASD elicit less brain activity when anticipating social rewards compared to their TD peers.

Previous ERP studies have also investigated electrophysiological correlates of reward processing in ASD. In studies examining reward processing in ASD, two studies have utilized a guessing game with monetary rewards. Both studies found similar activation patterns in children with ASD and TD [30,31], suggesting that children with ASD do not demonstrate deficits in reward feedback processing when the rewards are monetary. Our previous investigation of social versus non-social rewards revealed group differences in reward processing between TD children and those with ASD—especially for social stimuli [29].

Functional neuroimaging studies. Previous research on social versus nonsocial rewards in ASD has also utilized functional

magnetic resonance imaging (fMRI). The fMRI literature on social versus nonsocial rewards in ASD vs. TD is mixed. Some studies have suggested that individuals with ASD may elicit reduced neural activation for monetary rewards compared to TD children, but have similar neural activation for social rewards [32]; others have found reduced brain activity in response to social rewards in ASD [33].

Behavioral studies. One recent study has investigated reward responsiveness to both familiar versus unfamiliar faces, as well as nonsocial rewards, in both TD children and those with ASD using a modified go/no-go task [26]. Children either received auditory or visual indicators of reward after successful response inhibition. The authors found that both monetary and social (both familiar and unfamiliar faces) rewards increased performance versus a control (no-reward) condition. The authors did not find evidence of decreased responsiveness to social rewards in children with ASD, but found that parents' practices with rewards and contingencies at home strongly predicted performance in the ASD group [26].

Effects of Familiarity in ASD

Electrophysiological studies. We now turn to previous research investigating the effects of familiarity on face processing in ASD. Several ERP studies have measured responses to familiar and unfamiliar faces. Some investigations have found that individuals with ASD are less responsive to familiar faces compared to their typically developing peers [18,25], yet others have found that responsiveness to familiarity may be typical, but delayed, in ASD [24], or may increase after exposure to social skills groups [17]. Conversely, other investigations found no differences between adults with and without ASD in responsiveness to familiar faces [23], or in children at high versus low risk for ASD [20,34]. The ERP literature on the effects of familiarity on face processing in ASD is widely varied, and likely depends on a variety of factors, including cognitive functioning, age of participants, and the tasks utilized.

Functional Neuroimaging Studies. Two studies have investigated recognition of face familiarity using functional neuroimaging with individuals with and without ASD [13,22]. In a study of adults, both typical and ASD groups showed increased neural activation in response to familiar versus unfamiliar faces. [22]. In a study of school-aged children with and without ASD, children with ASD demonstrated similar brain activity to their TD peers when viewing pictures of children or familiar adults, but reduced activation when viewing pictures of unfamiliar adults [13]. In contrast to these findings, many studies in which brain responses are elicited to novel faces suggest that people with ASD do not activate face-processing brain areas to the same degree that TD controls do [16,35]. Thus, the results of recent face processing studies that have manipulated familiarity using fMRI measures suggest that brain responses might be normalized when familiar faces are used as stimuli.

Summary

Previous research on the *reward* system in ASD has been mixed, likely due to the wide variety of methodologies and procedures utilized. However, several studies have found that individuals with ASD have differences in the neural correlates of the reward system compared to TD individuals. Similarly, previous investigations of *familiar faces* on face processing have met with mixed findings. While previous literature has investigated the effects of familiar faces on face processing, as well as the effects of social versus nonsocial stimuli on the reward system in ASD, only one study has directly investigated the effect of familiar faces on reward responsiveness in ASD [26]. No previous studies have investigated the effects of familiarity on *neural correlates* of reward in TD versus ASD.

Current Study

The aim of the current study was to utilize electrophysiology to investigate the effect of familiarity on reward anticipation in response to faces versus non-faces in children with and without ASD. While previous studies have investigated the effects of familiarity on face processing, none have directly explored how the neural reward system is affected by familiarity in ASD. Specifically, we wanted to investigate reward anticipation for familiar versus unfamiliar faces, and scrambled versions of those images.

Previous investigations using electrophysiology to measure reward anticipation focused on the stimulus preceding negativity (SPN) component [29,36,37] The SPN is a component of the ERP that reflects brain activity occurring before expected feedback about one's performance [38]. SPN reflects the *expectation* of reward, and related activity of the dopaminergic reward system [39]. Our previous study of the SPN in children with ASD versus their TD peers revealed differences in how children with ASD anticipate social stimuli (pictures of faces) [29]. However, this previous study utilized a variety of unfamiliar faces.

The current study utilized one familiar and one unfamiliar face in order to determine whether familiar faces accompanying reward stimuli normalized reward anticipation in children with ASD. This design allowed us to gain information about both the effect of familiar faces on reward anticipation, and also whether the use of only one face in each condition may lead to habituation effects over time. In the current study, we also investigated whether brain activity and behavioral measures of ASD (via the SRS-2) were correlated, and whether children with more severe social impairments had reduced reward anticipation for face stimuli. We hypothesized that TD children would have an increased SPN response to face versus arrow stimuli—and that this effect would be most pronounced for familiar versus unfamiliar faces. We hypothesized that children with ASD would not have increased SPN responses to face versus arrow stimuli overall, but would have larger SPN responses to a familiar versus unfamiliar face. Lastly, we hypothesized that we would find a specific brain-behavior correlation—children with more severe social impairments (as measured with the SRS-2) would have decreased SPN amplitude to faces.

Methods

Participants

To estimate the needed sample size for the current study, we ran a power analysis on data from our previous study which used the same paradigm [29]. The resulting power value of .86 yielded a sample size of 26. Therefore, we recruited 28 participants for the current study: TD children ($N = 14$) and children with ASD ($N = 14$). Each child that was tested provided an adequate number of ERP trials for analysis and was included in the final sample. Exclusionary criteria for participants with ASD included history of seizures, brain injury, neurological disorders, genetic causes of ASD (e.g. Fragile X), or any concurrent psychiatric condition (other than ASD), based on parent report. Exclusionary criteria for TD participants included all of the above criteria, plus an immediate family history of ASD. None of the children in the TD group were taking psychoactive medications. One child in the ASD group was taking medication to improve concentration, and one was taking medication to decrease aggression and stabilize mood. Participants were recruited from a UC San Diego subject pool and through postings on websites for parents of children on the autism spectrum. All participants had normal hearing and normal or corrected to normal vision. Procedures were approved by the University of California, San Diego institutional review board, and written consent was obtained from caregivers. All children over 7 years of age signed an assent form.

Table 1 provides detailed participant information. IQ scores [40] were available for all participants. TD children were matched with children with ASD on mental age (full scale IQ/100 * chronological age). No differences were found between groups on mental age, $F(1,26) = .01$. Children in the ASD group had been previously diagnosed with ASD through various sources (e.g. formal evaluations through an autism center, or school diagnosis). Diagnosis was confirmed for the current study with Module 3 of the ADOS-2 [41]. The ADOS-2 was administered by an individual trained to research reliability on administration, scoring, and interpretation of the measure.

Behavioral Measures

Participants' caregivers completed the Social Responsiveness Scales (SRS-2) [42], which measures social responsiveness and behavior. We also tested for overt motivation or affective differences between groups for each condition. To accomplish this, children ($N = 9$ TD, 13 ASD) completed a 1–7 Likert rating scale of how much they enjoyed the game (1 = "I do not like this game", and 7 = "I love this game") after each block. This was used in order to gather more information about whether one group felt more or less motivated to engage in the task. Previous research suggests that the presence of reward versus no reward affects SPN amplitude—with greater SPN amplitude in reward versus no-reward conditions [43]—and we wished to assess whether both groups felt equally invested in the game. Participants also completed a 1–7 Likert scale about their perception of answering correctly (1 = "I never got correct answers", and 7 = "I always got correct answers"). In reality, the correct versus incorrect answers was predetermined, equated for individuals, and controlled by experimental design; the rating was used to verify that the groups did not differ in their perception that they were obtaining correct answers.

Stimuli and Task

The task was identical to that described in previous studies [29,37], but the stimuli differed in order to include different blocks of trials with a familiar or an unfamiliar face. The task was a guessing game that presented blocks of trials that used left and right visual stimuli (question marks). Participants were asked to indicate their guess via button press whether the left or right stimulus was "correct." After this choice, the left and right question marks were replaced with an arrow in the middle pointing towards whichever question mark the participant chose. This was done to reinforce the idea that participants had control over the task and their responses were being recorded.

There were four blocked feedback conditions: *familiar social, familiar nonsocial, unfamiliar social,* and *unfamiliar nonsocial.* The incidental stimulus in the familiar social condition was a picture of the child's caregiver that was smiling for "correct" answers and frowning for "incorrect" answers (photographs obtained via digital camera in our lab, and modeled after the NimStim stimulus set) [44]. The incidental stimulus in the unfamiliar social condition was a picture of another child's caregiver that was smiling for "correct" answers and frowning for "incorrect" answers. Incidental stimuli in the nonsocial conditions were composed of scrambled face elements from the social conditions formed into an arrow that pointed upwards for

Table 1. Participant characteristics including: IQ (WASI), chronological age, mental age (WASI/100 * chronological age), gender, SRS-2 T-score, and ADOS-2 severity scores for the ASD group.

Group	Participants	WASI (full-scale)	Chron. Age	Mental Age	Gender	SRS-2 SCI T-Score	SRS-2 RBB T-Score	ADOS-2 Severity Score
ASD	14	$M=99.42_a$ $SE=4.10$	$M=8.85$ $SE=.39$	$M=8.86$ $SE=.57$	11 M 3 F	$M=77.50_b$ $SE=1.94$	$M=80.07_c$ $SE=2.30$	$M=7.14$ $SE=.46$
TD	14	$M=112.64_a$ $SE=4.10$	$M=7.94$ $SE=.39$	$M=8.96$ $SE=.57$	11 M 3 F	$M=43.53_b$ $SE=2.01$	$M=46.38_c$ $SE=2.39$	N/A

$_a p=.03$, 95% CI [−1.28 −25.14].
$_b p<.0001$, 95% CI [39.72 28.20].
$_c p<.0001$, 95% CI [40.52 26.84].
WASI Wechsler Abbreviated Scale of Intelligence, SRS-2 Social Responsiveness Scale, second edition, SCI Social Communication and Interaction, RBB Restricted Interests and Repetitive Behavior, ADOS-2 Autism Diagnostic Observation Schedule Second Edition.

"correct" answers and downwards for "incorrect" answers (e.g. the stimulus in the familiar nonsocial condition was an arrow composed from the familiar social photograph, and stimulus in the unfamiliar nonsocial condition was an arrow composed from the unfamiliar social photograph). The face images and scrambled-face images were individually created from photographs taken in our lab with a digital camera. The face in the unfamiliar condition was chosen for each subject to match his or her caregiver's face on ethnicity, gender, and presence or absence of glasses. The use of scrambled faces to construct the arrow controlled for low-level visual features of the stimuli. Presented stimuli subtended a horizontal visual angle of 14.5 degrees, and a vertical visual angle of 10.67 degrees. The order in which children saw the four blocks of trials was counterbalanced between participants.

Participants were told that the reward for each correct answer was a goldfish cracker, or if they preferred, fruit snacks. They were told that if they guessed correctly, they would see a ring of intact goldfish crackers, and the goldfish would be crossed out for incorrect answers. Participants were told that the computer would sum their total of correct responses, and they would receive a goldfish cracker for each correct answer they gave, but would not lose any goldfish crackers for incorrect answers. Importantly, in both the familiar and unfamiliar social and nonsocial feedback trials, the face/arrow information was incidental. A computer program predetermined correct versus incorrect answers in pseudorandom order such that children got 50% "correct" and 50% "incorrect," with no more than three of the same answer in a row.

The four feedback conditions were tested in separate blocks, each composed of 60 trials. There were four conditions that composed the trials (familiar face/"familiar social"; unfamiliar face/"unfamiliar social"; familiar arrow/"familiar nonsocial"; and unfamiliar arrow/ "unfamiliar nonsocial" trials). Within each block of 60 trials, there were 10-s breaks every 15 trials. During breaks, participants were asked to relax, or move if they felt restless. Between blocks, a longer break (2–5 min.) was taken. To control for attentional effects, children were observed via webcam, and trials in which they were not attending to the stimulus were marked and discarded during analysis. Of the final sample, none of the children had any trials discarded for this reason.

EEG Recording

Participants wore a standard, fitted cap (Electrocap International) with 33 silver/silver-chloride (Ag/AgCl) electrodes placed according to the extended international 10–20 system. Continuous EEG was recorded with a NeuroScan 4.5 System with a reference electrode at Cz and re-referenced offline to the average activity at left and right mastoids. Electrode resistance was kept under 10 kOhms. Continuous EEG was amplified with a low pass filter (70 Hz), a directly coupled high pass filter (DC), and a notch filter (60 Hz). The signal was digitized at a rate of 250 samples per second via an Analog-to-Digital converter. Eye movement artifacts and blinks were monitored via horizontal electrooculogram (EOG) placed at the outer canthi of each eye and vertical EOG placed above and below the left eye. ERP trials were time locked to the onset of the feedback stimulus. The baseline period was −2200 to −2000 ms, and the data were epoched from −2200 to 100 ms. The interval between trials was varied between 1,800–2,000 ms. Trials with no behavioral response, or containing electrophysiological artifacts, were excluded from the averages.

Artifacts were removed via a four-step process. Data were visually inspected for drift exceeding +/−200 mV in all electrodes, high frequency noise visible in all electrodes larger than 100 mV, and flatlined data. Following inspection, data were epoched and eyeblink artifacts were identified using independent component analysis (ICA). Individual components were inspected alongside epoched data, and blink components were removed. To remove additional artifacts, we utilized a moving window peak-to-peak procedure in ERPlab [45], with a 200 ms moving window, a 100 ms window step, and a 150 mV voltage threshold. Participants with less than 10 artifact-free trials in any block of testing were excluded ($N=0$). Thus, our final analysis includes 14 children with ASD and 14 TD children.

Results

Data were analyzed using JMP (version 10.0). For our initial analysis, we separated familiarity (familiar, unfamiliar) from condition (face, arrow). We used mixed model (between and within subjects) analysis of variance (ANOVA) to test for differences between group, condition, familiarity, and caudality (anterior-posterior scalp locations).

Behavioral Measures

As expected, SRS-2 T-scores (which reflect more severe social impairments) were significantly higher for the ASD group than the TD group for the social communication subscale $F(1, 32) = 215$, $p<.0001$, and the repetitive and restricted behavior subscale $F(1,32)=158.55$, $p<.0001$. Means and standard deviations between groups on the SRS-2 are shown in *Table 1*. No significant differences were found between groups on children's Likert ratings of liking the game for any of the four conditions, (all $ps>.2$), or perception of generating correct answers, (all $ps>.1$)

ERP

SPN. The mean amplitude of the SPN was measured between -210 and -10 ms, prior to feedback onset, as defined in previous research [29,37,46]. Electrode sites F3/F4, C3/C4, P3/P4, and T5/T6, which are typically maximum amplitude sites for SPN [43], were analyzed. Artifact-free trials were analyzed for each of the four conditions between groups. No significant differences were found between groups for any of the four conditions (all $ps>.15$). Mean amplitude and trial numbers for each group in all 4 conditions are shown in *Table 2*.

A 2 (Group) ×2 (Condition) ×2 (Familiarity) ×4 (Electrode location) ANOVA did not reveal a significant effect of familiarity, $F(1, 32.06) = .23$, *n.s*, or any interactions with familiarity and other variables of interest. It is possible that over the course of each block, children's response to the single repeated stimulus habituated. In order to explore this possibility, we analyzed the first and second half of each participant's accepted trials for all four blocks in a 2 (Time) ×2 (Group) 2 (Familiarity) ×2 (Condition) ×4 (Electrode location) ANOVA. There was a marginal main effect of time such that the first half of trials elicited a larger SPN than the second half, regardless of group or condition $F(25.9) = 3.72$, $p=.064$, 95% CI [-2.31 to 4.99]. No other interactions with time were significant.

Given previous reports of differences in brain responses to familiar versus unfamiliar faces in TD children, but not those with ASD we conducted a planned 4 (Condition) ×2 (Group) ×4 (Electrode location) ANOVA for faces. We found a significant effect of group × electrode. Subsequent pairwise comparisons were non-significant. In order to better understand the effects of the different conditions on each group, a 4 (Condition) ×4 (Electrode location) ANOVA was conducted for the TD group and ASD groups separately. For TD children there was a main effect of condition, $F(3, 37.55) = 2.76$, $p=.055$, such that the familiar and unfamiliar face conditions elicited larger responses

Table 2. Descriptive statistics of trial numbers and amplitude of the SPN for typically developing (TD) individuals and those with autism spectrum disorder (ASD).

Group	Familiar Faces		Unfamiliar Faces		Familiar Arrows		Unfamiliar Arrows	
	Trials	Amplitude	Trials	Amplitude	Trials	Amplitude	Trials	Amplitude
TD	30.15 (2.67)	-6.58 (2.97)	30.21 (2.72)	-3.91 (2.89)	29.92 (3.01)	-.28 (2.97)	30.14 (2.31)	-.12 (2.89)
ASD	25.07 (2.57)	-3.65 (2.89)	30.28 (2.72)	-3.74 (2.89)	28.14 (2.90)	-2.21 (2.89)	25.21 (2.31)	-5.73 (2.89)

Means are displayed, followed by standard error in parentheses (SE). Amplitude is the average magnitude of the SPN over the last 200 ms before reward stimulus onset (measured in microvolts).

than the familiar and unfamiliar arrow conditions. Follow-up contrasts between the familiar face condition and the other three conditions (alpha corrected = .016) revealed marginally significant differences between the familiar face condition and the unfamiliar arrow condition ($p = .018$, 95% CI [1.15 to 11.82]) as well as a marginally significant difference between the familiar face and unfamiliar arrow conditions ($p = .02$, 95% CI [.90 to 11.82]). No other pairwise comparisons were significant. For the ASD group, there was no effect of condition $F(3, 36.24) = .53$, n.s. *Figure 1* shows grand averages of all four conditions for each group.

Because there was no main effect of familiarity within or between groups, nor interactions involving familiarity, we collapsed across familiarity for each condition (face, arrow) separately and conducted a 2 (Group) ×2 (Condition) ×4 (Electrode location) ANOVA. This analysis resulted in a significant group × condition interaction, $F(1, 26.03) = 5.97$, $p = .021$. Pairwise comparisons (alpha corrected = .012) revealed a significant effect of condition for the TD group, such that faces elicited a larger SPN than arrows for TD children, $F(1, 25.75) = 8.36$, $p > .01$, 95% CI [1.70 to 8.75], but not for children with ASD. *Figure 2* shows grand averages of the face and arrow conditions for each group.

There was a significant effect of electrode position, $F(3, 77.28) = 2.72$, $p = .05$, such the SPN was larger over central and parietal electrodes than frontal or temporal electrode sites. Follow-up Tukey's HSD showed that central electrode sites showed a significantly larger SPN than frontal electrode sites ($p = .04$, 95% CI [.1 to 7.67]). No other pairs of electrode sites were significantly different. There was a Condition × Electrode interaction, $F(3, 75.59) = 2.72$, $p = .05$. Pairwise comparisons (alpha corrected = .008) revealed that the significant effect of electrode was largely driven by the face condition, $F(3, 140.7) = 4.31$, $p = .006$, such that faces elicited a larger SPN than arrows differentially over various electrode sites. Pairwise comparisons also revealed a significant effect of the parietal electrode position, $F(1, 76.74) = 8.53$, $p = .004$ 95% CI [1.29 9.20], such that the face condition elicited a larger SPN than the arrow conditions at this electrode site regardless of group. There was a Group × Condition × Electrode interaction, $F(3, 75.59) = 3.40$, $p = .02$. In order to investigate the Group × Condition interaction at each electrode site, we performed contrasts at all four electrode sites. These contrasts showed a significant Group × Condition interaction (alpha corrected = .012) at both the central, $F(1, 78.57) = 6.51$, $p = .012$, 95% CI [1.07 to 8.20], and frontal electrodes, $F(1, 78.57) = 11.24$, $p = .001$, 95% CI [2.53 to 9.66], such that for the TD group, faces elicited a larger SPN than arrows, whereas for the ASD group arrows elicited a larger SPN than faces.

Nc. Visual inspection of our waveforms in *Figure 1* suggested a potential difference between groups in anticipation of face stimuli in a middle latency negative component (similar to an Nc) that occurred about 400 ms after the stimulus that signaled the choice of the participant in the guessing game. The Nc is traditionally thought to reflect attention and salience in frontal and central midline electrodes, and has previously been described as a response to a presented stimulus [47,48]. Our waveforms suggest an *anticipatory* Nc that occurred prior to the onset of face stimuli, but after children made their response. To investigate this possibility, we conducted a 2 (Group) ×2 (Familiarity) ×3 (Electrode) ANOVA for face stimuli between −1700 and −1550 ms (before the reward stimulus onset) in electrodes Fz, FCz, and Cz. Children's responses via button pad occur at −2000 ms— suggesting that this component occurred around 300 to 450 ms after the response. This time-frame (300 to 450 ms after response) is consistent with the time course of the Nc in previous

investigations [47]. The ANOVA revealed a marginally significant effect of electrode, $F(2, 52.47) = 3.10$, $p = .053$. However, Tukey HSD follow-up tests did not reveal any significant differences between electrode pairs. We found a significant main effect of group, $F(1, 26.06) = 4.91$, $p = .035$, 95% CI [2.50 to 10.81], such that the face stimulus elicited a larger Nc component for TD children compared to children with ASD. No significant effects of familiarity were found, $F(1, 25.66) = 1.8$, n.s. We re-ran the ANOVA collapsed across familiarity and our significant effects remained. Grand averages for both groups for the face condition are seen in *Figure 3*.

Brain-Behavior Correlations

We also investigated the relationship between brain activity and behavioral measures of ASD. Specifically, we asked whether magnitude of autism symptoms in the ASD group, as measured by the SRS-2, could predict the magnitude of SPN ERP response in the face condition (collapsed across familiarity). We found a significant correlation between T-scores on the SRS-2 and magnitude of SPN in response to faces, such that children with lower T-scores (and thus less severe social impairments as reported by caregivers), showed larger SPNs in response to faces, $F(1, 12) = 6.95$, $p = .021$, Cohen's $f^2 = .577$. *Figure 4* shows a scatter-plot of SRS-2 scores and amplitude in the face condition. However, it is can be noted that one subject elicited a particularly large SPN response, and thus may be considered an outlier, and when this subject was removed, the correlation no longer reached statistical significance, $F(1,11) = 1.5$, n.s.

Discussion

ERP

SPN. The current study suggests that there is not a significant difference in anticipation of a familiar versus an unfamiliar face for either children with ASD or their TD peers. However, TD children showed differences between conditions such that familiar faces elicited larger SPN compared to either of the arrow conditions, whereas unfamiliar faces were numerically larger (but not significantly different from) either arrow condition. This suggests that for TD children between the ages of 6–11 years old, familiar faces elicit a larger reward anticipation response compared to non-face stimuli. For children with ASD, we did not find any significant differences between conditions. Because we did not find the expected familiarity differences, we also explored whether the use of one repeated stimulus in each block would lead to habituation effects in either or both groups. We found a marginal effect of time, such that the first half of trials in each block elicited larger SPN responses than the second half, regardless of stimulus type or group. This suggests that although there is likely some habituation in the SPN response to a large number of repetitions of a single stimulus, it does not differ between groups or social versus nonsocial stimuli. Thus, it is unlikely that differences in the SPN response observed between groups are due to differences in how children with and without ASD habituate to stimuli, although habituation effects may explain the lack of familiarity effects in the present study.

Our results differ from several previous investigations [13,17,18,22,24,25]. Key differences in our task compared to previous studies may explain this. Whereas previous studies have utilized passive viewing tasks, or tasks in which participants attend directly to images and respond to a target stimulus, the current study was designed such that pictures of faces (and scrambled versions of those images) were incidental to the task. In other words, participants did not need to attend to the face or arrow

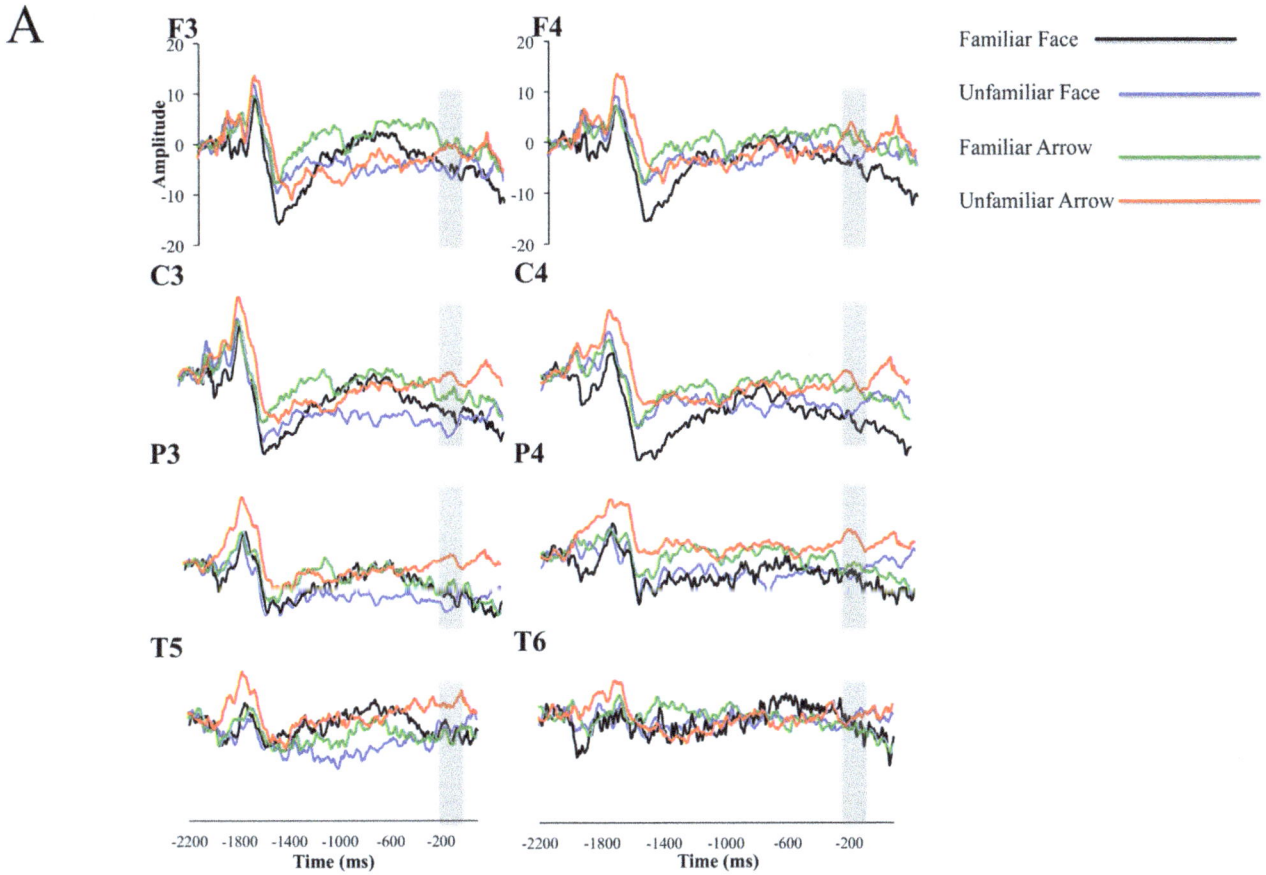

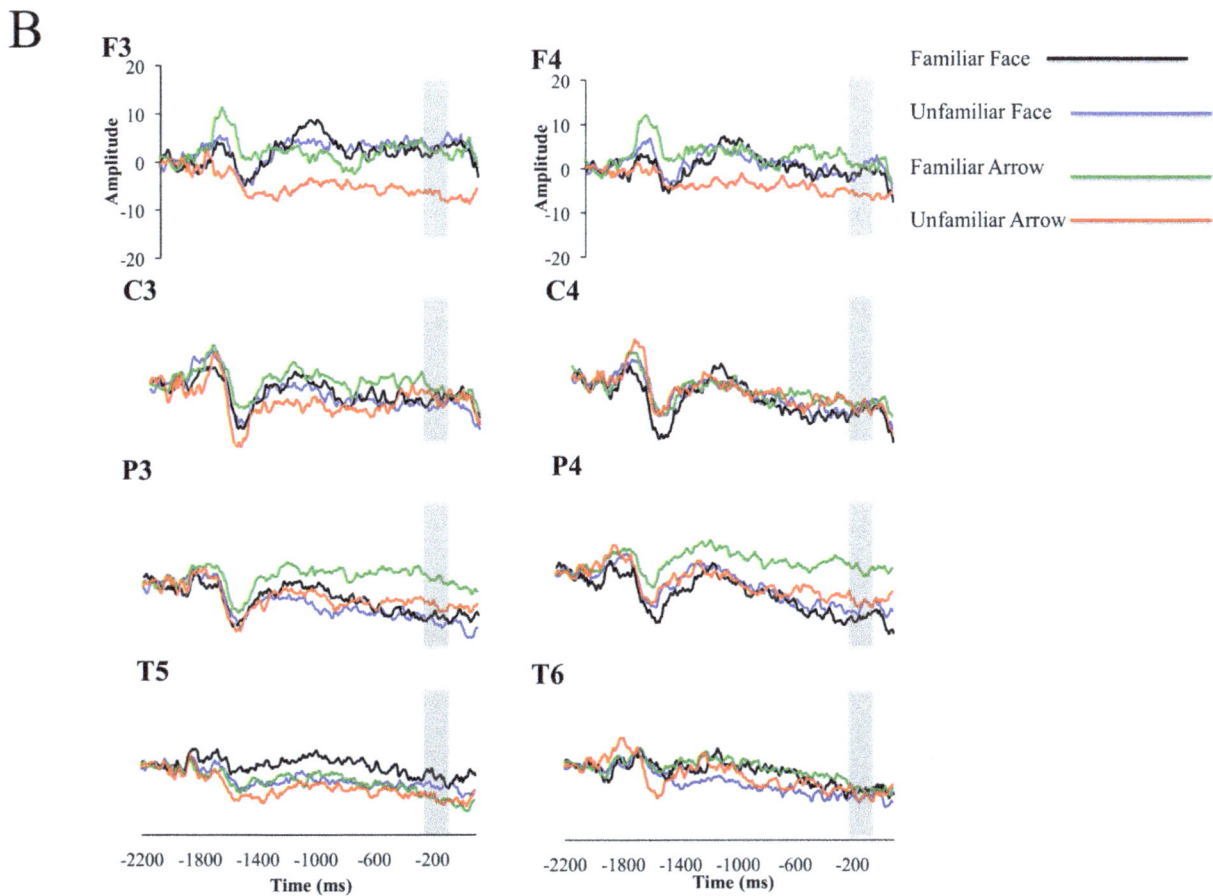

Figure 1. Grand averaged waveforms for the Stimulus Preceding Negativity (SPN). (A) Grand averaged waveforms for TD children from the Stimulus Preceding Negativity (SPN) prior to familiar faces, unfamiliar faces, familiar arrows, and unfamiliar arrows. (B) Grand averaged waveforms for children with ASD from the Stimulus Preceding Negativity (SPN) in ancitipation of familiar faces, unfamiliar faces, familiar arrows, and unfamiliar arrows. The area between −210 and −10 ms, used for statistical analysis, is highlighted with a grey box.

stimulus in order to gain information about whether their responses were "correct" or "incorrect." Although this paradigm allowed us to directly control for physical stimulus properties and tangibility between conditions, it is difficult to directly compare our results with those found in previous studies.

In previous research, one group of authors found that children with ASD showed differential neural activity in response to familiar versus unfamiliar faces [13], and another group of authors found that a small subset of children with ASD began to show differential neural activity in response to familiar face after social skills training [17]. One potential reason for this discrepancy in previous literature may be due to stimulus differences between studies. Previous studies used multiple familiar and unfamiliar faces (rather than just one familiar and one unfamiliar face) [13]. With the exception of [17], which investigated neural activation after social skills training, Pierce and Redcay [13] was the only study to find differences between familiar and unfamiliar faces in children with ASD. One possibility is that children with ASD are more likely to differentiate between familiar versus unfamiliar faces when viewing multiple exemplars from each category. The finding in the current study that there was a marginal tendency for children across groups to habituate to the repeated presentation of a single stimulus supports this idea. Previous research suggests the fusiform face area (FFA) may be involved in determining the identity of individual faces [49]—thus, presenting multiple different faces may activate the FFA to a greater degree than presentations of single faces. It is possible that in previous research, presentation of multiple different familiar faces was adequate to normalize brain responses to faces in ASD. This is an interesting direction for future research, and future studies may wish to compare within subjects whether children with ASD elicit differential neural activity when viewing multiple faces versus one face.

Importantly, although we did not find a main effect of familiarity or interactions between group and familiarity, when we collapsed across familiarity for both groups, we found a group by condition interaction such that TD children showed a larger SPN component in response to faces versus arrows, while children with ASD demonstrated the opposite pattern. This replicates our previous work [29] with a novel group of participants and novel stimuli. These results are in line with the social motivation hypothesis—that TD children are more rewarded by social versus nonsocial stimuli, while children with ASD do not demonstrate this pattern.

Our results are consistent with previous studies that examined reward anticipation in these populations [27,28], in that we found TD children and those with ASD elicited a statistically equivalent SPN response to *non*social feedback. Similarly, while the current study investigated reward anticipation of social versus nonsocial stimuli, and other ERP studies of the reward system in ASD have focused on reward processing of monetary stimuli only [30,31], our results are consistent with these investigations insofar as we found that children with ASD elicit similar reward anticipation to their TD peers for nonsocial stimuli. Our results differ with regards to TD children, however, because we found that TD children elicited a larger SPN response to social versus nonsocial stimuli, whereas [28] found the opposite pattern. Our results also differ from behavioral measures of response inhibition for social versus

monetary rewards [26], as those authors found that both TD children and those with ASD have increased performance for all reward types. However, the authors also found no difference in performance for familiar versus unfamiliar social stimuli in either group, which is consistent with the current findings [26].

One important difference between our current and previous findings is that current pairwise comparisons did not reveal a significant difference between the ASD and TD [29] groups for face stimuli. That is, while TD children had a significantly larger SPN to faces versus non-faces, there was not a significant difference between TD children and those with ASD for the face stimuli. This differs from our previous findings, where in addition to differences between face and non-face stimuli, TD children also had larger SPN responses to faces than children with ASD. One potential reason for this is stimulus variation. In our previous study, children saw a variety of unfamiliar faces, whereas in the current study they saw just one unfamiliar and one familiar face. When comparing our current results to our previous findings, TD children have a smaller SPN response in the face condition, while children with ASD have a larger SPN response in the face condition. In contrast, for the arrow condition, both groups are largely unchanged between studies. This raises the possibility that while TD children show larger SPN responses when viewing multiple faces, children with ASD demonstrate the opposite pattern. The current study was not designed to investigate this, and thus these possibilities remain conjecture, but future studies could manipulate the number of faces in the stimulus set, and measure resulting effects on the SPN.

Nc. We found an Nc-like component after participant's response, but before feedback. This component differentiated TD children from those with ASD. The component occurred at about the time (~400 msec after the participant's button press) and had a similar scalp distribution (prominent at frontal electrode sites) as the Nc component that has typically been investigated in response to visual stimuli [50]. These findings provide novel information about the Nc component—in effect that the Nc can act as an anticipatory waveform. Previous findings have examined the Nc as a component related to salience and attention in response to a stimulus in infants and young children (e.g. [25]). Our findings, however, suggest that the Nc is also sensitive to anticipation of upcoming stimuli and/or the testing context (i.e., blocks of familiar and unfamiliar faces vs. arrows), and differentiates between diagnostic groups. It is important to note, however, that the current study was not designed to investigate anticipatory effects of the Nc component, as most studies on the Nc do not involve overt responses by the participant. Thus, while our results have interesting implications for the Nc, it is necessary for future studies to look directly at the effect of anticipation on the Nc between children with and without ASD.

Brain and Behavior Correlations

The present results provide evidence that magnitude of reward anticipation response to faces in children with ASD can be predicted by reported levels of social impairments (as measured by the social responsiveness scales). This provides evidence that is in line with the social motivation hypothesis, insofar as children with lower levels of reported social impairments showed larger reward anticipation responses to faces compared to children with higher

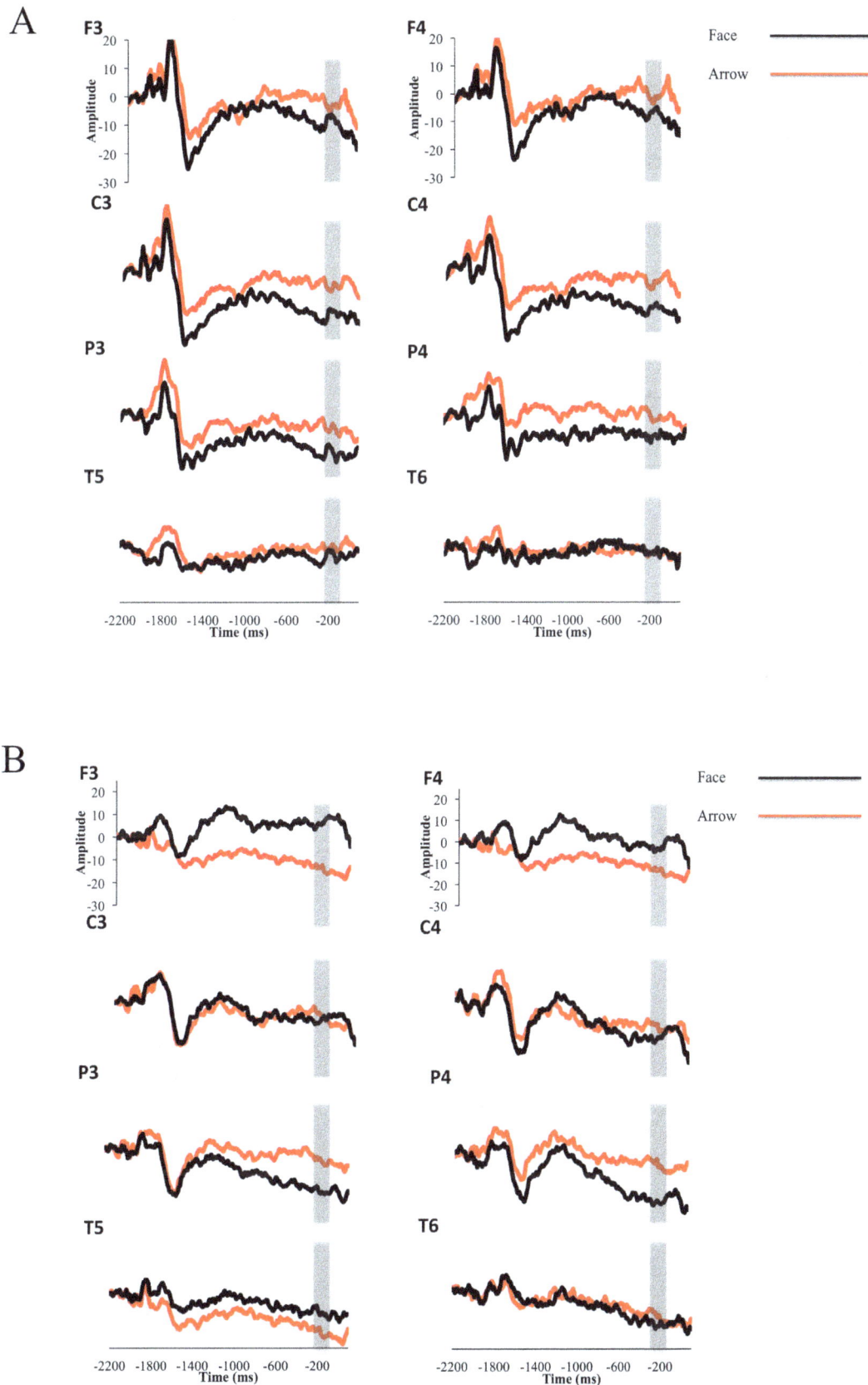

Figure 2. Grand averaged waveforms collapsed across familiarity. (A) Grand averaged waveforms for TD children from the Stimulus Preceding Negativity (SPN) prior to faces and arrows (collapsed across familiarity). The area between −210 and −10 ms, used for statistical analysis, is highlighted with a grey box. (B) Grand averaged waveforms for children with ASD from the Stimulus Preceding Negativity (SPN) prior to faces and arrows (collapsed across familiarity). The area between −210 and −10 ms, used for statistical analysis, is highlighted with a grey box.

Familiar Faces

Unfamiliar Faces

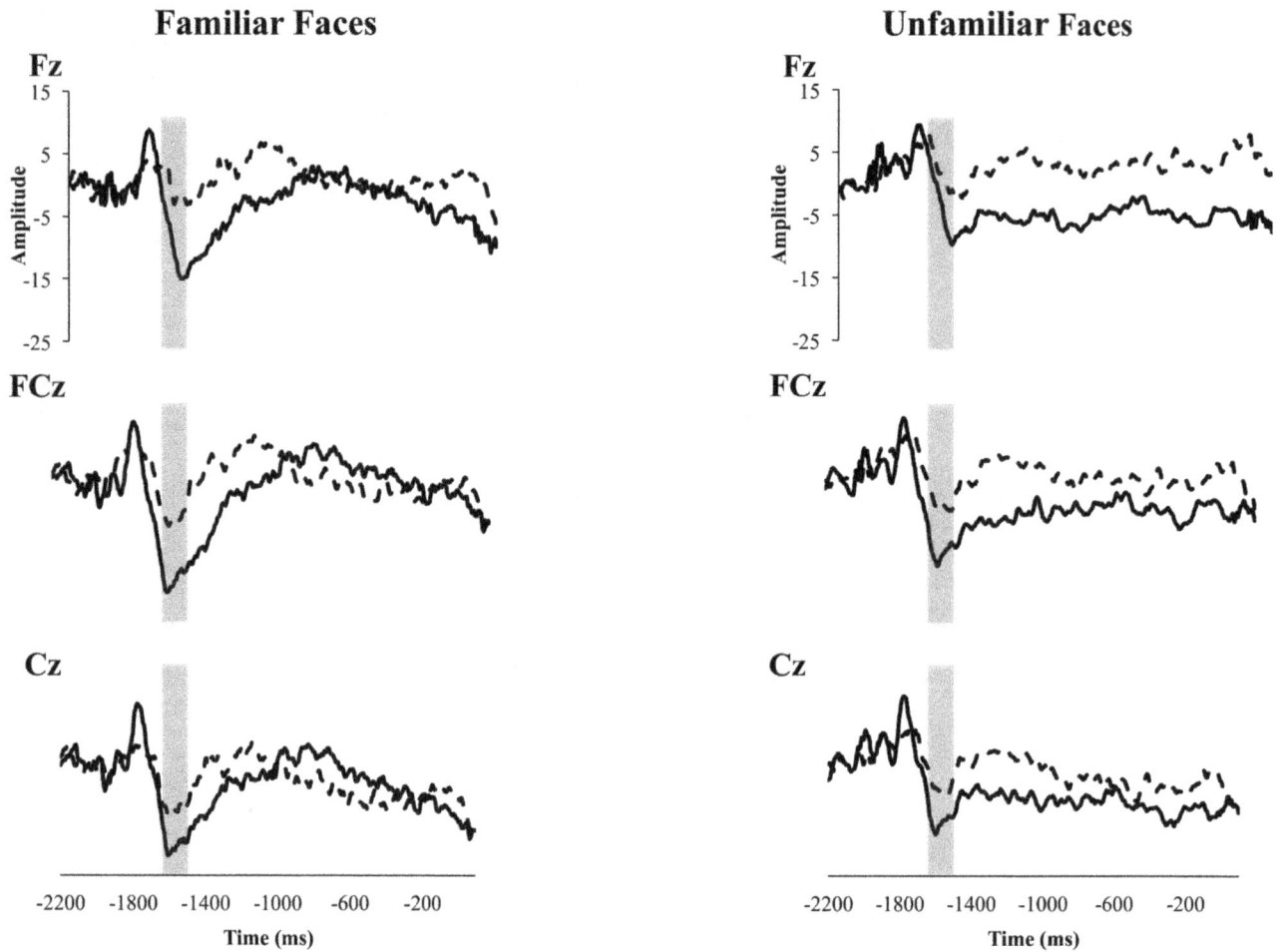

Figure 3. Grand averaged waveforms for both groups from the Nc component prior to familiar and unfamiliar faces. TD children are represented with a solid line, and children with ASD with a dashed line. The area between −1700 and −1550 ms, used for statistical analyses, is highlighted with a grey box.

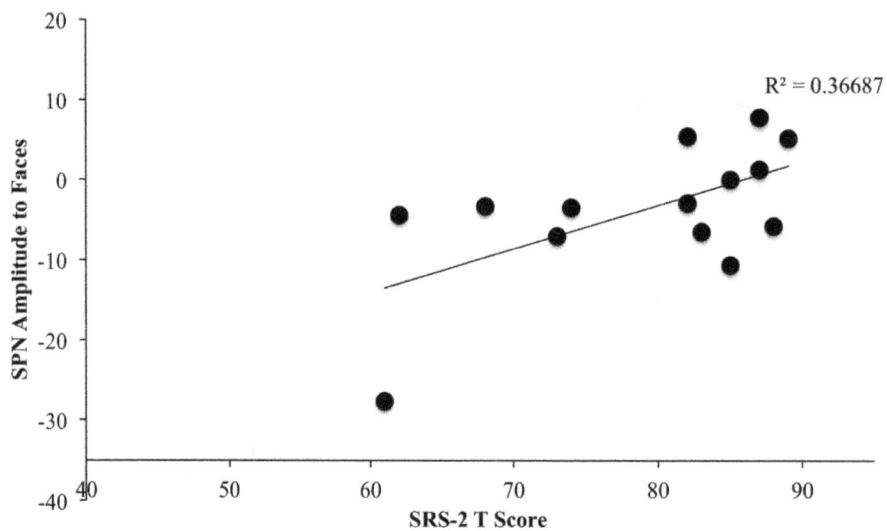

Figure 4. Scatter plot of SPN amplitude to faces (collapsed across familiarity) by SRS-2 T-score for children with ASD. Higher SRS-2 T-scores indicate more severe social impairments. As the SPN is a negative ERP component, more negative values indicate a larger response. Note that one participant had a particularly large SPN response and thus may be considered an outlier; and when this subject was removed, the correlation no longer reached statistical significance, $F(1,11) = 1.5$, *ns*.

levels of reported impairments. We note, however, that this effect may have been driven by a single participant in the current study, so it is not advisable to draw large-scale conclusions from this analysis. Future studies should look into these types of correlations with a larger sample of children with ASD.

The current study has some limitations that should be noted. First, our sample size ($N = 14$ in each of the TD and ASD groups) is relatively small (although within the estimates provided by our power analysis). This makes it difficult to draw broad and generalized inferences. Further, we did not obtain information about treatment history from participants. Given previous findings about the effect of social skills training on face processing [17], as well as parent attitudes towards reward contingencies on behavioral sensitivity to rewards [26], this limitation should be taken into consideration when interpreting the current findings.

Conclusions and Broader Implications

We examined reward anticipation of incidental familiar versus unfamiliar faces and scrambled versions of those images in children with and without ASD. Although we did not find evidence for an effect of familiar versus unfamiliar faces in either group, the current study adds to the body of literature supporting the social motivation hypothesis, and replicates previous findings using different stimuli and participants. The current study also provides evidence that magnitude of reward anticipation to faces is significantly correlated with levels of parent-reported social impairments. This suggests that our paradigm is sensitive to social impairments as measured by questionnaires, which provides evidence that we are accurately capturing social motivation in children with ASD.

Our findings provide interesting implications for future work on the Nc-like component, which we observed as a measure of anticipation in children, and suggest that for TD children, anticipation of face stimuli elicits a larger Nc-like component than for children with ASD. While our study was not designed to directly address this question, we feel it is an important future direction. The current study also suggests intriguing areas for

future research in regards to whether children with and without ASD are differentially affected by viewing one versus multiple unfamiliar faces. The current study and previous work suggest that perhaps TD children show larger reward anticipation for multiple unfamiliar faces, while children with ASD show the opposite pattern. However, because the current and previous studies utilized different participants and stimuli, we suggest this as an important future direction.

The current study suggests that social motivation deficits in ASD are not ameliorated by viewing familiar faces when face stimuli are incidental to the task. Future research is necessary to determine whether task specifications or number of faces within a stimulus set affects these findings. The current study provides further evidence for the social motivation hypothesis, and suggests that levels of social impairment in ASD are correlated with magnitude of reward anticipation to faces. This paradigm could be utilized as a biomarker of social motivation, and could be used before and after behavioral or pharmacological interventions designed to improve social motivation. In this way, individual children's levels of reward anticipation to faces could be tracked over time along with behavioral levels of social impairment, in order to see changes throughout the course of intervention.

Acknowledgments

We thank the children and their parents for their participation, and the members of the Developmental Neuroscience lab for their assistance. We thank Dr. Sara Webb for her recommendations about analysis strategies, and Kevin Smith, Dr. Julian Parris, and Dr. Mark Appelbaum, for assistance with statistics. We thank Dr. Eric Courchesne for assistance with study conceptualization, and Dr. Steven Hillyard for sharing his expertise concerning anticipatory ERP components.

Author Contributions

Conceived and designed the experiments: KKMS LJC. Performed the experiments: KKMS. Analyzed the data: KKMS. Contributed reagents/materials/analysis tools: KKMS LJC. Contributed to the writing of the manuscript: KKMS LJC.

References

1. Mundy P, Sigman M, Ungerer J, Sherman T (1986) Defining the social deficits of autism: the contribution of non-verbal communication measures. J Child Psychol Psychiatry 27: 657–669. doi: 10.1111/j.1469-7610.1986.tb00190.x.

2. Walters AS, Barrett RP, Feinstein C (1990) Social relatedness and autism: current research, issues, directions. Res Dev Disabil 11: 303–326. doi: 10.1016/0891-4222(90)90015-Z.

3. Charman T, Swettenham J, Baron-Cohen S, Cox A, Baird G, et al. (1998) An experimental investigation of social-cognitive abilities in infants with autism: Clinical implications. Infant Ment Health J 19: 260–275. doi: 10.1002/(SICI)1097-0355(199822)19:2<260::AID-IMHJ12>3.0.CO;2-W.

4. Chevallier C, Kohls G, Troiani V, Brodkin ES, Schultz RT (2012) The social motivation theory of autism. Trends Cogn Sci 16: 231–239. doi:10.1016/j.tics.2012.02.007.

5. Dawson G (2008) Early behavioral intervention, brain plasticity, and the prevention of autism spectrum disorder. Dev Psychopathol 20: 775–803. doi:10.1017/S0954579408000370.

6. Dawson G, Carver L, Meltzoff AN, Panagiotides H, McPartland J, et al. (2002) Neural correlates of face and object recognition in young children with autism spectrum disorder, developmental delay, and typical development. Child Dev 73: 700–717. doi: 10.1111/1467-8624.00433.

7. Dawson G, Webb SJ, Wijsman E, Schellenberg G, Estes A, et al. (2005) Neurocognitive and electrophysiological evidence of altered face processing in parents of children with autism: implications for a model of abnormal development of social brain circuitry in autism. Dev Psychopathol 17: 679–697. doi:10.1017/S0954579405050327.

8. Grelotti D, Gauthier I, Schultz RT (2002) Social Interest and the Development of Cortical Face Specialization: What Autism Teaches Us About Face Processing. Dev Psychobiol 40: 213–225. doi:10.1002/dev.10028.

9. Schultz RT (2005) Developmental deficits in social perception in autism: the role of the amygdala and fusiform face area. Int J Dev Neurosci 23: 125–141. doi:10.1016/j.ijdevneu.2004.12.012.

10. Sigman M, Mundy P (1989) Social attachments in autistic children. J Am Acad Child Adolesc Psychiatry 28: 74–81. doi: 10.1097/00004583-198901000-00014.

11. Sigman M, Ungerer JA (1984) Attachment behaviors in autistic children. J Autism Dev Disord 14: 231–244.

12. Rutgers AH, van Ijzendoorn MH, Bakermans-Kranenburg MJ, Swinkels SHN, van Daalen E, et al. (2007) Autism, attachment and parenting: a comparison of children with autism spectrum disorder, mental retardation, language disorder, and non-clinical children. J Abnorm Child Psychol 35: 859–870. doi:10.1007/s10802-007-9139-y.

13. Pierce K, Redcay E (2008) Fusiform function in children with an autism spectrum disorder is a matter of "who". Biol Psychiatry 64. 552–560. doi:10.1016/j.biopsych.2008.05.013.

14. McPartland J, Dawson G, Webb SJ, Panagiotides H, Carver LJ (2004) Event-related brain potentials reveal anomalies in temporal processing of faces in autism spectrum disorder. J Child Psychol Psychiatry 45: 1235–1245. doi:10.1111/j.1469-7610.2004.00318.x.

15. Dawson G, Webb SJ, Carver L, Panagiotides H, McPartland J (2004) Young children with autism show atypical brain responses to fearful versus neutral facial expressions of emotion. Dev Sci 7: 340–359. doi: 10.1111/j.1467-7687.2004.00352.x.

16. Schultz RT, Gauthier I, Klin A, Fulbright RK, Anderson AW, et al. (2000) Abnormal ventral temporal cortical activity during face discrimination among individuals with autism and Asperger syndrome. Arch Gen Psychiatry 57: 331–340. doi: 10.1001/archpsyc.57.4.331.

17. Gunji A, Goto T, Kita Y, Sakuma R, Kokubo N, et al. (2013) Facial identity recognition in children with autism spectrum disorders revealed by P300 analysis: a preliminary study. Brain Dev 35: 293–298. doi:10.1016/j.braindev.2012.12.008.

18. Gunji A, Inagaki M, Inoue Y, Takeshima Y, Kaga M (2009) Event-related potentials of self-face recognition in children with pervasive developmental disorders. Brain Dev 31: 139–147. doi:10.1016/j.braindev.2008.04.011.

19. Key APF, Stone WL (2012) Processing of novel and familiar faces in infants at average and high risk for autism. Dev Cogn Neurosci 2: 244–255. doi:10.1016/j.dcn.2011.12.003.

20. Kylliäinen A, Wallace S, Coutanche MN, Leppänen JM, Cusack J, et al. (2012) Affective-motivational brain responses to direct gaze in children with autism spectrum disorder. J Child Psychol Psychiatry 53: 790–797. doi:10.1111/j.1469-7610.2011.02522.x.

21. Luyster RJ, Wagner JB, Vogel-Farley V, Tager-Flusberg H, Nelson CA (2011) Neural correlates of familiar and unfamiliar face processing in infants at risk for autism spectrum disorders. Brain Topogr 24: 220–228. doi:10.1007/s10548-011-0176-z.

22. Pierce K, Haist F, Sedaghat F, Courchesne E (2004) The brain response to personally familiar faces in autism: findings of fusiform activity and beyond. Brain 127: 2703–2716. doi:10.1093/brain/awh289.

23. Webb SJ, Jones EJH, Merkle K, Murias M, Greenson J, et al. (2010) Response to familiar faces, newly familiar faces, and novel faces as assessed by ERPs is intact in adults with autism spectrum disorders. Int J Psychophysiol 77: 106–117. doi:10.1016/j.ijpsycho.2010.04.011.

24. Webb SJ, Jones EJH, Merkle K, Venema K, Greenson J, et al. (2011) Developmental change in the ERP responses to familiar faces in toddlers with autism spectrum disorders versus typical development. Child Dev 82: 1868–1886. doi:10.1111/j.1467-8624.2011.01656.x.

25. Dawson G, Carver L, Meltzoff AN, Panagiotides H, McPartland J, et al. (2002) Neural correlates of face and object recognition in young children with autism spectrum disorder, developmental delay, and typical development. Child Dev 73: 700–717. doi: 10.1111/1467-8624.00433

26. Pankert A, Pankert K, Herpertz-Dahlmann B, Konrad K, Kohls G (2014) Responsivity to familiar versus unfamiliar social reward in children with autism. J Neural Transm. doi:10.1007/s00702-014-1210-6.

27. Groen Y, Wijers AA, Mulder LJM, Waggeveld B, Minderaa RB, et al. (2008) Error and feedback processing in children with ADHD and children with Autistic Spectrum Disorder: an EEG event-related potential study. Clin Neurophysiol 119: 2476–2493. doi:10.1016/j.clinph.2008.08.004.

28. Kohls G, Peltzer J, Schulte-Rüther M, Kamp-Becker I, Remschmidt H, et al. (2011) Atypical brain responses to reward cues in autism as revealed by event-related potentials. J Autism Dev Disord 41: 1523–1533. doi:10.1007/s10803-011-1177-1.

29. Stavropoulos KKM, Carver LJ (2014) Reward anticipation and processing of social versus nonsocial stimuli in children with and without autism spectrum disorders. J Child Psychol Psychiatry. doi:10.1111/jcpp.12270.

30. McPartland JC, Crowley MJ, Perszyk DR, Mukerji CE, Naples AJ, et al. (2012) Preserved reward outcome processing in ASD as revealed by event-related potentials. J Neurodev Disord 4: 16. doi:10.1186/1866-1955-4-16.

31. Larson MJ, South M, Krauskopf E, Clawson A, Crowley MJ (2011) Feedback and reward processing in high-functioning autism. Psychiatry Res 187: 198–203. doi:10.1016/j.psychres.2010.11.006.

32. Dichter GS, Richey JA, Rittenberg AM, Sabatino A, Bodfish JW (2012) Reward circuitry function in autism during face anticipation and outcomes. J Autism Dev Disord 42: 147–160. doi:10.1007/s10803-011-1221-1.

33. Scott-Van Zeeland AA, Dapretto M, Ghahremani DG, Poldrack RA, Bookheimer SY (2010) Reward processing in autism. Autism Res 3: 53–67. doi:10.1002/aur.122.

34. Luyster RJ, Wagner JB, Vogel-Farley V, Tager-Flusberg H, Nelson CA (2011) Neural correlates of familiar and unfamiliar face processing in infants at risk for autism spectrum disorders. Brain Topogr 24: 220–228. doi:10.1007/s10548-011-0176-z.

35. Pierce K, Müller RA, Ambrose J, Allen G, Courchesne E (2001) Face processing occurs outside the fusiform "face area" in autism: evidence from functional MRI. Brain 124: 2059–2073. doi: 10.1093/brain/124.10.2059.

36. Ohgami Y, Kotani Y, Tsukamoto T, Omura K, Inoue Y, et al. (2006) Effects of monetary reward and punishment on stimulus-preceding negativity. Psychophysiology 43: 227–236. doi:10.1111/j.1469-8986.2006.00396.x.

37. Stavropoulos KKM, Carver LJ (2013) Reward sensitivity to faces versus objects in children: an ERP study. Soc Cogn Affect Neurosci. doi:10.1093/scan/nst149.

38. Brunia CHM, Hackley SA, van Boxtel GJM, Kotani Y, Ohgami Y (2011) Waiting to perceive: reward or punishment? Clin Neurophysiol 122: 858–868. doi:10.1016/j.clinph.2010.12.039.

39. Boxtel GJM Van, Böcker KBE (2004) Cortical Measures of Anticipation. J Psychophysiol 18: 61–76. doi:10.1027/0269-8803.18.2.

40. Wechsler D (1999) Wechsler Abbreviated Scale of Intelligence. San Antonio. TX: Pearson.

41. Lord C, Rutter M, DiLavore PC, Risi S, Gotham K (2012) ADOS-2: autism diagnostic observation schedule. Los Angeles: Western Psychological Services.

42. Constantino JN, Gruber CP (2012) Social Responsiveness Scale, Second Edition. Los Angeles: Western Psychological Services.

43. Kotani Y, Kishida S, Hiraku S, Suda K, Ishii M, et al. (2003) Effects of information and reward on stimulus-preceding negativity prior to feedback stimuli. Psychophysiology 40: 818–826. doi: 10.1111/1469-8986.00082.

44. Tottenham N, Tanaka JW, Leon AC, McCarry T, Nurse M, et al. (2009) The NimStim set of facial expressions: judgments from untrained research participants. Psychiatry Res 168: 242–249. doi:10.1016/j.psychres.2008.05.006.

45. Lopez-Calderon J, Luck SJ (2014) ERPLAB: an open-source toolbox for the analysis of event-related potentials. Front Hum Neurosci 8: 1–14. doi:10.3389/fnhum.2014.00213.

46. Kotani Y, Hiraku S, Suda K, Aihara Y (2001) Effect of positive and negative emotion on 10.1111/j.1467-7687.2005.00452.x.

47. Courchesne E (1978) Neurophysiological correlates of cognitive development: Changes in long-latency event-related potentials from childhood to adulthood. Electroencephalogr Clin Neurophysiol 45: 468–482. doi: 10.1016/0013-4694(78)90291-2.

48. Webb SJ, Long JD, Nelson CA (2005) A longitudinal investigation of visual event-related potentials in the first year of life. Dev Sci 8: 605–616. doi: 10.1111/j.1467-7687.2005.00452.x.

49. Haxby JV, Hoffman EA, Gobbini MI (2000) The distributed human neural system for face perception. Trends Cogn Sci 4: 223–233. doi:10.1111/j.1467-7687.2005.00452.x.

50. De Haan M, Johnson MH, Halit H (2003) Development of face-sensitive event-related potentials during infancy: a review. Int J Psychophysiol 51: 45–58. doi:10.1016/S0167-8760(03)00152-1.

17

An Efficient ERP-Based Brain-Computer Interface Using Random Set Presentation and Face Familiarity

Seul-Ki Yeom[1,9]**, Siamac Fazli**[1,9]**, Klaus-Robert Müller**[1,2]**, Seong-Whan Lee**[1]*

1 Department of Brain and Cognitive Engineering, Korea University, Seoul, Republic of Korea, **2** Machine Learning Group, Berlin Institute of Technology, Berlin, Germany

Abstract

Event-related potential (ERP)-based P300 spellers are commonly used in the field of brain-computer interfaces as an alternative channel of communication for people with severe neuro-muscular diseases. This study introduces a novel P300 based brain-computer interface (BCI) stimulus paradigm using a random set presentation pattern and exploiting the effects of face familiarity. The effect of face familiarity is widely studied in the cognitive neurosciences and has recently been addressed for the purpose of BCI. In this study we compare P300-based BCI performances of a conventional row-column (RC)-based paradigm with our approach that combines a random set presentation paradigm with (non-) self-face stimuli. Our experimental results indicate stronger deflections of the ERPs in response to face stimuli, which are further enhanced when using the self face images, and thereby improving P300 based spelling performance. This lead to a significant reduction of stimulus sequences required for correct character classification. These findings demonstrate a promising new approach for improving the speed and thus fluency of BCI-enhanced communication with the widely used P300-based BCI setup.

Editor: Nader N. Pouratian, UCLA, United States of America

Funding: This work was supported by National Research Foundation of Korea (NRF) funded by the Ministry of Science, ICT and Future Planning (No. 2012-005741). The funders had no role in study design, data collection and analysis, decision to publish, or preparation of the manuscript.

Competing Interests: The authors have declared that no competing interests exist.

* Email: sw.lee@korea.ac.kr

9 These authors contributed equally to this work.

Introduction

Brain-computer interface (BCI) systems provide a direct electronic interface to translate messages and commands from the brain of the user to external devices without muscular control. To date, a major part of BCI research is focused on the restoration of communication [1–3]. Therefore, BCI's have been particularly utilized for patients whose motor and communicative abilities have been impaired by severe neuromuscular diseases such as amyotrophic lateral sclerosis (ALS). Those affected suffer from a gradual loss of voluntary muscular control due to motor neuron degeneration [4–6].

The P300 is the ERP component with the strongest deflection and has been widely investigated over the past few years. P300-based BCIs constitute arguably the largest category of BCI research. The first P300-based matrix speller (aka P300 Speller) was introduced by Farwell and Donchin [7]. Since its introduction it has been studied extensively by many research groups. In this conventional paradigm, a letter-matrix consisting of the alphabet and digits, arranged in a 6×6 grid, is displayed on a computer screen and presented to the subject. While the subject attends to the specific letter they wish to spell, the rows and columns are flashed consecutively in a random order (the so-called classical Row-Column (RC) paradigm). When a row or column is flashed, that contains the attended letter, an elevated P300 can be detected in the subjects' EEG.

Since the publication of this paper in 1988 many extensions to the original RC paradigm have been proposed in order to improve its performance in terms of speed and accuracy (see [8] for a recent review). Some of the various configurations include: (1) electrode montages [9], (2) stimulus (or matrix) property alteration (i.e. color, size, rate and motion) [10–16], (3) variations of inter-stimulus intervals (ISIs) (or stimulus onset asynchrony (SOA)) and target-to-target intervals (TTIs) [10,17–19], (4) various pattern recognition/machine learning algorithms for feature extraction [20–22], and classification [9,23–25].

Furthermore, other groups have made a constant effort on the redesign of novel visual stimulus representation patterns for improving the P300 speller. Guger *et al.* [26] propose a single character (SC) speller, where characters are flashed individually in a randomized order. They compare the SC speller with the classical RC speller for 38 subjects and demonstrate that although the SC paradigm produces larger P300 responses than the RC paradigm, the RC paradigm still retains a higher performance than their novel SC paradigm. They attribute their findings to the increased fatigue as a result of the longer sequence of character selection. Two other research groups (Fazel-Rezai and Abhari [27] and Treder *et al.* [28]) propose a P300 speller, where the desired letter is chosen, based on a two-step process. Letters are grouped and randomly flashed, as opposed to the row and column intensification. The subject needs to identify and select the group containing the desired letter in the first step. During the second step the desired character is selected within that group. Treder *et al.* [29] further extends this two-step process by 3 alternatives (they are termed, "Hex-o-spell", "Cake-", and "Center- speller") using covert spatial attention and non-spatial feature attention modal-

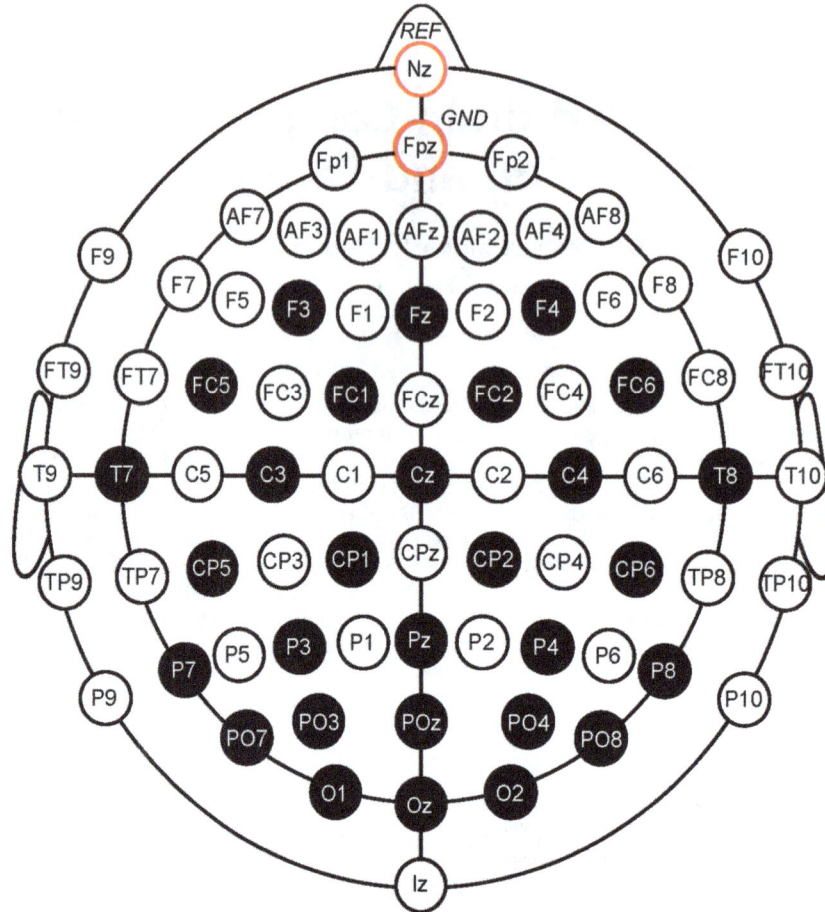

Figure 1. The selected electrode locations of the International 10–20 system (29 EEG recording electrodes (black circles), one ground and one reference electrode (red circles) used in this paper).

ities. Recently a series of papers has also considered online adaptation and unsupervised learning for BCI ERP spellers (see [30–32]).

Townsend *et al*. [33], (see also [34]) investigated a checkerboard paradigm (CBP) to overcome the following two issues: 1) adjacency-distraction errors which can occur when neighboring items flash with respect to target items and 2) double-flash errors, which occur when the same character flashes sequentially. The original CBP presents stimuli in an 8×9 matrix and then separates the letters into 2 groups (a white and a black group each in a 6×6 matrix). By disassociating the rows and columns, the CBP can overcome 'repetition blindness' [35] by introducing the constraint that a minimum of six intervening flashes (of non-targets) should be between targets and the 'flanker effect' [36] by only simultaneously flashing letters which are not in the same row or column.

Finally, Jin *et al*. [37,38] designed a novel stimulus presentation pattern that requires fewer flashes than RC and SC paradigms. They test a number of different flash patterns as well as adaptively detecting the necessary number of flashes to average. Their

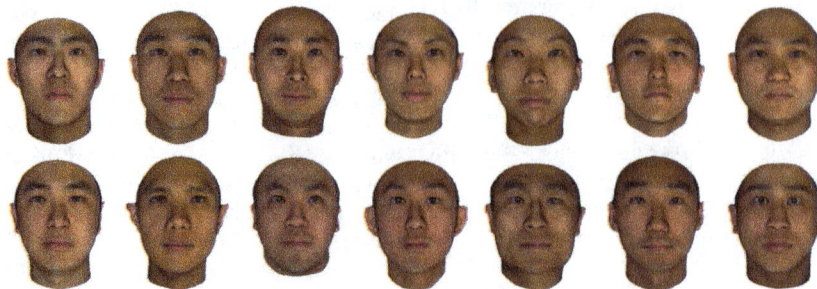

Figure 2. Examples of the face stimuli obtained by the 3dMD face capture system with the same illumination conditions. One self-face image and a number of non-self-face images are depicted here.

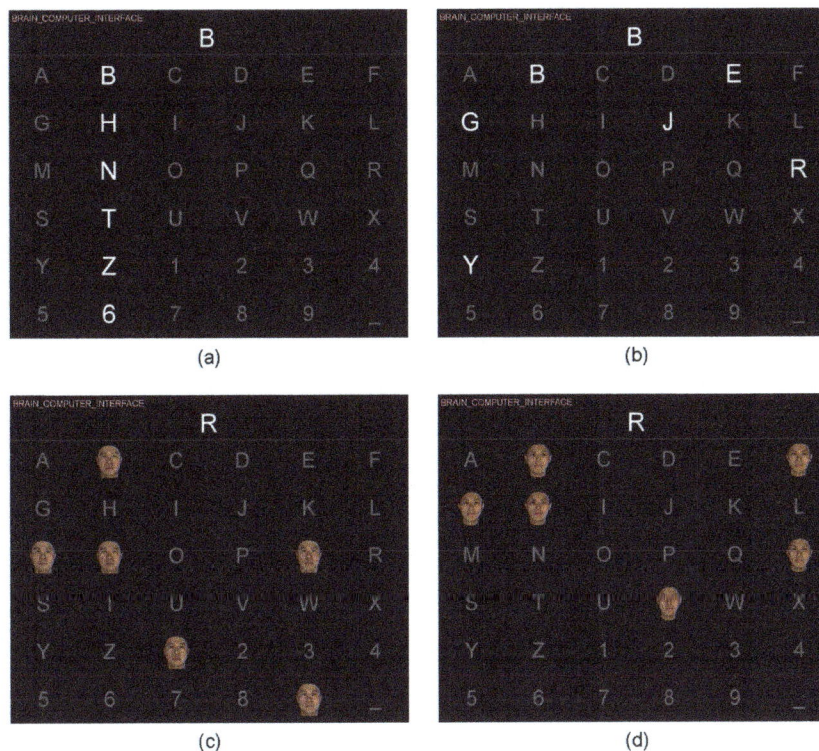

Figure 3. The different conditions of the paradigm. (a) The classical row-column (RC) paradigm, (b) The proposed random set presentation (RASP) paradigm, (c) RASP paradigm with flashing self-face in one row of the virtual matrix, (d) RASP paradigm with flashing non-self-face in one column of the virtual matrix. Both RASP and RASP-F stimuli were shown semi-transparently to the participants such that the characters were still visible. However, this is not shown here for illustration purposes.

findings indicate that they are able to reduce the numbers of flashes, as well as minimizing the interference from items adjacent to targets.

In recent years, a number of groups have focused on changing the stimuli from intensified characters to alternative stimuli such as faces. In particular, face stimuli based approaches elicit not only P300 responses, but also face-specific ERP components, namely N170 and N400f. N170, a negative deflection at around 140-200 ms after the onset of the stimulus presentation, is known to show a stronger deflection when faces are presented as compared to other stimuli [39]. When compared with unfamiliar faces, familiar faces elicit an enhanced negativity between 300 and 500 ms ('N400f).

Based on the above-mentioned face-specific temporal features, Kaufmann *et al.* [40] adopted famous face images and superimposed them with the letters of a P300 matrix speller. In their study, the face-sensitive ERPs show an enhanced accuracy due to the contribution of the N170 and N400f features, which are accompanied by the recognition of familiar faces. In addition, they could show in [41] that face stimuli can be helpful to avoid BCI inefficiency [42] for patients with neurodegenerative diseases. Zhang *et al.* [43] also utilized stimuli based on configural processing of human faces in an oddball paradigm. Also here, face configuration related ERP components such as N170 and vertex positive potentials (VPP) result in higher accuracies, as compared to the conventional P300-based BCI with stimuli of intensification patterns. A number of previous studies have investigated, whether face emotion has an effect on BCI performance, however to date no performance differences have been found for these type of stimuli [41,44].

In this paper, an offline study is performed, where two improvements to the above mentioned issues of P300 spelling are examined: 1) to minimize adjacency-distraction errors we adopted a random set-based stimulus representation pattern (RASP), similar to a previous study [33]. However, in this previous work, two factors were manipulated: Not only did they alter the (random) groups of letters flashed simultaneously, but also tried to minimize the double-flash related problems by ensuring a minimum of six intervening flashes between targets. As a result, it was not possible to determine, which of these factors were responsible for the increased performance and to which extent. In this study we did not define a static TTI and this enabled us to examine the effect of various TTIs. By isolating the two factors (i.e. the required minimum TTI as well as the random set-based stimulus representation pattern) it is now possible to more accurately quantify the benefit of the two individual approaches. 2) effects of face familiarity on P300-based BCIs: The present offline study is dedicated to further investigate the effects of face familiarity on the performance of BCIs using stimuli of facial images. In a previous study, we found that brain activity responses to one's own face are markedly unique and show stronger responses when compared to familiar or unfamiliar non-self faces and this phenomenon was defined as 'face-specific visual self-representation' in [45] for the neurophysiological basis thereof we refer to [46]. These results were obtained in a previous person authentication study [47]. Earlier studies have also shown that task complexity shows a strong positive correlation with the amplitude of the ERP responses [48], however habituation effects, which may be caused by repeated presentation of the same stimulus, could counteract this effect [10]. To this end we designed the

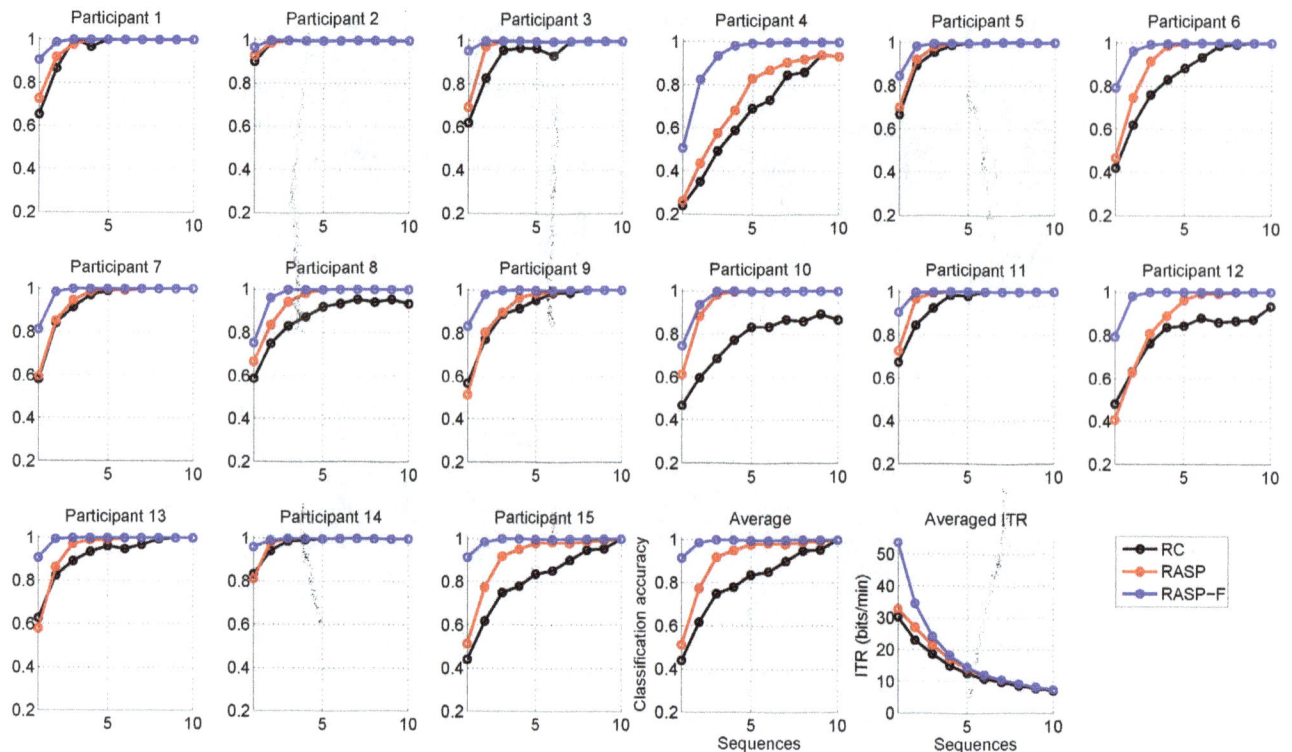

Figure 4. Classification accuracy curves of each subject for three conditions ('RC', 'RASP', and 'RASP-F') using one to ten sequences. Also, on the bottom right the averaged classification accuracy and ITR on all subjects are plotted.

paradigm, such that self-faces as well as non-self faces are presented in a randomized order.

Materials and Methods

Participants

Fifteen healthy university students who were between 26 and 32 years (mean 27.7 ± 1.5, right-handed, all males) took part in our experiments. All participants had normal or corrected-to-normal vision. None of the participants had a previous history of psychiatric, neurological, or other diseases that might otherwise affect the experimental results. All experiments were conducted according to the principles expressed in the Declaration of Helsinki. This study was reviewed and approved by the Institutional Review Board at Korea University and written informed consent was obtained from all participants before the experiments. Participants were seated comfortably in a chair with armrests in a quiet room at a distance of 60 ± 5 cm from a standard 19 inch LCD monitor (60 Hz refresh rate, 1280×1024 screen resolution) which corresponds to an angle range from $-10° \sim 10°$. During the experiment, they were asked to relax while remaining attentive and avoiding unnecessary movement.

Equipment and data acquisition

EEG signals were recorded with a sampling rate of 500 Hz with a BrainAmp multichannel EEG amplifier by Brain Products from the following 29 Ag/AgCl electrodes on a cap (actiCAP, Brain Products, Munich, Germany), according to the international 10–20 system: F3, F4, Fz, FC1, FC2, FC5, FC6, C3, C4, Cz, T7, T8, CP1, CP2, CP5, CP6, P3, P4, Pz, P7, P8, PO3, PO4, POz, PO7, PO8, O1, Oz, O2 (see Figure 1). Channels were nasion-referenced and grounded to electrode Fpz. EEG signals were then down-

sampled to 100 Hz with a 10th order digital Chebyshev filter. The impedances of the EEG electrodes were below 10 kΩ. EEG data was amplified and digitized using BrainAmp hardware (Brain Products, Munich, Germany).

For acquiring face images a 3dMD face capture system was used ensuring the same lighting conditions for all subjects (http://3dmd.com) making a neutral facial expression, while facing the camera. Face images were derived from front-view photographs using Adobe PhotoShop software. All the face images were processed to remove external features such as hair and then cropped into a common oval frame which was placed on a black uniform background. Face images were scaled to an image size of 400×500 pixels. These final face stimuli were presented as in Figure 2 (for further details, please refer to [47]).

Experimental stimuli and paradigm

Three different spellers, all derived from the original P300 speller, were examined. Each speller allowed the user to choose one out of 36 unique symbols, comprising the letters of the English alphabet (A to Z), digits (1 to 9) and underbar (_). All three matrix spellers were presented with a 6×6 matrix and highlighted characters or faces were flashed consecutively in random order. The three spellers were implemented with the Psychophysics Toolbox (http://psychtoolbox.org). The Row-Column (RC) condition corresponded to the traditional approach [7]. In the RC condition each sequence necessary to select a target (i.e. letter to spell) comprised 12 stimulus flashes of each row and each column.

In the first proposed variant, called random set-based stimulus representation pattern (RASP), letters were randomly shuffled in a virtual six-by-six matrix, prior to stimulus presentation and then 12 stimulus flashes were presented to the subject. As a result users saw a unique combination of letters in each stimulus during a

Table 1. F-values and significance of the repeated measures 3×10 ANOVA.

		accuracy	ITR
speller	F(2,28)	54.64***	92.24***
sequences	F(9,126)	270.65***	109.02***
speller × sequences	F(18,252)	14.1***	8.04***

speller stands for *type of speller* (RC, RASP, RASP-F) and *sequences* for *number of sequences* (1 to 10). *** corresponds to $p < 0.001$

given sequence. The number of stimuli were equal for the RC and RASP paradigms and the temporal distribution of TTIs was the same on average. Similar to the RC condition, each letter was flashed twice within a sequence. In other words, in a series of 12 flashes, the target letter (but also every other letter) was contained in two of the twelve flashes.

As a second variant, also based on RASP, the characters were overlaid with face stimuli. This variant was termed RASP-F. The face images were semi-transparent to allow for uninterrupted focusing on the target letter while the face stimuli were flashed. The types of face stimuli, which were used in the experiments can be divided into 2 categories. Self-face and non-self-face images were used for stimulation. A self-face image consisted of the image of the subject, while a non-self-face image consisted of a familiar face such as his/her friends or of unfamiliar faces whom he/she has never seen before. In the case of self-face presentation, the same face image was presented as a stimulus but in the case of non-self-faces different face images were presented each time in order to counter the effect of habituation. When a row was selected in the virtual 6 by 6 matrix, the letters contained in this row were flashed with self-faces in the speller. Similarly, when a column was selected, contained letters were flashed with non-self-faces. Therefore, the ratio between self-face and non-self-face presentation was 50:50. See Figure 3.

During the experiment, participants were instructed to sit still, relax their muscles and try to minimize eye movements. Each experiment consisted of 2 phases: a training phase and a test phase. Training and test phases were recorded on two separate days. Transfering classifiers from one session to another is known as *session-to-session* transfer and known to lead to (slightly) reduced classification rates. The presentation order of the spellers was randomized across participants. In each session, participants were provided with strings of letters they were supposed to spell. The whole string was displayed at the top left of the monitor and the next item-to-spell (the target letter) was displayed above the letter matrix (see Figure 3). During the initial training phase, subjects had to copy-spell one sentence 'BRAIN_COMPUTER_INTER-FACE'. There was no feedback and EEG was recorded for offline analysis. In the second phase subjects had to copy-spell another sentence 'KOREA UNIVERSITY' (without the space). The participant's task was to attend to (or count) the number of times the target character flashed. Each run started with a 2 s countdown. For all speller conditions, each set of characters flashed for 135 ms, followed by an ISI of 50 ms. When subjects were instructed to copy-spell, the spelling of each letter consisted of 10 sequences without a prolonged inter-sequence interval. One sequence consists of 12 flashes. For the RC case every column and every row was flashed once. For the RASP and RASP-F cases each letter was flashed twice, however groups of letters were shuffled after each flash. Note, that for all cases the target flashed twice.

Data analysis

We used the BBCI toolbox (http://bbci.de/toolbox) for our analysis. EEG data was band-pass filtered between 0.1 and 30 Hz with a 5th order Butterworth digital filter. In each experimental session, the data was epoched from -200 ms to 800 ms with respect to stimulus onset. Epoched EEG signals were baseline-corrected by subtracting the mean amplitudes in the -200 to 0 ms pre-stimulus interval from every epoch. Then, averaged features of the ERPs were extracted from 8 selected discriminative intervals, which were selected by a well established heuristic, which depends on signed r-values [23]. These subject-dependent intervals were located in the 100–600 ms poststimulus interval, thereby forming an averaged spatiotemporal feature vector with a dimension of 232 (i.e. 29 channels $\times$ 8 averaged temporal features). After that, these features from the training phase were validated with the data from the test phase with the help of a regularized linear discriminant analysis (RLDA) classifier with analytic shrinkage of the covariance matrix [23,49]. For the evaluation of the 3 matrix spellers classification accuracies (a 0–1 loss function was used) as well as Information Transfer Rates (ITRs) were computed. ITRs are commonly used as an evaluation measurement for BCIs. The unit of ITRs is given as *bits per unit time* [bits min^{-1}] and can be calculated as

$$ITR = M\{\log_2 N + P \log_2 P + (1-P) \log_2 (\frac{1-P}{N-1})\} \quad (1)$$

where M denotes the number of commands per minute and N indicates the number of the possible choices in which each choice is equally probable to be selected by the user. P is the accuracy of the BCI (i.e. the probability that the BCI selects what the user intends). In summary ITR corresponds to the amount of information received by the system.

To further examine the effect of self-face stimuli on classification performance, we separated all self-face stimuli from non-self stimuli in the RASP-F condition, where self-faces occured in rows and non-self faces in columns. For each session and subject we performed 8-fold chronological cross-validation employing an RLDA classifier. To evaluate whether classification accuracy of self-face stimuli outperforms accuracy of non-self stimuli significantly, we performed sign-tests. The sign-test is a non-parametric test, which relies on only very few assumptions [50,51]. Three statistical tests were performed on the cross-validated accuracies of RC vs. SF, RASP vs. SF and NSF vs. SF to test the hypothesis, whether the difference median is zero between the continuous distributions of the two random variables. Results of this test were then Bonferroni corrected [52].

Furthermore, a two way repeated measure ANOVA was performed in order to study *accuracy* and *ITR* (dependent variables) with respect to the within-subject factors *type of speller* and *number of sequences*. *Type of speller* contained three levels:

Table 2. Single-trial classification accuracy [%], based on 8-fold cross validation for each paradigm and subject.

Subject	RC	RASP	RASP-F	
			NSF	SF
1	93.7	88.8	86.8	90.6
2	96.1	96.6	98.0	98.6
3	90.8	89.6	91.8	94.8
4	79.1	76.5	81.6	85.2
5	89.8	89.3	88.8	91.9
6	89.2	82.8	91.7	94.3
7	88.3	86.1	81.9	89.9
8	87.4	87.3	90.1	90.4
9	90.1	82.2	91.7	97.7
10	80.1	89.0	92.8	95.2
11	89.8	93.4	96.4	97.4
12	76.0	87.1	85.8	92.6
13	85.4	87.6	95.2	95.8
14	90.8	89.9	96.9	97.9
15	79.2	79.6	91.9	93.4
Mean	87.1	87.1	90.7	93.7***

RC stands for Row Column, *RASP* for random set presentation, *RASP-F* for random set presentation with face stimuli, *NSF* stands for *non-self face stimuli*, while *SF* stands for *self-face stimuli*. The three stars indicates the level of significant improvement ($p<0.001$) for NSF vs. SF., based on a sign test with the hypothesis of equal means.

RC, RASP and RASP-F. The *number of sequences* contained 10 levels (from 1 to 10).

To examine, whether ERP components were significantly different for the three types of spellers, values were first averaged across time in the following intervals with respect to stimulus onset: 130–200ms for N170 (channel 'PO7'), 280–370ms for P300 (channel 'Cz') and 400–550ms for N400f (channel 'Cz'). The choice of intervals and electrode locations was based on previous publications in order to increase comparability of the analysis [29,33,43]. Then two-sample t-tests were performed with the null hypothesis of equal means. Results were then Bonferroni corrected (3 tests per ERP component were performed).

Results

Classification accuracy and ITR

Figure 4 depicts the classification accuracy for each subject as well as averaged accuracies and ITRs for all subjects. The number of sequences were varied from one to ten sequences (x-axis) for all three different spellers. In the RASP-F condition, on average fewer sequences ($M = 1.1 \pm 0.3$) were necessary for achieving an accuracy level of $\geq 70\%$ as compared to RC ($M = 2.5 \pm 1.3$) and RASP conditions ($M = 1.9 \pm 1.0$). This threshold has previously been argued to be the minimum accuracy level for meaningful communication [53]. To ensure an accuracy level of $\geq 90\%$, the number of sequences needed were $M = 1.6 \pm 0.6$, for the RASP-F condition, $M = 4.9 \pm 2.9$ for the RC condition and $M = 3.0 \pm 1.5$ for the RASP condition.

Offline selection accuracies for selecting one symbol out of 36 by using single sequence data were $58.4\% \pm 1.6\%$ for RC, $61.3\% \pm 1.6\%$ for RASP and $84.0\% \pm 1.2\%$ for RASP-F. In an offline analysis, we investigated classification performance and ITR as a function of the number of sequences (i.e. repetitions of the intensification). As expected, performance increased sharply with the number of repetitions.

Table 1 summarizes the results of the two-way repeated measures ANOVA. The ANOVA revealed an increase of accuracy with the number of sequences, and a difference in accuracy for the three spellers. Interaction between type of speller and number of sequences was significant. When we compared the RC and RASP conditions with single sequences, a paired t-test revealed that accuracies are not significantly different (RC < RASP, $t=1.95, p=0.07$). However, when increasing the number of sequences to 3, accuracies become significantly different (RC < RASP, $t=3.48, p=0.0037$). The difference between face-related stimuli and highlighted characters are significantly different for a single sequence (RC < RASP-F: $t=9.97, p<0.001$; RASP < RASP-F: $t=8.06$ *mmap*<0.001) as well as for 3 sequences (RC < RASP-F: $t=4.23, p<0.001$; RASP < RASP-F: $t=2.72, p=0.017$).

ITR among the three spellers was also significantly different. The best performance with an ITR of 53.7 ± 11.8 bits/min was achieved by RASP-F as compared to the 30.3 ± 13.3 bits/min for RC and 32.8 ± 13.8 bits/min for RASP. The difference between face-related stimuli and highlighted characters was significantly enhanced for single sequence data (RC < RASP-F: $t=10.60, p<0.001$; RASP < RASP-F: $t=8.64, p<0.001$) as well as for 3 repeated sequences (RC < RASP-F: $t=4.95, p<0.001$; RASP < RASP-F: $t=3.32, p=0.017$).

Table 2 shows the single-trial classification accuracy [%] of the 8-fold cross-validation for each paradigm and subject. *RC* stands for Row Column, *RASP* for random set presentation, *RASP-F* for random set presentation with face stimuli, *NSF* stands for *non-self face stimuli*, while *SF* stands for *self-face stimuli*. Average performance of SF was significantly higher, when compared to any of the other methods ($p<0.001$, Bonferroni corrected). The stars in the table indicate the comparison of SF to NSF.

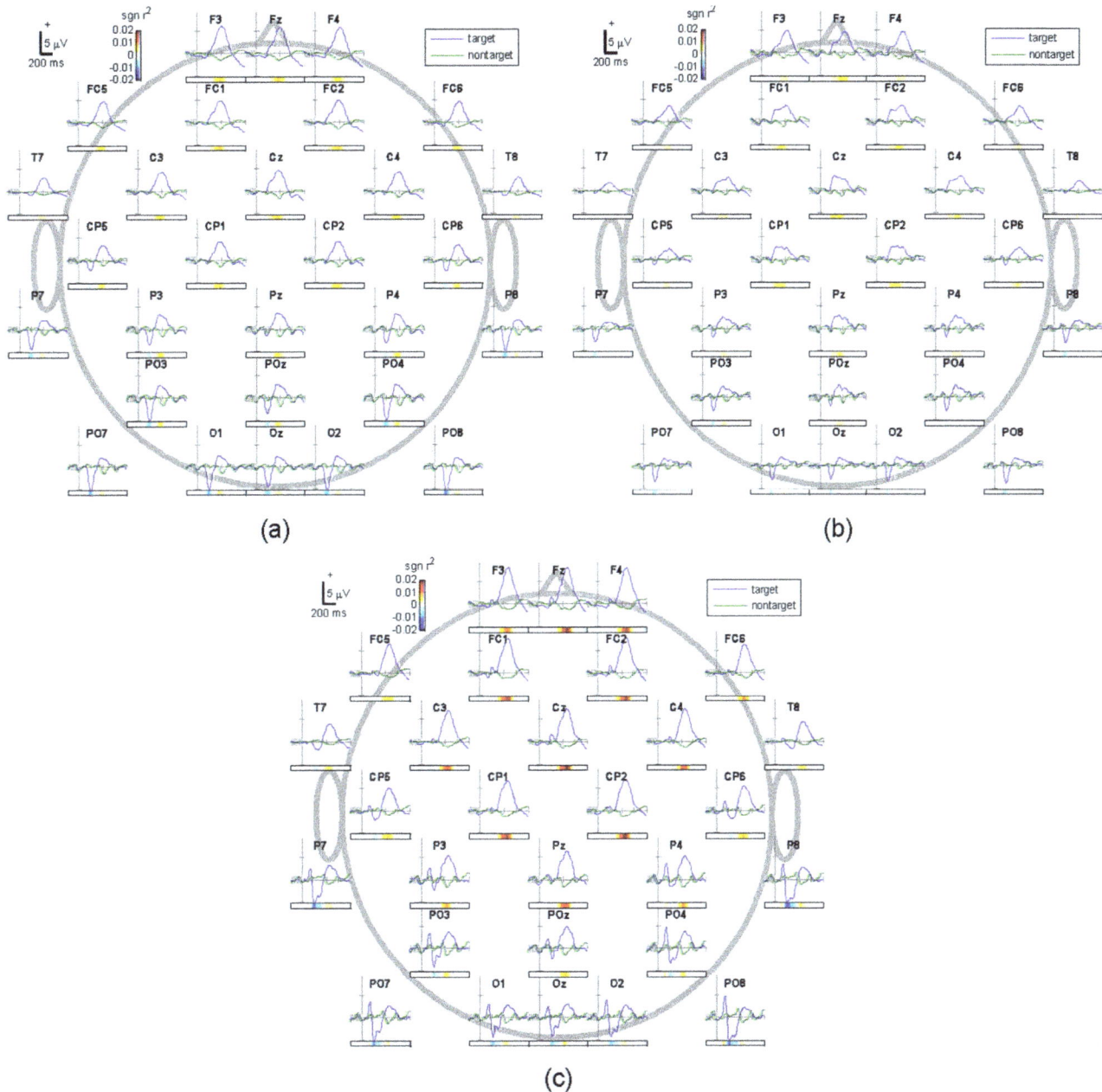

Figure 5. Topographic plots of grand average ERP waveform derived from the target and non-target stimuli for all 15 participants at 29 electrode channels ((a) RC, (b) RASP, (c) RASP-F). The scales of x and y axes for each channel are the same.

ERP analysis

Figure 5 depicts the grand average ERP waveforms for the target and non-target stimuli for each of the three spellers. Figure 6 shows grand average ERPs and scalp topographies at representative electrodes Cz and PO7.

Table 3 summarizes the differences of ERP components with respect to stimulus patterns. The ANOVA revealed significant N170 and N400f amplitude differences among spellers, especially at central and parieto-occipital sites (see also center of Figure 6). As can be seen in rows 3–4, face stimuli show significantly enhanced N170 as well as N400f components when compares to RC and RASP paradigms. Furthermore, and more interestingly self-face stimuli showed stronger deflections than non-self face

stimuli for P300 and N400f components (row 5; please also compare Figures 7 and 8).

Figure 8 shows statistical differences of brain responses due to the various stimulus presentation patterns as well as stimuli. While brain responses to target stimuli were similar for RC and RASP conditions (A), face-stimuli elicited an additional N170 and a N400f component, related to face-specific processing (B and C). Self-face stimuli showed a greatly enhanced central and parietal N400f component (D).

Error and variation on target-to-target interval analysis

Figure 9 illustrates the topographical distribution of errors in relation to the target item for the RC, RASP, and RASP-F based paradigms. All target items have been centered in this matrix for

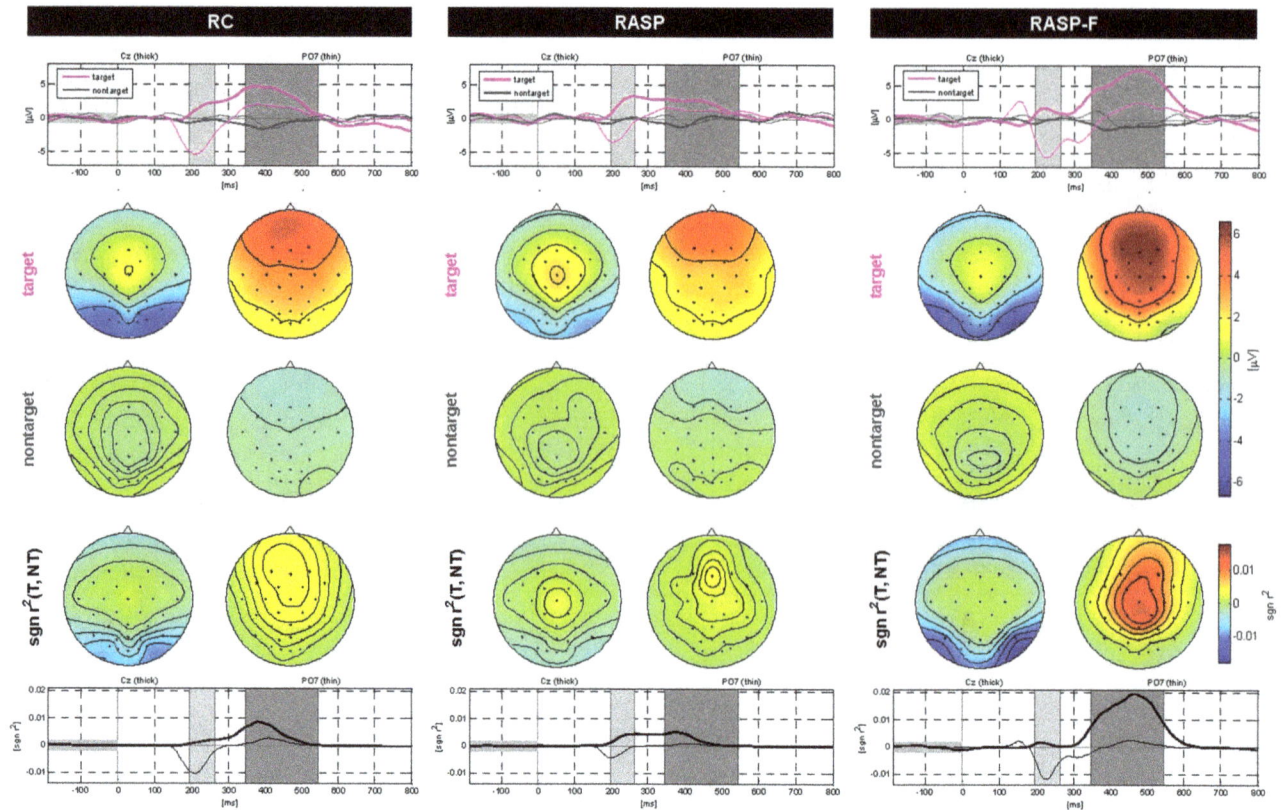

Figure 6. Grand average ERPs and scalp topographies for the three conditions RC, RASP, and RASP-F. Top row: ERPs for targets and nontargets at two selected electrodes Cz and PO7. The two shaded areas in each ERP plot mark the intervals for which scalp maps are shown underneath. Center: The first and second row of scalp plots indicate the ERP responses to the target and nontarget classes. Bottom row: Temporal distribution based on sgn r^2 at two selected electrodes Cz and PO7. The P300 component show a higher discriminability for RASP-F as compared to the two other spellers at the central and parieto-occipital sites.

display purposes; the numbers in the black cells represent the number of correct selections for each paradigm. The numbers in other cells correspond to the locations of errors relative to the target location. In the RC many errors occurred in the direct neighborhood. These non-targets were flashed simultaneously with the target item in the rows and columns. The upper matrices show the results if only one sequence is considered, the lower matrices consider three sequences. As can be seen, the RASP and RASP-F based paradigms successfully reduced the number of errors, because combinations of letters were shuffled within each sequence.

Additionally, we assessed the performance according to the variation of TTIs. Figure 10 depicts the performance with respect to increasing the number of the preceding non-targets between two targets. Value '0' on the x-axis indicates the 'double flashed target' which occured when the same character flashed sequentially. We found that the accuracy for all considered spellers is lower when target items were frequently flashed. This effect was most prominent for less than 3 preceding non-targets. The performance gradually increased when the temporal distance between two target flashes was expanded. A minimum of four TTIs is necessary to ensure optimal performance.

Table 3. Examines differences of ERP components with respect to *target stimuli*.

		N170	P300	N400f
RC - RASP - RASP-F	F(2,28)	6.39**	0.32	11.04***
RC - RASP	t	−3.98**	0.92	1.75
RC - RASP-F	t	−7.31***	0.92	−5.74***
RASP - RASP-F	t	−4.82***	0.46	−6.29***
NSF - SF	t	1.49	5.01***	5.03***

First row: F-values and significance of the repeated measures one-way ANOVA. Next three rows: Show statistical significance (p-values) of ERP components having different means for the three speller conditions (two-sample t-test with the hypothesis of equal means). Last row: Shows p-values of whether ERP components have different means for the non-self face and self-face stimuli.
* - $p < 0.05$ ** - $p < 0.01$ *** - $p < 0.001$

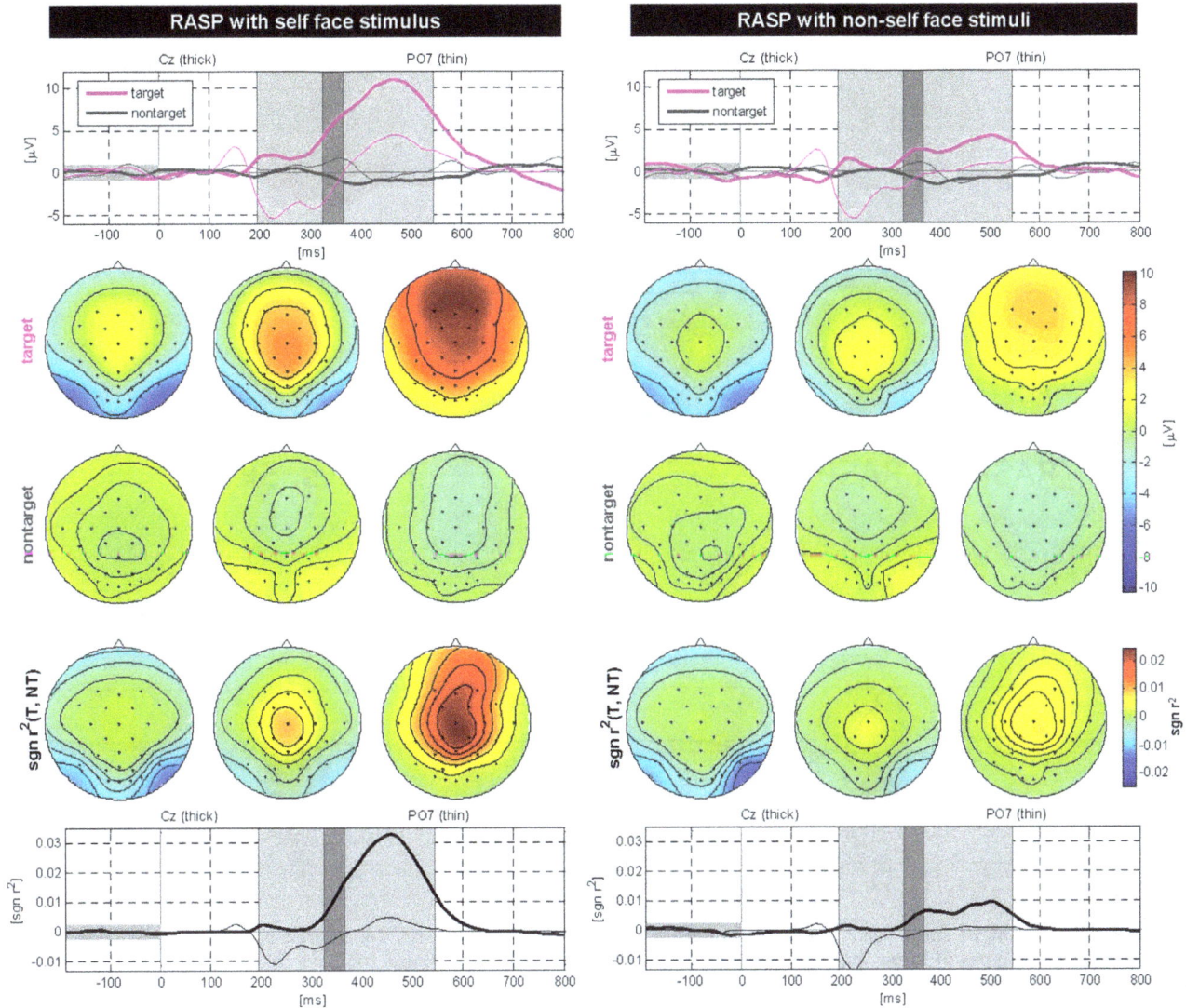

Figure 7. Grand average ERPs and scalp topographies for the self-face and non-self-face stimuli of the RASP-F condition. Top row: ERPs for targets and nontargets at two selected electrodes Cz and PO7. The three shaded areas extract 3 discriminative intervals. Scalp maps are shown underneath using these intervals. Center: The first and second row of scalp plots indicate the ERP responses to the target and nontarget classes. Bottom row: Temporal distribution based on sgn r^2 at two selected electrodes Cz and PO7. ERPs resulting from the self-face stimulus show stronger responses as those of the non-self face stimulus.

Concluding Discussion

Accurate target detection with shorter sequence data continues to be a challenging problem, since the P300 is relatively weak and usually occurs amid some ongoing background brain activities, such as spontaneous EEG as well as other task unrelated noise sources. For this reason the development of new paradigms with more effective 1) visual stimulus types, and 2) stimulus presentation patterns, which elicit stronger differential ERP responses, is considerably important for improving the performance of such BCI systems. In this study we firstly compared a recently proposed presentation method termed 'RASP' to the classic row-column P300-based paradigm and secondly compared (non-) self-face stimuli to the classical approach of simply flashing the characters. As mentioned earlier, related work for random stimulus presentation patterns have been proposed previously [33], however the insight from this previous approach was limited by the fact that two main factors were manipulated concurrently in order to avoid

adjacency-distraction errors as well as *double flash errors*. In this study we are able to confirm previous findings, that a random set presentation approach outperforms the classical row-column paradigm [33]. By following this type of approach the *adjacency-distraction problem* can be diminished to some degree, since now most of the times the neighbouring letters do not flash simultaneously with the target letter. However, this does not eliminate the *double flash problem*. This enables us to study the effects of these two issues independently (see Figure 10). While long TTIs will increase the time for each decision and thus limit ITRs, long TTIs will at the same time increase classification accuracy. A TTI below 3 will reduce accuracy decisively, while a TTI above 4 will not increase classification accuracies enough to justify the time delay this would cause (compare Figure 10).

While the effects of face specific self-representation on brain activity has been researched extensively in the field of cognitive neuroscience [45,54,55], to our knowledge these findings have not been applied to enhance P300-based BCIs. In this study, we

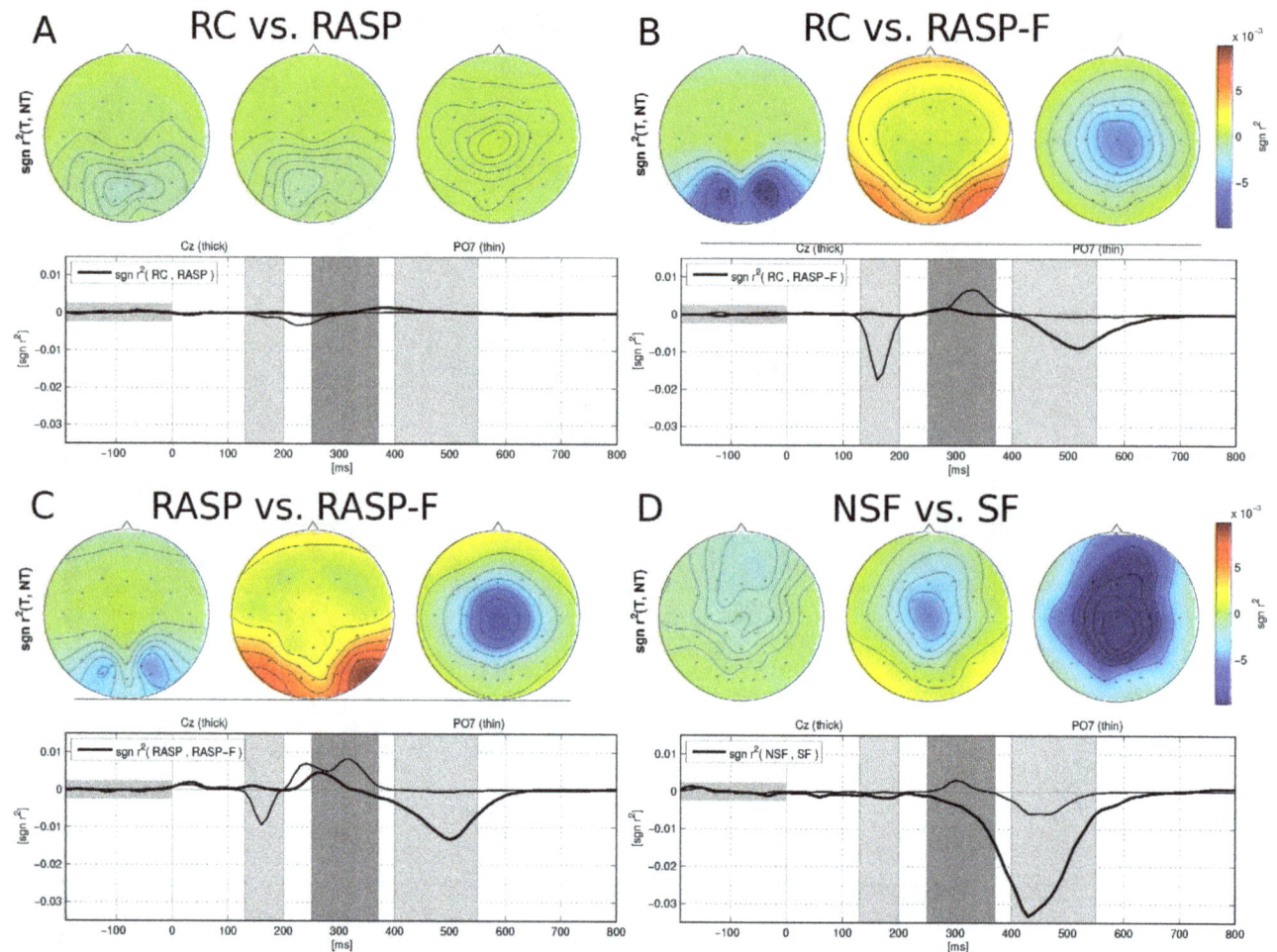

Figure 8. All scalp maps show sign(r^2) **values, comparing** *target stimuli* **for the three considered paradigms (A,B,C) as well as comparing the two types of target stimuli in RASP-F: non-self-face and self-face stimuli (D).** Time courses of sign(r^2) values are given below for two EEG channels (namely 'Cz' and 'PO7').

compared ERP resposes to self-face and non-self-face stimuli. Presentation of self-face stimuli produced ERPs with larger amplitudes (see Figures 5 and 8 as well as Table 3) which resulted in higher discriminability and thus lead to significantly higher classification accuracy between target and non-target characters as compared to non-self face stimuli (see Table 2). Similar findings have previously been obtained for a related setting where familiar and famous faces are compared to unfamiliar faces [40,41].

To further increase the speed of character selection one has to focus on reducing the number of stimulus sequences used for averaging. However, usually several P300 responses must be averaged for the response to be recognized due to the low signal-to-noise ratio [56,57]. By reshuffling and thus creating unique combinations of letters for each flash our findings indicate increased performance for the same number of sequences (see Figure 4). As can be seen from Figure 9 the performance of RASP and RASP-F increases with the number of sequences and significantly outperforms RC consistently. As can be seen from Table 1 interaction of the *type of speller* with respect to accuracy and ITR was significant, however only those subjects who performed considerably well with the RC matrix also performed well with the RASP. In those who did not, the RASP performance seemed to be visibly below that of RASP-F. Still unclear remains how the visual design of the BCI can be improved to meet

peculiarities of peripheral vision such as low spatial acuity and crowding for the RASP paradigm.

Face stimuli including self- and non-self-faces yielded significantly higher accuracies and ITRs than those of highlighted characters for all participants. This implies that stimuli with higher cognitive task requirements such as facial images, are more effective than the intensified stimuli of dull characters for a P300-based BCI system. As already discussed above, previous studies have shown that faces boost BCI performance [40,41,43,44]. Furthermore, familiar and famous faces have been shown to improve BCI performance even more, when compared to unknown faces [40,41]. In this study we have analyzed these finding further by specifically comparing self-face stimuli to non-self-face stimuli; here non-self-face stimuli include unfamiliar as well as familiar faces. Thus our study can ultimately not assess the full combinatorial plentitude of stimulus types previously proposed, namely, unfamiliar vs. familiar, famous vs. familiar, famous vs. unfamiliar, self-faces vs. unfamiliar etc., rather we have chosen a particular abstraction level, i.e. self-face vs. non-self-faces (cf. also a previous study [54], which showed very prominent ERP responses, specifically to self-face stimuli).

In this study, the noticeable offline performance with an accuracy of $84.0\% \pm 1.2\%$ and an ITR of 53.7 ± 11.8 bits/min, when considering single sequences, indicates that the proposed

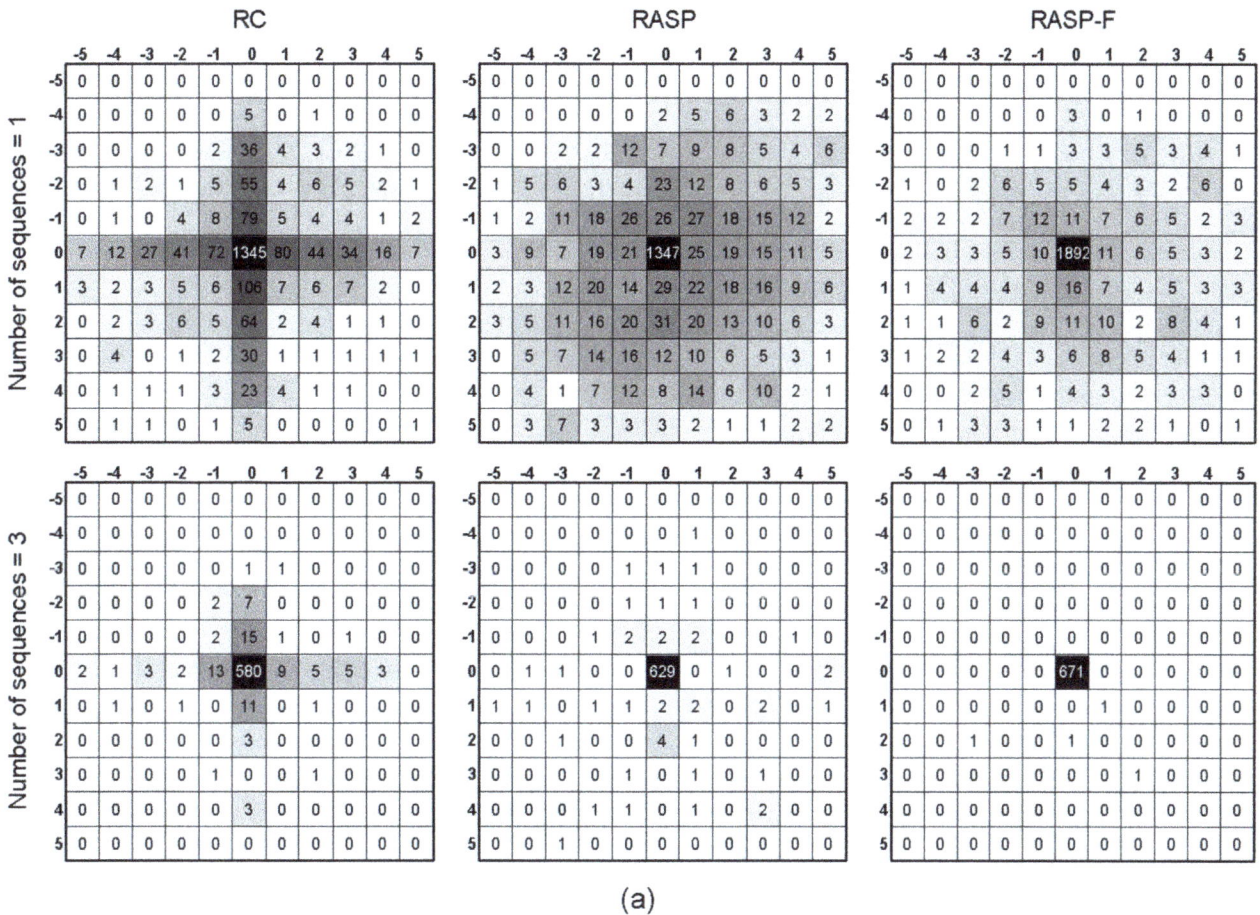

(a)

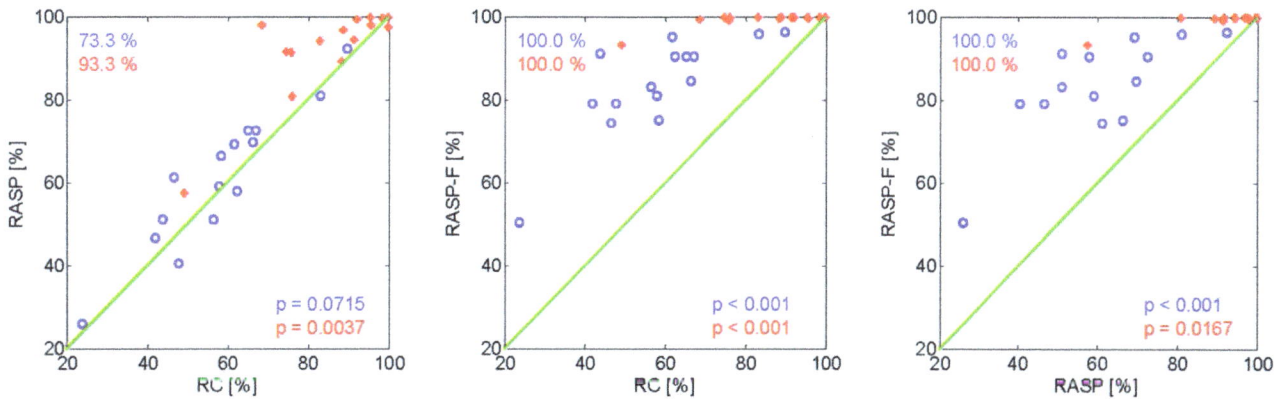

(b)

Figure 9. Performance comparison across spellers as number of sequences is increased. Blue circles used one repetition and red stars three repetitions. (a) Error distributions for the RC (left), RASP (center), and RASP-F (right). All target items have been centered in each matrix. The number in a black centered cell corresponds the number of correct selections and numbers in other cells represents the number of error corrected selections occurring in each cell relative to the target location for each speller. (b) Scatter plot comparing classification accuracies and significance values of various combinations of the three conditions. Each circle represents the classification accuracy of one subject.

paradigm is very promising (see Figure 4). For achieving a performance level of ≥70% (described as the minimum level for communication in the literature [53]) RASP-F can reduce the overall time needed to spell a character by a factor of 2.3 on average in comparison to RC and by a factor of 1.7 in comparison to RASP.

It may be possible to further improve the performance of the proposed BCI by adopting more advanced feature extraction techniques, such as kernel PCA [58] and/or non-linear machine learning techniques, such as logistic regression or support vector machines [59–61].

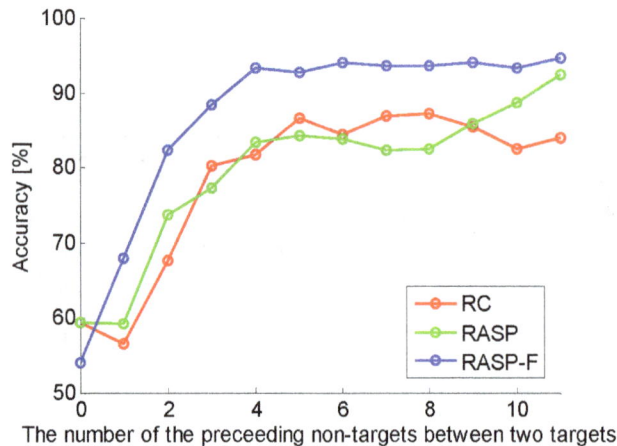

Figure 10. Compares the classification accuracy (y-axis) when increasing the number of non-targets preceding a target stimulus for the three conditions (x-axis). The value '0' of x-axis presents 'double flashed target'.

While some individual variation is evident, the individual participants' averaged ERPs conform to the grand mean shown in Figures 5 and 6, which shows that both the target and non-target ERPs differ in several respects across spellers. N170 amplitudes were significantly enlarged at parieto-occipital sites, when face stimuli were compared to highlighted characters. P300 tends to be more pronounced at the central sites for face stimuli, against those evoked by the highlighted character (RC and RASP). Face stimuli elicited significantly higher P300s than the highlighted character (see Figure 5 and 6). This suggests higher level of cognitive components in the central areas through the face perception task. Such cognitive components associated with face perception result in more discriminative features.

We also checked the neurophysiological phenomena associated with face-specific visual self-representation in a human brain. Our findings show class-discriminative ERP patterns between self-face and non-self-face stimuli (see Figures 7 and 8). Although individual differences of ERP patterns for the face processing exist, the amplitudes of N400f for self-face stimuli were significantly larger than those for non-self-face stimuli. Besides, the N170, which is related to cognitive processing, can show large amplitudes for both self- and non-self-face stimuli.

Summarizing, a novel BCI paradigm combining random set presentation with self-face stimuli has been proposed and developed. The proposed BCI can lead to higher classification accuracy and ITRs than the conventional RC-based paradigm. The performance of the RASP-F condition yielded a single-trial classification accuracy of $84.0\% \pm 1.2\%$ and an ITR of 53.7 ± 11.8 bits/min.

We would like to finally remark that our approach as virtually all other work on P300 spellers is gaze dependent. However, as pointed out in their contribution [28,29,62], a clear path to gaze independent BCI spellers can be pursued (see also a recent patient study contributing to the debate [63]). Future work will therefore extend the present paradigms towards gaze independency.

Acknowledgments

We gratefully acknowledge the use of the BBCI toolbox. The authors thank Benjamin Blankertz and Felix Bießmann for valuable discussions and helpful comments.

Author Contributions

Conceived and designed the experiments: SY KRM SF. Performed the experiments: SY. Analyzed the data: SY SF. Contributed reagents/materials/analysis tools: SY SF SL KRM. Wrote the paper: SY SF SL KRM.

References

1. Mak JN, Wolpaw JR (2009) Clinical applications of Brain–Computer Interfaces: Current state and future prospects. Biomedical Engineering, IEEE Reviews in 2: 187–199.
2. Wolpaw J, Wolpaw EW (2012) Brain–Computer Interfaces: Principles and practice. Oxford University Press.
3. Dornhege G, Millán JR, Hinterberger T, McFarland DJ, Müller KR (2007) Toward Brain–Computer Interfacing. MIT press.
4. Wolpaw JR, Birbaumer N, McFarland DJ, Pfurtscheller G, Vaughan TM (2002) Brain–Computer Interfaces for communication and control. Clinical Neurophysiology 113: 767–791.
5. Kübler A, Kotchoubey B, Kaiser J, Wolpaw JR, Birbaumer N (2001) Brain–Computer communication: Unlocking the locked in. Psychological Bulletin 127: 358.
6. Nijboer F, Sellers E, Mellinger J, Jordan M, Matuz T, et al. (2008) A P300-based Brain–Computer Interface for people with amyotrophic lateral sclerosis. Clinical Neurophysiology 119: 1909–1916.
7. Farwell LA, Donchin E (1988) Talking off the top of your head: Toward a mental prosthesis utilizing event-related brain potentials. Electroencephalography and Clinical Neurophysiology 70: 510–523.
8. Gao S, Wang Y, Gao X, Hong B (2014) Visual and auditory Brain–Computer Interfaces. Biomedical Engineering, IEEE Transactions on 61: 1436–1447.
9. Krusienski DJ, Sellers EW, Cabestaing F, Bayoudh S, McFarland DJ, et al. (2006) A comparison of classification techniques for the P300 speller. Journal of Neural Engineering 3: 299.
10. Sellers EW, Krusienski DJ, McFarland DJ, Vaughan TM, Wolpaw JR (2006) A P300 Event-Related Potential Brain–Computer Interface (BCI): The effects of matrix size and inter stimulus interval on performance. Biological Psychology 73: 242–252.
11. Gibert G, Attina V, Mattout J, Maby E, Bertrand O (2008) Size enhancement coupled with intensification of symbols improves P300 speller accuracy. In: 4th BCI Workshop and Training Course.
12. Martens S, Hill N, Farquhar J, Schölkopf B (2009) Overlap and refractory effects in a Brain–Computer Interface speller based on the visual P300 Event-Related Potential. Journal of Neural Engineering 6: 026003.
13. Takano K, Komatsu T, Hata N, Nakajima Y, Kansaku K (2009) Visual stimuli for the P300 Brain–Computer Interface: A comparison of white/gray and green/blue flicker matrices. Clinical Neurophysiology 120: 1562–1566.
14. Salvaris M, Sepulveda F (2009) Visual modifications on the P300 speller BCI paradigm. Journal of Neural Engineering 6: 046011.
15. Liu T, Goldberg L, Gao S, Hong B (2010) An online Brain–Computer Interface using non-flashing visual evoked potentials. Journal of Neural Engineering 7: 036003.
16. McFarland DJ, Sarnacki WA, Townsend G, Vaughan T, Wolpaw JR (2011) The P300-based brain–computer interface (BCI): Effects of stimulus rate. Clinical Neurophysiology 122: 731–737.
17. Allison BZ, Pineda JA (2006) Effects of SOA and flash pattern manipulations on ERPs, performance, and preference: Implications for a BCI system. International Journal of Psychophysiology 59: 127–140.
18. Jin J, Sellers EW, Wang X (2012) Targeting an efficient target-to-target interval for P300 speller Brain–Computer Interfaces. Medical & Biological Engineering & Computing 50: 289–296.
19. Polprasert C, Kukieattikool P, Demeechai T, Ritcey JA, Siwamogsatham S (2013) New stimulation pattern design to improve P300-based matrix speller performance at high flash rate. Journal of Neural Engineering 10: 036012.
20. Xu N, Gao X, Hong B, Miao X, Gao S, et al. (2004) BCI competition 2003-data set IIb: Enhancing P300 wave detection using ICA-based subspace projections for BCI applications. Biomedical Engineering, IEEE Transactions on 51: 1067–1072.
21. Serby H, Yom-Tov E, Inbar GF (2005) An improved P300-based Brain–Computer Interface. Neural Systems and Rehabilitation Engineering, IEEE Transactions on 13: 89–98.
22. Rivet B, Souloumiac A, Attina V, Gibert G (2009) xDAWN algorithm to enhance evoked potentials: application to Brain–Computer Interface. Biomedical Engineering, IEEE Transactions on 56: 2035–2043.
23. Blankertz B, Lemm S, Treder M, Haufe S, Müller KR (2011) Single-trial analysis and classification of ERP components–A tutorial. NeuroImage 56: 814–825.

24. Krusienski DJ, Sellers EW, McFarland DJ, Vaughan TM, Wolpaw JR (2008) Toward enhanced P300 speller performance. Journal of Neuroscience Methods 167: 15–21.

25. Rakotomamonjy A, Guigue V (2008) BCI competition III: Dataset II-ensemble of SVMs for BCI P300 speller. Biomedical Engineering, IEEE Transactions on 55: 1147–1154.

26. Guger C, Daban S, Sellers E, Holzner C, Krausz G, et al. (2009) How many people are able to control a P300-based Brain–Computer Interface (BCI)? Neuroscience Letters 462: 94–98.

27. Fazel-Rezai R, Abhari K (2009) A region-based P300 speller for Brain–Computer Interface. Electrical and Computer Engineering, Canadian Journal of 34: 81–85.

28. Treder MS, Blankertz B (2010) (C)overt attention and visual speller design in an ERP-based Brain–Computer Interface. Behavioral and Brain Functions 6: 28.

29. Treder MS, Schmidt NM, Blankertz B (2011) Gaze-independent Brain–Computer Interfaces based on covert attention and feature attention. Journal of Neural Engineering 8: 066003.

30. Kindermans PJ, Verschore H, Verstraeten D, Schrauwen B (2012) A P300 BCI for the masses: Prior information enables instant unsupervised spelling. In: Advances In Neural Information Processing Systems 25.

31. Kindermans PJ, Tangermann M, Müller KR, Schrauwen B (2014) Integrating dynamic stopping, transfer learning and language models in an adaptive zero-training ERP speller. Journal of Neural Engineering 11: 035005.

32. Spüler M, Rosenstiel W, Bogdan M (2012) Online adaptation of a c-VEP Brain–Computer Interface (BCI) based on Error-related potentials and unsupervised learning. PloS One 7: e51077.

33. Townsend G, LaPallo B, Boulay C, Krusienski D, Frye G, et al. (2010) A novel P300-based Brain–Computer Interface stimulus presentation paradigm: Moving beyond rows and columns. Clinical Neurophysiology 121: 1109–1120.

34. Townsend G, Shanahan J, Ryan DB, Sellers EW (2012) A general P300 Brain–Computer Interface presentation paradigm based on performance guided constraints. Neuroscience Letters 531: 63–68.

35. Kanwisher NG (1987) Repetition blindness: Type recognition without token individuation. Cognition 27: 117–143.

36. Sanders A, Lamers J (2002) The Eriksen flanker effect revisited. Acta Psychologica 109: 41–56.

37. Jin J, Allison BZ, Sellers EW, Brunner C, Horki P, et al. (2011) Optimized stimulus presentation patterns for an Event-Related Potential EEG-based Brain–Computer Interface. Medical & Biological Engineering & Computing 49: 181–191.

38. Jin J, Allison BZ, Sellers EW, Brunner C, Horki P, et al. (2011) An adaptive P300-based control system. Journal of Neural Engineering 8: 036006.

39. Bentin S, Allison T, Puce A, Perez E, McCarthy G (1996) Electrophysiological studies of face perception in humans. Journal of Cognitive Neuroscience 8: 551–565.

40. Kaufmann T, Schulz S, Grünzinger C, Kübler A (2011) Flashing characters with famous faces improves ERP-based Brain–Computer Interface performance. Journal of Neural Engineering 8: 056016.

41. Kaufmann T, Schulz SM, Köblitz A, Renner G, Wessig C, et al. (2013) Face stimuli effectively prevent Brain–Computer Interface inefficiency in patients with neurodegenerative disease. Clinical Neurophysiology 124: 893–900.

42. Blankertz B, Sannelli C, Halder S, Hammer EM, Kübler A, et al. (2010) Neurophysiological predictor of SMR-based BCI performance. Neuroimage 51: 1303–1309.

43. Zhang Y, Zhao Q, Jin J, Wang X, Cichocki A (2012) A novel BCI based on ERP components sensitive to configural processing of human faces. Journal of Neural Engineering 9: 026018.

44. Jin J, Allison BZ, Kaufmann T, Kübler A, Zhang Y, et al. (2012) The changing face of P300 BCIs: A comparison of stimulus changes in a P300 BCI involving faces, emotion, and movement. PloS One 7: e49688.

45. Miyakoshi M, Kanayama N, Iidaka T, Ohira H (2010) EEG evidence of face-specific visual selfrepresentation. NeuroImage 50: 1666–1675.

46. Ninomiya H, Onitsuka T, Chen CH, Sato E, Tashiro N (1998) P300 in response to the subject's own face. Psychiatry and Clinical Neurosciences 52: 519–522.

47. Yeom SK, Suk HI, Lee SW (2013) Person authentication from neural activity of face-specific visual self-representation. Pattern Recognition 46: 1159–1169.

48. Wintink AJ, Segalowitz SJ, Cudmore LJ (2001) Task complexity and habituation effects on frontal P300 topography. Brain and Cognition 46: 307–311.

49. Lemm S, Blankertz B, Dickhaus T, Müller KR (2011) Introduction to machine learning for brain imaging. NeuroImage 56: 387–399.

50. Wilcoxon F (1945) Individual comparisons by ranking methods. Biometrics 1: 80–83.

51. Siegel S (1956) Nonparametric statistics for the behavioral sciences. McGraw-hill.

52. Bonferroni CE (1936) Teoria statistica delle classi e calcolo delle probabilita. Libreria internazionale Seeber.

53. Kübler A, Birbaumer N (2008) Brain–Computer Interfaces and communication in paralysis: Extinction of goal directed thinking in completely paralysed patients? Clinical Neurophysiology 119: 2658–2666.

54. Keyes H, Brady N, Reilly RB, Foxe JJ (2010) My face or yours? Event-Related Potential correlates of self-face processing. Brain and Cognition 72: 244–254.

55. Uddin LQ, Kaplan JT, Molnar-Szakacs I, Zaidel E, Iacoboni M (2005) Self-face recognition activates a frontoparietal "mirror" network in the right hemisphere: An event-related fMRI study. NeuroImage 25: 926–935.

56. Polich J (2007) Updating P300: An integrative theory of P3a and P3b. Clinical Neurophysiology 118: 2128–2148.

57. Pritchard WS (1981) Psychophysiology of P300. Psychological Bulletin 89: 506.

58. Schölkopf B, Smola A, Müller KR (1998) Nonlinear component analysis as a kernel eigenvalue problem. Neural Computation 10: 1299–1319.

59. Müller KR, Anderson CW, Birch GE (2003) Linear and nonlinear methods for Brain–Computer Interfaces. Neural Systems and Rehabilitation Engineering, IEEE Transactions on 11: 165–169.

60. Bishop CM (2006) Pattern Recognition and Machine Learning, volume 1. springer.

61. Vapnik V (1995) The Nature of Statistical Learning Theory. Springer.

62. Riccio A, Mattia D, Simione L, Olivetti M, Cincotti F (2012) Eye-gaze independent EEG-based Brain–Computer Interfaces for communication. Journal of Neural Engineering 9: 045001.

63. Kaufmann T, Holz EM, Kübler A (2013) Comparison of tactile, auditory, and visual modality for brain-computer interface use: a case study with a patient in the locked-in state. Frontiers in neuroscience 7.

iTBS-Induced LTP-Like Plasticity Parallels Oscillatory Activity Changes in the Primary Sensory and Motor Areas of Macaque Monkeys

Odysseas Papazachariadis[1]*, **Vittorio Dante**[2], **Paul F. M. J. Verschure**[3], **Paolo Del Giudice**[2,4], **Stefano Ferraina**[1]

1 Department Physiology & Pharmacology, Sapienza University Rome, Rome, Italy, **2** Istituto Superiore di Sanità (ISS), Rome, Italy, **3** Laboratory for Synthetic, Perceptive, Emotive and Cognitive Systems, Center of Autonomous Systems and Neurorobotics, ICREA-Universitat Pompeu Fabra, Barcelona, Spain, **4** INFN, Rome, Italy

Abstract

Recently, neuromodulation techniques based on the use of repetitive transcranial magnetic stimulation (rTMS) have been proposed as a non-invasive and efficient method to induce *in vivo* long-term potentiation (LTP)-like aftereffects. However, the exact impact of rTMS-induced perturbations on the dynamics of neuronal population activity is not well understood. Here, in two monkeys, we examine changes in the oscillatory activity of the sensorimotor cortex following an intermittent theta burst stimulation (iTBS) protocol. We first probed iTBS modulatory effects by testing the iTBS-induced facilitation of somatosensory evoked potentials (SEP). Then, we examined the frequency information of the electrocorticographic signal, obtained using a custom-made miniaturised multi-electrode array for electrocorticography, after real or sham iTBS. We observed that iTBS induced facilitation of SEPs and influenced spectral components of the signal, in both animals. The latter effect was more prominent on the θ band (4–8 Hz) and the high γ band (55–90 Hz), de-potentiated and potentiated respectively. We additionally found that the multi-electrode array uniformity of β (13–26 Hz) and high γ bands were also afflicted by iTBS. Our study suggests that enhanced cortical excitability promoted by iTBS parallels a dynamic reorganisation of the interested neural network. The effect in the γ band suggests a transient local modulation, possibly at the level of synaptic strength in interneurons. The effect in the θ band suggests the disruption of temporal coordination on larger spatial scales.

Editor: Robert Chen, University of Toronto, Canada

Funding: OP was supported by a doctoral fellowship of the Sapienza University in Neurophysiology. PDG, SF and VD were supported by the ISS-USA project "Brain reorganization under cortical stimulation - BRUCOS". The funders had no role in study design, data collection and analysis, decision to publish, or preparation of the manuscript.

Competing Interests: The authors have declared that no competing interests exist.

* Email: odysseas.papazachariadis@gmail.com

Introduction

At the basis of the ability of the nervous system to generate adaptive behaviour lie mechanisms of synaptic plasticity such as Long-Term Potentiation (LTP). A clear link between LTP-inducing protocols and the oscillatory activity of neural populations has been reported first in slice preparation and later at a macroscopic level, showing the involvement of θ and γ rhythms in LTP [1,2,3,4,5,6,7,8]. Recently, a similar phenomenon has been observed at a macroscopic level, commonly referred to as LTP-like conditioning. LTP-like conditioning refers mainly to aftereffects of repetitive transcranial magnetic stimulation (rTMS) [9]. Applying rTMS over a cortical area transiently enhances or diminishes the excitability of the area, often with behavioural correlates [9,10]. So far, in vivo evidence of induced oscillatory changes after LTP-like conditioning in a neocortical interconnected neural population is scattered and controversial [11,12,13,14].

A promising methodology to directly characterize stimulation-induced brain response at a cortical level is the combination of TMS with electroencephalography (EEG) [16]. By combining TMS with EEG, we can directly and non-invasively stimulate a cortical area and measure the effects produced by this perturbation both in amplitude and in frequency domains [15,16]. By doing so it has been discovered that single pulse TMS induces short lasting field potential modulations of the neural activity while high-intensity rTMS pulses, induce modulations that last several minutes [17,18,19]. Though neural oscillatory activity is often related to cortical excitability [17,20,21], the relationship between LTP-like induced long-term excitability modulations and continuous neural rhythmic activity remains open.

Intermittent theta burst stimulation (iTBS) constitutes a non-invasive recently developed rTMS stimulation protocol able to induce lasting aftereffects commonly attributed to local LTP-like plasticity mechanisms [10]. The iTBS paradigm consists of repetitive, low intensity TMS pulses, unable to generate a Motor Evoked Potential (MEP) when applied over the primary motor cortex (M_1). iTBS over both the primary somatosensory cortex (S_1) or M_1 leads to an increase in cortical excitability that corresponds to increased-amplitude somatosensory evoked potentials (SEP) [22,23] and MEP [10] respectively, for approximately 30 minutes.

Still, in order to study subtle rhythmic modulations in continuous recordings a more sensitive technique than EEG is needed. Electrocorticography (ECoG) [24,25] has the advantage of having a higher signal to noise ratio over EEG. Additionally, due to the lack of the skull barrier, high frequencies are less attenuated than in EEG studies [26] and recordings can be made from smaller electrodes with denser distribution, thus finely isolating neural populations and delivering greater spatial resolution. In humans, ECoG recordings are applied almost exclusively pre-surgically in epilepsy patients in order to better define the surgical site. As a consequence, the advantage is nulled by the unnecessary risk of applying iTBS over potential epileptic sites and would not be ethically justified [27,28].

We used a monkey model to investigate iTBS-induced aftereffects at the mesoscopic level in the hand region of both S_1 and M_1, a highly interconnected network [29]. We addressed a relatively simple issue: whether and in what way does the network dynamics change between two states, an iTBS-conditioned and an unconditioned state.

Materials and Methods

We used an iTBS protocol to stimulate the sensorimotor area in a non-human primate model and recorded induced oscillatory activity at high spatial and temporal resolution using a custom-made ECoG array. Stimulation intensity was chosen based on MEP evoked using single pulse TMS during preliminary tests. SEP modulation was evaluated during conditioning protocols to probe the effect of iTBS and confirm that rhythm modulations were attributable to iTBS after-effects.

Animal model and Ethics Statement

We performed the experiments in two Macaca mulatta monkeys. Under general anesthesia (isoflurane 1–3% to effect), we surgically mounted a permanent frontal headpost approximately over Fz and circular recording chamber (18 mm in diameter) for chronic neural activity recording over the right hemisphere granting access to the M_1, the central sulcus and the S_1 (Figure 1a). Surgical locations were measured stereotaxically and confirmed by visual inspection after dura opening at the end of the experiment in both animals.

All efforts were made to minimize suffering. Ten minutes prior each experimental session each monkey was sedated with a single shot of Metedomidine (0.02 mg/kg) which ensured approximately 45 minutes of sedation. During the experiments the monkeys were seated on a primate chair in a dimly lit room with their head, arms and legs immobilized. Animal care, housing and surgical procedures were in conformity with the European (Directive 2010/63/UE) and Italian (DD.LL. 116/92 and 26/14) laws on the use of non-human primates in scientific research and were approved (no. 132/2012-C) by the Italian Ministry of Health. The housing conditions and the experimental procedures were in accordance with the recommendations of the Weatherall report (for the use of non-human primates in research). Purpose-bread monkeys were pair-housed in primate cages (Tecniplast, Italy) in an illumination and temperature controlled ambient, and their health and welfare was monitored daily by the researchers and a designated veterinarian. We routinely introduced in the home cage environment, toys to promote their exploratory behaviour. Both monkeys have been used in other experimental protocols at the end of the experimental procedures here described.

Transcranial Magnetic Stimulation Technique

We first applied test stimulations consisting of single pulse TMS delivered through a biphasic high-power magnetic stimulator (Magstim Rapid[2], The Magstim Company Ltd, Whitland, South West Wales, UK) connected to a custom-made figure-of-eight coil with mean loop external and internal diameters of 7 cm and 2 cm, respectively and center-to-center loop distance of 6 cm, (Magstim Company Ltd). The magnetic stimulus had a biphasic waveform with a pulse width of ~300 μs. During the first phase of the stimulus, the current in the centre of the coil flowed toward the handle. The coil was placed over the recording chamber on the optimum scalp position (hot spot) to elicit MEPs in the contralateral first dorsal interosseus muscle. In contrast to human studies, the optimal coil position over the monkey scalp in order to evoke MEPs was found to be tangentially to the scalp with the coil midline pointing away from the scalp midline at 72° inducing postero-anterior followed by antero-posterior (PA-AP) current in the brain (Figure 2). The distance between the coil surface and the brain was, because of the presence of the recording chamber, 17 mm ca. in both monkeys. However, this value is not different of the average coil-cortex distance reported in previous studies in humans [30].

Conditioning stimulation consisted of iTBS delivered over the recording chamber using the above experimental setup. iTBS was applied according to the technique described by Huang et al. (2005) [10] with the coil positioned as described earlier. iTBS consisted of a 2-sec train of magnetic stimulation with triplets of 50 Hz in a 5 Hz rhythm repeated every 10 sec for a total of 190 s (600 pulses) at 80% of the intensity necessary to evoke a 1 mV MEP [10]. It is important to stress that in the studied monkeys during sedation the intensity necessary to evoke a 1 mV MEP increased from an average of 33% to an average of 54% of the maximum stimulator output. Considering the difficulty in measuring active motor threshold in the awake monkey we chose to modify the original iTBS [10] protocol by setting the stimulator intensity slightly lower than the intensity necessary to evoke a 1 mV MEP in the awake monkey, but significantly lower from the intensity necessary to evoke a 1 mV MEP in the sedated monkey, at 27% of the maximum stimulator output. Sham iTBS was delivered with the coil placed orthogonally over the 'hot spot' defined earlier. Experimental sessions were performed with at least 7 days of interval between sessions.

Electromiographic Recording

During test stimulation, in each animal we recorded surface electromyography (EMG) from the first dorsal interosseus muscle using a belly-tendon montage, with two gold plated Ag/AgCl recording electrodes and a ground electrode on the wrist (see Figure 2). The EMG signal was acquired with the notch filter on (45–55 Hz) and a bandpass filter implemented at the 20–1000 Hz band (Magstim Rapid[2], The Magstim Company Ltd, Whitland, South West Wales, UK). The amplitude of MEPs recorded was measured peak to peak (mV) and then averaged. Test TMS pulses over the hot spot for the first dorsal interosseus muscle were applied in order to identify the intensity necessary to evoke a 1 mV MEP average out of 10 consecutive test TMS pulses.

Electrocorticographic Recordings

We recorded continuous epidural ECoG from a custom-made multi-electrode grid, designed and implemented in collaboration with the ISS Lab (Rome) composed of sixteen 2 mm round gold plated electrodes with a 2.5 mm step on a Kapton substrate commonly referenced to the headpost, which ensured a Fz-like reference [31]. The impedance between the electrodes and the reference was kept below 5 kOhm. All recordings with impedance measurements above 5 kOhm were discarded, as high signal to noise ration was considered a key element of the study. Generally, impedance values remained bellow 1 kOhm. A grounding electrode was used on the ipsilateral auricular point. The signal

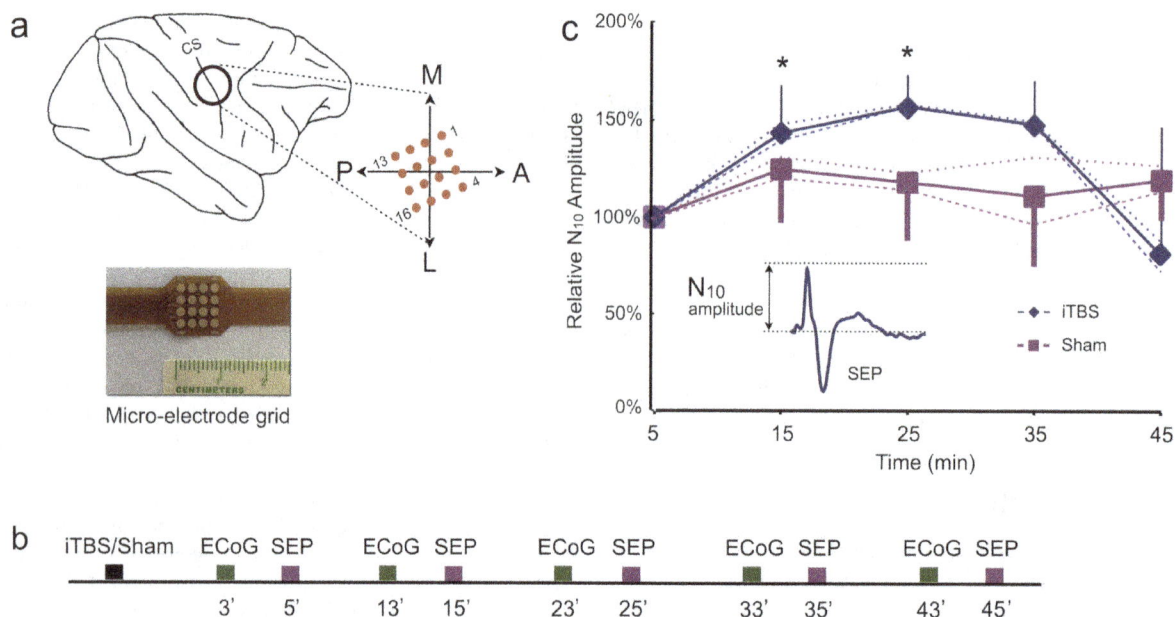

Figure 1. Effect of iTBS-induced LTP-like potentiation, a) schematic electrode distribution over the central sulcus (CS) and the actual epidural grid used during the experiments, b) experimental paradigm timeline, c) iTBS and sham stimulation effect on SEP amplitude. Amplitude is reported as ratios of the first time point (5th min) minute after real or sham iTBS stimulation. N_{10} indicates the signal's negative deflection observed at a latency of about 10 ms in SEP responses (inset). Error bars are standard deviations. Dotted lines represent individual monkeys while continuous lines their average (*p<.01).

from each electrode was amplified, digitised and optically transmitted to a digital signal processing unit were it was acquired at 6 kHz together with the stimulation trigger (Tucker-Davis Technologies, Alachua, FL).

Median Nerve Electrical Stimulation and SEP Recordings

The median nerve was electrically stimulated using a pair of ring electrodes at the left index finger at the level of the collateral ligament between the 1st–2nd and 2nd–3rd phalanx with the cathode proximal and an inter-electrode distance of approximately 1 cm (Figure 2). Square wave pulses (width 0.15 ms; current 15 mA) were delivered with an S88 dual output square pulse stimulator paired to a PSIU6 photoelectric stimulus isolation unit (Grass Technologies, Astro-Med Inc, West Warwick, RI). A ground electrode was placed on the wrist of the hand that was stimulated to minimise the stimulus artifact. Each test experimental block consisted of 300 electric pulses delivered at 10 Hz.

For each conditioning session, the median nerve was stimulated every 10 minutes from 5 to 45 minutes after real or sham iTBS (Figure 1b). To extract evoked potentials from the signal, we selected epochs of 100 ms starting from the time of stimulus onset. The raw signal for each electrode was filtered using a bi-directional FIR bandpass filter (0.3–300 Hz, notch filter 45–55 Hz) and re-referenced to the average of all electrodes. For each electrode we removed the mean value and the linear trend of each epoch and then averaged the signal across epochs. Evoked components were identified as deflections of the signal amplitude that exceeded 2 standard deviations. The amplitude of the first negative deflection in the signal (N_{10}; see Figure 1c, inset), used for statistical analysis, was measured using the electrode over S_1 that presented the least variable signal during the first block and persisted during the session. Electrode location, over M_1 or S_1, was identified according to the phase inversion of the principal SEP components [32] and further confirmed by visual inspection (after

surgically opening the dura at the end of the experiment) of the position of recording chamber vs the central sulcus.

Time-Frequency Analysis

To extract iTBS-induced modulations we focused on five segments of the ECoG signal lasting 1 minute each, obtained every 10 minutes from 3 to 43 minutes after real or sham iTBS (Figure 1b). These segments where free of SEP and stimulation artifacts as SEPs where acquired with an offset of 2 minutes, from 5 to 45 minutes of the experimental session (see *Median Nerve Electrical Stimulation and SEP Recordings*). We calculated the modulations of the power spectral density (PSD) using Welch's averaged modified periodogram method of spectral estimation. We applied the fast Fourier transform over chunks of 8192 points (1.34 sec), with Hanning windowing and 50% overlapping (0.67 sec) and averaged the modulus of the resulting time-frequency coefficient matrix, that is throughout the whole minute to get the mean power estimate (frequency resolution of 0.73 Hz) for each electrode [33]. In order to reduce the complexity of analysis and interpretation, we grouped the electrodes in $M_{1\ (1-8)}$, $S_{1\ (9-16)}$ and S_1–$M_{1\ (1-16)}$ and calculated the arithmetical mean of the power in each group to get the average power for the underlying cortical areas.

We also calculated a coefficient of variation (C_V) for the power of the signal, C_V, across selected electrodes, for every Fourier chunk considered.

$$C_v = \frac{1}{N} \sum_i^N \frac{\sigma_{pow}(i)}{\mu_{pow}(i)}$$

N (ca 90) stands for the number of chunks examined over the one minute period, σ is the variance of the values and μ the mean value across the electrodes encompassed in each group. C_V

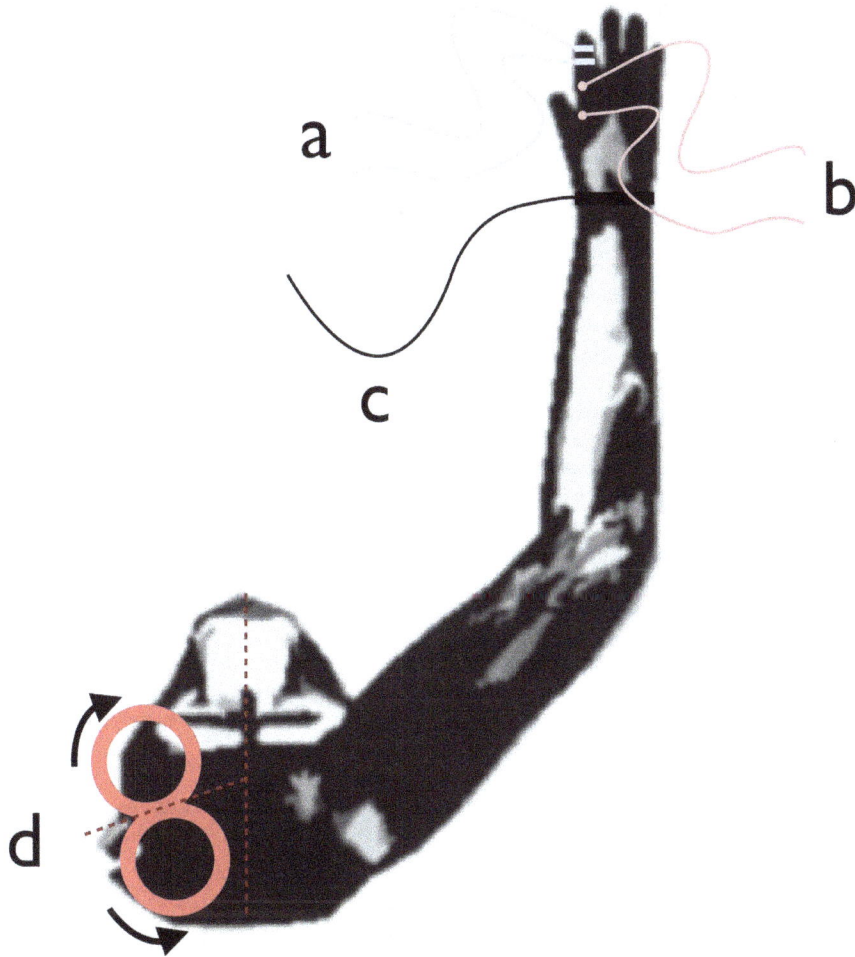

Figure 2. Schematic representation of peripheral nerve stimulation ring electrodes (a), surface electromyographic electrodes on the first dorsal interosseus muscle (b), ground electrode (c) and coil positioning (d) with arrows indicating the current flow.

discloses the spatial constrains of the various oscillatory drives affected and studied. More autonomous activity of the underlying neural population should result in higher C_V values.

Statistical Analysis

We first averaged the band power of the signals and the C_V for δ (1–4 Hz), θ (4–8 Hz), α (9–12 Hz), β (13–26 Hz) low γ (27–45 Hz) and high γ (55–90 Hz) bands.

In order to study the time evolution of iTBS aftereffects we expressed the SEP-N_{10} amplitude, the power spectral distribution and C_V values for each time point as ratios of the first time point values. We applied a repeated-measures ANOVA, with 'Time' (time point after real or sham iTBS) and 'Stimulation' (real iTBS, sham iTBS) as within-subject factors to compare the effect of stimulation on SEP-N_{10} amplitude. We also applied a repeated-measures ANOVA, with 'Time' (time point after real or sham iTBS), 'Site' (M_1, S_1, S_1–M_1) and 'Stimulation' (real iTBS, sham iTBS) as within-subject factors to compare the effect of stimulation on frequency band power and C_V modulations for each band (δ, θ, α, β, low γ, high γ). To disclose differences between subjects, we repeated the above statistics after adding the factor 'Monkey' (Tables S1–S3).

A Pearson rank correlation test was used to assess all possible correlations between TBS-induced changes in SEP-N_{10} ampli-

tudes at all time points, significant power modulations and C_V across bands and sites.

All Post hoc comparisons were performed using Fisher's Least Significant Difference test with the Bonferroni adjustment for multiple comparisons, as in all multiple comparisons here presented. In cases where Mauchly's sphericity test was violated, Greenhouse-Geisser corrected P values where used. All data analysis procedures were implemented with custom routines using Matlab (Mathworks©, MA) and PASW© Statistics.

Results

We performed a total of nine iTBS (five for monkey A and four for monkey I) and six sham experimental sessions (three for each monkey). Results were consistent across monkeys (Tables S1–S3). We observed that the SEP N_{10} component significantly increased in amplitude (Figure 1c) after real but not after sham iTBS [main effect for Time: $F_{1.566,20.353} = 5.499$, $p = .017$; main effect for Stimulation: $F_{1,13} = 1.582$, $p = .231$; Interaction Time*Stimulation: $F_{1.566,20.353} = 6.103$, $p = .012$] (Figure 1c). Post-hoc analysis (Bonferroni $P = .01$) revealed that the stimulation effect was significant at 15 ($p = .005$) and 25 ($p = .3e\text{-}5$) minutes after iTBS.

We observed similar effects after iTBS over the different bands independently of the spatial location of the electrodes (Figure 3), animal (Figure 4) and electrodes (Figure 5). Repeated measures

ANOVA disclosed a significant time trend in both real and sham iTBS sessions for the δ and β band power. We found significant Time-Stimulation interaction differences between real and sham iTBS sessions for the θ, α, low and high γ bands. Detailed results can be found in Table 1. Post-hoc analysis disclosed that real iTBS blocked the activity increase in the θ band, observed during the sham iTBS, at 13 (p = .0001), 23 (p = .005), 33 (p = .0007) and 43 (p = .0005) minutes and in the α band at 23 (p = .009), 33 (p = .001) and 43 (p = .00005) minutes. Conversely, iTBS promoted an activity increase in the low γ band at 13 (p = .000003), 23 (p = .003), 33 (p = .0006) and 43 (p = .0002) minutes after iTBS and high γ band at 13 (p = .000001), 23 (p = .000003) 33 (p = .00005) and 43 (p = .00007) minutes after iTBS. These results were Site independent (see Table 1), thus iTBS induces aftereffects on the signal power of both S_1 and M_1 neural oscillatory activity.

Repeated measures ANOVA with 'Time' (time point after real or sham iTBS), 'Site' (M_1, S_1, S_1–M_1) and 'Stimulation' (real iTBS, sham iTBS), as within-subject factors for each band (δ, θ, α, β, low γ, high γ) disclosed significant C_V modulation after iTBS for the β band for Time-Stimulation interaction and for the high γ band for Time, Stimulation and Time-Stimulation interaction (details in Table 2). Post-hoc analysis disclosed that C_V for the β band decreased significantly at 23 minutes (p = .009), 33 minutes (p = .001) and 43 minutes (p = .003) after real stimulation, as compared to the sham stimulation and C_V for the high γ band increased significantly at 13 minutes (p = .0004), 23 minutes

(p = .001) and 33 minutes (p = .001) after real stimulation, as compared to the sham stimulation (Figure 6).

Pearson correlation test showed that the C_V decrease of the β band was correlated to the β band power decrease in the S_1 (r = .979, p = .004), while the C_V increase of the high γ band was correlated to the transient increase of the high γ band power in S_1 (r = .974, p = .005) and M_1–S_1 (r = .993, p = .001). No significant correlation was found with SEP-N_{10} amplitude and band power or C_V (Table S4).

Discussion

In our study, we explored the iTBS induced neural activity modulation obtained from a custom miniaturised ECoG grid, surgically placed over the sensorimotor region in two sedated monkeys. Our results show that LTP-like aftereffects induced by iTBS modulate the spectral imprint of rhythmic activity both locally and in the interconnected network. iTBS induced changes of local neural interactions, attested by the significant modulation of the power spectrum, and distributed changes attested by the C_V. Regarding the iTBS-induced aftereffects on N_{10}, we confirm the previously reported observations made on humans [22,23].

Several authors reported that TMS pulses over the scalp modulate cortical activity. In a co-registration EEG-TMS study Paus and colleagues (2001) [17], reported that single pulse TMS applied over M_1 induced highly synchronous oscillatory activity in

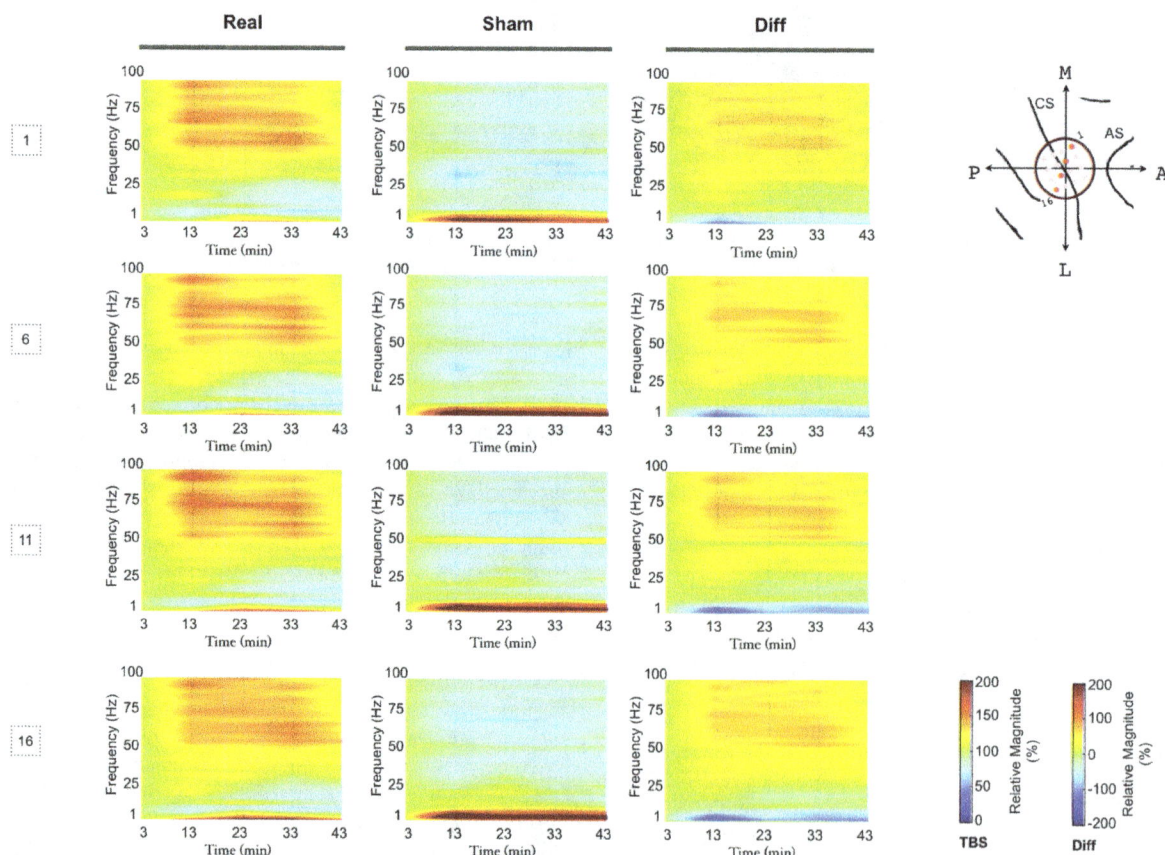

Figure 3. Power spectral density modulation of the signal from M_1 (1 and 6) and S_1 electrodes (11 and 16), as highlighted in the figure (CS: Central Sulcus, AS: Arcuate Sulcus), after iTBS and sham stimulation. Average values of nine sessions of real iTBS (Real) and six sessions of sham iTBS (Sham) are presented, as well as their spectral difference (Diff). Frequency power values for each time point are expressed as ratios of the first time point (3rd min) frequency power values. We interpolated the missing time in the figure by calculated isolines from the time points analysed.

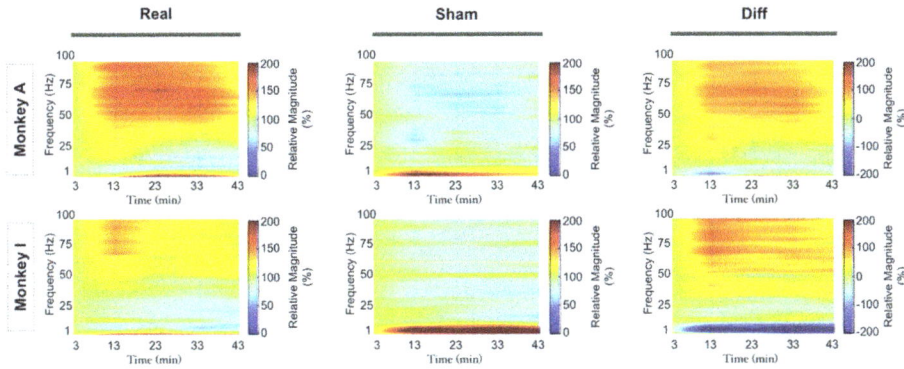

Figure 4. Power spectral density modulation for the signal obtained in the two animals. Real iTBS (Real), sham iTBS (Sham) and spectral difference (Diff) spectrograms for each monkey. Average values of all the electrodes are presented. Frequency power values for each time point are expressed as ratios of the first time point (3rd min) frequency power values. We interpolated the missing time in the figure by calculated isolines from the time points analysed.

the β band that lasted several hundred milliseconds, a finding confirmed by Fuggetta and colleagues (2005) [18] who further showed that single TMS pulses produced neural synchronisation both in α and β range which increased linearly with the TMS intensity within 500 ms. In extracellular recordings, Allen and colleagues [19] observed that immediately after a TMS pulse, oscillatory activity in the γ band tends to increase while lower bands tend to decrease in power. These oscillatory modulations are probably linked to the resetting of the ongoing oscillatory activity and could be considered part of a wider, recently conceived neurophysiological measurements applied to study cortical connectivity and excitability, termed transcranial evoked potentials (TEPs, [36]). However, long lasting modulations of naturally occurring cortical rhythms may require long-term local cortical activity modulation as well as functional reorganization of the neural connections involved. Thus further study of continuous brain rhythmic activity modulation induced by TMS is opportune to clarify the long term aftereffects attributed to LTP-like plasticity.

To our knowledge there are only two published studies that explored the influence of TBS in naturally occurring rhythms, one by Saglam and colleagues (2008) and one by McAllister and colleagues (2012) [11,12]. Both studies, present EEG activity from healthy humans after having applied the continuous TBS paradigm and conclude that though TBS seems to influence rhythmic activity, power modulation never reaches statistical significance. Contrary to trial-averaged event-related studies, continuous EEG recordings do not contain a persistent and recurrent signal that blends with a noisy background and can be brought to light by averaging several trials, but a subtle, more variant signal that is virtually indistinguishable from the noisy background [24,25]. Thus, the lower signal to noise ratio and the spatial blurring of EEG within and between subjects could be responsible for the negative results.

An important difference with respect to previous studies is that in our study subjects were examined in a sedated state. In a sedated state, pulse propagation is compromised, cortical response is amplified, and rhythmic activity is shifted towards slower

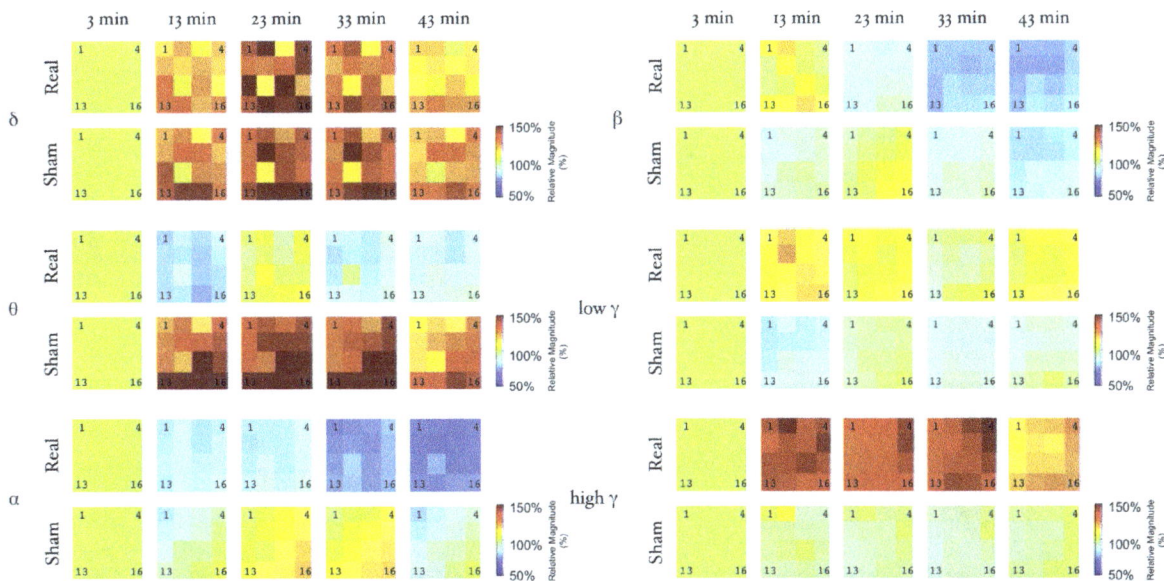

Figure 5. Topographic distribution of power modulation. We present in a grid representation, color-coded power modulation for each electrode of the 16, in every band considered and for every time point as refereed to the baseline period (3 min after iTBS stimulation).

Table 1. RM-ANOVA results for band power modulation in Time (3 min, 13 min, 23 min, 33 min, 43 min) Stimulation (iTBS, Sham) and Site (M_1, S_1, M_1–S_1). Bonferroni corrected P values<.008 (values in bold) were considered significant.

	δ (1–4 Hz)	θ (5–7 Hz)	α (8–12 Hz)	β (13–26 Hz)	low γ (27–45 Hz)	high γ (55–90 Hz)
Time	**F(2.648, 103.2)=12.141, p=2e-6**	F(2.591, 101.05)=4.031, p=.013	F(2.583, 100.72)=3.297 p=.03	**F(2.126, 82.9)=11.157, p=5e-8**	F(2.664, 103.9)=4.422, p=.008	F(2.661, 103.78)=1.354, p=.252
Time *Stimulation	F(2.648, 103.2) =1.228, p=.3	**F(2.591, 101.05)=8.653, p=8e-6**	**F(2.583, 100.72)=5.432, p=.003**	F(2.126, 82.9)=1.905, p=.153	**F(2.664, 103.9)=10.036, p=1e-5**	**F(2.661, 103.78)=12.99, p=8e-7**
Time*Site	F(5.296, 103.2) =.015, p=1	F(5.182, 101.05)=.026, p=1	F(5.165, 100.72)=.065, p=.998	F(4.251, 82.9)=.035, p=.998	F(5.328, 103.9)=.032, p=1	F(5.322, 103.78)=.034, p=1
Time*Site *Stimulation	F(5.296, 103.2) =.11, p=1	F(6.295, 101.05)=.032, p=1	F(5.165, 100.72)=.065, p=.997	F(4.251, 82.9)=.023, p=.999	F(5.328, 103.9)=.009, p=1	F(5.322, 103.78)=.014, p=1
Stimulation	F(1,39)=.979., p=.33	**F(1,39)=14.536, p=4e-4**	**F(1,39)=0.2, p=.004**	F(1,39)=.164, p=.688	**F(1,39)=20.433, p=5e-5**	**F(1,39)=30.693, p=2e-6**
Site	F(2,39)=.003, p=.997	F(2,39)=.044, p=.95	F(2,39)=.15, p=.861	F(2,39)=.107, p=.898	F(2,39)=.06, p=.942	F(2,39)=.019, p=.981
Stimulation *Site	F(2,39)=.02, p=.98	F(2,39)=.051, p=.95	F(2,39)=.146, p=.864	F(2,39)=.057, p=.945	F(2,39)=4e-4, p=1	F(2,39)=.016, p=.984

oscillations [37]. Metedomedine, the administered sedative, is an α_2-agonist that induces a sleep-like state, promoting reliable sedation and anxiolysis [38,39,40]. These effects are mediated by α_2 receptors located primarily in locus coeruleus neurons on the pons and lower brainstem [38,39,40]. Thus, Metedomedine does not disrupt the local cortical network, nor it interferes directly with NMDA or GABA transmission, but it probably provides a state of lesser inputs to the S_1 and M_1 [38,39], which could make the neural populations of these cortical areas more susceptible to external influence by means of TBS. In fact, noradrenergic activity in the thalamus has a blocking effect on the relay cells through α-2 adrenoceptors located on the thalamocortical neurons [38].

Interestingly, the muscle relaxation effect that accompanies sedation is due to inhibition of α_2-receptors at the interneuron level of the spinal cord, which is in line with the significant difference in the intensity necessary to evoke a 1 mV MEP that we found between sedated and awake states [40]. Additionally, significant modulations in time observed for δ and β bands can be related to different stages of sedation that evolves from deep to superficial at the end of the experimental session, when Metedomedine washes off.

A less critical difference between the experimental paradigm here described and other similar paradigms [22,23] is the assumption of a baseline immediately after instead of before the

Table 2. RM-ANOVA results for the coefficient of variability (C_V) modulation in Time (3 min, 13 min, 23 min, 33 min, 43 min) Stimulation (iTBS, Sham) and Site (M_1, S_1, M_1–S_1).

	δ (1–4 Hz)	θ (5–7 Hz)	α (8–12 Hz)	β (13–26 Hz)	low γ (27–45 Hz)	high γ (55–90 Hz)
Time	F(3.215, 125.395) =2.153, p=.092	F(3.028, 118.111) =2.058, p=.109	F(2.610, 101.8)=2.506, p=.071	F(2.478, 96.623)=4.465, p=.009	F(2.101, 81.928)=2.654, p=.074	**F(3.221, 125.62)=5.978, p=.001**
Time *Stimulation	F(3.215, 125.395) =1.814, p=.144	F(3.028, 118.111) =2.135, p=.099	F(2.610, 101.8)=4.044, p=.013	**F(2.478, 96.623)=5.035, p=.005**	F(2.101, 81.928)=2.080, p=.129	**F(3.221, 125.62)=4.999, p=.002**
Time*Site	F(6.430, 125.395) =.377, p=.902	F(6.057, 118.111) =.688, p=.661	F(5.220, 101.8) =.532, p=.759	F(4.955, 96.623)=.227, p=.949	F(4.201, 81.928)=.457, p=.776	F(6.442, 125.62)=.256, p=.963
Time*Site *Stimulation	F(6.430, 125.395) =.479, p=.834	F(6.057, 118.111) =.322, p=.926	F(5.220, 101.8) =.090, p=.995	F(4.955, 96.623)=.084, p=.994	F(4.201, 81.928)=.435, p=.792	F(6.442, 125.62)=.450, p=.855
Stimulation	F(1, 39)=1.109, p=.299	F(1, 39)=.172, p=.680	F(1, 39)=6.801, p=.013	F(1, 39)=6.880, p=.012	F(1, 39)=.012, p=.914	**F(1, 39)=12.691, p=.001**
Site	F(2, 39)=.649, p=.528	F(2, 39)=1.431, p=.251	F(2, 39)=2.166, p=.128	F(2, 39)=.624, p=.541	F(2, 39)=.828, p=.444	F(2, 39)=.082, p=.922
Stimulation *Site	F(2, 39)=.416, p=.662	F(2, 39)=.608, p=.549	F(2, 39)=.004, p=.996	F(2, 39)=.295, p=.746	F(2, 39)=.634, p=.536	F(2, 39)=.526, p=.595

Bonferroni corrected P values<.008 (values in bold) were considered significant.

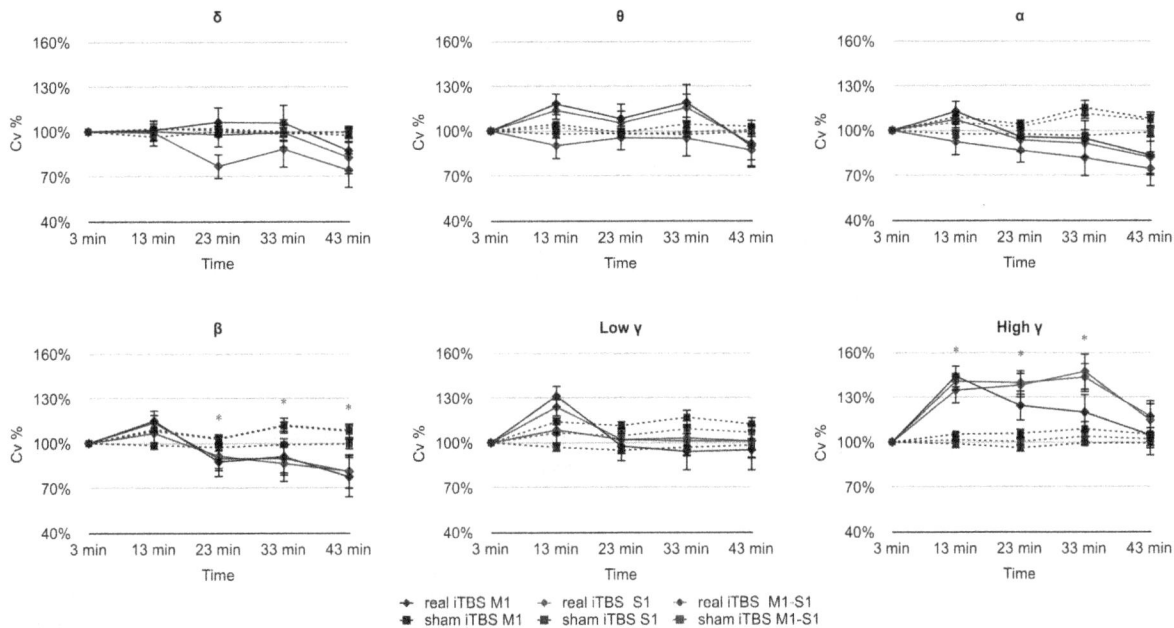

Figure 6. Modulation of the C_V for the bands considered. Real iTBS aftereffects are marked by continuos lines while dashed lines indicate sham iTBS aftereffects. Note the raise of the high γ band C_V in M_1, S_1 and M_1–S_1 after real iTBS and the small but significant fall of the β band (*p<.01).

iTBS conditioning. We adopted the former approach for two main reasons. Firstly, we decided not to stimulate through the multi-electrode grid in order to avoid magnetic line deformation and exposure of the animal to possible risks due to heating of the metal elements. Secondly, though multi-electrode grid positioning was controlled by anatomical landmarks, manipulation of the multi-electrode grid during testing sessions occasionally resulted in failure to maintain precise adherence and position, that we considered to be crucial in order to compare the different time points during each session. Thus, the multi-electrode grid was applied immediately after each iTBS conditioning protocol and removed daily at the end of the experimental session.

Classically, iTBS aftereffects grow from 3–15 min and maximum aftereffects are observed at 15–25 min interval after iTBS conditioning [10,22,23]. Additionally, iTBS aftereffects tend to recede at 35–45 min after iTBS conditioning. Hence, in our experimental paradigm we included most of the expected iTBS-induced modulated neural activity.

A crucial parameter of the iTBS protocol is the TMS stimulation intensity. A single high-intensity TMS pulse induces massive cortical activation lasting seconds, distributed across layers, with interneurons showing the shortest latency to respond, followed by axonal activation of thalamo-cortical and cortico-cortical afferent fibers [41,42]. In M_1, the resulting indirect activation of pyramidal cells, often generated by long polysynaptic networks or recurrent synaptic networks, induces the propagation of a cortico-spinal action potential and an observable MEP [41]. It has been suggested that iTBS, delivered at comparatively low intensities, unable to evoke a MEP, targets mainly interneurons, in contrast to high-intensity TMS pulses [10].

Interneuronal involvement in the iTBS aftereffects is also supported by the modulation of the power spectral density in our data. Interneuron activity is closely related to both θ and γ band activity [1,43,44]. In vivo, in vitro and simulation data portray the interneurons as the principal neural population involved in γ band oscillatory activity modulation [1,44,45,46]. In the neocortex, γ band activity has been observed to originate form superficial layers

2/3 that mainly include interneurons [47], while recently Ahmed and Mehta (2012) [48] proposed that γ band modulations are correlated with changes in the firing rate of individual interneurons also in the hippocampus. Thus, the γ band power modulation we observed in sensorimotor cortex further supports the hypothesis that iTBS increases cortical excitability by affecting interneurons.

We found modulations in both high and low frequency band power in both monkeys (Figure 4). Field potentials from epidural electrodes highlight the common action of neurons because of neural topographical arrangement combined with the dynamic coordination of neurons and depend on the underlying functional network [34]. As higher frequency oscillatory activity are thought to reflect the coordination of smaller ensembles of cortical neurons [51,52], the rise in γ power is consistent with the activation of local cortical loops [35], also supported by the global rise of the C_V. Lower oscillation frequencies on the other hand reflect long-range coupling [2,4,50], so that diminished θ and α power may indicate the disruption of a large-scale distributed network, possibly involving thalamo-cortical couplings. In summary, the results we report here suggest that after iTBS conditioning, local sets of neurons are brought together into coherent ensembles, while remote connections are inhibited, thereby establishing a long-lasting reorganisation [35,52].

To measure whether the ECoG activity observed simultaneously in selected electrodes was clustered or dispersed after real iTBS, with respect to sham iTBS, for each considered electrode group (S_1, M_1, S_1–M_1) we computed the C_V measure (see Methods). For each time segment, the more inhomogeneous the electrical activity was, the higher was the C_V. After real iTBS high γ band C_V increased transiently and fell back towards the end of the experimental session, while after sham iTBS high γ band C_V remained globally uninfluenced (Figure 6). Conversely, iTBS aftereffects on β band C_V decreased after real iTBS and never completely recovered during the experimental session, while after sham iTBS, again, β band C_V remained uninfluenced globally. Thus, regional activity in the β band was more homogeneous while the activity in the γ band was increased and more irregular.

One explanation may come from the local origin of both bands. In the neocortex, γ band oscillations are prominent in layers 2/3, which contains cells of similar properties that mainly project horizontally, while beta-band oscillations seem to originate from layers 5/6 [47,49]. It has been proposed that a regulating network between these two neural populations exists [47,49]. Neuronal populations situated in layers 2/3 generate synchronous oscillations in the γ band that propagate information to layers 5/6, which generate oscillations in the β band, under some circumstances [47,49]. The role of the layers 2/3 neural populations in this network is feed-forward, while layers 5/6 populations have a feed-back role [47,49]. We believe that rise in magnitude and irregularity of the γ band is consistent with a feed-forward mechanism that evolves in local synchronisation, while more regular β band activity reflects a broader feed-back process. It should also be noted that while high γ band C_V modulations have an early onset, β band C_V modulations arise only after γ band modulations reach significant levels. While more experiments are needed to provide an accurate accounting of our results, our data indicate that iTBS also modulates local cortical activity distributions.

Our study had some limitations. Although iTBS induces mainly focal LTP-like aftereffects and we used a small focal figure-of-eight coil, we found significant modulation in most of the electrodes, spanning from M_1 to S_1, as the topographical distribution of induced currents comprises the whole recording chamber. Moreover, a distant epicortical or deep brain recording would be of extreme usefulness in interpreting our data. Finally, it is difficult to generalize the outcome of our study in non-human primates to humans.

In conclusion, we found that iTBS modulated the spectral imprint of the area studied. We propose that spectral modulation is achieved by transiently reorganising the synaptic strength of interneurons promoting local cortical high-frequency oscillation and inducing a transient "deafferentation" of the targeted neural population. The down-modulation in the θ band (quite homogeneous among electrodes) suggests that this reorganisation could disrupt large-scale coordination. Our findings are in line with the accepted view that LTP phenomena underlie iTBS aftereffects. The similarity of our results to the θ and γ oscillatory activity modulation found in the hippocampus circuitry during LTP protocols [2] may point to a common plasticity backbone in both

the neocortex and the hippocampus. Recently Siebner and Ziemann (2010) [53] cautiously drew a relationship between the frequency of naturally occurring neural oscillatory activity and those induced by external stimuli, speculating on the role the latter have in effectively boosting cortical oscillations. Further studies will establish the exact mechanism through which iTBS induces plastic after-effects. The lack of invasive studies examining the mechanism underlying TMS-induced LTP-like plasticity is remarkable. Considering that TMS techniques are routinely applied on humans, knowledge gaps should be filled for safety, methodological and neurophysiological reasons.

Supporting Information

Table S1 RM-ANOVA results for SEP N_{10} modulation in Time (3 min, 13 min, 23 min, 33 min, 43 min), Stimulation (iTBS, Sham) and Monkey (Monkey I vs Monkey A).

Table S2 RM-ANOVA results for band power modulation in Time (3 min, 13 min, 23 min, 33 min, 43 min), Stimulation (iTBS, Sham), Site (M1, S1, M1–S1) and Monkey (Monkey I vs Monkey A).

Table S3 RM-ANOVA results for coefficient of variation (C_v) modulation in Time (3 min, 13 min, 23 min, 33 min, 43 min), Stimulation (iTBS, Sham), Site (M_1, S_1, M_1–S_1) and Monkey (Monkey I vs Monkey A).

Table S4 Correlation coefficient between SEP N_{10} amplitude, band power and coefficient of variation Cv for each Site (M_1, S_1, M_1–S_1).

Author Contributions

Conceived and designed the experiments: OP. Performed the experiments: OP. Analyzed the data: OP SF. Contributed reagents/materials/analysis tools: SF VD PFMJV OP PDG. Wrote the paper: OP SF PDG PFMJV. Designed and tested the custom epidural grid: VD PDG SF OP.

References

1. Buzsáki G (1996) The hippocampo-neocortical dialogue. Cereb Cortex 6: 81–92.
2. Buzsáki G (2010) Neural syntax: cell assemblies, synapsembles, and readers. Neuron 68: 362–385.
3. Diba K, Buzsáki G (2007) Forward and reverse hippocampal place-cell sequences during ripples. Nat Neurosci 10: 1241–1242.
4. Buzsáki G, Draguhn A (2004) Neuronal oscillations in cortical networks. Science 304: 1926–1929.
5. Girardeau G, Benchenane K, Wiener SI, Buzsáki G, Zugaro MB (2009) Selective suppression of hippocampal ripples impairs spatial memory. Nat Neurosci 12: 1222–1223.
6. Izaki Y, Akema T (2008) Gamma-band power elevation of prefrontal local field potential after posterior dorsal hippocampus-prefrontal long-term potentiation induction in anesthetized rats. Exp Brain Res 184: 249–253.
7. Kahana MJ, Seelig D, Madsen JR (2001) Theta returns. Curr Opin Neurobiol 11: 739–744.
8. Rutishauser U, Ross IB, Mamelak AN, Schuman EM (2010) Human memory strength is predicted by theta-frequency phase-locking of single neurons. Nature 464: 903–907.
9. Bütefisch CM, Davis BC, Wise SP, Sawaki L, Kopylev L, et al. (2000) Mechanisms of use-dependent plasticity in the human motor cortex. Proc Natl Acad Sci U.S.A. 97: 3661–3665.
10. Huang Y, Edwards M, Rounis E, Bhatia K, Rothwell JC (2005) Theta burst stimulation of the human motor cortex. Neuron 45: 201–206.
11. Saglam M, Matsunaga K, Murayama N, Hayashida Y, Huang YZ, et al. (2008) Parallel inhibition of cortico-muscular synchronization and cortico-spinal excitability by theta burst TMS in humans. Clin. Neurophysiol 119: 2829–2838.
12. McAllister SM, Rothwell JC, Ridding MC (2011) Cortical oscillatory activity and the induction of plasticity in the human motor cortex. Eur J Neurosci 33: 1916–1924.
13. Noh NA, Fuggetta G, Manganotti P, Fiaschi A (2012) Long lasting modulation of cortical oscillations after continuous theta burst transcranial magnetic stimulation. PLoS ONE. 7: e35080.
14. Thut G, Pascual-Leone A (2010) A Review of combined TMS-EEG studies to characterize lasting effects of repetitive TMS and assess their usefulness in cognitive and clinical neuroscience. Brain Topogr 22: 219–232.
15. Ilmoniemi RJ, Virtanen J, Ruohonen J, Karhu J, Aronen HJ, et al. (1997) Neuronal responses to magnetic stimulation reveal cortical reactivity and connectivity. Neuroreport 8: 3537–3540.
16. Komssi S, Kähkönen S (2006) The novelty value of the combined use of electroencephalography and transcranial magnetic stimulation for neuroscience research. Brain Res Rev 52: 183–192.
17. Paus T, Sipila P, Strafella A (2001) Synchronization of neuronal activity in the human primary motor cortex by transcranial magnetic stimulation: an EEG study. J Neurophysiol 86: 1983–1990.
18. Fuggetta G, Fiaschi A, Manganotti P (2005) Modulation of cortical oscillatory activities induced by varying single-pulse transcra- nial magnetic stimulation intensity over the left primary motor area: A combined EEG and TMS study. Neuroimage 27: 896–908.

19. Allen EA, Pasley BN, Duong T, Freeman RD (2007) Transcranial magnetic stimulation elicits coupled neural and hemodynamic consequences. Science 317: 1918–1921.
20. Mehring C, Rickert J, Vaadia E, Cardosa de Oliveira S, Aertsen A, et al. (2003) Inference of hand movements from local field potentials in monkey motor cortex. Nat Neurosci 6: 1253–1254.
21. van Elswijk G, Maij F, Schoffelen JM, Overeem S, Stegeman DF, et al. (2010) Corticospinal Beta-Band Synchronization Entails Rhythmic Gain Modulation. J Neurosci 30: 4481–4488.
22. Katayama T, Rothwell JC (2007) Modulation of somatosensory evoked potentials using transcranial magnetic intermittent theta burst stimulation. Neurophysiol Clin 118: 2506–2511.
23. Katayama T, Suppa A, Rothwell JC (2010) Somatosensory evoked potentials and high frequency oscillations are differently modulated by theta burst stimulation over primary somatosensory cortex in humans. Clin Neurophysiol 121: 2097–2103.
24. Crone NE, Miglioretti DL, Gordon B, Lesser RP (1998) Functional mapping of human sensorimotor cortex with electrocorticographic spectral analysis. II. Event-related synchronization in the gamma band. Brain 121: 2301–2315.
25. Gevins A, Cutillo B, Desmond J, Ward M, Bressler S, et al. (1994) Subdural grid recordings of distributed neocortical networks involved with somatosensory discrimination. Electroencephalogr Clin Neurophysiol 92: 282–290.
26. Pfurtscheller G, Cooper R (1975) Frequency dependence of the transmission of the EEG from cortex to scalp. Electroencephalogr Clin Neurophysiol 38: 93–96.
27. Bae EH, Schrader LM, Machii K, Alonso-Alonso M, Riviello JJ Jr, et al. (2007) Safety and tolerability of repetitive transcranial magnetic stimulation in patients with epilepsy: a review of the literature. Epilepsy Behav. 10: 521–528.
28. Oberman L, Edwards D, Eldaief M, Pascual-Leone A (2011) Safety of theta burst transcranial magnetic stimulation: a systematic review of the literature. J Clin Neurophysiol 28: 67–74.
29. Kaas JH (2004) Evolution of somatosensory and motor cortex in primates. Anat Rec A Discov Mol Cell Evol Biol 281: 1148–1156.
30. Kozel FA, Nahas Z, deBrux C, Molloy M, Lorberbaum JP, et al. (2000) How coil-cortex distance relates to age, motor threshold, and antidepressant response to repetitive transcranial magnetic stimulation. J Neuropsychiatry Clin Neurosci 12: 376–384.
31. Papazachariadis O, Dante V, Ferraina S (2013) Median nerve stimulation modulates extracellular signals in the primary motor area of a macaque monkey. Neuroscience Letters, 550: 184–188.
32. Allison T, McCarthy G, Wood CC, Jones SJ (1991) Potentials evoked in human and monkey cerebral cortex by stimulation of the median nerve. A review of scalp and intracranial recordings. Brain 114: 2465–2503.
33. Halliday DM, Rosenberg JR, Amjad AM, Breeze P, Conway BA, et al. (1995) A framework for the analysis of mixed time series/point process data–theory and application to the study of physiological tremor, single motor unit discharges and electromyograms. Prog Biophys Mol Biol 64: 237–278.
34. Buzsáki G, Anastassiou C, Koch C (2012) The origin of extracellular fields and currents–EEG, ECoG, LFP and spikes. Nat Rev Neurosci 13: 407–420.
35. Varela F, Lachaux JP, Rodriguez E, Martinerie J (2001) The brainweb: phase synchronization and large-scale integration. Nature Rev Neurosci 2: 229–239.
36. Casali AG, Casarotto S, Rosanova M, Mariotti M, Massimini M (2010) General indices to characterize the electrical response of the cerebral cortex to TMS. Neuroimage 49: 1459–1468.
37. Alkire MT, Hudetz AG, Tononi G (2008) Consciousness and anesthesia. Science 5903: 876–880.
38. Nasrallah FA, Lew SK, Low ASM, Chuang KH (2014) Neural correlate of resting-state functional connectivity under α2 adrenergic receptor agonist, medetomidine. NeuroImage 84: 27–34.
39. Buzsáki G, Kennedy B, Solt VB, Ziegler M (1991) Noradrenergic control of thalamic oscillation: the role of α-2 receptors. Eur J Neurosci 3: 222–229.
40. Sinclair M (2003) A review of the physiological effects of α2-agonists related to the clinical use of medetomidine in small animal practice. Can Vet J 44: 885–897.
41. Hallett M (2007) Transcranial magnetic stimulation: a primer. Neuron 55: 187–199.
42. Huerta PT, Volpe BT (2009) Transcranial magnetic stimulation, synaptic plasticity and network dynamics. J Neuroeng Rehabil 2: 6–7.
43. Buzsáki G (1998) Memory consolidation during sleep: a neurophysiological perspective. J Sleep Res 7 Suppl 1: 17–23.
44. Wang XJ, Buzsáki G (1996) Gamma oscillation by synaptic inhibition in a hippocampal interneuronal network model. J Neurosci 16: 6402–6413.
45. Traub RD, Whittington MA, Colling SB, Buzsáki G, Jefferys JG (1996) Analysis of gamma rhythms in the rat hippocampus in vitro and in vivo. J Physiol 493: 471–484.
46. Buia CI, Tiesinga PH (2008) Role of interneuron diversity in the cortical microcircuit for attention. J Neurophysiol 99: 2158–2182.
47. Arnal LH, Giraud AL (2012) Cortical oscillations and sensory predictions. Trends Cogn Sci 16: 390–398.
48. Ahmed OJ, Mehta MR (2012) Running speed alters the frequency of hippocampal gamma oscillations. J Neurosci 32: 7373–7383.
49. Wang X (2010) Neurophysiological and computational principles of cortical rhythms in cognition. Physiol Rev 90: 1195–1268.
50. Engel AK, Fries P, Singer W (2001) Dynamic predictions: oscillations and synchrony in top-down processing. Nature Rev Neurosci 2: 704–716.
51. von Stein A, Sarnthein J (2000) Different frequencies for different scales of cortical integration: from local gamma to long range alpha/theta synchronization. Int J Psychophysiol 38: 301–313.
52. Ray S, Crone NE, Niebur E, Franaszczuk PJ, Hsiao SS (2008) Neural correlates of high-gamma oscillations (60–200 Hz) in macaque local field potentials and their potential implications in electrocorticography. J Neurosci 45: 11526–11536.
53. Siebner HR, Ziemann U (2010) Rippling the cortex with high-frequency (> 100 Hz) alternating current stimulation. J Physiol 15: 4851–4852.

19

A Simple ERP Method for Quantitative Analysis of Cognitive Workload in Myoelectric Prosthesis Control and Human-Machine Interaction

Sean Deeny[1,2], Caitlin Chicoine[1¤], Levi Hargrove[1], Todd Parrish[2], Arun Jayaraman[1,2]*

1 Rehabilitation Institute of Chicago, Center for Bionic Medicine, Chicago, IL, United States of America, **2** Northwestern University, Feinberg School of Medicine, Chicago, IL, United States of America

Abstract

Common goals in the development of human-machine interface (HMI) technology are to reduce cognitive workload and increase function. However, objective and quantitative outcome measures assessing cognitive workload have not been standardized for HMI research. The present study examines the efficacy of a simple event-related potential (ERP) measure of cortical effort during myoelectric control of a virtual limb for use as an outcome tool. Participants trained and tested on two methods of control, direct control (DC) and pattern recognition control (PRC), while electroencephalographic (EEG) activity was recorded. Eighteen healthy participants with intact limbs were tested using DC and PRC under three conditions: passive viewing, easy, and hard. Novel auditory probes were presented at random intervals during testing, and significant task-difficulty effects were observed in the P200, P300, and a late positive potential (LPP), supporting the efficacy of ERPs as a cognitive workload measure in HMI tasks. LPP amplitude distinguished DC from PRC in the hard condition with higher amplitude in PRC, consistent with lower cognitive workload in PRC relative to DC for complex movements. Participants completed trials faster in the easy condition using DC relative to PRC, but completed trials more slowly using DC relative to PRC in the hard condition. The results provide promising support for ERPs as an outcome measure for cognitive workload in HMI research such as prosthetics, exoskeletons, and other assistive devices, and can be used to evaluate and guide new technologies for more intuitive HMI control.

Editor: Blake Johnson, ARC Centre of Excellence in Cognition and its Disorders (CCD), Australia

Funding: This research was supported by the National Institute on Disability and Rehabilitation Research (NIDRR) (H133F120017), and the American Orthotic and Prosthetic Association (AOPA) (EBP-043012). The funders had no role in the study design, data collection and analysis, decision to publish, or preparation of the manuscript.

Competing Interests: The authors have declared that no competing interests exist.

* Email: a-jayaraman@northwestern.edu

¤ Current address: University of Chicago, Pritzker School of Medicine, Chicago, IL, United States of America

Introduction

The fields of rehabilitation and medical technology have seen significant recent advances that incorporate human-machine interaction (HMI), including the use of exoskeletons designed to enable ambulation in patients with spinal cord injury (SCI) and stroke [1,2], robotic aids for surgery [3], and myoelectric control of prostheses using electromyographic (EMG) signals from residual muscles [4]. As the field of HMI in rehabilitation and medicine rapidly evolves, so do attempts to increase the ease of use and decrease the cognitive demand on the user. A recent example includes incorporating haptic feedback in robotic surgery designed to reduce cognitive overload [5].

In the field of prosthetics, the past decade has seen advances in human interaction for controlling prosthetic limbs with improved myoelectric control strategies [6], improved prosthesis design [7], and implantable electrodes for high-performance neural control of robotic limbs [8,9]. Surgical techniques such as targeted muscle reinnervation (TMR), which allows transfer of residual limb nerves to alternative muscle sites for facilitation of EMG signals have been pioneered to enhance prosthesis control [10]. TMR has even

been shown to enable the potential for somatosensory feedback in amputee patients [11,12,13], which may significantly reduce the attentional demands of using a prosthesis since users currently rely on visual feedback for tasks such as grasping [14]. All of these advances are intended to make prosthesis control as intuitive and functional as possible since basic activities of daily living, such as dressing, toileting, and ambulation can be very challenging for individuals with amputations. As such, calls for future research have included studies on cognitive workload in conjunction with development of new technologies to improve performance [15].

Researchers and clinicians in prosthetics have made recent efforts to review, improve, and validate outcome measures for prosthetic limb users [16,17], however, most assessments currently used are qualitative, relying on subjective observations from clinicians or self-reports from subjects [18]. More broadly, in the field of HMI, some studies have employed self-report scales such as the NASA Task Load Index (NASA-TLX), however, such scales are also subjective [19]. Despite efforts to improve prosthetics and HMI by reducing the attentional burden, standardized methods for objectively quantifying cognitive workload in the field of HMI, rehabilitation, and prosthetics have not been established. More objective approaches to understanding cognitive strategies and workload in prosthetics and rehabilitation have included efforts to measure eye gaze [20,21]. Although gaze behavior, blinking rate, and pupil dilation can reflect cognitive workload, they can also reflect other environmental and task factors such as ambient light [21,22]. Such applications of eye tracking behavior remain promising, especially when used in conjunction with measures of cortical dynamics [23].

The electroencephalogram (EEG) offers the potential to examine cognitive effort with precise temporal resolution and freedom of movement during data collection, facilitating adaptability to clinical, operational, or real-world settings [24,25,26,27]. Remarkably, although efforts to use measures of cortical dynamics such as EEG are increasingly abundant in the literature for control of assistive devices [28,29,30,31,32,33,34], EEG measures of cognitive workload for evaluation of new HMI technologies have not been adapted and applied to this field.

One EEG approach is based on the allocation of neural resources to a primary task, and the subsequent "attentional reserve" available for the processing of any additional demands [35]. Event-related potentials (ERPs) are EEG peaks averaged in the time domain and time-locked to discrete stimuli. ERPs have been used to examine cognitive workload during task performance based on the inverse relationship between cognitive workload of the primary task, and the amplitude of ERPs elicited by the secondary task or probe. When cognitive demand on the primary task is high, ERP amplitudes to a secondary stimulus are low, reflecting the reduced available neural resources allocated to process the distractor under high cognitive workload [30].

Early ERP studies employed dual-task paradigms, whereby the participants were engaged in a primary cognitive task while simultaneously attending to a secondary auditory or visual target-detection task [35,36,37,38]. However, secondary discrimination tasks can alter the nature of the primary task [39], leading some researchers to adopt a strategy of using an irrelevant probe to elicit ERPs during primary task performance [40,41,42]. The irrelevant probe method is more conducive to preserving the ecological validity of the primary task, and more generalizable to naturalistic situations [43]. To maximize the saliency of the probe stimuli and optimize the attentional response, recent studies have used of rare novel sounds in place of common tones [42,44]. Miller and colleagues [42] combined this approach with graded manipulation of task difficulty to examine cognitive workload while participants played the video game Tetris. The graded difficulty included three conditions: passively watching (view), playing at level 1 (easy), and playing at level 8 (hard). The authors found that four ERP components, including the N100, P200, P300, and late positive potential (LPP), significantly distinguished cognitive workload in the three conditions, all exhibiting an inverse relationship between amplitude and level of difficulty. The early ERP components are thought to reflect obligatory perceptual processing of the auditory stimulus (N100, P200), and later ERP components are thought to reflect cognitive evaluation of the stimulus [45,46]. However, the early components have also been shown to be sensitive to attention and cognitive workload [41,42,44].

Myoelectric Limb Control: Direct Control (DC) and Pattern Recognition Control (PRC)

Several advanced prosthetic limbs have recently reached the market [47] and several more are in development. The most promising approach to controlling such advanced devices is myoelectric control, or use of EMG signals from residual muscles. The conventional method of myoelectric control, called direct control (DC), uses the amplitude of the EMG signal from a single muscle to control a single movement. As such, DC requires a pair of agonist/antagonist muscles (e.g. biceps/triceps) to control a single degree of freedom (DOF), such as hand open/close. Control of two DOFs would require either four separate muscle sites for control (two sets of agonist/antagonist muscles), or a mechanism for switching between DOFs while using the same two muscles. A newer method of myoelectric control, called pattern recognition control (PRC) extracts features from the EMG signal associated with the intended movement of the patient, and passes them to a classifier, which outputs them as a movement class label (e.g. hand close). The algorithms can be trained for multiple DOFs (e.g. hand open/close, wrist extension/flexion, and wrist pronation/supination) enabling the patient to make movements in all three DOFs just by thinking about making the natural movement in the phantom limb. As such, researchers have speculated that PRC is more intuitive and lower in cognitive burden than DC. However, this has not been empirically tested using an objective measure of cognitive workload.

Statement of Purpose

The purpose of this study was to establish the efficacy and potential of a new outcome measure for cognitive workload in prosthetics research, and to compare the relative cognitive workload of two different prosthetic control approaches using the new measure. EEG/ERPs have been shown to reflect cognitive workload in previous studies, while allowing the participant to execute ecologically valid tasks such as baggage screening [23] or video gaming [48], and were explored here for application to clinical studies examining prosthetic limb use. Healthy control participants engaged in a myoelectrically controlled virtual arm task under three conditions: simply watching the arm move (view), moving the hand in 1 DOF (easy), and moving the hand in 3 DOF (hard). Participants were trained and tested using DC, the most successful clinically available method, and a state-of-the-art PRC approach. ERPs were examined for differences in amplitude between the three levels of difficulty, and compared between DC and PRC conditions. Based on previous reports, we expected the amplitude of the ERPs to exhibit an inverse relationship to the level of difficulty of the virtual arm task, which would confirm the potential for this as a measure of cognitive workload in future prosthetic and rehabilitation technology research.

Materials and Methods

Participants

Twenty intact-limb individuals were recruited to participate in the study. All participants were inexperienced in using myoelectric control strategies. The sample size was determined based on a power analysis from previously published data [42]. Two participants were excluded from analysis following data collection due to excessive noise in the EEG signal, therefore, 18 participants (7M/11F) ranging in age from 21–38 years (mean = 26.6) were included in the analysis.

Ethics Statement

Written, informed consent was provided by all participants to participate in the study. The study was specifically approved by the Northwestern University institutional review board (IRB) (Ref no.: STU00062490).

Procedures

Participants were trained and tested using both DC and PRC, with the order counter balanced. Participants made four visits to the Rehabilitation Institute of Chicago (RIC) over two weeks. The first visit was to train on one of the two myoelectric control strategies (DC or PRC), and the second visit during the same week was for testing during collection of EEG. The same procedure was followed the next week on the other myoelectric control strategy.

Myoelectric Control of the Virtual Arm

Myoelectric control of the virtual arm was accomplished using a software suite developed at the RIC called Control Algorithms for Prosthetic Systems (CAPS). CAPS was designed for clinical testing and training of patients using myoelectric inputs to control real-time avatar motion with both DC and PRC algorithms, and supports communication with external programs. The use of CAPS for target acquisition testing in 3 DOF has been previously reported in patients with transradial amputation [49], and was used in the current paper. EMG inputs for virtual arm control were acquired using six bipolar EMG electrodes placed in predetermined positions on the forearm (Figure 1a). Only Channels 1 and 2 were used to control the virtual arm in the DC condition, and all six channels were used in the PRC condition. Electrodes 1 and 2 were placed to optimize amplitude acquired during wrist flexion and extension, respectively. Channels 3 and 4 were placed equidistant to channels 1 and 2 on the medial and lateral sides of the forearm. Channels 5 and 6 were placed distally on the dorsal and ventral aspects of the wrist. Signals were amplified and high-pass filtered at 20 Hz, and data were sampled at 1 kHz by an analog-to digital converter (USB-1616FS; Measurement Computing Corp, Norton, Massachusetts). For the DC condition, gains were set to optimize control of the hand, and to optimize switching between DOFs. Switching was accomplished in DC using a co-contraction of the flexor and extensor muscles by making a fist and relaxing in quick succession. In the PRC condition, participants performed movements to train the algorithms for the appropriate DOFs.

Training. All six electrodes were applied to the non-dominant arm during training in both conditions for consistency. After the electrodes were applied, the signals were viewed and checked for quality using a signal viewing tool within CAPS. Participants then performed 20 trials in each single DOF (wrist extension/flexion, wrist pronation, supination, hand open/close) for a total of 60 trials to practice for the easy condition. Participants then completed a total of 40 trials in the hard condition, which required moving the virtual arm in all 3 DOFs to complete the trial (Figure 1).

Testing. The virtual limb was presented on a 17″ monitor connected to a computer that ran the CAPS software integrated with Matlab for presentation of sounds and associated EEG triggers. Testing consisted of three conditions: 1) passively viewing the virtual hand execute the 3DOF condition; 2) performing the 1DOF task for 24 trials in each of the three degrees of freedom (easy); 3) performing 32 trials of the the 3DOF task (hard). Participants received the view condition first 50% of the time (view, easy, hard), and last 50% of the time to counterbalance the novelty of the sounds across conditions (easy, hard, view); participants always completed the easy task prior to the hard task. Trials consisted of a "+" in the center of the screen as a visual prompt prior to start of the trial, followed by presentation of the task cue, consisting of the current position of the hand in gray, superimposed over the flesh colored target position of the hand. Participants had four seconds to plan the movement prior to receiving a "Go" stimulus to start moving. Moving prior to the

"Go" stimulus would result in no movement of the virtual hand. Successfully moving the virtual hand over the target position resulted in the hand turning green and completion of the trial. If they did not successfully reach the target position within 24 seconds, the trial ended and the hand turned yellow before beginning the next trial. Participants received auditory probes at random intervals during the trials (0–3 probes per trial) (Figure 1). The novel distractor sounds were the same as those used in Miller et al., (2011), which were selected from Fabiani et al., (1996) [50].

EEG. Continuous EEG was recorded during testing using a lycra cap, (Electro-Cap International Inc.). Data were acquired from 16 sites adapted from the 10–20 system [51] and referenced to the left earlobe (A1). Eye channels were place above and below the left eye, and on the outer canthi of both eyes to record eyeblinks. Impedances were kept below 10 KΩ, and channels were amplified 1000 times using Neuroscan Synamps^2 with a sampling rate of 1000 Hz. Online bandpass filters were set from .01–100 Hz. ERPs were obtained by extracting epochs from 100 ms pre-stimulus onset to 10 00 ms post-stimulus onset, baseline correcting on the pre-stimulus interval, and bandpass filtering from 1–15 Hz. Each epoch was visually inspected for artifact, and trials with excessive movement or blinks were deleted ("trials" in the ERP analysis refers to the number of auditory probes, and subsequent single-trial ERPs, not the number of task trials). At least 30 trials in each condition were used for averaging; in the event that 30 clean trials were not available for each condition, the participant was excluded from analysis. The mean amplitude for each ERP component at sites Fz, Cz, and Pz (frontal, central, and parietal midline sites, respectively) was calculated using the method reported by Handy [52], and used in Miller et al., [42]. Narrow time windows for each peak were centered around the grand average peak, and average amplitude was calculated in the following time windows: N100 = 105–120 ms; P200 = 190–205 ms; P300 = 295–330 ms; LPP = 570–590 ms.

Performance. The target acquisition testing in CAPS generates log files during testing for performance analysis. The percentage of trials successfully completed in each condition, and time to complete successful trials (seconds) was examined.

Self-report. Immediately after completion of testing in the DC condition and the PRC condition participants filled out a self-report questionnaire indicating the perceived difficulty of controlling the arm. The questions were taken from questionnaires commonly administered by clinicians at the RIC (Appendix Survey S1). It consisted of 7 questions on a five-point Likert scale, with questions 1, 3, and 7 reverse scored such that a high score reflected a high level of perceived difficulty.

Statistical Design. Our primary hypothesis was that the ERPs would reveal differences in cognitive workload between the view, easy, and hard conditions, and that those ERPs that reflected cognitive workload as a main effect would also distinguish PRC and DC during the hard condition. To assess the efficacy of the ERPs for delineating cognitive workload, main effects on the cognitive workload factor were analyzed using 3 (view, easy, hard) ×2 (DC, PRC) repeated measures ANOVAs. Separate ANOVAs were conducted on average amplitude for each peak reported to reflect cognitive workload previously using this paradigm [Miller et al., [42]]: N1 (Cz), P2 (Fz, Cz, Pz), P3 (Pz), and LPP (Pz). To compare differences between myoelectric control conditions, two-tailed paired-samples t-tests were conducted in the easy and hard conditions on peaks that exhibited main effects for cognitive workload in both the current analysis, and in Miller et al. Performance results (% correct, time to complete trials) were compared between DC and PRC in each condition (easy, hard) using two-tailed paired-samples t-tests. Self-report was compared

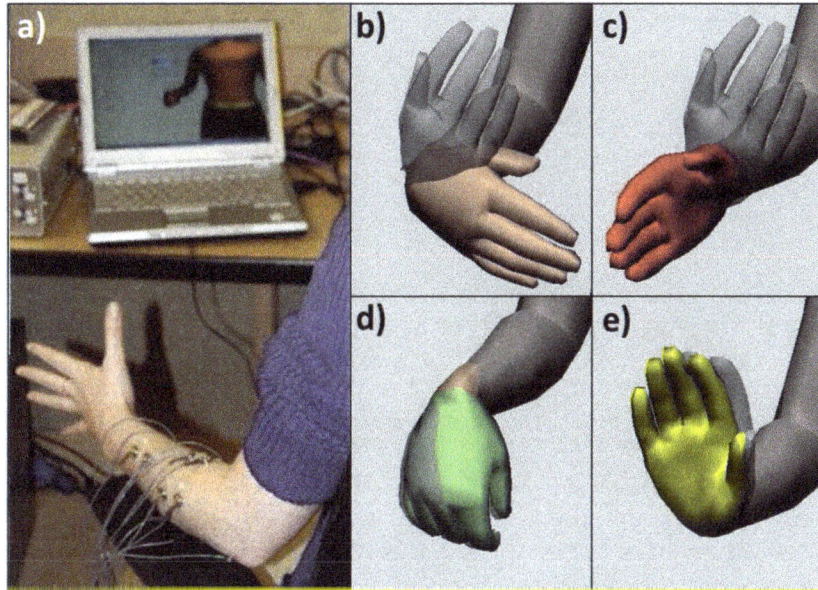

Figure 1. Electrode setup and virtual arm task in CAPS. a) Participant controlling the virtual arm using six bipolar electrodes (three visible in image) affixed to the non-dominant forearm. The small "go" text box above the virtual hand signals when the trial begins. b) The flesh-colored hand indicates the current hand position, and the gray hand indicates the target position. c) In the DC condition, a red hand flash indicates successful switching of the DOF through co-contraction of electrodes 1 and 2. d) Successfully acquiring the hand position results in the hand turning green and the end of the trial. e) If the target position is not successfully acquired within 24 sec, the hand turns yellow and a new trial begins.

between DC and PRC using a two-tailed paired samples t-test. Simple correlations were also examined between ERPs exhibiting cognitive workload effects and performance, ERPs and self-report, and self-report and performance.

Results

EEG analysis

Figure 2 illustrates the strong general inverse relationship between ERP amplitudes and cognitive workload for P200, P300, and LPP. Main effects and ERPs are pictured for electrodes Cz and Pz, where most of the effects occurred. No significant main effects or interactions emerged for cognitive workload on the N1 component. Consistent with Miller et al. (2011) [42], the main effects for cognitive workload were significant at all three electrode sites (Fz, Cz, Pz) for P200: Fz ($F_{2,34} = 5.15$; p = 0.011), Cz ($F_{2,34} = 12.90$; p<0.001), and Pz ($F_{2,34} = 5.03$; p = 0.012). P200 effects at Cz and Pz are pictured in Figure 2 (a–d). Post-hoc tests revealed that for P200 at Cz, the view condition differed from both the easy and hard conditions. For P200 at Fz and Pz, the hard conditions differed from the view conditions. Significant main effects emerged on P300 at Pz ($F_{2,34} = 7.67$; p = 0.002) and LPP at Pz ($F_{2,34} = 5.61$; p = 0.008), and are pictured in Figure 2 (b, e, f). For both P300 and LPP, pots-hoc testing revealed that the hard conditions were significantly different from the view conditions.

To compare DC and PRC, two-tailed paired samples t-tests were run on hard conditions for P200 (Fz, Cz, Pz), P300 (Pz), and LPP (Pz), which all showed main effects for cognitive workload. Because t-tests do not control for multiple comparisons like Tukey HSD, the number of analyses was limited to only the peaks that exhibited significant main effects in the current study, and were also reported to be significant in Miller et al. [42]. A significant difference in average amplitude in the hard condition emerged for LPP ($t_{17} = -2.35$, p = 0.031), with PRC exhibiting a higher LPP

amplitude relative to DC. Figure 3 illustrates the ERPs at Pz for DC and PRC in the hard condition.

Performance

Figure 4 illustrates the results for trials completed (4a), and time to complete trials (4b). No significant performance differences for percent correct emerged between DC and PRC in either the easy or hard conditions. Mean completion time was significantly lower for DC (2.4 sec, SD = 0.81) relative to PRC (2.8 sec, SD = 0.81) in the easy condition ($t_{17} = -2.34$, p = 0.031), however, it was significantly higher for DC (15.1 sec, SD = 2.18) relative to PRC (12.5 sec, SD = 2.19) in the hard condition ($t_{17} = 3.66$, p = 0.002). The results indicate that DC may be more effective relative to PRC for simple (1 DOF) tasks, but more challenging for complex (3 DOF) tasks.

Self-report

Self-report was not obtained from one participant, so the analyses reflect scores from 17 participants. There were no differences between DC (mean = 15.1, SD = 3.8) and PRC (mean = 16.3, SD = 4.4) on the self-report questions examining difficulty.

Correlations

ERPs exhibiting a cognitive workload effect (P200, P300, LPP) did not correlate significantly with performance in either the DC condition or the PRC condition. This suggests that cortical effort during the tasks was independent of performance. Self-report did correlate significantly with mean completion time in the hard condition for both the DC (r = 0.70, p = 0.002) and PRC (r = 0.64, p = 0.006), however, it did not correlate with ERPs in either the DC or PRC conditions. This result suggests that participants self-rated the difficulty consistent with their performance, and not consistent with the cortical effort required for task completion.

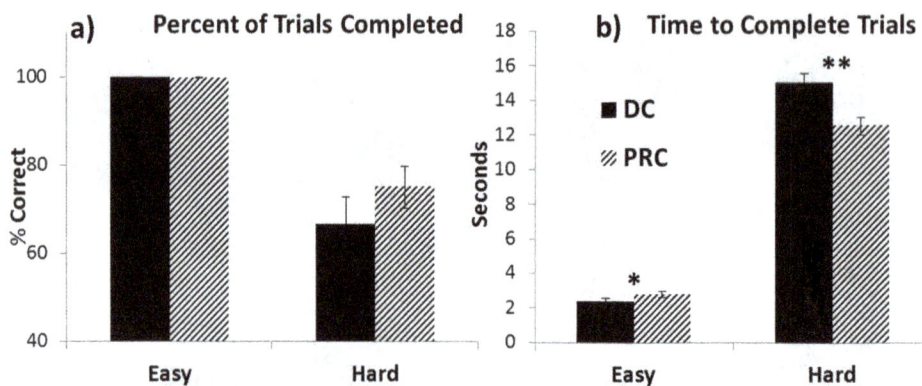

Figure 2. Virtual arm task performance. a) Percentage of trials completed within 24 seconds. b) Average time to complete successful trials; participants performed significantly faster in the easy condition using DC, and significantly faster in the hard condition using PRC (*p<0.05; **p< 0.01.).

Discussion

EEG/ERPs have been explored as measures of cognitive workload during performance of real-world, ecologically valid tasks ranging from flight simulation [37], to video games [42,48], to baggage screening [23], and even soldiers in operational settings [25]. The current study adapted one such approach to examine the use of ERPs as a cognitive workload outcome measure for HMI, specifically, during myoelectric prosthetic limb control. Consistent with previous research, the results indicated an inverse

relationship between ERP amplitude and task difficulty, supporting the efficacy of this measure.

ERPs and Cognitive Workload

Significant main effects of cognitive workload were demonstrated in the omnibus tests for P200, P300, and for LPP. The results are remarkably consistent with the results of Miller et al., [42], who employed the same paradigm to examine cognitive workload during play of the video game Tetris. Consistent with the previous report, P200 exhibited cognitive workload effects across all three sites (Fz, Cz, Pz), with the strongest effect over the vertex (Cz).

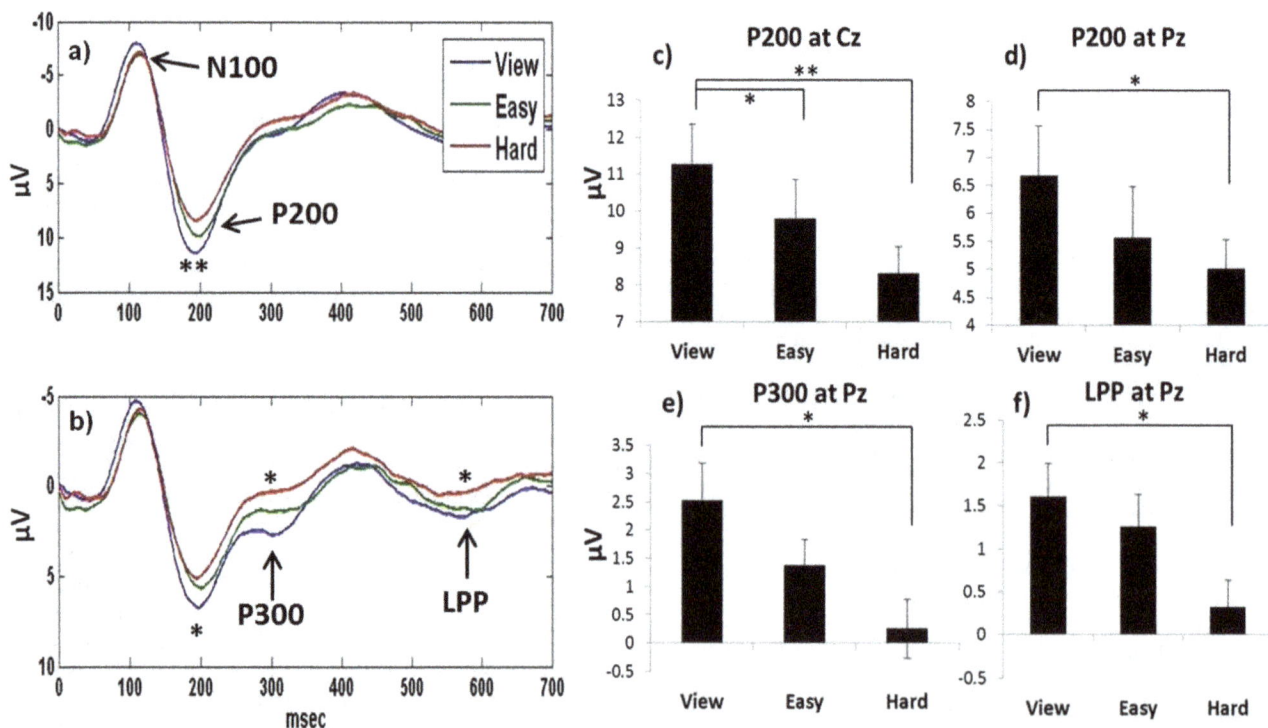

Figure 3. ERPs and main effects for the cognitive workload measure on the view, easy, and hard conditions for DC and PRC combined. Note that positive and negative on the y-axis are traditionally reversed for ERP graphs; as such positive is graphed down. a) Electrode Cz, where the P200 effect was most prominent. b) Electrode Pz, where the P200, P300, and LPP all exhibited cognitive workload effects. c–f) Average amplitude graphs for P200 at Cz and Pz, P300, and LPP (*p<0.05, **p<0.01.).

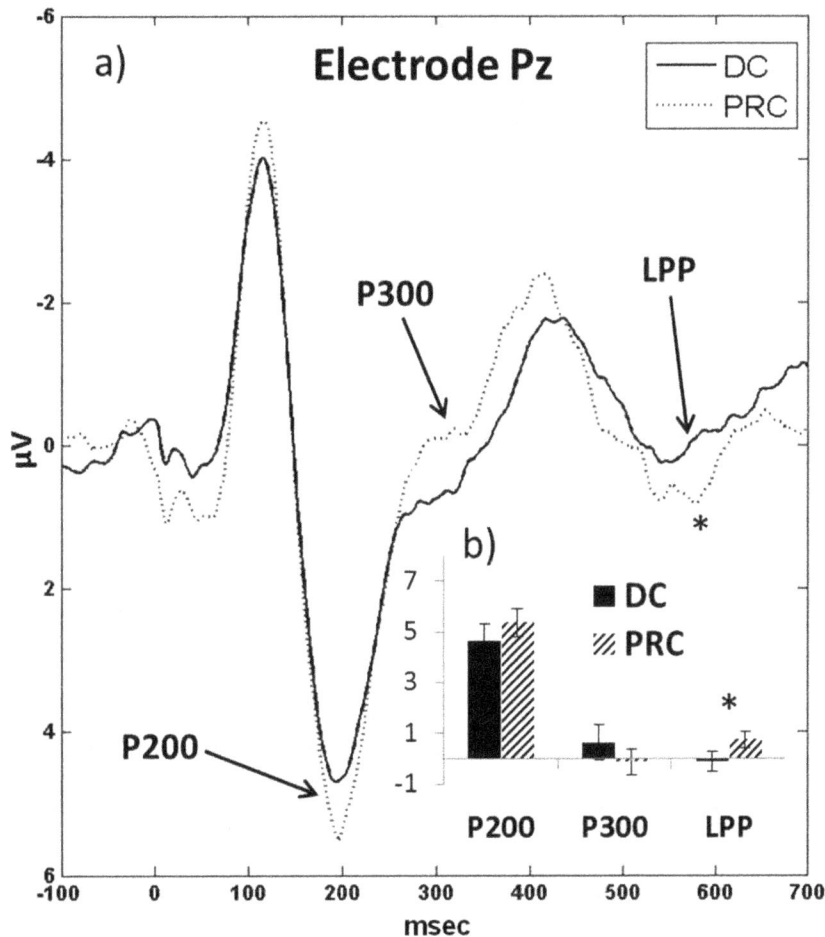

Figure 4. DC and PRC ERPs and amplitudes for electrode Pz in the hard condition. a) Visual inspection of the ERP shows that in the hard condition the P300 was not visually prominent, and close to zero. b) Although LPP was not visually prominent, the difference was significant between DC and PRC, with higher amplitude for PRC (*p<0.05.).

Main effects were also found for P300 and LPP at electrode Pz. No significant cognitive workload effects were found in the current study for N100. Although the N100 component is believed to reflect early sensory auditory processing, it has been shown to be sensitive to attention in previous studies [41,42,44].

The P300 is one of the most commonly studied cognitive ERP components over the last several decades [for a review, see [53]]. In the current study the P300 exhibited a strong cognitive workload effect, however, in the hard condition for both DC and PRC, the P300 was virtually absent in the grand average across all subjects. The P200 and LPP components have received less examination in cognitive neuroscience in general, and in the cognitive workload literature relative to P300, yet both P200 and LPP exhibited strong effects in the current paper, and a previous paper using a very similar paradigm [42], and identical novel auditory tones [50]. Although the P200 was considered by some researchers in early studies to be the tail end of the N100-P200 complex, more recent studies have demonstrated that the P200 is an independent component that can be elicited through visual, somatosensory, and auditory modalities, and is maximal over the vertex [for a review see [54]]. It has been suggested to represent early processing of emotionally or motivationally relevant stimuli [55]. The LPP, often referred to as the late positive component or complex (LPC), has been proposed to reflect continued or

enhanced elaborate processing of emotional or arousing stimuli [55,56], and has been suggested to exhibit positivity with latencies ranging from 300 milliseconds to several seconds [57]. In the current study, the grand average across all subjects was used to identify the LLP peak in a relatively narrow time window for analysis [52], from 570–590 milliseconds, which is temporally consistent with the LLP reported in Miller et al., [42].

Direct Control vs Pattern Recognition

The second goal of the present study was to compare DC and PRC using the ERP measures. Because the PRC method allows the user to make natural movements (in the case of non-amputee controls) or imagine natural movements (in amputee patients) to accomplish the tasks, PRC has been speculated to be more intuitive and lower in cognitive demand than DC, although this notion had not previously been examined empirically.

Having exhibited significant cognitive workload effects across both DC and PRC conditions, P200, P300, and LPP were compared between DC and PRC conditions in the hard and easy tasks. Only LPP exhibited a significant difference between DC and PRC, and only in the hard condition. Amplitude was higher in the PRC condition than the DC condition, consistent with lower cognitive workload for a complex task using PRC relative to DC.

This is interpreted cautiously however, since the P200 and P300 components were not different between DC and PRC.

Although PRC has been speculated to be lower in cognitive workload relative to DC in the absence of previous empirical evidence, many aspects of the cognitive workload required to complete the tasks are inherent to both DC and PRC, and were held constant in this study. One of the more challenging aspects of the task was the mental visual rotation necessary to see the current hand position, and decipher the hand movements in 3 DOFs required to achieve the target position. This aspect of the cognitive burden was consistent between DC and PRC, and was very challenging for the participants. Beyond deciphering how the virtual hand needed to move, the participants then had to complete the appropriate sequence of contractions to accomplish the proper movement. In DC, this required frequent switching between DOFs, and the mental conversion of remembering how to use movements in 1 DOF (wrist extension/flexion) to control 3 DOFs (e.g. extending the wrist to supinate the wrist and open the hand, and flexing the wrist pronate and close the hand). Although the pattern of contractions for DC may be less intuitive, the participants learned fairly quickly. Yet, despite subtle differences in the cognitive burden between DC and PRC on the hard task in this study, the significant difference in LPP amplitude indicates the sensitivity of ERP studies for detecting subtle differences in cognitive workload.

Self-report

One of the most important features of EEG as an outcome measure is objectivity. Researchers in the prosthetics field currently rely on observation by trained clinicians, and self-report from patients or family members to evaluate the mental workload of using a prosthesis, both of which are subjective and prone to bias. The self-report questions administered here correlated with task performance in the hard condition for DC and PRC, but did not correlate with the ERP measures of cognitive effort. This suggests that the participants' perceived effort reflected knowledge of their own performance rather than the actual cortical resources required for the task. In retrospect, this was likely influenced by the sequence of the procedures and the immediate feedback they received. The questionnaire was administered immediately after seeing the performance results for the hard task at the end of testing. As such, knowledge of their performance was fresh in their mind as the participants completed the questionnaire. Although future studies can be designed to administer brief self-reports more frequently, or prior to such salient feedback on the task, the correlation of the self-report with performance rather than cortical activation during task execution in this study illustrates the subjectivity of self-report, and the need for an objective outcome measure of cognitive workload to supplement self-reports in the rehabilitation and prosthetics field. Such a measure will be informative for evaluating current technology, and guiding efforts for new technology.

Advantages of EEG/ERPs

This study represents the first attempt to quantify cognitive workload in myoelectric limb control, and the results are promising. Three separate ERP components exhibited significant cognitive workload effects illustrating the inverse relationship between ERP amplitude to the novel sounds and task difficulty. The paradigm is easily adaptable to research on a variety of HMI tasks where cognitive workload is relevant, including control of exoskeletons or surgical robots. Wireless EEG caps can enable real-time and offline EEG analysis for ecologically valid movements and ambulatory tasks. By examining the cortical resources

available during task engagement for processing of additional stimuli, the paradigm is agnostic to strategy, and allows objective examination of cognitive workload when strategy and cortical activation patterns for two tasks may be different, as in the two myoelectric prosthesis control strategies examined here. Other approaches to measuring cognitive workload with EEG, such as pattern recognition and neural networks [26,58,59,60], are optimal for monitoring workload for a specific task in an individual, but may introduce bias when comparing cognitive workload between two similar, but different tasks. However, more sophisticated signal processing approaches may increase the sensitivity of the ERP approach used in this study.

An additional advantage of the approach presented here is the sensitivity of the information acquired through a small number of electrodes. Although 16 channels of EEG data were obtained in this study, the results could have been obtained using only three or fewer midline electrodes (Fz, Cz, Pz), a few eye channels, a ground, and a reference. Newer EEG caps are being designed to be donned and doffed with ease, and without gel. Furthermore, other EEG measures where additional electrodes are employed can simultaneously address task difficulty, regional activation, and functional communication between different cortical regions to examine sensory, motor, and cognitive demands of a task such as prosthesis use [61,62].

Limitations and Future Studies

The current study was limited to healthy participants with intact limbs, and conducted using a virtual environment. As such, future efforts will extend to upper and lower limb amputee patients, and should be adapted to activity of daily living tasks such as object manipulation and stair climbing. The advantage of the attentional reserve paradigm of assessing cognitive workload is the broad adaptability of the approach for comparison of different tasks and strategies in a range of HMI environments.

Although the results in this study pertain only to healthy control participants, and the specific virtual task in this study, the ERP approach as an outcome measure is a promising technique to evaluate new emerging prosthetic technologies and clinical approaches. For instance, the PRC method tested here required making one DOF movement at a time. In other words, the hand could not be supinated and closed simultaneously. However, studies are underway to adapt PRC measures for multiple simultaneous movements [63], which may continue to improve efficiency and decrease cognitive demand. Other ongoing research efforts address the lack of sensory feedback from a prosthesis, requiring a prosthesis user to rely solely on visual information to control tasks such as grasping. Studies exploring tactile and other forms of feedback seek to enhance performance while reducing the attentional demands [11,12,13,14]. Even surgical techniques such as targeted muscle reinnervation [TMR; [10]], designed to optimize the EMG signal in the residual muscle, have been developed with the goal of making prosthetic limb control more natural and intuitive. The ERP method described here can be adapted to evaluate cognitive workload with these or other emerging rehabilitation technologies.

Conclusions

The goal of this study was to examine the efficacy of using ERPs as an outcome measure for cognitive workload in HMI, specifically, during myoelectric prosthesis control. Secondly, to use the ERP measures exhibiting main effects for cognitive workload to compare two myoelectric strategies, DC and PRC. The results indicated an inverse relationship between cognitive workload and amplitude on P200, P300, and LPP following presentation of novel auditory probes. LPP amplitude was higher on the complex task using PRC compared to DC, suggesting a subtle difference in cognitive workload between DC and PRC.

The current study examined only a virtual arm task in healthy participants with in-tact limbs, and requires replication in patients with amputations, and adaptation to manipulation and mobility tasks using a prosthesis. However, the ERP approach, and other

EEG measures are adaptable to a variety of HMI tasks as objective outcome measures of cortical and attentional effort.

Author Contributions

Conceived and designed the experiments: SD AJ LH CC. Performed the experiments: SD CC. Analyzed the data: SD CC LH TP AJ. Contributed reagents/materials/analysis tools: SD LH TP. Wrote the paper: SD LH AJ. Designed software for data analysis: CC SD.

References

1. Pons JL (2010) Rehabilitation exoskeletal robotics. The promise of an emerging field. IEEE Eng Med Biol Mag 29: 57–63.
2. Sale P, Franceschini M, Waldner A, Hesse S (2012) Use of the robot assisted gait therapy in rehabilitation of patients with stroke and spinal cord injury. Eur J Phys Rehabil Med 48: 111–121.
3. Simorov A, Otte RS, Kopietz CM, Oleynikov D (2012) Review of surgical robotics user interface: what is the best way to control robotic surgery? Surg Endosc 26: 2117–2125.
4. Parker P, Englehart K, Hudgins B (2006) Myoelectric signal processing for control of powered limb prostheses. J Electromyogr Kinesiol 16: 541–548.
5. Diaz I, Gil JJ, Louredo M (2013) A haptic pedal for surgery assistance. Comput Methods Programs Biomed.
6. Dawson MR, Carey JP, Fahimi F (2011) Myoelectric training systems. Expert Rev Med Devices 8: 581–589.
7. Behrend C, Reizner W, Marchessault JA, Hammert WC (2011) Update on advances in upper extremity prosthetics. J Hand Surg Am 36: 1711–1717.
8. Collinger JL, Wodlinger B, Downey JE, Wang W, Tyler-Kabara EC, et al. (2013) High-performance neuroprosthetic control by an individual with tetraplegia. Lancet 381: 557–564.
9. Hochberg LR, Bacher D, Jarosiewicz B, Masse NY, Simeral JD, et al. (2012) Reach and grasp by people with tetraplegia using a neurally controlled robotic arm. Nature 485: 372–375.
10. Kuiken TA, Li G, Lock BA, Lipschutz RD, Miller LA, et al. (2009) Targeted muscle reinnervation for real-time myoelectric control of multifunction artificial arms. JAMA 301: 619–628.
11. Marasco PD, Kim K, Colgate JE, Peshkin MA, Kuiken TA (2011) Robotic touch shifts perception of embodiment to a prosthesis in targeted reinnervation amputees. Brain 134: 747–758.
12. Marasco PD, Schultz AE, Kuiken TA (2009) Sensory capacity of reinnervated skin after redirection of amputated upper limb nerves to the chest. Brain 132: 1441–1448.
13. Schultz AE, Marasco PD, Kuiken TA (2009) Vibrotactile detection thresholds for chest skin of amputees following targeted reinnervation surgery. Brain Res 1251: 121–129.
14. Witteveen HJ, de Rond L, Rietman JS, Veltink PH (2012) Hand-opening feedback for myoelectric forearm prostheses: performance in virtual grasping tasks influenced by different levels of distraction. J Rehabil Res Dev 49: 1517–1526.
15. Resnik L, Meucci MR, Lieberman-Klinger S, Fantini C, Kelty DL, et al. (2012) Advanced upper limb prosthetic devices: implications for upper limb prosthetic rehabilitation. Arch Phys Med Rehabil 93: 710–717.
16. Hill W, Kyberd P, Hermansson N, Hubbard S, Stavdahl O, et al. (2009) Upper Limb Prosthetic Outcome Measures (ULPOM): a working group and their findings. Journal of Prosthetics and Orthotics 21: 69–82.
17. Lindner HY, Natterlund BS, Hermansson LM (2010) Upper limb prosthetic outcome measures: review and content comparison based on International Classification of Functioning, Disability and Health. Prosthet Orthot Int 34: 109–128.
18. Metcalf C, Adams J, Burridge J, Yule V, Chappell P (2007) A review of clinical upper limb assessments within the framework of the WHO ICF. Musculoskeletal Care 5: 160–173.
19. Mazur LM, Mosaly PR, Hoyle LM, Jones EL, Marks LB (2013) Subjective and objective quantification of physician's workload and performance during radiation therapy planning tasks. Pract Radiat Oncol 3: e171–177.
20. Sobuh MM, Kenney LP, Galpin AJ, Thies SB, McLaughlin J, et al. (2014) Visuomotor behaviours when using a myoelectric prosthesis. J Neuroeng Rehabil 11: 72.
21. Tokuda S, Obinata G, Palmer E, Chaparro A (2011) Estimation of mental workload using saccadic eye movements in a free-viewing task. Conf Proc IEEE Eng Med Biol Soc 45: 23–29.
22. Goldberg JH, Wichansky AM (2003) Eye tracking in usability evaluation: A practitioner's guide. In In: Hyönä J, Radach, R., & Deubel, H. (Eds.), editor. The mind's eye: Cognitive and applied aspects of eye movement research. The Netherlands: North-Holland.
23. Soussou W, Rooksby M, Forty C, Weatherhead J, Marshall S (2012) EEG and eye-tracking based measures for enhanced training. Conf Proc IEEE Eng Med Biol Soc 2012: 1623–1626.
24. Casson AJY, Smith S, Duncan JS, Rodriguez-Villegas E (2010) Wearable Electroencephalography: What is it, why is it needed, and what does it entail? IEEE Eng Med Biol Mag 29: 44–56.
25. Kruse AA (2007) Operational neuroscience: neurophysiological measures in applied environments. Aviat Space Environ Med 78: B191–194.
26. Lan T, Erdogmus D, Adami A, Mathan S, Pavel M (2007) Channel selection and feature projection for cognitive load estimation using ambulatory EEG. Comput Intell Neurosci: 74895.
27. Seneviratne U, Mohamed A, Cook M, D'Souza W (2013) The utility of ambulatory electroencephalography in routine clinical practice: a critical review. Epilepsy Res 105: 1–12.
28. Agashe HA, Contreras-Vidal JL (2013) Decoding the evolving grasping gesture from electroencephalographic (EEG) activity. Conf Proc IEEE Eng Med Biol Soc 2013: 5590–5593.
29. Do AH, Wang PT, King CE, Abiri A, Nenadic Z (2011) Brain-computer interface controlled functional electrical stimulation system for ankle movement. J Neuroeng Rehabil 8: 49.
30. Do AH, Wang PT, King CE, Schombs A, Cramer SC, et al. (2012) Brain-computer interface controlled functional electrical stimulation device for foot drop due to stroke. Conf Proc IEEE Eng Med Biol Soc 2012: 6414–6417.
31. Gollee H, Volosyak I, McLachlan AJ, Hunt KJ, Graser A (2010) An SSVEP-based brain-computer interface for the control of functional electrical stimulation. IEEE Trans Biomed Eng 57: 1847–1855.
32. Kilicarslan A, Prasad S, Grossman RG, Contreras-Vidal JL (2013) High accuracy decoding of user intentions using EEG to control a lower-body exoskeleton. Conf Proc IEEE Eng Med Biol Soc 2013: 5606–5609.
33. King CE, Wang PT, Chui LA, Do AH, Nenadic Z (2013) Operation of a brain-computer interface walking simulator for individuals with spinal cord injury. J Neuroeng Rehabil 10: 77.
34. Pascual J, Velasco-Alvarez F, Muller KR, Vidaurre C (2012) First study towards linear control of an upper-limb neuroprosthesis with an EEG-based Brain-Computer Interface. Conf Proc IEEE Eng Med Biol Soc 2012: 3269–3273.
35. Wickens C, Kramer A, Vanasse L, Donchin E (1983) Performance of concurrent tasks: a psychophysiological analysis of the reciprocity of information-processing resources. Science 221: 1080–1082.
36. Isreal JB, Chesney GL, Wickens CD, Donchin E (1980) P300 and tracking difficulty: evidence for multiple resources in dual-task performance. Psychophysiology 17: 259–273.
37. Kramer AF, Sirevaag EJ, Braune R (1987) A psychophysiological assessment of operator workload during simulated flight missions. Hum Factors 29: 145–160.
38. Sirevaag EJ, Kramer AF, Wickens CD, Reisweber M, Strayer DL, et al. (1993) Assessment of pilot performance and mental workload in rotary wing aircraft. Ergonomics 36: 1121–1140.
39. Kramer AF, Wickens CD, Donchin E (1985) Processing of stimulus properties: evidence for dual-task integrality. J Exp Psychol Hum Percept Perform 11: 393–408.
40. Bauer LO, Goldstein R, Stern JA (1987) Effects of information-processing demands on physiological response patterns. Hum Factors 29: 213–234.
41. Kramer AF, Trejo LJ, Humphrey D (1995) Assessment of mental workload with task-irrelevant auditory probes. Biol Psychol 40: 83–100.
42. Miller MW, Rietschel JC, McDonald CG, Hatfield BD (2011) A novel approach to the physiological measurement of mental workload. Int J Psychophysiol 80: 75–78.
43. Papanicolaou AC, Johnstone J (1984) Probe evoked potentials: theory, method and applications. Int J Neurosci 24: 107–131.
44. Ullsperger P, Freude G, Erdmann U (2001) Auditory probe sensitivity to mental workload changes - an event-related potential study. Int J Psychophysiol 40: 201–209.
45. Parasuraman R, Beatty J (1980) Brain events underlying detection and recognition of weak sensory signals. Science 210: 80–83.
46. Fabiani M, Gratton G, Coles MGH (2000) Event-related brain potentials: Methods, theory, and applications. In: In J. Cacioppo LT, & G. Berntson (Eds.), editor. Handbook of Psychophysiology. New York, NY: Cambridge University Press.
47. Belter JT, Segil JL, Dollar AM, Weir RF (2013) Mechanical design and performance specifications of anthropomorphic prosthetic hands: a review. J Rehabil Res Dev 50: 599–618.

48. Allison BZ, Polich J (2008) Workload assessment of computer gaming using a single-stimulus event-related potential paradigm. Biol Psychol 77: 277–283.

49. Simon AM, Hargrove LJ, Lock BA, Kuiken TA (2011) Target Achievement Control Test: evaluating real-time myoelectric pattern-recognition control of multifunctional upper-limb prostheses. J Rehabil Res Dev 48: 619–627.

50. Fabiani M, Kazmerski VA, Cycowicz YM, Friedman D (1996) Naming norms for brief environmental sounds: effects of age and dementia. Psychophysiology 33: 462–475.

51. Jasper HH (1958) The ten-twenty system of the international system federation. Electroencephalogr Clin Neurophysiol 10: 371–375.

52. Handy TC (2005) Event-Related Potentials: A methods handbook. Cambridge, MA: MIT Press.

53. Polich J (2007) Updating P300: an integrative theory of P3a and P3b. Clin Neurophysiol 118: 2128–2148.

54. Crowley KE, Colrain IM (2004) A review of the evidence for P2 being an independent component process: age, sleep and modality. Clin Neurophysiol 115: 732–744.

55. Paulmann S, Bleichner M, Kotz SA (2013) Valence, arousal, and task effects in emotional prosody processing. Front Psychol 4: 345.

56. Kanske P, Kotz SA (2007) Concreteness in emotional words: ERP evidence from a hemifield study. Brain Res 1148: 138–148.

57. Hajcak G, Dunning JP, Foti D (2009) Motivated and controlled attention to emotion: time-course of the late positive potential. Clin Neurophysiol 120: 505–510.

58. Kothe CA, Makeig S (2011) Estimation of task workload from EEG data: new and current tools and perspectives. Conf Proc IEEE Eng Med Biol Soc 2011: 6547–6551.

59. Mathan S, Smart A, Ververs T, Feuerstein M (2010) Towards an index of cognitive efficacy EEG-based estimation of cognitive load among individuals experiencing cancer-related cognitive decline. Conf Proc IEEE Eng Med Biol Soc 2010: 6595–6598.

60. Wilson GF, Russell CA (2003) Real-time assessment of mental workload using psychophysiological measures and artificial neural networks. Hum Factors 45: 635–643.

61. Gentili RJ, Bradberry TJ, Hatfield BD, Contreras-Vidal JL (2009) Brain biomarkers of motor adaptation using phase synchronization. Conf Proc IEEE Eng Med Biol Soc 2009: 5930–5933.

62. Rietschel JC, Miller MW, Gentili RJ, Goodman RN, McDonald CG, et al. (2012) Cerebral-cortical networking and activation increase as a function of cognitive-motor task difficulty. Biol Psychol 90: 127–133.

63. Young AJ, Smith LH, Rouse EJ, Hargrove LJ (2013) Classification of simultaneous movements using surface EMG pattern recognition. IEEE Trans Biomed Eng 60: 1250–1258.

20

Metrical Presentation Boosts Implicit Learning of Artificial Grammar

Tatiana Selchenkova[1]*, Clément François[2,3,4], Daniele Schön[5,6], Alexandra Corneyllie[1], Fabien Perrin[1], Barbara Tillmann[1]

[1] Lyon Neuroscience Research Center, Auditory Cognition and Psychoacoustics Team, Centre National de la Recherche Scientifique, Unité Mixte de Recherche 5292, Institut National de la Santé et de la Recherche Médicale, Unité 1028, University Lyon 1, Lyon, France, [2] Cognition and Brain Plasticity Group, Bellvitge Biomedical Research Institute, L'Hospitalet de Llobregat (Barcelona), Barcelona, Spain, [3] Department of Basic Psychology, University of Barcelona, Barcelona, Spain, [4] Attention, Perception and Acquisition of Language Lab, Hospital Sant Joan de Déu, Barcelona, Spain, [5] Aix-Marseille Université, Institut de Neurosciences des Systèmes, Marseille, France, [6] Institut National de la Santé et de la Recherche Médicale, Unité 1106, Marseille, France

Abstract

The present study investigated whether a temporal hierarchical structure favors implicit learning. An artificial pitch grammar implemented with a set of tones was presented in two different temporal contexts, notably with either a strongly metrical structure or an isochronous structure. According to the Dynamic Attending Theory, external temporal regularities can entrain internal oscillators that guide attention over time, allowing for temporal expectations that influence perception of future events. Based on this framework, it was hypothesized that the metrical structure provides a benefit for artificial grammar learning in comparison to an isochronous presentation. Our study combined behavioral and event-related potential measurements. Behavioral results demonstrated similar learning in both participant groups. By contrast, analyses of event-related potentials showed a larger P300 component and an earlier N2 component for the strongly metrical group during the exposure phase and the test phase, respectively. These findings suggests that the temporal expectations in the strongly metrical condition helped listeners to better process the pitch dimension, leading to improved learning of the artificial grammar.

Editor: Todd W. Troyer, University of Texas at San Antonio, United States of America

Funding: This research was supported by a grant from EBRAMUS ITN (Europe BRAin and MUSic) (Grant Agreement number 238157). The team "Auditory cognition and psychoacoustics" is part of the LabEx CeLyA ("Centre Lyonnais d'Acoustique", ANR-10-LABX-60). The funders had no role in study design, data collection and analysis, decision to publish, or preparation of the manuscript.

Competing Interests: The authors have declared that no competing interests exist.

* Email: tatiana.selchenkova@gmail.com

Introduction

Humans develop expectations about regularities occurring in structures encountered in everyday life (e.g., language, music). Expectations about future events facilitate the processing of expected events in comparison to unexpected events. Humans can learn structural regularities implicitly by mere exposure, that is, in an unconscious way. Implicit learning (IL) is the acquisition of knowledge without the intention to learn [1,2]. Three main paradigms to study IL are the serial reaction time task (SRTT) [3], artificial language learning (ALL) [4,5] and artificial grammar learning (AGL) [2]. Of interest here is the AGL paradigm. Participants are first exposed to grammatical sequences, and then, in the test phase they successfully provide grammaticality judgments that distinguish between new grammatical sequences and ungrammatical sequences without being able to explain their choice, suggesting implicit grammar knowledge acquired during the exposure phase.

In addition to behavioral measures (i.e. number of correct responses and response times) in IL experiments, neurophysiological methods, such as electroencephalography (EEG), functional magnetic resonance imaging and transcranial magnetic stimula-

tion have been used to investigate neural correlates underlying IL (e.g., [6–10]). For example, the IL studies using EEG have shown that violations to newly learned sequence structures alter event-related potential (ERP) components, such as the N1, N2, N2/P3 complex, P300, N400, P600 components (e.g., [6,7,11–15]). Using the AGL paradigm, Carrión and Bly [6] demonstrated that ill-formed test sequences elicited a larger N2b/P3 complex (time-locked to the event that violates the grammar) in comparison to well-formed sequences. The N2/P3 complex has been also shown in studies that compared IL and explicit learning [12,16,17]. These studies suggested that the N2/P3 complex arises when explicit knowledge was acquired. However, when participants were unaware of the sequential presentation (i.e. implicit knowledge), only the N2 component showed the difference between well-formed and ill-formed sequences.

While most AGL studies presented the events of the artificial sequences simultaneously in the visual modality, some studies used a sequential presentation in the auditory modality, keeping the temporal presentation of the material constant. However, it is well known that the temporal structure of event presentation can influence auditory processing, notably leading to facilitated event processing when presented in isochronous patterns or regular temporal patterns in comparison to irregular temporal patterns [18–23]. Temporal expectations appear to facilitate not only auditory event perception (see above), but also event discrimination [18,19] and implicit learning [24,25].

The influence of temporal presentation on auditory processing may be explained in the framework of the Dynamic Attending Theory (DAT) [26,27]. The DAT postulates that external temporal regularities between events can entrain internal oscillators that guide attention over time and help listeners to develop temporal expectations for future events. In line with the DAT, Schmidt-Kassow et al. [22] showed that the temporal predictability of the occurrence of a deviant stimulus leads to larger amplitude and shorter latency of the P3b than deviants in temporally random sequences. Schwartze et al. [23] further compared the influence of isochronous and random presentations of tone sequences on ERPs related to an oddball paradigm in pre-attentive (participants did not pay attention to the stimuli) and attentive conditions (participants performed a task related to the tone sequences). As in Schmidt-Kassow et al. [22], Schwartze et al. [23] found that deviant tone processing elicited a larger P3b in the isochronous presentation than in the random presentation in the attentive condition, but no influence of temporal structure was found in the pre-attentive condition.

According to the DAT and the metric binding hypothesis [28], meter may modulate attentional resources over time and thus influence temporal expectations for future events. Meter can be conceived as a cognitive construct that has a hierarchical structure with stressed and unstressed elements superimposed on an underlying regular pulse. Selchenkova et al. [25] investigated whether temporal regularities influence the learning of pitch structures based on an artificial grammar. Two different sets of temporal patterns, i.e. regular and irregular, were created to be associated with artificial grammar of tone sequences in the exposure phase. Regular patterns were constructed to allow for the abstraction of a clear metrical framework. In contrast, irregular patterns were constructed by reorganizing the same temporal intervals to disrupt this metrical framework. This study revealed that the learning of the artificial grammar was facilitated by the regular presentation (i.e. strongly metrical) of the tone sequences in the exposure phase in comparison to the irregular presentation. Interestingly, results in the strongly metrical condition were highly similar to the results of Tillmann and Poulin-Charronnat [29], wherein the same artificial grammar was presented isochronously. However, on the basis of the DAT and its metrical binding hypothesis [28], one would expect a greater attentional peak at expected points in the strongly metrical presentation, leading to a more pronounced benefit compared to the isochronous presentation.

Our present study aimed to compare directly the IL of an artificial pitch grammar presented with two different regular temporal structures. The tone sequences were associated either with strongly metrical patterns or with an isochronous pattern and presented each to a different group of participants. Combining behavioral and ERP measurements allows studying whether a metrical framework may provide an additional benefit for learning in comparison to an isochronous presentation. In line with other studies on implicit learning (e.g., [6]), the difference in amplitude and/or latency of ERP components between ungrammatical target events versus grammatical target events might be an indicator of perceived grammatical violations and thus a marker of the acquired grammar knowledge. We made the hypothesis that if the strongly metrical presentation in the exposure phase helps developing stronger temporal expectations than the isochronous

presentation, this should lead to enhanced grammar learning, as revealed in the test phase: correct responses should be more numerous and/or ERP differences between ungrammatical and grammatical target tones should be larger and/or start earlier for the participant group with the strongly metrical presentation than for the group with the isochronous presentation.

In addition, the advantage for event processing thanks to the metrical structures may also be reflected in the exposure phase. To keep participants attentive, we introduced some mistuned tones in the exposure phase and participants had to detect them. We hypothesized that the strongly metrical presentation should facilitate pitch processing and thus facilitate mistuned-tone processing in comparison to an isochronous presentation.

Materials and Methods

Participants and ethics statement

Thirty-one university students participated in this experiment (10 men). Five participants were discarded from EEG analyses due to major artifacts, resulting in two groups of 13 participants. Age ranged from 21 to 29 years, with a mean of 23.54 ($SD = 2.44$). Participants were randomly assigned to one of the two experimental groups listening either to the isochronous material (referred to as the Iso group hereafter) or the strongly metrical material (referred to as the SM group hereafter). All participants signed informed consent before the experiment. The present experimental paradigm and the written informed consent were approved by the French ethics committee, Comité de Protection de Personnes Sud-Est II. After the experiment, they were asked to fill out a questionnaire about musical experience (including years of dancing, singing, playing musical instruments (if any) and a self estimation of their sense of rhythm on a 5-point scale where "1" = "I don't have any sense of rhythm" and "5" = "yes, I have very good sense of rhythm"). One additional participant in the Iso group was discarded from the analyses of the exposure phase due to major EEG artifacts.

The two groups of participants did not differ in their musical, dancing and singing experience (musical experience: 0.85 years ($SD = 1.28$) for the Iso group, 0.40 years ($SD = 1.38$) for the SM group, $p = .40$; dancing experience: 3.46 years ($SD = 1.19$) for the Iso group and 2.69 years ($SD = 1.32$) for the SM group, $p = .13$; singing experience: 1.31 years ($SD = 3.09$) for the Iso group and 1.15 years ($SD = 2.82$) for the SM group, $p = .89$). The groups also did not differ in their self-reported sense of rhythm (2.85 ($SD = 0.89$) for the Iso group and 3.0 ($SD = 0.82$) for the SM group, $p = .46$). Participants had self-reported normal hearing and none of them reported to have absolute pitch.

Stimuli

Exposure phase. The material was based on the artificial grammar from Tillmann and Poulin-Charronnat [29], which was adapted from previously used grammars (e.g., [30]). For this finite-state grammar, five pitches were used: a3, a#3, c4, d4, f#4.

For the exposure phase, thirteen 10- and twenty-two 12-tone grammatical sequences (thirty-five grammatical sequences in total) were coupled to fourteen different strongly metrical patterns in such way that each grammatical sequence was associated with four different 10-item and 12-item strongly metrical patterns. In the isochronous condition, the thirty-five 10- and 12-tone grammatical sequences were all coupled to an isochronous pattern. This allowed us to create 140 sequences for the strongly metrical exposure phase and 140 sequences for the isochronous exposure phase.

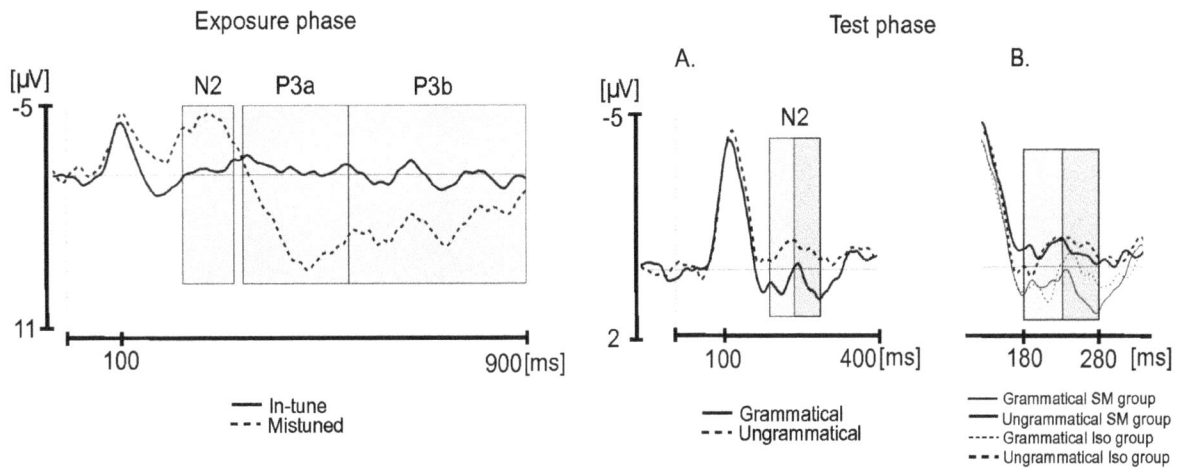

Figure 1. Presentation of the time windows for analyses of ERP components in the exposure phase (left) and the test phase (right) on the Cz electrode. Grey rectangles indicate time windows chosen for the analyses. Exposure phase: Time windows of N2, P3a and P3b for in-tune and mistune tones averaged over participant groups. Test phase: Subdivision of the N2 into ascending (light grey rectangle) and descending (dark grey rectangle) parts for grammatical and ungrammatical target tones averaged over participant groups (A) and separated for SM and Iso groups (B).

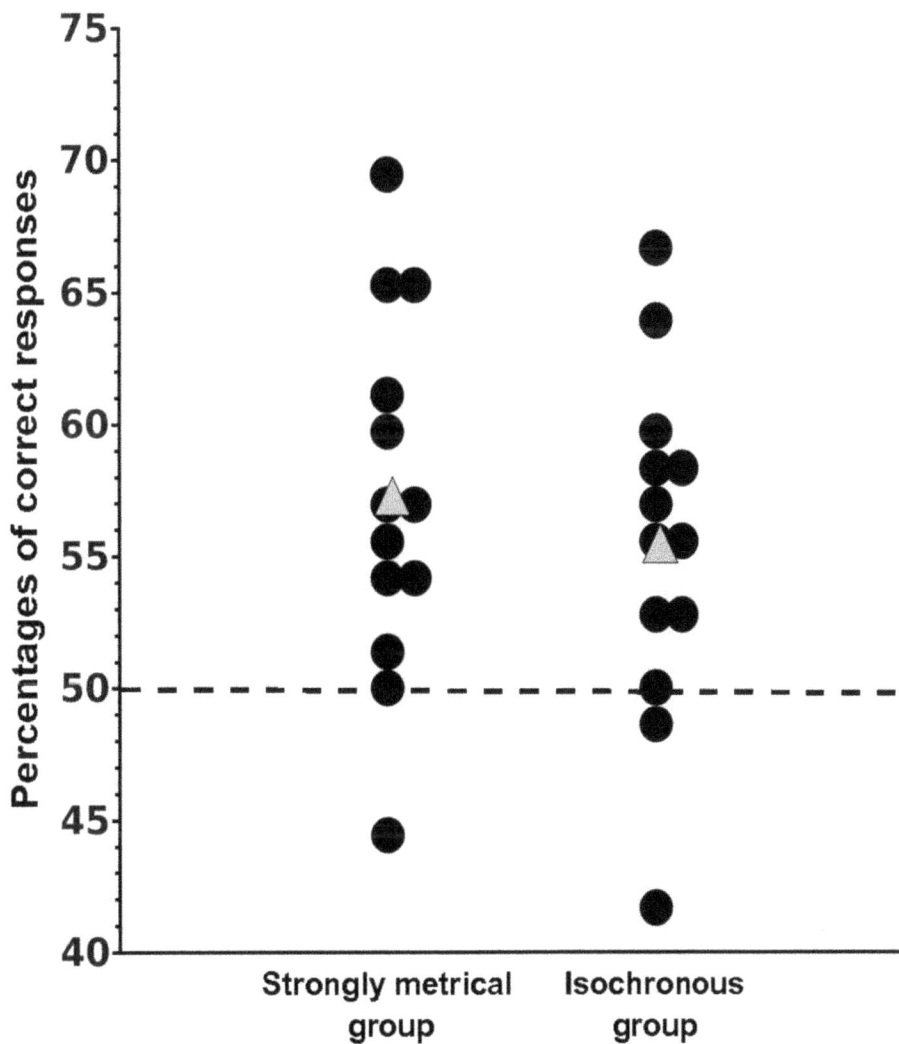

Figure 2. Percentages of correct responses for strongly metrical and isochronous exposure groups for each participant represented by a black dot. Grey triangles represent the average performance for each group, the dotted line represents chance level performance.

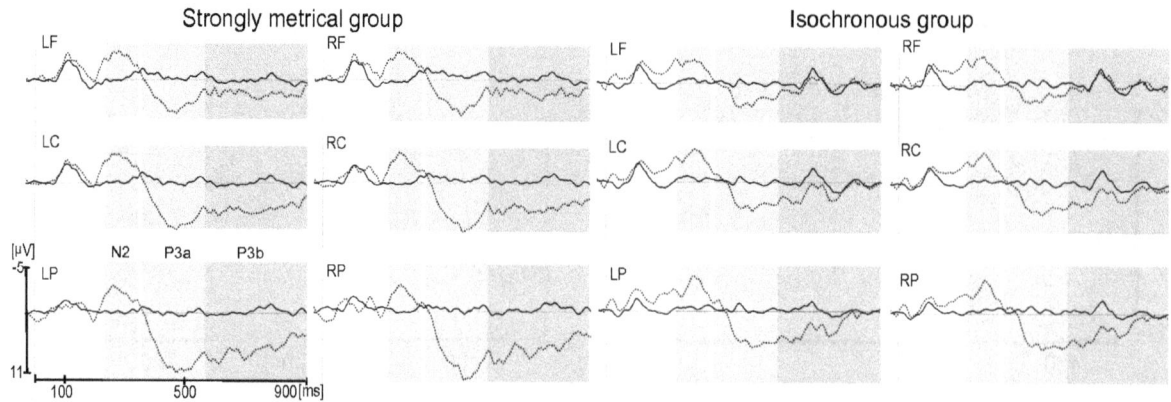

Figure 3. Exposure phase: Grand-average ERPs for in-tune (solid line) and mistuned (dashed line) target tones in the Strongly Metrical group (left) and Isochronous group (right). Each site represents the mean of the five electrodes included in the ROI (LF, left frontal; LC, left central; LP, left parietal; RF, right frontal; RC, right central; RP, right parietal). Grey rectangles indicate time windows of the N2 (230–330 ms), P3a (350–550 ms) and P3b (550–900 ms) chosen for the analyses.

Each tone lasted 220 ms. The inter-onset-intervals (IOIs) were 220, 440, 660 or 880 ms for the strongly metrical patterns and 570 ms for the isochronous pattern. Thus, the sequences in both temporal conditions had similar durations: the 10- and 12-tone exposure sequences with strongly metrical presentation lasted for 5,500 and 6,380 ms and the 10- and 12-tone sequences with the isochronous presentation lasted for 5,350 and 6,490 ms, respectively.

During the exposure phase, one mistuned tone (-52 cents) was inserted in 25% of the 140 sequences. The serial position of this mistuned tone varied across sequences from the second to the ninth tone position.

The strongly metrical patterns (taken from [25]) were constructed to ensure the establishment of a strong metrical framework. For this, IOIs were organized to respect oscillatory cycles at two levels, i.e. with a period of 440 ms and a period of 880 ms. The temporal structure of each temporal pattern had

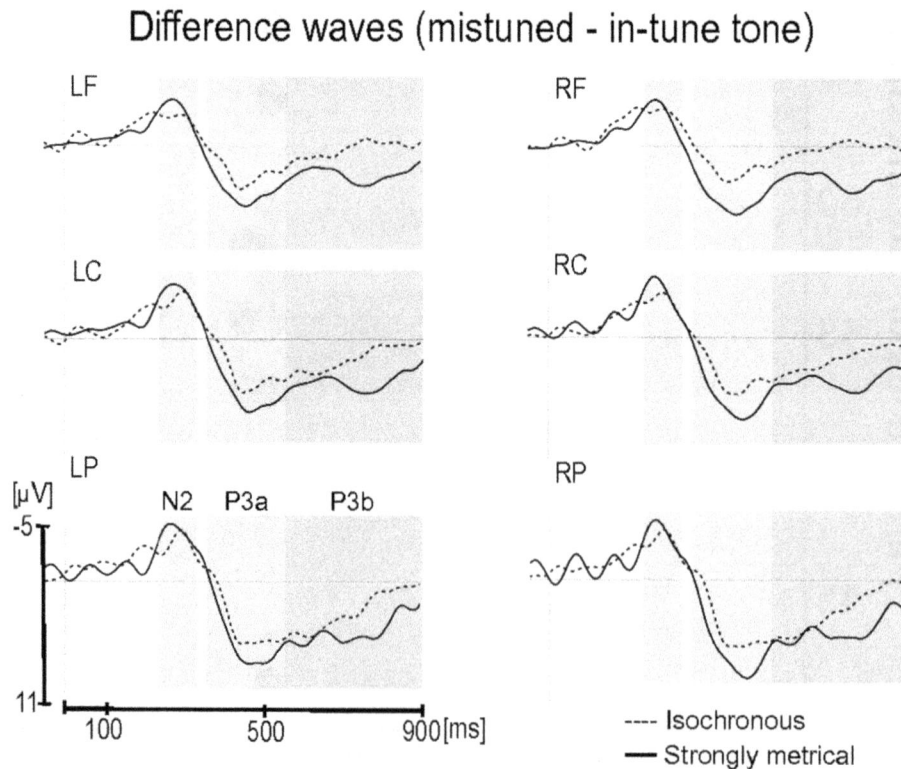

Figure 4. Exposure phase: Difference waves (mistuned minus in-tune target tones) for the Isochronous group (dashed line) and Strongly Metrical group (solid line). Each site represents the mean of the five electrodes included in the ROI (LF, left frontal; LC, left central; LP, left parietal; RF, right frontal; RC, right central; RP, right parietal). Only for visualization purposes waveforms are presented with a 10 Hz low-pass filter. Grey rectangles indicate time windows of the N2 (230–330 ms), P3a (350–550 ms) and P3b (550–900 ms) chosen for the analyses.

Strongly metrical group   Isochronous group

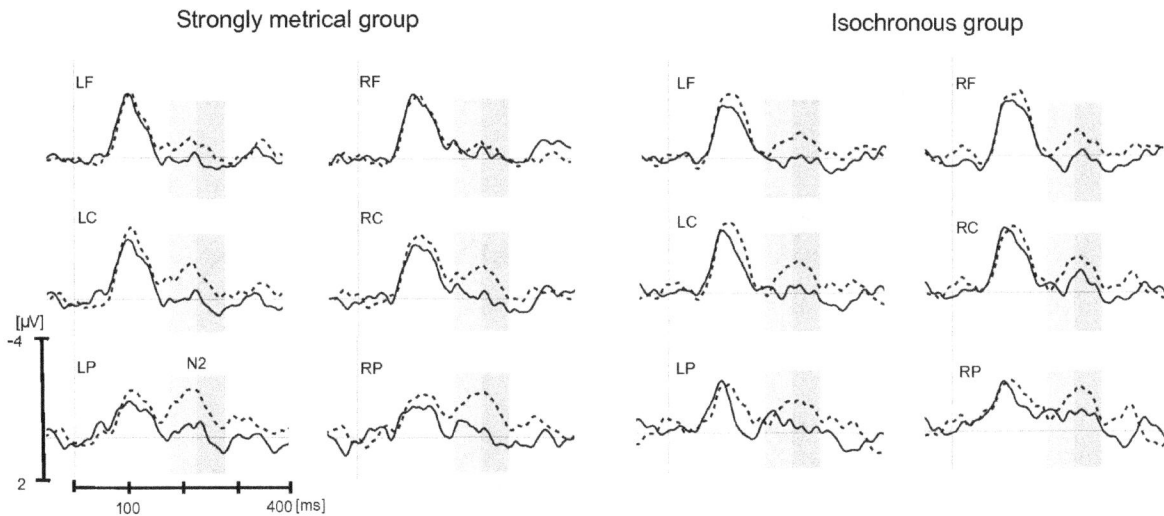

Figure 5. Test phase: Grand-average ERPs for grammatical (solid line) and ungrammatical (dashed line) target tones in the Strongly Metrical (left side) group and Isochronous group (right side). Each site represents the mean of the five electrodes included in the ROI (LF, left frontal, LC, left central, LP, left parietal, RF, right frontal, RC, right central, RP, right parietal). Grey rectangles indicate time windows of ascending (light grey) and descending (dark grey) part of the N2 chosen for the analyses.

been analyzed at global and local levels. Global metric structure was assessed using two indices provided by Povel and Essens's Clock model [31] (a C-score indicating the best internal clock for the smallest obtained values) and the DAT theory (a DAT index; developed in [25] based on [26]), respectively. For the Clock model, a C-score of 0, which thus indicates strongest metric regularity, was found for all strongly metrical patterns. The DAT index reflects the difference between the number of accented and the number of unaccented tones in a sequence. Calculating this index for our patterns also confirmed high metric regularity of the strongly metrical patterns. Local temporal structure features (e.g., rhythmic groupings and frequency analyses of IOI co-occurrences) demonstrated low variability and relatively high repetitions of IOI pairs (local temporal structure within three successive tones) and IOI triplets (local temporal structure within four successive tones), thus further highlightening the temporal regularity of the strongly metrical patterns. In sum, global and local metric analyses confirmed the metrical characteristics of the patterns (see [25] for analyses and more details about patterns construction). Audio examples of the exposure and test sequences (Sound examples S1–S5) and temporal patterns (Table S1) are available in Supporting information.

Test phase. The test phase comprised thirty-six new grammatical sequences and thirty-six ungrammatical sequences. The ungrammatical test sequences differed by one tone from the grammatical sequences. This tone was part of the finite-state grammar, but created controlled subtle grammatical violations; for example, the ungrammatical tone did not create new bigrams (see [29] for more details). Sequences were played with either strongly metrical patterns for the SM group or isochronously for the Iso group. In all sequences, each tone lasted 220 ms.

Procedure and Equipment

For the present study, we have developed an adaptation of previously used implicit learning paradigms that aimed to avoid informing participants about the rule-governed nature of the grammatical melodies during the entire experiment (exposure phase and test phase) and thus allowing for a more direct investigation of implicit learning processes (see also [29]).

In the exposure phase, participants were told that a beginner pianist played all melodies and that after recording we randomly introduced a mistuned tone. They were asked to indicate whether each sequence contained a mistuned tone or not. This mistuned tone-detection task aimed to keep participants' attention to the stimuli during the exposure phase, and in particular to the pitch dimension of the stimuli (that is, the dimension of the to-be-learned grammatical structures). This task was adapted from [29] (Experiment 2).

During the test phase, the sequences were presented by pairs. Each pair contained one new grammatical sequence and one ungrammatical sequence (order was counterbalanced). Participants were asked to indicate which melody was played by the same pianist than the one of the exposure phase. With this instruction, we made the hypothesis (even though we did not explicitly say so) that the pianist beginner was playing melodies of a specific style or repertoire. After having given this judgment, participants rated the confidence of their decision on a 5-point Likert scale (where "1" was not confident at all, "5" was highly confident and "0" was guessing). The test phase contained 72 trials presented in random order for each participant and in two blocks with a small break between them.

The experiment was run using the software Presentation (Neurobehavioural Systems). Stimuli were delivered binaurally using air-delivery headphones (ER-2, Etymotic).

Data acquisition and analyses

Behavioral analyses. For the exposure phase, correct responses for mistuned tones (Hits) and false alarms (mistuned tone responses for in-tune sequences) were calculated for each participant. For the test phase, correct responses for grammatical and ungrammatical target tones were calculated for each participant. The one-sample Wilcoxon signed rank test was used to test whether participants' performance was above chance, and the Mann-Whitney U test was used to compare groups' performance. To obtain an index of explicit vs. implicit acquired knowledge, confidence ratings were calculated separately for correct and incorrect responses, and analyzed with a 2×2 ANOVA with responses (correct/incorrect) as within-participant

Difference waves
(Ungrammatical - Grammatical targets)

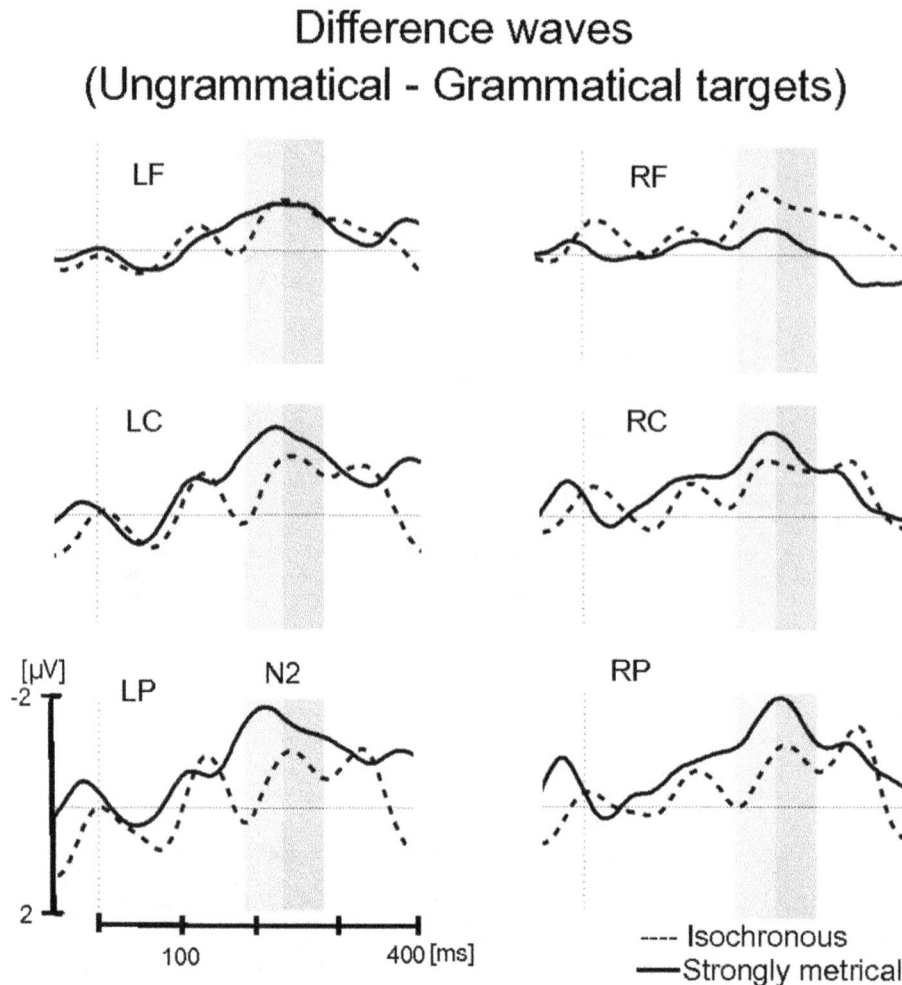

Figure 6. Test phase: Difference waves (ungrammatical minus grammatical target tones) for the Isochronous group (dashed line) and Strongly Metrical group (solid line). Each site represents the mean of the five electrodes included in the ROI (LF, left frontal; LC, left central; LP, left parietal; RF, right frontal; RC, right central; RP, right parietal). Only for visualization purposes waveforms are presented with a 10 Hz low-pass filter. Grey rectangles indicate time windows of ascending (light grey) and descending (dark grey) part of the N2 chosen for the analyses.

factor and group (SM, Iso) as between-participants factor. Difference between confidence ratings to correct and incorrect responses suggests explicit knowledge, whereas no difference suggests that learning was implicit. Note that participants were not informed about grammatical rules of the sequences and this index thus indicated knowledge related to the cover story of the pianist.

ERP acquisition and analyses. Participants were comfortably seated in a sound-attenuated booth in front of a monitor. The EEG signal was recorded from 95 active scalp electrodes (Acticap, Munich) located at standard positions (10-5 montage) via BrainAmp amplifier (BrainProduct, Munich) setup with a nose reference and ground placed at AFz. The vertical electro-oculogram (EOG) was recorded from one electrode placed to the right of the external canthus located below Fp2 electrode. Sampling rate was 500 Hz.

Continuous EEG data collected during exposure and test phases were filtered offline with a bandpass filter of 0.1–30 Hz, the slope of the filters was 24 dB/octave. In the exposure phase, eye blink artifacts were removed using Independent Component Analysis decomposition [32]. ERP data were analyzed by computing the mean amplitude, starting 100 ms before the onset of the tone and

ending 1000 ms after the onset of the tone. In the test phase, epochs exceeding +/−60 μV at midline electrodes were discarded. Remaining trials with movement artifacts in both phases and with blink artifacts and/or eyes saccades in the test phase were excluded using a semi-automatic artifact-rejection procedure. ERP data were analyzed by computing the mean amplitude, starting 100 ms before the onset of the tone and ending 600 ms after the onset of the tone. Epochs were averaged for each condition (mistune/in-tune; grammatical/ungrammatical) and each participant and then averaged across participants to compare groups. Regions of interest (ROI) were defined as follow: left-frontal (F7, F5, F3, FC5, FC3), left-central (C5, C3, CCP5h, CP5, CP3), left-parietal (P7, P5, P3, PO7, PO3), right-frontal (F8, F6, F4, FC6, FC4), right-central (C6, C4, CCP6h, CP6, CP4) and right-parietal (P8, P6, P4, PO8, PO4) regions.

In the exposure phase, the mistuned tones elicited a large N2, followed by large P3a and P3b. The time windows for the analysis of the potentials amplitude were chosen according to visual inspection of grand averages (Figure 1). The N2 was defined as the mean peak amplitude within the post-stimulus time window 230–330 ms. The P3a and P3b were defined as the mean amplitudes within the post-stimulus time windows 350–550 ms and 550–

900 ms, respectively. For each of these three main time windows, a repeated measure ANOVA with item type (mistuned vs. in-tune), hemisphere (left vs. right), region (frontal vs. central vs. parietal) and electrode (5 electrodes in each ROI) as within-participant factors and group as between-participants factor was performed.

In the test phase, the ungrammatical tones elicited a large N2 peaking at approximately 230 ms. The N2 was defined as the mean peak amplitude within the post-stimulus time window 180–280 ms (peak value ±50 ms) (Figure 1). Because visual inspection revealed a group difference in the ascending part of the N2, we also ran additional analyses on the ascending part and the descending part of the N2 (180–230 ms and 230–280 ms, respectively). These analyses used the same ANOVA model with item type (grammatical vs. ungrammatical), hemisphere (left vs. right), region (frontal vs. central vs. parietal) and electrodes (5 electrodes in each ROI) as within-participant factors and group as between-participants factor. All p-values reported below were adjusted using the Greenhouse-Geisser correction for nonsphericity, when appropriate, and Tukey tests were used in post-hoc comparisons. Statistical analyses were performed using Statistica software (version 10).

Results

Behavioral data

Exposure phase. The SM group detected more mistuned tones (88.57%) than did the Iso group (80.47%; $U = 32.0$, $z = 2.475$, $p = .01$, Mann-Whitney test). However, the two groups did not differ in their false alarm rate (21.03% and 23.45% for SM and Iso groups, respectively, $p = .98$).

Test phase. Percentages of correct responses were above chance level for participants in both groups, 55.45% ($SD = 6.55$) for the Iso group ($p = .02$, Wilcoxon test) and 57.26% ($SD = 6.90$) for the SM group ($p < .01$, Wilcoxon test) (Figure 2). Performance of the two groups did not differ significantly ($p = .56$; Mann-Whitney test).

For the confidence ratings, the ANOVA revealed a main effect of response, $F(1,24) = 10.38$, $MSE = 0.800$, $p = .004$: The confidence ratings for correct responses were higher than for incorrect responses (2.55 ($SD = 0.79$) and 2.30 ($SD = 0.73$), respectively). The main effect of group was marginally significant showing that the SM group tended to be more confident in their responses (2.68 ($SD = 0.57$) than the Iso group (2.16 ($SD = 0.85$), ($F(1,24) = 3.61$, $MSE = 3.54$, $p = .06$). The interaction between response and group was not significant ($p > .56$).

Electrophysiological data

Exposure phase. For the N2 component, the main effect of item type was significant, $F(1,23) = 24.33$, $p < .0001$, with a larger negativity for mistuned tones than for in-tune tones, (in-tune, −0.30 μV; mistuned, −3.74 μV) (Figures 3 and 4). The interaction between item type and group was not significant, $p > .76$).

For the P3a component, the main effect of item type was significant, $F(1,23) = 28.82$, $p < .0001$, with a larger positivity for mistuned tones than in-tune tones, (in-tune, −0.36 μV; mistuned, 3.75 μV). No interaction was found between item type and group, $p > .13$.

For the P3b component, the main effect of item type was significant, $F(1,23) = 26.77$, $p < .0001$, with a larger positivity for mistuned tones than for in-tune tones, (in-tune, −0.14 μV; mistuned, 2.68 μV). The main effect of region was also significant, $F(2,46) = 37.68$, $p < .0001$, that is larger in the parietal region in comparison to central ($p < .001$) and frontal regions ($p < .001$). Importantly, the interaction between item type and group was

significant, $F(1,23) = 5.74$, $p = .025$: the mistuned tones elicited a larger positivity than did the in-tune tones, and this difference was larger for the SM group than for the Iso group ($p = .0002$ and $p = .25$, respectively; effect size (mistuned − in-tune tone): SM group, 4.14 μV; Iso group, 1.52 μV).

Test phase. For the N2 component, the main effect of grammaticality was significant, $F(1,24) = 11.06$, $p = .003$, with a larger negativity for ungrammatical target tones than for grammatical target tones (grammatical, −0.22 μV, ungrammatical, −1.15 μV) (Figures 5 and 6). The interaction between grammaticality, group and region was significant, $F(2,48) = 4.91$, $p = .031$: The effect of grammaticality was stronger for the SM group than for the Iso group, and this was modified by region. The separate analyses of ascending (180–230 ms) and descending (230–280 ms) parts of the N2 revealed an interaction between grammaticality, group and region only for the ascending part ($F(2,48) = 4.99$, $p = .031$): While the SM group showed an effect of grammaticality over central and parietal regions (all $ps < .003$), no differences due to grammaticality were visible in the Iso group (all $ps > .08$). The analysis of the descending part revealed only a main effect of grammaticality ($F(1,24) = 9.42$, $p = .005$), with a larger negativity for ungrammatical tones than for grammatical tones. The main effect of group and the interactions involving group were not significant ($ps > .18$). Note that we also performed a statistical analysis in the N1 time window (85–125 ms), but neither the main effect of grammaticality ($p > .42$) nor the interaction between grammaticality and group ($p > .97$) were significant.

Discussion

The present study aimed to investigate the influence of temporal structures on the learning of an artificial grammar. For this aim, we compared learning of the same artificial pitch grammar in two temporal contexts: Participants were exposed to tone sequences presented either isochronously or with rhythmic patterns that had a strongly metrical structure. Both groups learned the artificial grammar. With the behavioral measurement, no difference was found between the performance of the two groups. Interestingly, ERPs in the exposure and the test phases revealed a benefit of the strongly metrical presentation over the isochronous presentation. We first discuss the results of the test phase and then those of the exposure phase.

The grammatical violations in the test phase elicited a negativity between 180 and 280 ms for both participant groups, suggesting that participants had learned the grammatical structure of the tone sequences and detected the ungrammaticality. This result is in line with previous implicit learning studies showing that violations to newly learned sequence structures alter the N2: this has been observed in a different implementation of the AGL paradigm with verbal material [6], as well as in the SRTT [12,16,17,33]. In addition, in music perception, violations of tone expectations – that is, expectations based on tonal structures learned over long term in every day life - have also been shown to affect early negativities, such as the N1 (e.g, [34]), the ERAN (early right anterior negativity) (e.g, [35]) and the right antero-temporal negativity (e.g., [36]).

In our study, the observed negativity (which could be also labelled as N2) was earlier for the SM group than for the Iso group. The N2 may represent working memory processes that are associated with template mismatch [37]. Sams et al. assumed that participants need to maintain a good mental template in order to be able to discriminate between standard and deviant stimuli, and this would be reflected by the N2. In our study, the newly acquired artificial grammar and the expectations developed on the basis of this structured system might thus represent the new mental template to which the incoming events (here tones) are compared. The N2 may indicate a mismatch between the newly acquired implicit knowledge (and notably the expectations for the next upcoming tones) and the incoming tone. Thus, the earlier N2 amplitude to grammatical violations in the SM group (in comparison to the Iso group) might suggest that the artificial pitch material was better acquired by the SM group, allowing participants to develop stronger pitch expectations and to reach an earlier mismatch with the ungrammatical event.

Our results extend previously reported data from verbal to nonverbal materials, from isochronous to complex temporal structures and to an improved test phase (i.e., use of more subtle grammatical violations and an implicit task) [6]. First, we provide evidence for the learning of nonverbal pitch material embedded in an isochronous structure as well as in more complex temporal structures (i.e., the strongly metrical presentations). Second, Carrión and Bly [6] tested unexpected events that were allover quite strong violations. In particular, they used context violations, which introduced, for example, a novel letter and grammatical violations, in which a trained letter was placed in a new position. However, even these "grammatical violations" are strong violations because they create new unseen bigrams (local violations), which can be detected without more general grammar learning. In contrast, in our study, the N2 was elicited by well-controlled, subtle grammar violations and thus suggests the acquisition of new grammar knowledge during the exposure phase. Third, in contrast to Carrión and Bly who asked participants for direct grammaticality judgments, our participants were never told about the rule-governed nature of the experimental material, that is the task remained implicit even in the test phase. Consequently, the ERP response observed for grammatical violations with this type of task might indicate that this difference in the N2 component reflects implicit knowledge acquisition. This result extends SRTT data that showed an appearance of the N2 at deviant targets in implicit learners, while a N2/P3 complex emerged in explicit learners [12,16,17].

In the exposure phase, we investigated how different temporal presentations may influence pitch processing, notably the processing of mistuned tones. Based on the DAT, both temporal presentations, i.e. the isochronous and strongly metrical ones, allow developing temporal expectations, but to a different extent, as suggested by the metric binding hypothesis [28]. As the isochronous pattern contains only one oscillatory level (equal to the IOI), listening to sequences with an isochronous presentation allows for the development of equal expectations for all forthcoming events (though see [38] for a different perspective). In contrast, the strongly metrical patterns incorporate at least two oscillatory levels, i.e. a lower oscillatory level with a period of 440 ms (as does the isochronous pattern) and a higher oscillatory level with a period of 880 ms. Binding these two oscillatory levels should lead to the creation of metric clusters that hierarchize and strengthen temporal expectations [28]. These stronger expectations may help listeners to better process the incoming information, and notably, here in our material, allow for better processing of the pitch dimension. Indeed, ERPs and behavioral measures of the exposure phase demonstrated better mistuned-tone processing, as reflected in increased accuracy and a larger P3 for the SM group than for the Iso group. This enhanced processing of the pitch dimension might then improve pitch structure learning as revealed by the test phase with an earlier negativity to grammatical violations for the SM group than for the Iso group.

In the exposure phase, the mistuned tones elicited a larger N2/P3 complex than the in-tune tones for both participant groups.

This result is in agreement with previous findings observed for the processing of pitch deviations. In Marmel et al. [39], out-of-tune tones elicited a larger N2/P3 complex than in-tune tones. Furthermore, incongruities in pitch contour have been also reported to elicit a larger negative component that ended around 200 ms followed by a large positivity between 200 and 800 ms [40]. In our study, the difference between the two groups in mistune-tone processing was observed in the P3. Mistuned target tones elicited a significantly larger P3 in the SM group than in the Iso group. Interpreting this result according to the metric binding hypothesis suggests that the strongly metrical presentation allows guiding more precisely attention to the next expected events than does the isochronous presentation, resulting in enhanced pitch processing. Similarly, previous studies reported more effective deviant tone processing when embedded in highly predictable temporal structures, as reflected in a larger and early P3b [22,23]. In line with the DAT, Schwartze et al. [23] suggested that this P3b effect might reflect stimulus-driven synchronization of attention that leads to facilitation of tone processing.

The parietal P3b activity may be also related to context updating operation and subsequent memory storage [41]. The findings thus suggest that working memory operations can be improved when the artificial grammar was presented strongly metrically rather than isochronously. When participants work on the mistune tone detection task, they might do real-time comparisons of the previous tones with the present tone. When listening to a melody, all previous tones are held in memory buffer in order to be compared with the next incoming tone. In line with the metric binding hypothesis, we assume that the stronger metrical presentation may help to direct attention more precisely in time (due to the two oscillatory levels binding), helping to compare more easily the current tone with the previous tones in the memory buffer. This may facilitate perceptual and cognitive processing (i.e. mistuned tone processing and implicit learning) during the exposure phase.

In sum, our present study showed that a strongly metrical presentation benefits the learning of an artificial grammar in comparison to an isochronous presentation. This facilitation might be related to better temporal processing in a subcortico-cortical network involving the basal ganglia, the frontal cortex and the cerebellum [42]. In line with the DAT, this network helps to extract temporal regularities of external events, and to generate temporal expectations, thus leading to facilitated perceptual and cognitive processes. Future studies are needed to investigate whether patients with lesions in either the basal ganglia or the inferior frontal cortex (with previously reported deficits in IL, [43,44]) might benefit from the strongly metrical presentation and show learning of an artificial grammar.

Supporting Information

Table S1 Strongly metrical patterns used to create the artificial pitch sequences.

Sound example S1 An exposure sequence with the strongly metrical presentation.

Sound example S2 An exposure sequence with the isochronous presentation.

Sound example S3 A test sequence with the strongly metrical presentation.

Sound example S4   A test sequence with the isochronous presentation.

Sound example S5   An exposure sequence with mistuned tone.

References

1. Perruchet P (2008) Implicit Learning. Cognitive psychology of memory. Vol.2 of Learning and memory: A comprehensive reference, Ed. J. Byrne. 597–621.
2. Reber AS (1967) Implicit Learning of Artificial Grammars. J Verbal Learning Verbal Behav 6: 855–863.
3. Nissen MJ, Bullemer P (1987) Attentional Requirements of Learning: Evidence from Performance Measures. Cogn Psychol 19: 1–32.
4. Saffran JR, Johnson EK, Aslin RN, Newport EL (1999) Statistical learning of tone sequences by human infants and adults. Cognition 70: 27–52. Available: http://www.ncbi.nlm.nih.gov/pubmed/10193055.
5. Saffran JR, Aslin RN, Newport EL (1996) Statistical learning by 8-month-old infants. Science (80−) 274: 1926–1928. Available: http://www.ncbi.nlm.nih.gov/pubmed/19489896.
6. Carrión RE, Bly BM (2007) Event-related potential markers of expectation violation in an artificial grammar learning task. Neuroreport 18: 191–195.
7. Francois C, Schön D (2010) Learning of musical and linguistic structures: comparing event-related potentials and behavior. Neuroreport 21: 928–932. Available: http://www.ncbi.nlm.nih.gov/pubmed/20697301. Accessed 2013 Nov 26.
8. Petersson KM, Hagoort P (2012) The neurobiology of syntax: beyond string sets. Philos Trans R Soc Lond B Biol Sci 367: 1971–1983. Available: http://www.pubmedcentral.nih.gov/articlerender.fcgi?artid=3367693&tool=pmcentrez&rendertype=abstract. Accessed 2013 Sep 24.
9. Petersson KM, Forkstam C, Ingvar M (2004) Artificial syntactic violations activate Broca's region. Cogn Sci 28: 383–407. Available: http://doi.wiley.com/10.1016/j.cogsci.2003.12.003. Accessed 2011 July 18.
10. Uddén J, Folia V, Forkstam C, Ingvar M, Fernandez G, et al. (2008) The inferior frontal cortex in artificial syntax processing: an rTMS study. Brain Res 1224: 69–78. Available: http://www.ncbi.nlm.nih.gov/pubmed/18617159. Accessed 2012 Nov 13.
11. Baldwin KB, Kutas M (1997) An ERP analysis of implicit structured sequence learning. Psychophysiology 34: 74–86. Available: http://www.ncbi.nlm.nih.gov/pubmed/9009811.
12. Ferdinand NK, Mecklinger A, Kray J (2008) Error and deviance processing in implicit and explicit sequence learning. J Cogn Neurosci 20: 629–642. Available: http://www.ncbi.nlm.nih.gov/pubmed/18052785.
13. François C, Schön D (2011) Musical Expertise Boosts Implicit Learning of Both Musical and Linguistic Structures. Cereb cortex 21: 2357–2365. Available: http://www.ncbi.nlm.nih.gov/pubmed/21383236. Accessed 2011 Aug 23.
14. Friederici AD, Steinhauer K, Pfeifer E (2002) Brain signatures of artificial language processing: evidence challenging the critical period hypothesis. PNAS 99: 529–534. Available: http://www.pubmedcentral.nih.gov/articlerender.fcgi?artid=117594&tool=pmcentrez&rendertype=abstract.
15. Schankin A, Hagemann D, Danner D, Hager M (2011) Violations of implicit rules elicit an early negativity in the event-related potential. Neuroreport 22: 642–645. Available: http://www.ncbi.nlm.nih.gov/pubmed/21817929. Accessed 2013 Jun 20.
16. Eimer M, Goschke T, Schlaghecken F, Stürmer B (1996) Explicit and implicit learning of event sequences: evidence from event-related brain potentials. J Exp Psychol Learn Mem Cogn 22: 970–987. Available: http://www.ncbi.nlm.nih.gov/pubmed/8708606.
17. Fu Q, Bin G, Dienes Z, Fu X, Gao X (2013) Learning without consciously knowing: evidence from event-related potentials in sequence learning. Conscious Cogn 22: 22–34. Available: http://www.ncbi.nlm.nih.gov/pubmed/23247079. Accessed 2013 May 24.
18. Geiser E, Notter M, Gabrieli JDE (2012) A Corticostriatal Neural System Enhances Auditory Perception through Temporal Context Processing. J Neurosci 32: 6177–6182. doi:10.1523/JNEUROSCI.5153-11.2012.
19. Jones MR, Moynihan H, MacKenzie N, Puente J (2002) Temporal aspects of stimulus-driven attending in dynamic arrays. Psychol Sci 13: 313–319. Available: http://www.ncbi.nlm.nih.gov/pubmed/12137133.
20. Lange K (2009) Brain correlates of early auditory processing are attenuated by expectations for time and pitch. Brain Cogn 69: 127–137. Available: http://www.ncbi.nlm.nih.gov/pubmed/18644669. Accessed 2011 Sep 28.
21. Schmidt-Kassow M, Kotz SA (2008) Entrainment of syntactic processing? ERP-responses to predictable time intervals during syntactic reanalysis. Brain Res 1226: 144–155. Available: http://www.ncbi.nlm.nih.gov/pubmed/18598675. Accessed 2010 Oct 7.
22. Schmidt-Kassow M, Schubotz RI, Kotz SA (2009) Attention and entrainment: P3b varies as a function of temporal predictability. Neuroreport 20: 31–36. Available: http://www.ncbi.nlm.nih.gov/pubmed/18987559.
23. Schwartze M, Rothermich K, Schmidt-Kassow M, Kotz SA (2011) Temporal regularity effects on pre-attentive and attentive processing of deviance. Biol Psychol 87: 146–151. Available: http://www.ncbi.nlm.nih.gov/pubmed/21382437. Accessed 2012 Mar 12.
24. Hoch L, Tyler MD, Tillmann B (2013) Regularity of unit length boosts statistical learning in verbal and nonverbal artificial languages. Psychon Bull Rev 20: 142–147. Available: http://www.ncbi.nlm.nih.gov/pubmed/22890871. Accessed 2013 Jun 1.
25. Selchenkova T, Jones MR, Tillmann B (2014) The influence of temporal regularities on the implicit learning of pitch structures. Q J Exp Psychol. In press.
26. Jones MR (1976) Time, Our Lost Dimension: Toward a New Theory of Perception, Attention, and Memory. Psychol Rev 83: 323–355.
27. Jones MR, Boltz M (1989) Dynamic attending and responses to time. Psychol Rev 96: 459–491. Available: http://www.ncbi.nlm.nih.gov/pubmed/2756068.
28. Jones MR (2009) Musical time. Oxford Handbook of Music Psychology, Ed. Susan Hallam, Ian Cross, Michael Thaut. 81–92.
29. Tillmann B, Poulin-Charronnat B (2010) Auditory expectations for newly acquired structures. Q J Exp Psychol 63: 1646–1664. Available: http://www.ncbi.nlm.nih.gov/pubmed/20175025. Accessed 2010 Dec 20.
30. Altmann GTM, Dienez Z, Goode A (1995) Modality Independence of Implicitly Learned Grammatical Knowledge. J Exp Psychol Learn Mem Cogn 21: 899–912.
31. Povel D-J, Essens P (1985) Perception of Temporal Patterns. Music Percept 2: 411–440.
32. Delorme A, Makeig S (2004) EEGLAB: an open source toolbox for analysis of single-trial EEG dynamics including independent component analysis. J Neurosci Methods 134: 9–21.
33. Rüsseler J, Rösler F (2000) Implicit and explicit learning of event sequences: evidence for distinct coding of perceptual and motor representations. Acta Psychol (Amst) 104: 45–67. Available: http://www.ncbi.nlm.nih.gov/pubmed/10769939.
34. Schön D, Besson M (2005) Visually induced auditory expectancy in music reading: a behavioral and electrophysiological study. J Cogn Neurosci 17: 694–705. Available: http://www.ncbi.nlm.nih.gov/pubmed/15829088.
35. Koelsch S, Gunter T, Friederici AD, Schröger E (2000) Brain indices of music processing: "nonmusicians" are musical. J Cogn Neurosci 12: 520–541. Available: http://www.ncbi.nlm.nih.gov/pubmed/10931776.
36. Patel AD, Gibson E, Ratner J, Besson M, Holcomb PJ (1998) Processing syntactic relations in language and music: an event-related potential study. J Cogn Neurosci 10: 717–733. Available: http://www.ncbi.nlm.nih.gov/pubmed/9831740.
37. Sams M, Alho K, Näätänen R (1983) Sequential effects on the ERP in discrimination two stimuli. Biol Psychol 17: 41–58.
38. Brochard R, Abecasis D, Potter D, Ragot R, Drake C (2003) THE "TICKTOCK" OF OUR INTERNAL CLOCK: Direct Brain Evidence of Subjective Accents in Isochronous Sequences. Psychol Sci 14: 362–366.
39. Marmel F, Perrin F, Tillmann B (2011) Tonal expectations influence early pitch processing. J Cogn Neurosci 23: 3095–3104. Available: http://www.ncbi.nlm.nih.gov/pubmed/21265601.
40. Schön D, Magne C, Besson M (2004) The music of speech: music training facilitates pitch processing in both music and language. Psychophysiology 41: 341–349. Available: http://www.ncbi.nlm.nih.gov/pubmed/15102118. Accessed 2013 May 28.
41. Polich J (2007) Updating P300: An Integrative Theory of P3a and P3b. Clin Neurophysiol 118: 2128–2148. doi:10.1016/j.clinph.2007.04.019.Updating.
42. Kotz SA, Schwartze M (2010) Cortical speech processing unplugged: a timely subcortico-cortical framework. Trends Cogn Sci 14: 392–399. Available: http://www.ncbi.nlm.nih.gov/pubmed/20655802. Accessed 2013 Sep 19.
43. Christiansen MH, Louise Kelly M, Shillcock RC, Greenfield K (2010) Impaired artificial grammar learning in agrammatism. Cognition 116: 382–393. Available: http://www.ncbi.nlm.nih.gov/pubmed/20605017. Accessed 2010 Aug 12.
44. Goschke T, Friederichi A, Kotz S, van Kampen A (2001) Procedural learning in Broca's Aphasia: Dissociation between the implicit acquisition of spatio-motor and phoneme sequences. J Cogn Neurosci 13: 370–388.

Acknowledgments

We thank Brian Mathias, Melodie Faguet et Maïté Castro for their help in EEG recordings.

Author Contributions

Conceived and designed the experiments: TS BT FP. Performed the experiments: TS AC. Analyzed the data: TS CF DS BT. Contributed to the writing of the manuscript: TS CF DS AC FP BT.

21

A Supplementary System for a Brain-Machine Interface Based on Jaw Artifacts for the Bidimensional Control of a Robotic Arm

Álvaro Costa*, Enrique Hortal, Eduardo Iáñez, José M. Azorín

Brain-Machine Interface Systems Lab, Miguel Hernández University, Elche, Spain

Abstract

Non-invasive Brain-Machine Interfaces (BMIs) are being used more and more these days to design systems focused on helping people with motor disabilities. Spontaneous BMIs translate user's brain signals into commands to control devices. On these systems, by and large, 2 different mental tasks can be detected with enough accuracy. However, a large training time is required and the system needs to be adjusted on each session. This paper presents a supplementary system that employs BMI sensors, allowing the use of 2 systems (the BMI system and the supplementary system) with the same data acquisition device. This supplementary system is designed to control a robotic arm in two dimensions using electromyographical (EMG) signals extracted from the electroencephalographical (EEG) recordings. These signals are voluntarily produced by users clenching their jaws. EEG signals (with EMG contributions) were registered and analyzed to obtain the electrodes and the range of frequencies which provide the best classification results for 5 different clenching tasks. A training stage, based on the 2-dimensional control of a cursor, was designed and used by the volunteers to get used to this control. Afterwards, the control was extrapolated to a robotic arm in a 2-dimensional workspace. Although the training performed by volunteers requires 70 minutes, the final results suggest that in a shorter period of time (45 min), users should be able to control the robotic arm in 2 dimensions with their jaws. The designed system is compared with a similar 2-dimensional system based on spontaneous BMIs, and our system shows faster and more accurate performance. This is due to the nature of the control signals. Brain potentials are much more difficult to control than the electromyographical signals produced by jaw clenches. Additionally, the presented system also shows an improvement in the results compared with an electrooculographic system in a similar environment.

Editor: Mikhail A. Lebedev, Duke University, United States of America

Funding: This research has been funded by the Commission of the European Union under the BioMot project - Smart Wearable Robots with Bioinspired Sensory-Motor Skills (Grant Agreement number IFP7-ICT- 2013-10-611695). The funders had no role in study design, data collection and analysis, decision to publish, or preparation of the manuscript.

Competing Interests: The authors have declared that no competing interests exist.

* Email: acosta@umh.es

Introduction

In our society there is an increasing concern about helping and assisting people who suffer from motor disabilities. Emerging from this concern, each day, different areas of research are focusing their efforts on developing Human-Machine systems to help people suffering from these conditions [1,2]. Brain-Machine Interfaces (BMIs) are a clear example of these systems. Depending on the nature of the neural phenomenons analyzed, these systems can be classified as evoked or spontaneous. On the one hand, spontaneous BMIs study those brainwaves that can be voluntarily controlled by a subject. To achieve this control it is usually necessary to have a training period during which the users learn how to control their brain potentials. On the other hand, evoked BMIs rely on the analysis of brain potentials that cannot be controlled by the users. These potentials appear in response to a external stimulus like flashlights or sounds among others [3,4]. Spontaneous systems are usually focused on generating commands to control a device taking advantage of the users capability to

control their EEG signals [5–7]. Regarding evoked systems, there are studies focused on generating control commands [8,9] and also on the evaluation of the brain response to different external stimulus with diagnosis purposes [10–12]. Besides, BMIs (both spontaneous and evoked) are used on other topics in the field of human health, such as the measurement of the mental state of a patient (workload, attention level, emotional state,...) [13] or as support systems on rehabilitation processes [14].

BMI systems can also be divided into two big groups depending on the invasion level needed to register signals. Invasive BMI systems register signals directly from the brain using electrodes implanted inside the cortex [15,16]. This method provides an excellent signal to noise ratio because the electrodes used are placed much closer to the source of the electrical signals. However, their use is limited due to the risk and ethical questions associated to the surgery needed to implant the electrodes under the scalp. On the other hand, for non-invasive BMIs, surgery is not needed. Instead, a set of electrodes is placed over the scalp in order to register the EEG signals. Nowadays, there are many studies

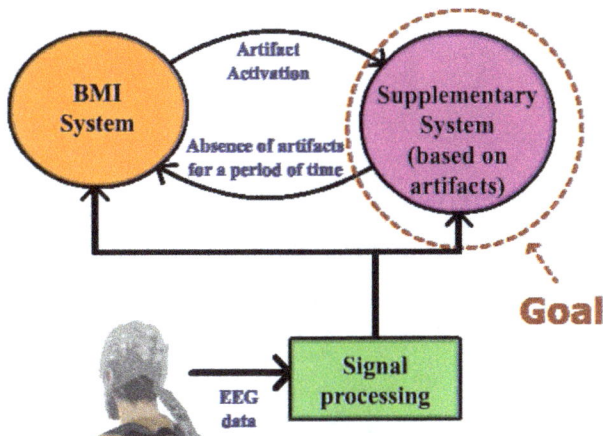

Figure 1. Block interconnection diagram. EEG data from the scalp is acquired, processed and classified in real time. The classification results are used as control commands for 2 different systems. The Supplementary System block is the main goal of the present work. It should be activated and controlled with EMG signals registered from a BMI set of electrodes. If no EMG signals are detected in the EEG data, the BMI system is used. When the user wants to use the Supplementary System, he/she has to generate an EMG signal.

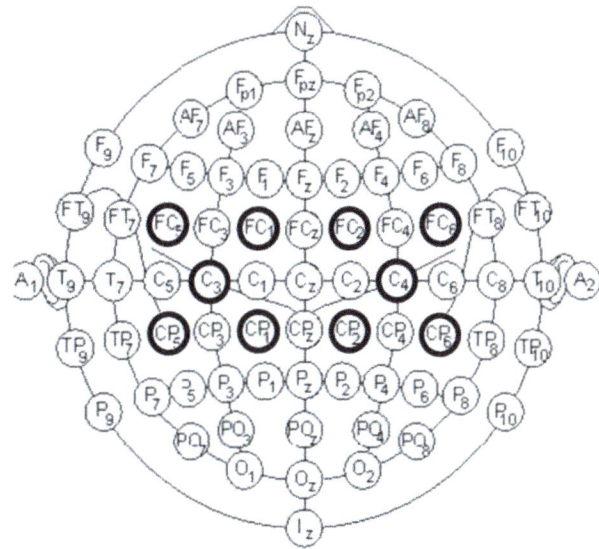

Figure 2. Electrode distribution. FC5, FC1, FC2, FC6, C3, C4, CP5, CP1, CP2 and CP6 (darker circles) according to the International 10/10 System.

focused on helping people with motor diseases based on non-invasive BMI systems, like [17–19]. The main disadvantage of non-invasive BMI systems is the quality of the registered signals. Due to volume conduction which is defined as the property, associated to biological tissues, of transmiting electric and magnetic fields from an electric primary source current, the scalp filters electric signals from the brain and there is mixing of signals from different sources. This makes difficult to isolate the signals produced in a single brain area. Due to the localization of those electrodes, EEG signals are also contaminated by several noise sources produced by other physiological factors like blood pressure, skin tension, muscular and ocular movements, etc. All of these unwanted signals are considered artifacts when the goal of the study is to evaluate how EEG signals behave. For that reason, on non-invasive systems, the signal to noise ratio is a critical factor and detecting and filtering artifacts is a fundamental part of the data analysis [20–22].

Some signals (usually considered artifacts on BMI systems) can be controlled by users, like those produced by voluntary movements of the eyes (electrooculographic (EOG)) and muscles (electromyographic (EMG)). In this work, the use of EMG signals generated voluntarily by subjects is proposed in order to implement a supplementary system for a BMI. The architecture that appears in Figure 1 shows how this system and the BMI system will coexist. The main advantage of this architecture is that they share the same set of EEG electrodes, instead of including EMG electrodes or other sensors.

The supplementary system proposed uses EMG signals (extracted from the EEG signals of the BMI), which are generated by the users clenching their jaws, in order to control the 2-dimensional movement of a robotic arm. These clench signals affect a wide range of frequencies (1–128 Hz) according to [23]. For that reason is not possible to use this system simultaneously with a BMI system. However, it is possible to freely alternate between both systems (non-simultaneous control). The proposed system, controlled voluntarily by the user as in a spontaneous BMI, has a decreased training time, improved classifier stability and accuracy, and an increased number of the detected tasks.

Since this system allows users a better control of a device, it could be used as a complement for a BMI focused on solving other problems also related with the improvement of the quality of life of people with disabilities. For example, internet browsers based on evoked potentials [24] can be complemented with the supplementary system described on this article. Thus the evoked BMI could be used to write text in the browser, while our system could be used to control the cursor.

Materials and Methods

Data Acquisition

EEG signals are acquired using an amplifier (g.USBamp, g.Tec, GmbH, Austria) with active electrodes to increase their signal/noise ratio by introducing a pre-amplification stage (g.GAMMA-box, g.Tec, GmbH, Austria). The acquisition of EEG signals is done using 10 electrodes placed over the scalp with the following distribution: FC5, FC1, FC2, FC6, C3, C4, CP5, CP1, CP2 and CP6 (see Figure 2) according to the International 10/10 System, with a monoauricular reference in the right earlobe and ground in AFz. Information is digitalized at 1200 Hz. A bandpass filter from 0.1 to 100 Hz has been applied. Also, a 50 Hz Notch filter to remove the power line interference is used. Finally, all the data are sent to a computer system where the processing and classification algorithms are applied. Figure 3 shows an image of the equipment used for the EEG recordings. Electrodes C3 and C4 are the main goal of our analysis. Their readings show the best classification results compared to the other electrodes analyzed. These electrodes are also associated with the sensorimotor areas where right and left motor imagery tasks are detected. The other electrodes shown in Figure 2 (FC5, FC1, FC2, FC6, CP5, CP1, CP2, CP6) are used in the processing stage to remove their power contribution from electrodes C3 and C4.

Data analysis

The signals are processed in real time as in [25]. To do that, the time between data windows must be small enough for the algorithm to provide feedback to the user in real time. Also, the

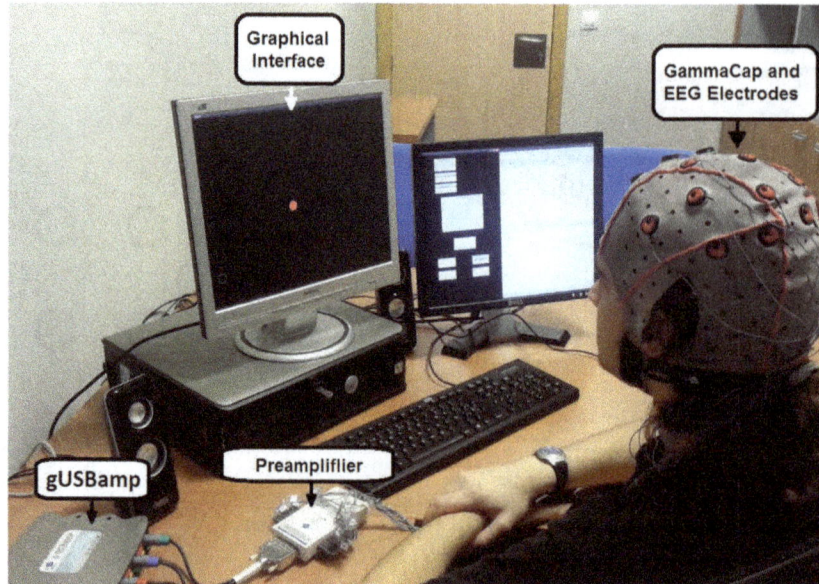

Figure 3. Equipment. Amplifier and GammaCap from g.Tec are used to register EEG Signals. Data are processed and classified in the computer, which is also used to provide visual feedback to the user.

window length should not be too long to avoid delays in the feedback. Every 50 ms a data window of 400 ms is stored, resulting in a 350 ms overlap between the windows. This overlap increases the stability of the classification results by using the information of previous data windows. Then, a four nearest neighbor Laplacian algorithm [26] is applied to the temporal data from electrodes C3 and C4. This algorithm uses the information received from the four nearest electrodes of C3 and C4 and their distances from them in order to reduce the unwanted signal contribution that these electrodes have on C3 and C4. The result is a smoother time signal where the main contribution comes from the electrode of interest. The Laplacian is computed according to the formula,

$$V_i^{LAP} = V_i^{CR} - \sum_{j \epsilon S_i} g_{ij} V_j^{CR} \qquad (1)$$

where V_i^{LAP} is the result of applying this algorithm to the electrode i, V_i^{CR} is the electrode i signal before the transformation and,

$$g_{ij} = \frac{\dfrac{1}{d_{ij}}}{\displaystyle\sum_{j \epsilon S_i} \dfrac{1}{d_{ij}}} \qquad (2)$$

where S_i is the set of electrodes that surround electrode i and d_{ij} is the distance between i and j electrodes.

Then, the power spectral density of the Laplacian waveforms is computed through the maximum entropy method (MEM) [27]. To differentiate between left and right clenches a frequency analysis is made. For each frequency from 1 to 100 hz, the power spectral density (PSD) of electrodes C3 and C4 is calculated. The difference between these 2 values (C4-C3) is computed when the user clenches the left side of the jaw (C4-C3)L and when the clench is produced on the right side (C4-C3)R. After that, the difference (C4-C3)L - (C4-C3)R is calculated and represented on Figure 4. This initial analysis shows that most differences in the

signal power for left and right clenches were present between 57 and 77 Hz and for algorithm only the integral of power spectrum between 57 and 77 Hz was calculated.

Classification

We have developed a classifier based on the application of different thresholds. First of all, each incoming feature is stored in the first position of a 10 position vector (at first filled with zeros) and the rest of the vector is shifted so the oldest value is lost. Every 50 ms, when a new data window (400 ms length with 350 ms overlap with the previous window) arrives, the average of this vector is compared with four thresholds in order to classify the signals. Five tasks have been established according to the power levels received from this average. Each task is associated with a jaw area and the level of clench pressure, and they are defined as follows:

- HardR: Hard right clench
- SoftR: Soft right clench
- Relax: Not clenching
- SoftL: Soft left clench
- HardL: Hard left clench

These tasks are classified through the comparison of 4 thresholds defined as HRthr, SRthr, SLthr and HLthr. Horizontal lines on Figure 5 show a representation of these thresholds, and the areas represent the 5 possible tasks. In Figure 6, PSD levels of tasks SoftR, Relax and SoftL are shown. The central graph shows two vectors of the classifier input from a subject who is not clenching the jaw (Relax). The right and left graphs display the waveforms caused by clenching right and left jaw areas respectively (SoftR and SoftL). This analysis shows that PSD levels from electrode C3 are higher than PSD levels from C4 when the clenching occurs on the left side of the jaw. In a similar way, C4 levels become dominant when clenching is produced on the right side. On the relax task, the PSD from C3 and C4 are similar so the absolute value of the factor C4-C3 is considerably lower. The absolute value of C4-C3 becomes higher when the clench pressure is higher. If the subjects clench the jaw in such a way that the thresholds HRthr or HLthr are exceeded, tasks HardR and

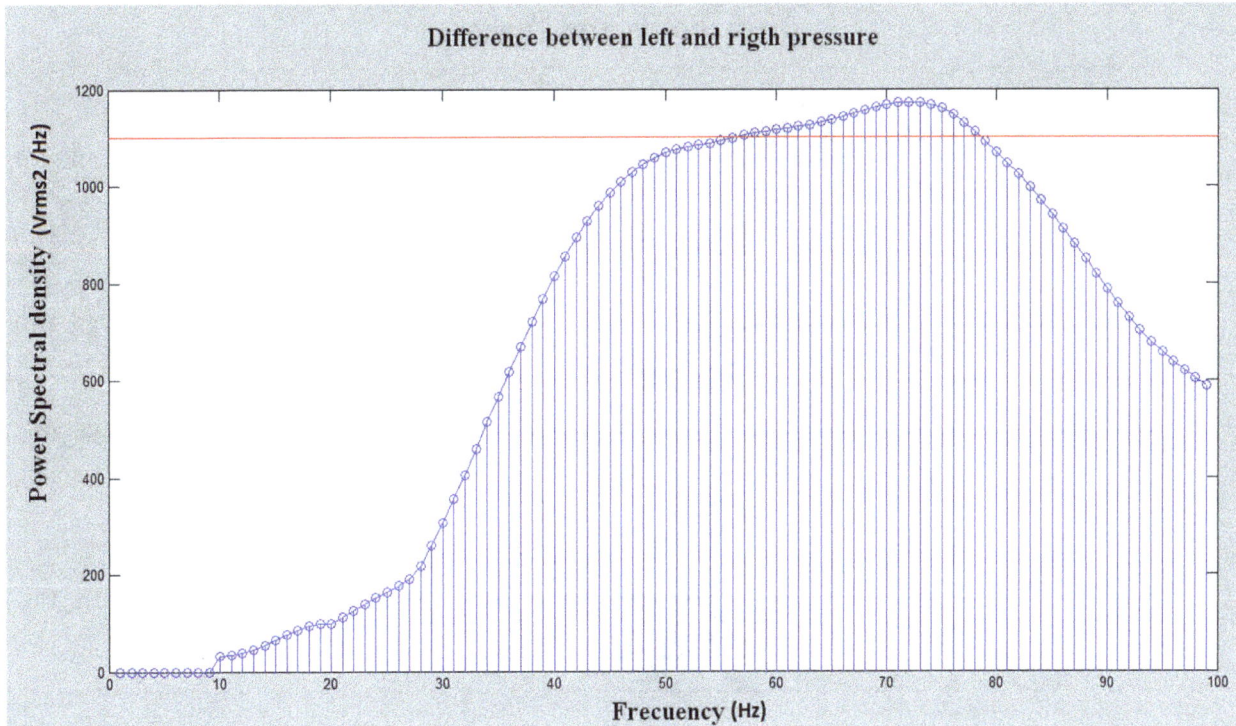

Figure 4. Frequency analysis results. The blue line represent the average Power Spectral Density(PSD) difference between electrodes C3 and C4 for each frequency. The red line represents the minimum spectral level required for a frequency to be target of analysis. These results were obtained from the user 2 (system developer) and compared with the other 3 volunteers to confirm that the optimum range of frequencies does not experience huge changes between users.

HardL (depending on the jaw side) are detected. If the subjects clench the jaw in such a way that the thresholds SRthr or SLthr are exceeded without reaching HRthr or HLthr, tasks SoftR or SoftL are detected depending, again, on the jaw area where the clench is produced. Finally, if the subject is not clenching his/her jaw, no threshold is exceeded and the relax task is detected.

User Training

In order to learn how to control the 2-dimensional movement of a cursor on a screen, two graphical interfaces and a three steps training program have been defined. Training steps 1 and 2 use the first graphical interface, while training step 3 uses the second one. Real time data are processed during all three steps and the interfaces provide visual feedback to the users. This way, the users know how the training is progressing in order to improve their results by adapting the way they clench the jaw. In next section, both graphical interfaces are described. The model used through the training is further described on the section Training Steps.

Graphical Interfaces. Two graphical interfaces are designed. Both of them show a red cursor with a diameter of 25 pixels (about 1.2 cm with a screen size of 38.5×33 cm). The 2-dimensional movement of this cursor is controlled by the user. Depending on the interface, training step and task, the feedback will be different. This is properly explained on each training step on the section Training Steps.

First Interface. This interface is shown on Figure 7. A white cross is shown for 3 seconds on the screen. During this time, the user rests. Afterwards, an image is shown for 2 seconds to indicate the required task to the user. During these seconds, the user is asked to start performing the task. Finally, a red cursor appears on the screen for 10 seconds. This cursor provides feedback of the task

detected by making different movements (in this case only left and right movement are used as feedback, which are further explained in the Training Step section). The control of the cursor depends on the training step. Over one run, this sequence is repeated 15 times making each run 4 minutes long. This interface is used to register data of concrete tasks and create a model adapted to each user.

Second Interface. Figure 8 shows how the second interface works. First, a white cursor appears on the screen for 3 seconds. After that, a target appears randomly on the screen and both the target and the white cursor remain on the screen for 2 more seconds. Finally, the cursor starts moving depending on the users commands generated by jaw clenches. The main goal of this interface is to simulate the bidimensional movement of the cursor controlled by the user. To do that, the model defined during the training is used. If the user reaches the target, the cursor becomes white and blinks several times as a reward.

Training Steps. During these three steps, the user is going to gradually learn how to control the two dimensional cursor movement by clenching the jaw. Each step uses one of the graphical interfaces previously described. All data are processed in real time. From the beginning of the training, the interfaces provide visual feedback to the user by generating cursor movements. In order to produce these movements, a model must exist along the three steps. At first, a default model is defined. During the training, this model is modified to be adapted to the signals of each user.

Step 1: Getting used to the clench. The first step starts with the default model (set of thresholds) [10000 100 -100 -10000] (HRthr, SRthr, SLthr and HLthr, respectively from Figure 6). The first graphical interface is used in order to provide visual feedback. The user is asked randomly by the interface to clench softly the

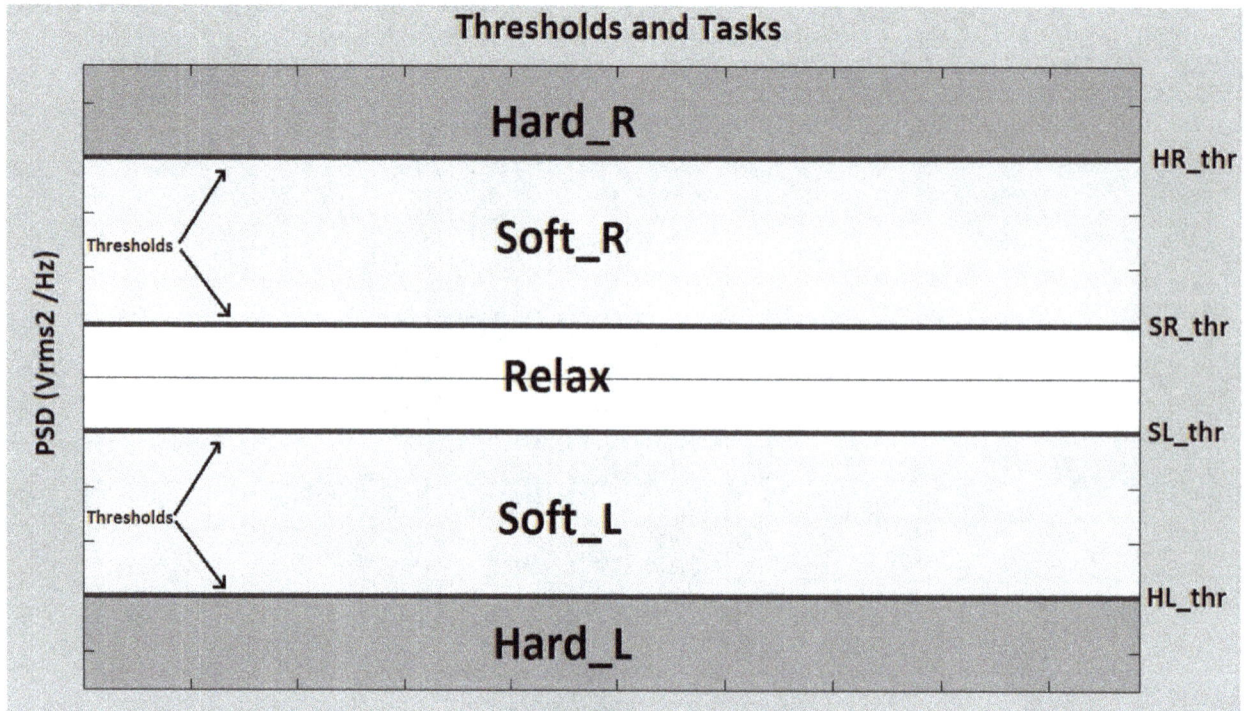

Figure 5. Thresholds and Tasks. Horizontal lines represent the set of thresholds used as model to classify the processed signals. Each threshold represents a level of Power Spectral Density (PSD). Each value on X-axis represents one processed data window. Each data window is classified depending their position on the Y-axis (PSD). Each area delimited by the thresholds represents one of the 5 possible tasks.

right and left jaw areas (tasks SoftR and SoftL). The model is not modified along this step. If the tasks are correctly classified, the red cursor moves right if the clench is produced on the right side, and left if it is produced on the left side. If the clench exceeds thresholds HRthr or HLthr, tasks HardR and HardL are detected and the cursor becomes blue and stops moving. If no threshold is reached, task Relax is detected and the cursor remains red and stopped. During this step, the user gets used to the kind of clench which feels more comfortable with. It has been found that by using this default threshold set, after one 4-minutes run, a user who has never used the system before, is able to control right and left cursor movements. The fact that this default model provides similar

results in different users means that the signals do not experience big changes between users.

Step 2: Creating the model. The second step also starts with the default threshold set [10000 100 -100 -10000]. The same interface from step 1 is used but, this time, tasks SoftR, SoftL and Relax are randomly asked. As in step 1, the user has to clench right and left jaw areas softly when tasks SoftR and SoftL are asked (respectively) and keeps the jaw released when the system asks for Relax task. The visual feedback provided by the interface is the same provided in step 1. Tasks SoftR and SoftL move the cursor right and left, respectively, task Relax makes the cursor stop, and tasks HardR and HardL stop the cursor and makes it blue. In this step, after each 10 seconds performed task by the user, a matrix

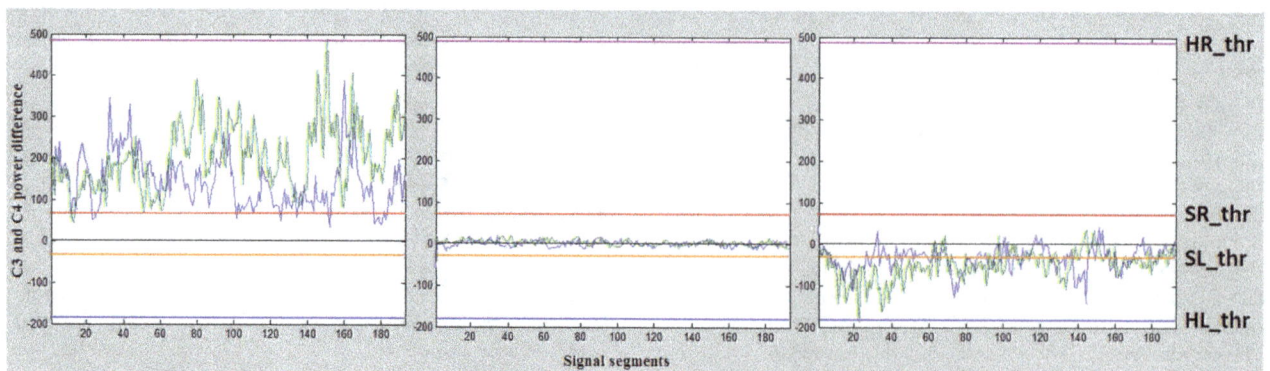

Figure 6. Results obtained for three different tasks during two trials. Signals from the right graph represent two trials (blue and green) where the user clenches the right area of the jaw (SoftR). Signals from the left graph represent two trials where the user clenches the left area of the jaw (SoftL). Signals from the center graph represent two trials where the user releases the jaw (Relax). These signals were recorded from user 2.

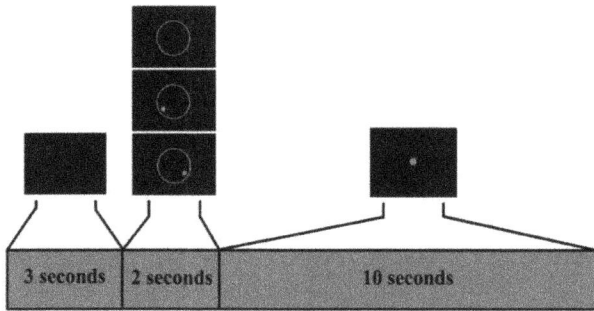

Figure 7. First Interface Protocol. The user is asked to relax during the first 3 seconds, after that, an image appears for 2 seconds to show the task (one of three possible ones) that the user has to perform. For the next 10 seconds, the cursor moves left, right or remains stopped depending on the classified task. After these 10 seconds, the sequence is repeated.

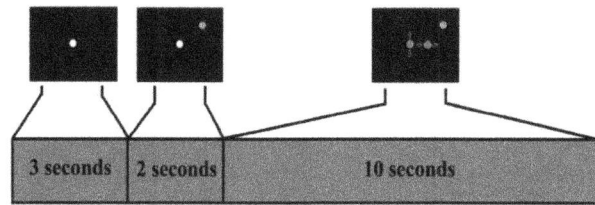

Figure 8. Second Interface Protocol. The user is asked to relax during the first 3 seconds, after that, the user is asked to reach a target. The cursor moves left, right, up, down or remains stopped depending on the classified task until it reaches the target.

like the one shown in Figure 9 is modified. It is a 3×5 matrix whose rows represent each requested task, while the columns represent the number of classified data windows according to the established set of thresholds (there are three rows because only tasks SoftR, SoftL and Relax are requested while there are five columns because tasks HardR and HardL can be also classified). Each 50 ms a new data window is classified, and the matrix is updated by increasing in one the value of the position indicated by the row requested and the column classified. This way, every 10 seconds it is possible to know which tasks were requested and which tasks were classified by looking at the matrix. According to the amount of wrong classified data windows, thresholds are modified to adjust each task area to the users' skills. If the success rate is 100%, those thresholds that delimit the requested task are reduced by 30%. This way, it is possible to reduce the strength of the clench if the user is able to achieve the same results with softer clenches. Also, reducing the area of the tasks performed could allow the inclusion of new tasks above HardR and below HardL in future works. Otherwise, the thresholds will be increased according to the percentage of misclassified tasks. This process makes threshold values converge to their optimal point. However, this process is endless. Therefore, when thresholds are close to their optimal values, they oscillate around them. After five 4-minutes runs, thresholds reach their oscillation point around their optimal values. The final values are decided by seeing the thresholds evolution and manually selecting them. On Figure 10 this evolution and the final set of thresholds selected are shown for all the users. These final thresholds become the model that best fits the signals produced by each user.

Step 3: 2-dimensional movement. In the last step, the starting model is the one obtained from step 2 and it does not evolve during this training step. This time, the second interface is used. Eight targets (with the same cursor size) are defined in eight fixed positions and they appear randomly during this step. The user is requested to reach them by controlling the movement of a two dimensional cursor before a time limit is reached. A target is successfully reached when there is less that 15 pixels (0.72 cm) on each axis (X and Y) between the cursor and the target position. Figure 11 shows a state machine that describes the behavior of the cursor depending on the tasks performed by the user. The 2-dimensional axes are not simultaneously controlled by the user but he/she is able to alternate between movement axis using HardR and HardL tasks. This axis alternation is represented by the change of the color of the cursor from red to blue and viceversa.

When the cursor turns red, the horizontal dimension is controlled and when it becomes blue, the vertical dimension is controlled. Tasks HardR and HardL are achieved by making a strong clench for a short period of time (less than 0.5 seconds, like a quick bite) on right or left areas of the jaw, respectively. The cursor movement is controlled by tasks SoftR and SoftL (right and left, or up and down according to the current selected axis, respectively). Tasks SoftR and SoftL are achieved by clenching softly the respective area of the jaw. Task Relax stops the cursor movement.

During this step, the user gets used to the 2-dimensional movement of the cursor and learns how to control it. Figure 12 shows the signals produced by a user when the two dimensional movement is being controlled. It clearly shows the difference between tasks SoftR, SoftL, HardR and HardL. Eight sessions are performed during this step and in each run, 10 targets appear. The user has 25 seconds to reach each target. Otherwise, the target counts as not reached and a new target appears.

Protocol Summary

Each run is approximately four minutes long, taking one minute break between them. The total training time needed to control the two dimensions with the cursor can be computed as:

- Step 1: One start up run to get used to the kind of jaw movements the system requires.
- Step 2: Five runs where a model is defined for the user (selection of thresholds).
- Step 3: Eight final runs where the user learns how to control the two dimensional movement.

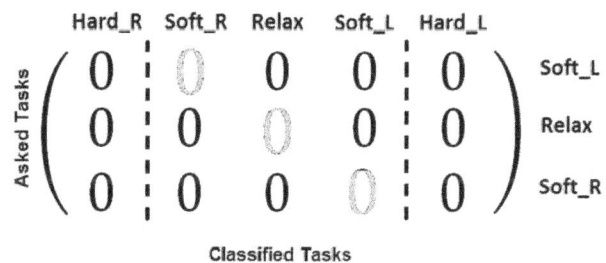

Figure 9. Task classification matrix. Rows represent the tasks requested by the interface and columns represent the tasks classified by the system. Only tasks SoftR, SoftL and Relax are requested while all five tasks (HardR, SoftR, Relax, SoftL and HardL) can be detected. The matrix is initialized with zeros at the beginning of each run and these values are updated with every classification. The thresholds are modified trying to get a diagonal matrix.

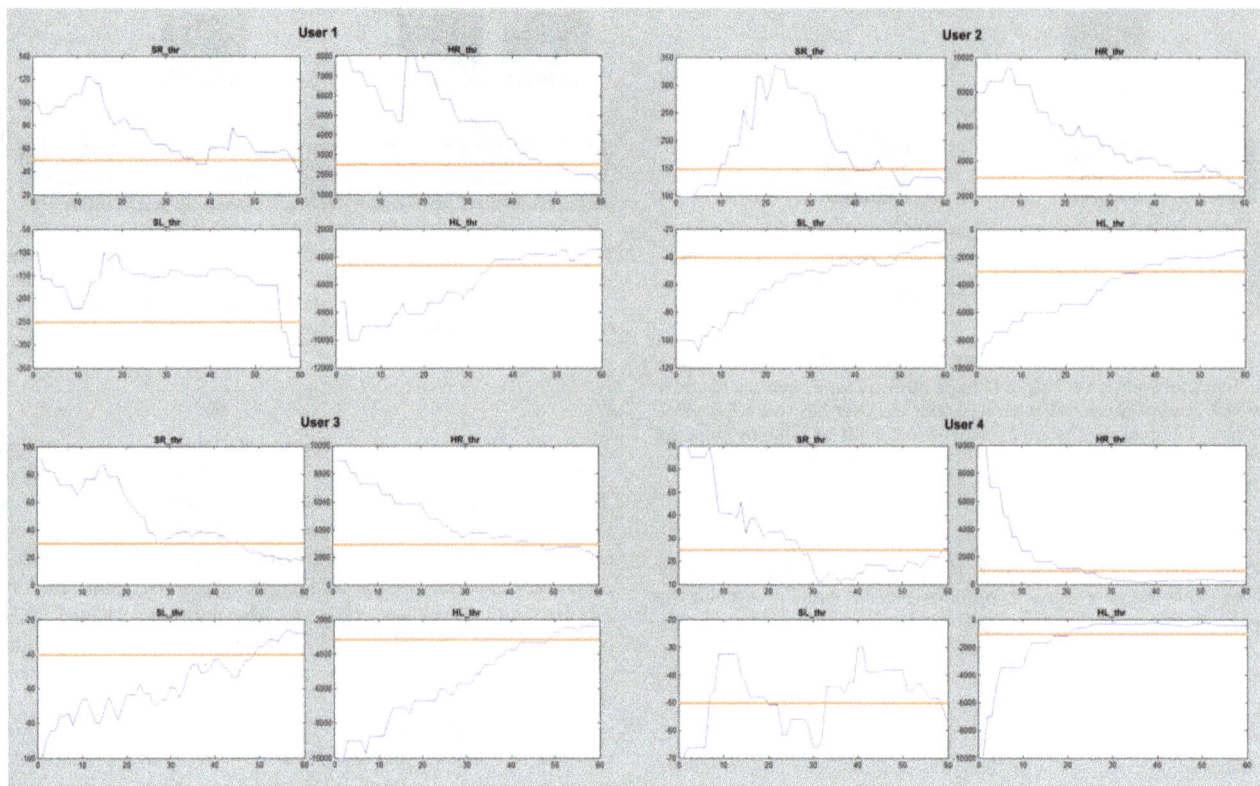

Figure 10. Threshold convergence. The evolution of HRthr, SRthr, SLthr and HLthr are shown for all users. Also the final value selected for each threshold and user is represented with a horizontal line. Y-axis represents the Power Spectral Density and the X-axis represents the number of tasks requested to the user along the 5 runs.

The training process takes approximately 70 minutes. After that, the user has an accurate control of the system and he/she is ready to start controlling the robotic arm as it is shown on the next section.

Robot Control System

After the user is trained in the 2-dimensional control of the cursor, the system is going to be adapted to control the end-effector of a robotic arm on a 2-dimensional plane. Two different

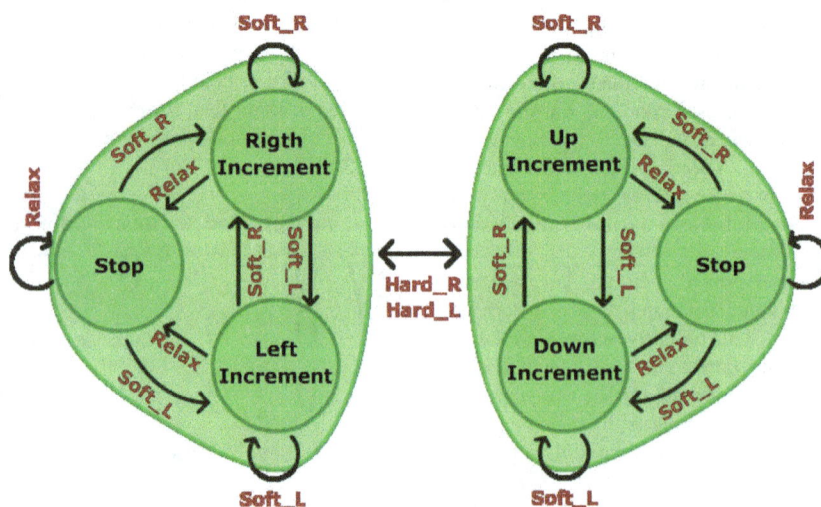

Figure 11. Cursor State Machine. Each group of 3 states represents one of the dimensions. The left group represents the horizontal dimension and the right group represents the vertical dimension. Tasks HardL and HardR are used to alternate between horizontal and vertical dimensions. Once the dimension is selected, tasks SoftR and SoftL control the direction of the movement (on the horizontal dimension, SolfR moves the cursor to the right and SoftL moves the cursor to the left, on the vertical dimension, SoftR moves the cursor up and SoftL moves the cursor down). Relax task stops the cursor no matter the dimension selected.

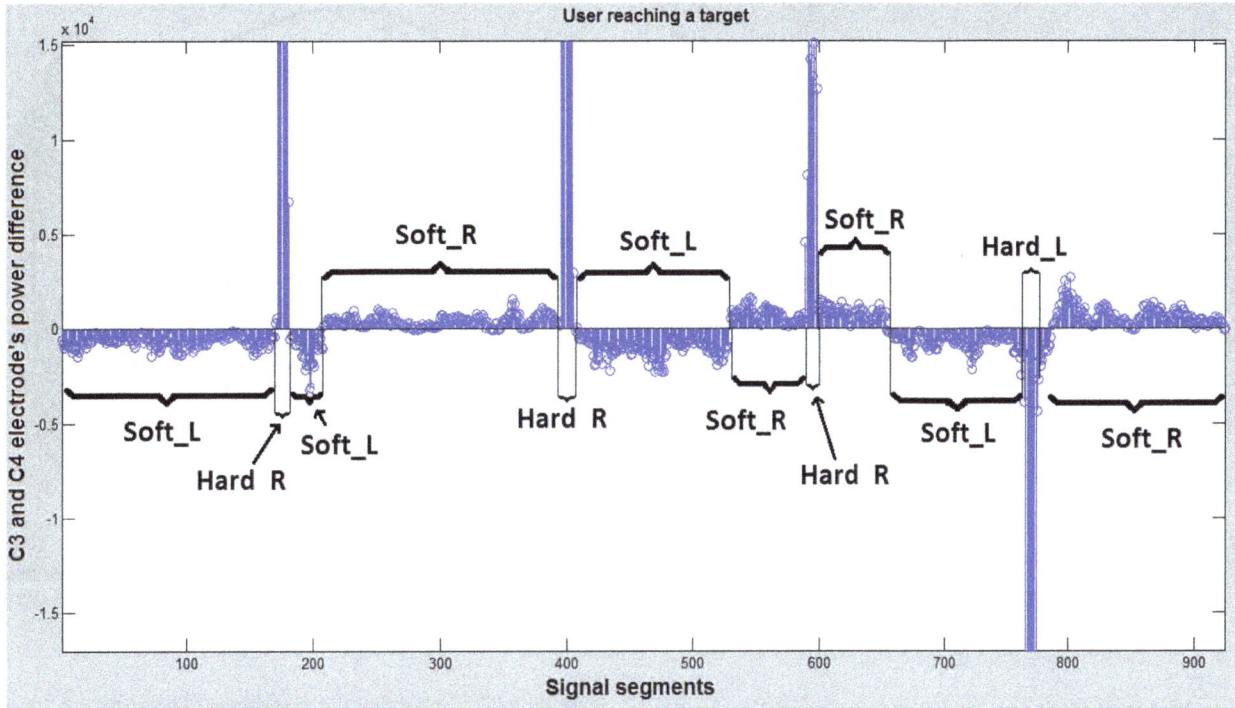

Figure 12. Online results from a user reaching a target (3rd step). SoftR corresponds to the low positive values, SoftL to the low negative values, HardR to the high positive values, and HardL to the high negative values. Relax task is not used (its power level is lower than SoftR and SoftL). Y-axis represents the PSD difference between C3 and C4. X-axis represents the number of analyzed data windows (each 50 ms a new data window is analyzed).

processes are running simultaneously to achieve this goal. A Matlab function is in charge of the processing and classification of signals and it also provides a simple graphical interface to help the users on their first contact with the robotic arm. A C++ program translates the classification results into control commands and sends them to the robotic arm.

Robotic Arm. For the kind of movements wanted on this research, a 2.5D plotter robot may be a more suitable option but due to equipment already available in the research facility, the robotic arm used is the Fanuc LR Mate 200iB. It is a six degrees of freedom robot that can be moved in a three dimensional workspace. Figure 13 shows the robot appearance. The robotic arm is controlled using a C++ program through a local computer network. This program is used to send movement instructions to the LR Mate 200iB. It also receives information about the current position of the robot. Moreover, the C++ program runs a control panel whose main goal is to provide a set of simple instructions to control the interaction with the robot [1]. Through this panel, it is possible to connect and disconnect the robot. It also implements a function to send the robot to a home position and another function is in charge of sending movement instructions to the robot in real time according to the classification results provided by Matlab.

Graphical Interface. A Matlab-based application algorithm registers, processes and classifies the information recorded from the sensorimotor scalp areas. The C++ program uses the final data provided by Matlab in order to send movement instructions to the robotic arm. A communication system has been implemented to make possible the interaction between both processes. This communication introduces a small delay (less than 0.5 seconds) between the moment when the user executes the task and the moment when the robotic arm starts moving. For that reason, a graphical interface has been designed to provide visual feedback of

each classified direction. This visual feedback uses the image shown in Figure 14. Each circle represents a direction in a two dimensional plane. This way, it is possible for a user to move the robotic arm to one of these directions. The full circle corresponding to the direction where the robot is moving gets coloured blue while the others remain empty. This interface is only used on the

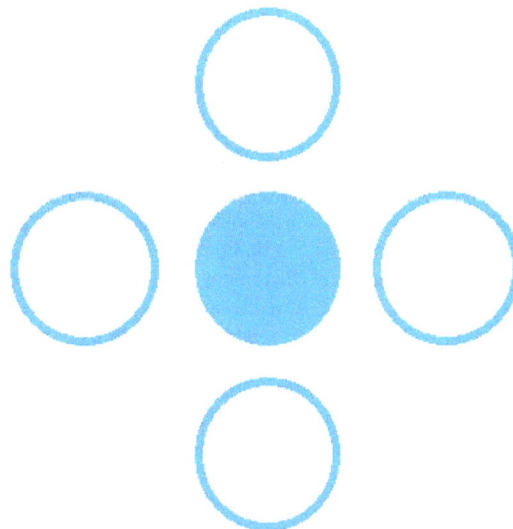

Figure 13. Robotic Arm Environment. It allows movements in a three dimensional workspace. Z-axis remains fixed during tests. The spots show the position of the 8 targets defined.

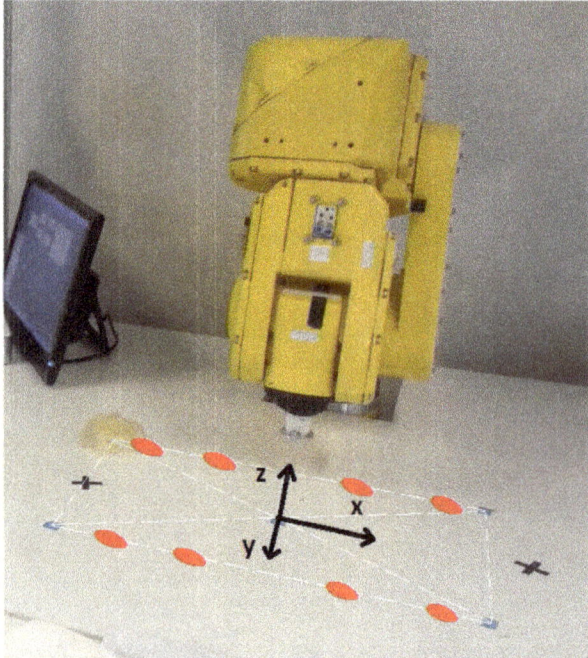

Figure 14. Visual feedback. The full circle represents the direction identified by the algorithm. The robotic arm moves according to the direction shown on this interface.

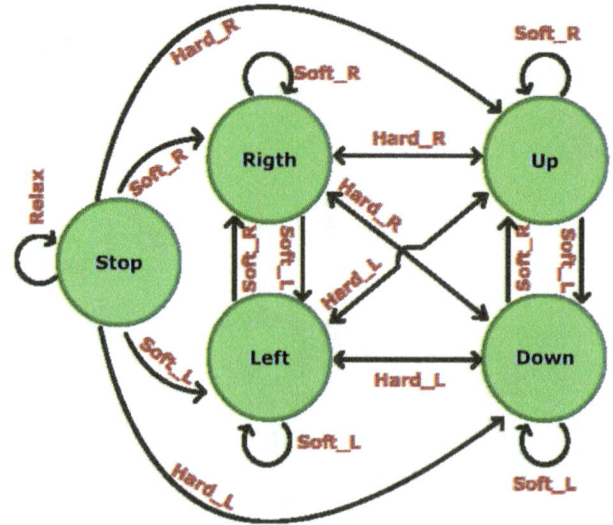

Figure 15. Robotic Arm State Machine. When a state changes, a continuous movement starts in the direction indicated by the current state.

first run performed with the robotic arm. After that, the user gets used to the small delay and the interface can be removed.

Real Time Test. Tests have been made over a two dimensional workspace. Z-axis is fixed and X-axis and Y-axis are restricted to a rectangle area DIN-A3 size. This way, the users who trained on a computer screen are familiar with the movement area. Figure 13 shows the mentioned workspace. As it can be seen, 8 targets have been placed on the workspace. The users were requested to reach these targets by controlling the robotic arm. Each user has performed nine runs. In the first run no target is requested. The user uses this run to get used to the system delay. The eight remaining runs are used to reach the eight possible targets shown on Figure 13. On each run, a different target is requested and the robotic arm movement stops when the target is reached. Robotic arm movement is controlled by the user through the five tasks previously described. In order to keep HardR and HardL as short duration tasks, a state machine (Figure 15) is designed. As it can be seen, the control of the two dimensional movement is similar to the one used on training step 3. The differences are due to the delay limitations introduced by the robot. Although the movement increment is detected by the system each 50 ms, the robotic arm cannot respond with such speed. For this reason, movement commands are sent only when a change of direction is detected in order to reduce the delay times. For instance, if a right movement state is detected, the robotic arm starts a right continuous movement until a new state is detected. At that moment, the current robot movement is stopped and a new movement begins.

Results and Discussion

The system was tested with four healthy volunteers (capable of moving their jaws) with ages between 22 and 28 (24.25 ± 2.62) (three men with previous experience with this kind of tests and one woman without any, all of them right-handed). All the volunteers

were sat while performing the experiment. They were told not to blink nor perform neck movements, except in rest periods indicated during the tests. The results presented on this work were obtained over a period of 3 months. The data of the cursor movement were registered in the first month and the robot arm control data in the third month. Human data presented in this article have been acquired under an experimental protocol approved by the ethics committee for experimental research of the Miguel Hernández University of Elche, Spain. Written consent according to the Helsinki declaration was obtained from each subject. Also the participants shown in Figure 3 and on referred videos have given written informed consent (as outlined in PLOS consent form) to publish these case details.

Cursor Movement Results

During step 1, all users got used to the kind of clenching that the system is able to identify. They also achieved a successful threshold convergence during the 5 runs from step 2. On the third step, users 1, 2 and 4 noticed that tasks SoftR and SoftL are correctly detected by making a small jaw movement to the side the user wants to move the cursor without the need of clenching their teeth. User 3 kept clenching the jaw. All the users achieved tasks HardR and HardL by making a quick bite with the right or left side of the jaw. Table 1 shows the success and fail rate depending on the number of targets reached by a user in each run. User 2 is the system developer so it has more experience than the rest. As a consequence, he reached all the targets under the time limit. As it has been mentioned, the learning process takes place from runs 1 to 3. During these 3 runs, success rate experiences a huge improvement and after that it remains constant. The control that the user achieves after the third run is very similar to the control anyone can achieve using a joystick or other manual control as shown on video S1. In section Protocol Summary, the training time was estimated as 70 minutes, but by seeing these results, in 3 runs the control of the system is really close to its optimum. Thus it is reasonable to say that the training process could be reduced to 45 min. Table 2 shows the time efficiency in the reaching of targets where the time efficiency coefficient has been defined as follows:

Table 1. Targets Reached.

	Run 1	Run 2	Run 3	Run 4	Run 5	Run 6	Run 7	Run 8
User 1	30	70	90	90	100	90	100	90
User 2	100	100	100	100	100	100	100	100
User 3	40	80	90	90	100	100	80	100
User 4	80	80	100	100	90	90	100	100

Percentage (%) of targets reached by the user on each run.

Table 2. Coefficient of Spent Time to Reach the Target with the Cursor.

		1	2	3	4	5	6	7	8	Avg
	1	0.636	0.688	0.815	0.790	0.784	0.824	0.733	0.801	0.759
	2	0.868	0.915	0.891	0.927	0.856	0.802	0.900	0.914	0.884
Users	3	0.657	0.768	0.812	0.740	0.739	0.791	0.825	0.784	0.765
	4	0.834	0.742	0.838	0.814	0.727	0.801	0.767	0.820	0.793
	Avg	0.749	0.778	0.839	0.818	0.777	0.804	0.806	0.830	**0.800**

The values show the C_{opT} for each user to reach every target.

Table 3. Robotic Arm Time Percentage.

		1	2	3	4	5	6	7	8	Avg
Users	1	0.856	0.768	0.931	0.894	0.680	0.904	0.833	0.816	0.835
	2	0.904	0.955	0.707	0.669	0.904	0.899	0.855	0.859	0.844
	3	0.879	0.990	0.837	0.946	0.837	0.938	0.821	0.911	0.895
	4	0.994	0.837	0.890	0.755	0.788	0.764	0.988	0.622	0.830
	Avg	0.908	0.890	0.841	0.816	0.802	0.876	0.874	0.802	**0.851**

The values shown indicate the C_{opT} for each user to reach every target.

$$C_{opT} = \frac{Optimum\ Time}{Time\ used} \qquad (3)$$

The *time used* is the time spent for the user to reach the target, and *optimum time* is the time needed to reach the target if the cursor is controlled manually. To obtain the optimum time, an algorithm that allows a subject to control the cursor by using the key arrows is implemented. All users were asked to reach each target using this manual control. The *optimum time* for each target is calculated as the average of the time employed by all users using this manual control (this average presents a very small deviation meaning that the optimum times are very similar between users). The non-reached targets were not computed to obtain these results. C_{opT} is in average 0.8 throughout the 8 runs for all subjects. In order to prove the efficiency of this system, the average value of the obtained C_{opT} is compared with the average C_{opT} of a BMI system based on motor imagery tasks and a system based in electrooculography (which usually provides better results than motor imagery systems). The optimum time is calculated on these systems according to the methodology previously explained. Analyzing the results from [27,28] (which are previous works done by our group in a similar environment with a hieralchical motor imagery BMI system and a electrooculographic system) the average C_{opT} obtained in the BMI system is 0.033, which is 30.30 times worse than the optimum time, and the average C_{opT} obtained in the electrooculographic system is 0.588, which is 1.7 times worse than the optimum time. Using our system to move a cursor on a screen, the average C_{opT} for all runs and users is 0.8, which is 24.24 times quicker than the motor imagery BMI system (0.033) and 1.36 times quicker than the electrooculographic system (0.588).

Robotic Arm Movement Trials Results

After the training section, users are ready to control the robotic arm in two dimensions. They are requested to reach eight different targets. Time required to reach each target is measured. Table 3 shows the values of C_{opT} obtained by the users to reach each target referred to the minimum time needed by the robot to reach them (manually controlled) under the same conditions. The strategy used in the previous section was applied here to obtain the values of the *optimum time*. All users were also requested to reach the targets using the arrow keys. In this case, there is no improvement along runs due to the similarities between the cursor movement system (Training section) and the robot movement system. Results are also compared with the needed time percentages to reach targets using a system based on motor imagery tasks seen on the last section (0.033). This time, the improvement is, in average, 0.818, which is 24.78 times better than a motor imagery BMI system and 1.4 times better than the electrooculographic system. On videos S2 and S3 are shown 2 subjects who have completed the training in a free movement test reaching a target with and without obstacles in the workspace.

System Limitations

The number of states able to be detected on this system is limited by the behavior of the measured signals. For soft clenching, the PSD increment can be easily controlled by the user, but when the clench is higher, the PSD behaves similar to an exponential function, increasing considerably the control difficulty. Also, thresholds have been defined in order to benefit tasks SoftR, SoftL, HardR and HardL, but making hard for some users the

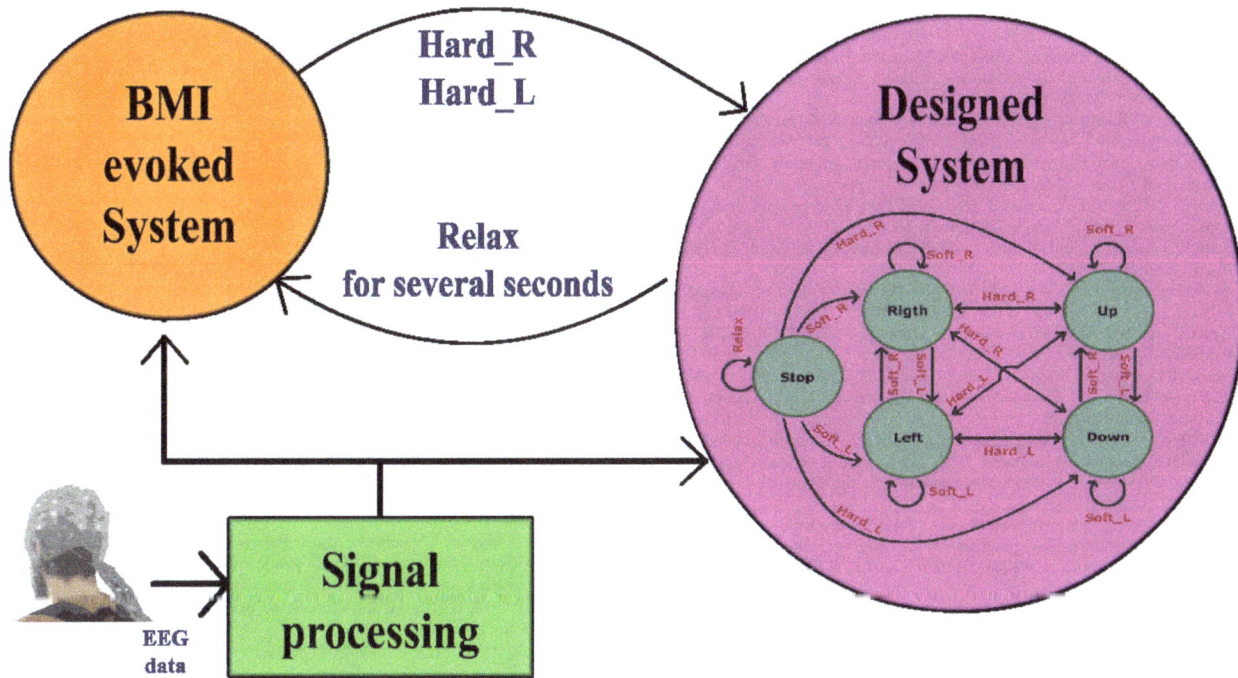

Figure 16. Block interconnection diagram. The supplementary system is activated with tasks HardR or HardL, while the control is returned to the BMI system when the user stays on the Relax state for several seconds.

control of the Relax state. This point should be further studied in future works.

Conclusion

A supplementary application for a BMI system has been designed. A very similar system could also be implemented placing a couple of electromyographic electrodes on both cheeks or placing pressure sensors on the teeth. However, the goal of this research is to use the electrodes of a BMI system in order to implement a supplementary system based on the skill of a user to control EMG signals produced by clenching different areas of the jaw. Results prove that the control acquired by users who can move their jaws is close to the control that a healthy user can acquire using a joystick or the movement arrows of a keyboard.

On the basis of this study, the architecture shown on Figure 16 is proposed as a future work. A BMI system would work while the jaw is relaxed. At the moment the user wants to alternate to jaw control, a quick bite (tasks HardR or HardL) would activate the jaw control algorithm. The change to the BMI system should be produced when the user remains several consecutive seconds on the Relax state. Our supplementary system should be complemented with an appropriate BMI system, i.e. a menu application that allows a patient to select the rehabilitation strategy desired while a BMI system measures the mental state of the patient in order to evaluate how the selected strategy affects the mental workload of the patient. It is also proposed its use in combination with a BMI system previously developed by our group [24], where visual evoked potentials were used to control an internet browser, allowing a user to write and move the cursor on the screen. The BMI system provides a quick and fluid writing but the cursor control can be improved by using the supplementary system designed. On the same work, the BMI system is used to control a robot arm in 3 dimensions. For that purpose, the user first selects

the movement plane and then, a 2-dimensional control also based on evoked potentials is used. Using the 2-dimensional control implemented in the current work, it would be possible to improve the performance of the 3-dimensional control described in [24], by combining the plane selection algorithm of the evoked BMI system and the 2-dimensional control implemented in our supplementary system. As a conclusion, this supplementary system allows us to implement a control system in combination with a BMI system using the same set of sensors. This system is oriented to help people who suffer from motor disabilities which deprive them from moving their arms or legs but still have mobility on the jaw. In the future, this system should be tested on this kind of patients. The system might be also adapted for 3-dimensional movement by alternating between three space axes instead of two. Another research line would be to compare a third electrode from a central position (like Cz or CPz) with C3 and C4 in order to measure separately the level of clench from left and right areas of the jaw so both dimensions, X and Y, would be simultaneously controlled.

Author Contributions

Conceived and designed the experiments: AC EI JMA. Performed the experiments: AC EH. Analyzed the data: AC. Contributed reagents/materials/analysis tools: EI JMA. Wrote the paper: AC EI EH JMA.

References

1. Iáñez E, Úbeda A, Hortal E, Azorín JM, Fernández E (2013) Empirical analysis of the integration of a bci and an eog interface to control a robot arm. In: IWINAC (1)'13. pp. 151–160.
2. Takahashi K, Kashiyama T (2005) Remarks on multimodal nonverbal interface and its application to controlling mobile robot. In: Mechatronics and Automation, 2005 IEEE International Conference. volume 2, pp. 999–1004 Vol. 2. doi:10.1109/ICMA.2005.1626688.
3. Sokol S (1976) Visually evoked potentials: Theory, techniques and clinical applications. Survey of Ophthalmology 21: 18–44.
4. Ruth R, Lambert P (1991) Auditory evoked potentials. Otolaryngologic clinics of North America 24: 349370.
5. Volosyak I, Guger C, Graser A (2010) Toward bci wizard - best bci approach for each user. In: Engineering in Medicine and Biology Society (EMBC), 2010 Annual International Conference of the IEEE. pp. 4201–4204. doi:10.1109/ IEMBS.2010.5627390.
6. Marshall D, Coyle D, Wilson S, Callaghan M (2013) Games, gameplay, and bci: The state of the art. Computational Intelligence and AI in Games, IEEE Transactions on 5: 82–99.
7. Hamadicharef B (2010) Brain-computer interface (bci) literature - a bibliometric study. In: Information Sciences Signal Processing and their Applications (ISSPA), 2010 10th International Conference on. pp. 626–629. doi:10.1109/ ISSPA.2010.5605421.
8. Bi L, Fan X, Jie K, Teng T, Ding H, et al. (2014) Using a head-up display-based steady-state visually evoked potential brain; computer interface to control a simulated vehicle. Intelligent Transportation Systems, IEEE Transactions on 15: 959–966.
9. Trejo L, Rosipal R, Matthews B (2006) Brain-computer interfaces for 1-d and 2-d cursor control: designs using volitional control of the eeg spectrum or steady-state visual evoked potentials. Neural Systems and Rehabilitation Engineering, IEEE Transactions on 14: 225–229.
10. Dasey T, Micheli-Tzanakou E (2000) Detection of multiple sclerosis with visual evoked potentials - an unsupervised computational intelligence system. Information Technology in Biomedicine, IEEE Transactions on 4: 216–224.
11. Fujita T, Yamasaki T, Kamio Y, Hirose S, Tobimatsu S (2011) Parvocellular pathway impairment in autism spectrum disorder: Evidence from visual evoked potentials. Research in Autism Spectrum Disorders 5: 277–285.
12. Nakamae T, Tanaka N, Nakanishi K, Fujimoto Y, Sasaki H, et al. (2010) Quantitative assessment of myelopathy patients using motor evoked potentials produced by transcranial magnetic stimulation. European Spine Journal 19: 685–690.
13. Roy R, Bonnet S, Charbonnier S, Campagne A (2013) Mental fatigue and working memory load estimation: Interaction and implications for eeg-based passive bci. In: Engineering in Medicine and Biology Society (EMBC), 2013 35th Annual International Conference of the IEEE. pp. 6607–6610. doi:10.1109/EMBC.2013.6611070.
14. Duvinage M, Castermans T, Petieau M, Seetharaman K, Hoellinger T, et al. (2012) A subjective assessment of a p300 bci system for lower-limb rehabilitation purposes. In: Engineering in Medicine and Biology Society (EMBC), 2012 Annual International Conference of the IEEE. pp. 3845–3849. doi:10.1109/ EMBC.2012.6346806.
15. Carmena JM, Lebedev MA, Crist RE, O'Doherty JE, Santucci DM, et al. (2003) Learning to control a brainmachine interface for reaching and grasping by primates. PLoS Biol 1: e42.
16. Velliste M, Perel S, Spalding MC, Whitford AS, Schwartz AB (2008) Cortical control of a prosthetic arm for self-feeding. Nature 453: 1098–1101.
17. Huang D, Qian K, Fei DY, Jia W, Chen X, et al. (2012) Electroencephalography (eeg)-based brain-computer interface (bci): A 2-d virtual wheelchair control based on event-related desynchronization/synchronization and state control. Neural Systems and Rehabilitation Engineering, IEEE Transactions on 20: 379–388.
18. Frisoli A, Loconsole C, Leonardis D, Banno F, Barsotti M, et al. (2012) Systems, man, and cybernetics. part c: Applications and reviews. IEEE Transactions 42: 1169–1179.
19. Postelnicu CC, Talaba D (2013) P300-based brain-neuronal computer interaction for spelling applications. Biomedical Engineering, IEEE Transactions on 60: 534–543.
20. Fatourechi M, Bashashati A, Ward RK, Birch GE (2007) Emg and eog artifacts in brain computer interface systems: A survey. Clinical Neurophysiology118: 480–494.
21. Daly I, Billinger M, Scherer R, Muller-Putz G (2013) On the automated removal of artifacts related to head movement from the Neural Systems and Rehabilitation Engineering, IEEE Transactions on 21: 427–434.
22. Savelainen A (2010) An introduction to eeg artifacts. Independent research projects in applied mathematics.
23. Yong X, Ward R, Birch G (2008) Facial emg contamination of eeg signals: Characteristics and effects of spatial filtering. In: Communications, Control and Signal Processing, 2008. ISCCSP 2008. 3rd International Symposium on. pp. 729–734. doi:10.1109/ISCCSP.2008.4537319.
24. Blasco JS, Iez E, beda A, Azorn J (2012) Visual evoked potential-based brainmachine interface applications to assist disabled people. Expert Systems with Applications 39: 7908–7918.
25. Guger C, Ramoser H, Pfurtscheller G (2000) Real-time eeg analysis with subject-speci c spatial patterns for a brain-computer interface (bci). Rehabilitation Engineering, IEEE Transactions on 8: 447–456.
26. Hjorth B (1975) An on-line transformation of fEEGg scalp potentials into orthogonal source derivations. Electroencephalography and Clinical Neurophysiology 39: 526–530.
27. Hortal E, Úbeda A, Iáñez E, Azorín JM (2014) Control of a 2 dof robot using a brainmachine interface. Computer Methods and Programs in Biomedicine
28. Úbeda A, Iáñez E, Azorín J (2011) Wireless and portable eog-based interface for assisting disabled people. Mechatronics, IEEE/ASME Transactions on 16: 870–873.

22

The Neural Response to Maternal Stimuli: An ERP Study

Lili Wu[1], Ruolei Gu[2], Huajian Cai[2*], Yu L. L. Luo[2], Jianxin Zhang[1*]

1 Key Laboratory of Mental Health, Institute of Psychology, Chinese Academy of Sciences, Beijing, China, **2** Key Laboratory of Behavioral Science, Institute of Psychology, Chinese Academy of Sciences, Beijing, China

Abstract

Mothers are important to all humans. Research has established that maternal information affects individuals' cognition, emotion, and behavior. We measured event-related potentials (ERPs) to examine attentional and evaluative processing of maternal stimuli while participants completed a Go/No-go Association Task that paired *mother* or *others* words with *good* or *bad* evaluative words. Behavioral data showed that participants responded faster to *mother* words paired with *good* than the *mother* words paired with *bad* but showed no difference in response to these *others* across conditions, reflecting a positive evaluation of mother. ERPs showed larger P200 and N200 in response to *mother* than in response to *others*, suggesting that *mother* attracted more attention than *others*. In the subsequent time window, *mother* in the *mother + bad* condition elicited a later and larger late positive potential (LPP) than it did in the *mother + good* condition, but this was not true for *others*, also suggesting a positive evaluation of mother. These results suggest that people differentiate *mother* from *others* during initial attentional stage, and evaluative *mother* positively during later stage.

Editor: Michael A. Motes, Center for BrainHealth, University of Texas at Dallas, United States of America

Funding: This work was supported by the National Natural Science Foundation of China [Grants No. 31200789 and 31070919], the Knowledge Innovation Program of the Chinese Academy of Sciences [Grants No. KSCX2-EW-J-8], Hundred Talents Program [Y0C2024002] as well as the Scientific Foundation of Institute of Psychology, Chinese Academy of Sciences [Grants No. Y0CX363S01 and Y2CQ013005]. The funders had no role in study design, data collection and analysis, decision to publish, or preparation of the manuscript.

Competing Interests: The authors have declared that no competing interests exist.

* Email: caihj@psych.ac.cn (HC); zhangjx@psych.ac.cn (JZ)

Introduction

The mother is important for human beings throughout their lifetime. A mother's physiological and mental state during the pregnancy contributes substantially to her child's physical and psychological health in both early and late infancy (e.g., [1–4]). In early childhood, the mother regulates the physiological state and behaviors of her child [5]. Attachment to their mothers is the start of children's socialization, which facilitates social and affective development [6]. Later, mothers' parenting behavior affects adolescents' emotional regulation ability and problem behaviors [7,8]. Finally, for adults, mothers are still an essential part of individuals' attachment networks [9]. Furthermore, the perceived quality of the parent-child relationship during childhood predicts adults' psychological and physical well-being throughout the lifespan [10,11]. In short, the significance of mothers is difficult to overestimate.

Given this physical and psychological significance, a large number of empirical studies have focused on how stimuli related to the mother, such as a mother's face or name, affect information processing. Findings from studies using behavioral (e.g., [12–14]), electrophysiological (e.g., [15]) and neuroimaging measures (e.g., [16]) show that maternal stimuli affect people's attention and evaluative responses. From the attentional perspective, individuals show a tendency to attend more to maternal stimuli than other kinds of stimuli across different ages. For instance, newborns (4 hours to 72 hours after birth) stare at their mother's face longer than at a stranger's face [12–14,17,18]. Furthermore, an electrophysiological study showed that mothers' faces elicited a larger negative component (Nc, occurring 400 to 800 ms,

indexing attentional response) compared with a stranger's face, indicating that infants allocate increased attention to the mother's face [15]. For adults, the faces of mothers elicited greater activation in facial-specific regions than the faces of others, including strangers, celebrities or even fathers [16]. From an evaluative perspective, maternal stimuli are perceived more positively than other stimuli. For instance, people favor their mother's name [19], show a higher retrieval rate for favorable traits than for unfavorable traits after a mother-reference task [20], and are inclined to interpret their mother's neutral faces as cheerful faces [21].

Although these studies highlight attentional preference and evaluative positivity when processing maternal stimuli, two issues still remain unclear. First, the attentional bias to maternal information usually has been attributed to familiarity [e.g., 15, 16], but a recent study showed that the preference for maternal information was strongly affected by the intense attachment to mother, rather than just reflecting familiarity [21]. However, it is difficult to rule out the familiarity effect because previous studies on the mother/stranger distinction used pictures of mothers and strangers as material. Thus, effectively controlling for the familiarity of material is necessary when evaluating whether the preference for mother is due to the intense attachment. Second, previous studies have found that individuals have positive evaluations of their mothers [19,20,21], but this tendency might be affected by a social desirability bias, influencing participants to show favoritism to their mother over others. However, combining an implicit task with measurements of neural responses that index online mental operations independent of behavioral response processes would reduce the impact of social desirability bias on maternal evaluations.

The present study sought to examine the attentional and evaluative processing of maternal stimuli using event-related potentials (ERPs). ERPs are particularly well-suited for examining these two processes, because the ERP waveform, measured in response to a stimulus, contains a number of components that are temporally linked to the emergence of different mental operations, including perception, attention, and evaluation [22]. This property of the ERP technique makes it particularly useful for examining attentional and evaluative processes by assessing different components.

Previous research used various types of maternal stimuli, including faces, names, and basic word descriptions (e.g., "mother") [15,16,19,20]. In the present study, we used words for *mother* and *others* as stimuli. We used words instead of pictures as maternal stimuli because the evaluative dimensions in the task were described by words (good or bad). This effectively eliminated the potential effect of switching between word and picture processing during the experiment. Most importantly, words are more effective for controlling for the familiarity, because the familiarity of word stimuli could be indexed by objective measures such as frequency.

We selected the Go/No-go Association Task (GNAT, [23]) because of its suitability for ERP studies (e.g., [24,25]). More importantly, this paradigm is suitable for examining the attentional and evaluative processing of maternal stimuli by creating contrasts between different experimental blocks. In particular, we used two blocks to explore the processing of maternal stimuli (*mother + good* and *mother + bad*) and two further blocks to explore the processing of non-specific *others* (*others + good* and *others + bad*). For all four blocks, we focused on the behavioral and neural responses to *mother* and *others* stimuli and compared them between the different conditions to test for difference in attentional and evaluative processes. The contrast between *mother* blocks and *others* blocks allowed for examining differences in attentional resource allocation between *mother* and *others*. Furthermore, the evaluative processing of maternal stimuli was examined by contrasting the *mother + good* and *mother + bad* conditions, where the evaluation of *mother* was operationalized as the associative strength of maternal stimuli with positive or negative attributes in the GNATs.

To examine the attentional processing of maternal stimuli, two ERP components, the P200 and N200 were measured and analyzed. Enhanced amplitudes of these two components are assumed to reflect increased attention to information with intrinsic personal relevance, such as self-related information [26,27,28–31]. Thus, we assessed whether participants differentiated *mother* from non-specific *others* at an early attentional stage by examining the amplitudes of these two ERP components across the four conditions. Specifically, we hypothesized that *mother* would draw more attention than *others*, as indicated by increased P200 and N200 components, because of the mother's critical role in a child's life.

In addition, to further explore the evaluative processing of maternal stimuli, the late positive potential (LPP) that is generally found to be maximal around the posterior region of the scalp (for reviews, see [32–35]) was examined. This component has been associated with evaluative processing [36–39]. Its peak latency could be used as a neural indicator of the speed of categorization and evaluation (for a review, see [33]). Inconsistency between the current stimulus representation and a previous expectation or evaluation enhances LPP amplitude [36,37]. In the area of social cognition, the LPP has been used to assess the evaluation of

specific social groups. For instance, the LPP amplitude is larger for counter-stereotype associations than stereotype-consistent associations, reflecting a violation of a previously established evaluation and implicit racial attitude [40,41]. Meanwhile, compared with stereotype-consistent information, the LPP latency is longer when counter-stereotype information is processed [40]. In the present study, we hypothesized that the LPP would reflect participants' evaluations of maternal stimuli. Specially, *mother* words would elicit a larger and later LPP in the *mother + bad* condition than in the *mother + good* condition due to the violation of the positive attitude towards the mother in the former condition. By contrast, people usually hold neutral attitudes towards non-specific others [42,43]. Therefore, we expected that the LPP amplitude or its latency would not differ between the *others + good* and *others +bad* conditions.

In short, we investigated the neural correlates underlying maternal stimulus processing. We hypothesized that the attentional bias for maternal stimuli would be reflected in the P200 and N200 components and the positive evaluation bias for maternal stimuli would be reflected in the LPP.

Method

Ethics statement

The experimental protocol was approved by the Institutional Review Board (IRB) at the Institute of Psychology, Chinese Academy of Sciences. We explained the experimental procedure to each participant after he or she arrived at the lab. Moreover, informed written consent was obtained from each participant before the experiment.

Participants

Twenty-seven college students (19–25 years old, 12 males, all right-handed) participated in this study as paid volunteers. None had a history of neurological or psychiatric disorders. All had normal or corrected-to-normal vision. Data from 4 participants (3 males) were not included in final analysis because of technical problems during data acquisition. As a result, the final sample consisted of twenty-three participants (9 males; age, $M = 21.8$ years, $SD = 1.7$ years).

Materials

We selected 170 Chinese words as stimuli: 5 *mother* words (ma, mother, mama, ama ("阿妈", means mom) and niang ("娘", means mom), 5 *others* words (he, him, his, other ("他人", means other people) and other ("别人", means other people), 80 *good* or *positive* and 80 *bad* or *negative* attributes. Most attributes were selected from the Chinese version of personal trait words provided by Anderson [44]. The remaining attributes were selected from a Chinese attribute list developed for a prior study examining implicit and explicit self-enhancement [45].

The familiarity of the target category was manipulated from three perspectives. First, all the characters we used are frequently used in daily life (i.e., they were among the top 8% of the 10,241 characters in the "Combined character frequency list of Classical and Modern Chinese, see the link http://lingua.mtsu.edu/chinese-computing/statistics/char/list.php?Which=TO"). Second, the frequency of *mother* words is not significantly different from that of *others* words (8,001 vs. 321,369, $t_{(4.002)} = 2.44$, $p = .071$) in the Chinese language, according to the word frequency Dictionary of Chinese characters and words (developed by the International R&D Center for Chinese Education, http://nlp.blcu.edu.cn). Third, to make sure that participants were familiar with both the *mother* and *others* words before the formal experiment, we required them to achieve response accuracy higher than 85% in the practice task.

Procedure

Two GNATs consisted of four blocks: *mother + good*, *mother + bad*, *others + good* and *others + bad*, measuring processing of *mother* (*mother + good* and *mother + bad*) and *others* (*others + good* and *others + bad*), respectively. In each block, four identical types of stimuli were presented randomly on the computer screen one by one. Different blocks, however, required participants to respond to different pairs of stimuli (targets) but ignore other stimuli (distracters). For instance, in the *mother + good* block, participants needed to press the space bar if a stimulus was a *mother* word or a *good* word (e.g., *mother* or *delight*), but did nothing if a stimulus was an *others* word or a *bad* word (e.g., *he* or *bragging*). The order of the blocks was counterbalanced across participants. Before each experimental block, participants worked through pilot trials to become familiar with the task.

Each block included 320 trials. The stimulus presented in each trial was selected from four types of concepts with equal probability. Each of the five target category words (*mother* and *others*) was presented 16 times. The attribute words (*good* and *bad*) were presented without repetition. Therefore, there were 160 trials that presented target category words and the other 160 trials presented attributed words. The ratio of signal to noise was 1:1 in each block.

Figure 1 shows an example of the trial stimulus presentations. Each trial started with a fixation (a cross "+") on the center of the screen appearing for a random duration between 500 and 1500 ms. After that, the stimulus word was presented on the center of the screen for 1000 ms, and the participants were required to press the SPACE bar if the stimulus word was a target item. Finally, the second fixation was presented for 500 ms. Thereafter, a new trial then started with a fixation.

EEG Data Recording and Analysis

The continuous electroencephalogram (EEG) was recorded from 64 scalp sites using Ag/AgCl electrodes mounted in an elastic cap (NeuroScan Inc.), with an online reference to the right mastoid and off-line algebraic re-reference to the average of left and right mastoids. The vertical electrooculogram (VEOG) and horizontal electrooculogram (HEOG) were recorded from two pairs of

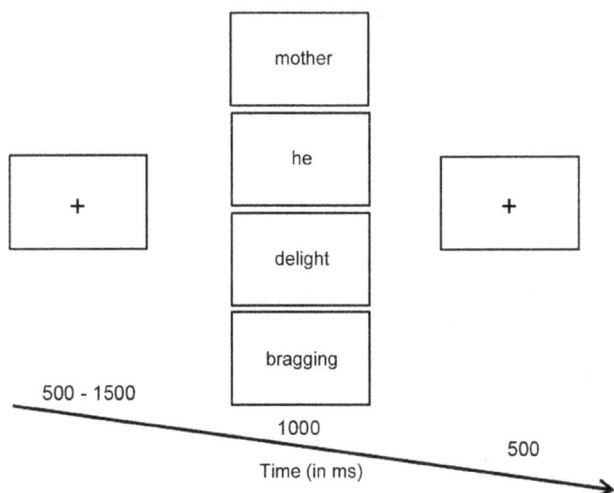

Figure 1. Illustration of the experimental procedure.

electrodes, with one placed above and below the left eye, and another 10 mm from the outer canthi of each eye. All interelectrode impedances were maintained below 5 kΩ. The EEG and EOG were amplified using a 0.05–100 Hz bandpass and continuously sampled at 500 Hz/channel.

During the off-line analysis, the EEG data were digitally filtered with a 30 Hz low-pass filter. Ocular artifacts were removed from the filtered EEG data using a regression procedure implemented in the Neuroscan software [46]. The onsets of the stimuli were set as the zero points, and the continuous EEG data were epoched into periods of 1000 ms including a 200-ms pre-stimulus baseline. Trials with artifacts due to eye blinks, amplifier clipping, and electromyographic (EMG) activity exceeding ±100 μV were excluded from averaging. In addition, trials where a participant had responded incorrectly were excluded from the final averaging. The mean percentage of trials excluded from averaging across the four blocks was less than 2% ($M = 1.8\%$, $SD = 2.1\%$). After that, the ERPs for category words (*mother* or *others*) with a Go response from the four blocks were averaged separately. Finally, two types of ERPs for each of the category words were obtained.

To examine attentional processing of maternal information, two ERP components, the P200 (within 140–210 ms) and N200 (within 250–350 ms), were examined. Previous studies showed that the P200 is generally found to be maximal around the frontal region of the scalp (e.g., [26,27]). Empirical evidence suggests that the anterior N200 may reflect attentional allocation processes, including the attentional selection of salient physical properties of items made by task manipulations [47,48] and the properties of social stimuli that are of inherent motivation/salience, such as out-group membership information (for a review, see [49]). Therefore, the peak amplitudes of P200 and N200 from 9 anterior sites (F3, FZ, F4, FC3, FCZ, FC4, C3, CZ and C4) and analyzed, respectively. These amplitudes from two components were entered into a four-way ANOVA (target category (*mother* vs. *others*) × attribute (*good* vs. *bad*) × Anterior-Posterior (F vs. FC vs. C) × Laterality (left vs. midline vs. right)), respectively.

To examine the evaluative processing of maternal stimuli, the peak latency and mean amplitude of LPP was measured. As this component is generally found to be maximal around the posterior area of the scalp (for reviews, see [32–35]), we selected 12 central parietal sites (C3, CZ, C4, CP3, CPZ, CP4, P3, PZ, P4, PO3, POZ and PO4) to measure its mean amplitude from 400 ms to 600 ms. These peak latencies and mean amplitudes were entered into a four-way ANOVA (target category (*mother* vs. *others*) × attribute (*good* vs. *bad*) × Anterior-Posterior (C vs. CP vs. P vs. PO) × Laterality (left vs. midline vs. right)), respectively.

Additionally, to check the physical properties differences between maternal stimuli and *others* stimuli, P100 and anterior N100 were assessed and analyzed. Peak amplitude of P100 (within 80–120 ms) was measured from 3 occipital sites (O1, OZ and O2) and then entered into a three-way ANOVA (target category (*mother* vs. *others*) × attribute (*good* vs. *bad*) × Laterality (left vs. midline vs. right)). Meanwhile, peak amplitude of N100 (within 90–130 ms) were measured from 9 anterior sites (F3, FZ, F4, FC3, FCZ, FC4, C3, CZ and C4) and then submitted into a four-way ANOVA (target category (*mother* vs. *others*) × attribute (*good* vs. *bad*) × Anterior-Posterior (F vs. FC vs. C) × Laterality (left vs. midline vs. right)).

For all the analyses listed below, the significance level was set at 0.05. Greenhouse–Geisser correction was used to compensate for sphericity violations when appropriate. Post-hoc analyses were conducted to explore the interaction effects. Partial eta-squared (η^2) was reported to demonstrate the effect sizes of significant results in the ANOVA tests.

Results

Behavioral Results

To examine whether attentional and evaluative factors contribute to the behavioral response, we performed an ANOVA on accuracy and reaction time to *mother* and *others* words in Go trials with target category (*mother* vs. *others*) and attribute (*good* vs. *bad*) as two within-subject factors, respectively. Regarding accuracy, participants performed at 96.63% accuracy in four conditions, and no significant difference was found across conditions, all $Fs < 0.11$ and all $ps > .35$. Regarding reaction time, the category effect was not significant, $F_{(1, 22)} = 2.31$, $p = .143$, *partial* $\eta^2 = 0.095$, but the attribute effect was significant, $F_{(1, 22)} = 5.48$, $p = .029$, *partial* $\eta^2 = 0.20$. Targets paired with *good* words elicited faster responses ($M = 474$ ms, $SD = 44$) than targets paired with *bad* words ($M = 490$ ms, $SD = 52$). More importantly, the interaction between category and attribute was highly significant, $F_{(1, 22)} = 12.76$, $p = .002$, *partial* $\eta^2 = 0.37$. Participants responded faster to *mother* words in the *mother + good* condition ($M = 461$ ms, $SD = 41$) than in *mother + bad* condition ($M = 492$ ms, $SD = 50$), $t_{(22)} = -4.13$, $p < .001$, but the reaction times for *others* words, between *others + good* ($M = 488$ ms, $SD = 47$) and *others + bad* ($M = 487$ ms, $SD = 54$), were not significantly different, $t_{(22)} = .07$, $p = .945$. These findings suggested that participants had positive attitudes to mother, which is consistent with previous findings [19–21].

ERP Results

P100 and N100 amplitude. No significant difference was detected in peak amplitudes of the P100 (peaks at 98.33 ms) and anterior N100 (peaks at 98.50 ms), all $Fs < 3.90$, and all $ps > .05$. Therefore, we concluded that *mother* and *others* words were processed similarly in terms of physical properties, thus not affecting early visual processing.

P200 amplitude. The peak amplitudes of the P200 (peaks at 165.62 ms) within 140–210 ms were entered into a four-way ANOVA. Main effect of target category was significant, $F_{(1, 22)} = 30.46$, $p < .001$, *partial* $\eta^2 = 0.58$, with *mother* words eliciting larger P200 ($M = 8.14$ µV, $SD = 4.45$) than *others* words ($M = 6.34$ µV, $SD = 3.72$) (see Figure 2). Neither the main effect of attribute nor the interaction effect was significant, $F_{(1, 22)} = 1.06$, 0.61, $p = .315, .442$, *partial* $\eta^2 = 0.05$, 0.03, respectively.

N200 amplitude. The peak amplitudes of the anterior N200 (peaks at 279.67 ms) within 250–350 ms were entered into a four-way ANOVA. Main effect of target category was significant, $F_{(1, 22)} = 14.86$, $p = .001$, *partial* $\eta^2 = 0.40$, with *mother* words eliciting larger N200 ($M = -1.92$ µV, $SD = 4.80$) than *other* words ($M = -0.53$ µV, $SD = 4.71$) (see Figure 2). Neither the main effect of attribute nor the interaction effect was significant, $F_{(1, 22)} = 0.01$, 0.52, $p = .932, .481$, *partial* $\eta^2 = 0.001, .023$, for valence and interaction, respectively.

LPP amplitude. The grand averaged ERPs to *mother* and *others* words from Go trials are shown in Figure 3a and Figure 3b, respectively. Mean amplitude of LPP was measured and submitted to a four-way ANOVA. The main effect of target category was significant, $F_{(1, 22)} = 20.41$, $p < .001$, *partial* $\eta^2 = 0.48$, with *mother* words eliciting larger LPP than *others* words (*mother*: $M = 10.24$ µV vs. *others*: $M = 8.90$ µV). The main effect of attribute was not significant, $F_{(1, 22)} = 1.79$, $p = .195$, *partial* $\eta^2 = 0.08$. The interaction effect for category and attribute was significant, $F_{(1, 22)} = 8.86$, $p = .007$, *partial* $\eta^2 = 0.29$. Further analyses showed that *mother* in the *mother + bad* condition ($M = 10.90$ µV) elicited larger LPP than in the *mother + good*

condition ($M = 9.59$ µV), $F_{(1, 22)} = 7.21$, $p = .014$, *partial* $\eta^2 = 0.25$. By contrast, no significant difference was found in LPP mean amplitude between the *others + bad* ($M = 8.75$ µV) and *others + good* conditions ($M = 9.06$ µV), $F_{(1, 22)} = 0.49$, $p = .493$, *partial* $\eta^2 = 0.02$.

LPP latency. Peak latencies of LPP were measured and submitted to a four-way ANOVA. The main effect of target category was not significant, $F_{(1, 22)} = 2.73$, $p = .113$, *partial* $\eta^2 = .11$. The main effect of attribute was significant, $F_{(1, 22)} = 6.22$, $p = .021$, *partial* $\eta^2 = .22$, with target category words paired with *good* words eliciting an earlier LPP ($M = 428$ ms) than those paired with *bad* words ($M = 441$ ms). The category by valence interaction was significant, $F_{(1, 22)} = 13.15$, $p = .001$, *partial* $\eta^2 = 0.37$. Further analyses showed that *mother* in the *mother + bad* condition ($M = 447$ ms) elicited a later LPP than in the *mother + good* condition ($M = 414$ ms), $F_{(1, 22)} = 26.26$, $p < .001$, *partial* $\eta^2 = .54$. By contrast, no significant difference was found in LPP latency between the *others + bad* ($M = 435$ ms) and *others + good* conditions ($M = 442$ ms), $F_{(1, 22)} = 0.54$, $p = .471$, *partial* $\eta^2 = 0.024$.

Results of the two gender neutral "others" items

One potential concern with the current results was the "woman are wonderful" effect, in which both males and females have a general tendency to associate women with more positive attributes and expectations than men [50]. It is possible that the *mother / others* manipulation was confounded with female/male in our findings, seeing that three of the *others* stimuli were masculine (he, him, his). One way to rule out this possibility was to directly compare the *mother* stimuli with the two non-masculine *others* stimuli. Specifically, we selected the trials elicited by the two gender-neutral words ("他人" and "别人") under *others + bad* and *others + good* conditions, respectively. Then, we compared the reaction time and the ERP components elicited by *mother* words with those elicited by these two *others* words, respectively. The results were similar to those reported above. Specifically, participants showed positive bias to *mother* at behavioral level. ERP results showed that they allocated more attentional resources to maternal stimuli, and they held positive evaluations of *mother*. The detailed results are listed below.

Behavioral result

The result showed that participants made faster responses to *mother* words ($M = 476$ ms, $SD = 42$) than to *others* words ($M = 500$ ms, $SD = 50$), $F_{(1, 22)} = 8.04$, $p = .01$, *partial* $\eta^2 = 0.27$. More importantly, the category × attribute interaction effect was significant, $F_{(1, 22)} = 11.13$, $p = .003$, *partial* $\eta^2 = 0.34$. Further tests showed that participants responded faster to *mother* words in the *mother + good* condition ($M = 461$ ms, $SD = 41$) than in the *mother + bad* condition ($M = 492$ ms, $SD = 50$), $t_{(22)} = -4.13$, $p < .001$; whereas the reaction times for *others* words, between *others + good* ($M = 501$ ms, $SD = 47$) and *others + bad* ($M = 499$ ms, $SD = 63$), were not significantly different, $t_{(22)} = .168$, $p = .868$.

ERP results

P200. The peak amplitudes of the P200 within 140–210 ms were entered into a four-way ANOVA. The main effect of category was significant, $F_{(1, 22)} = 20.23$, $p < .001$, *partial* $\eta^2 = 0.479$, with *mother* words eliciting larger P200 than *others* words (*mother*: $M = 8.14$ µV vs. *others*: $M = 6.70$ µV). Neither the main effect of attribute nor the interaction effect were significant, $F_{(1, 22)} = 0.465$, 0.716, $p = .503, .406$, *partial* $\eta^2 = 0.021$, 0.032, respectively.

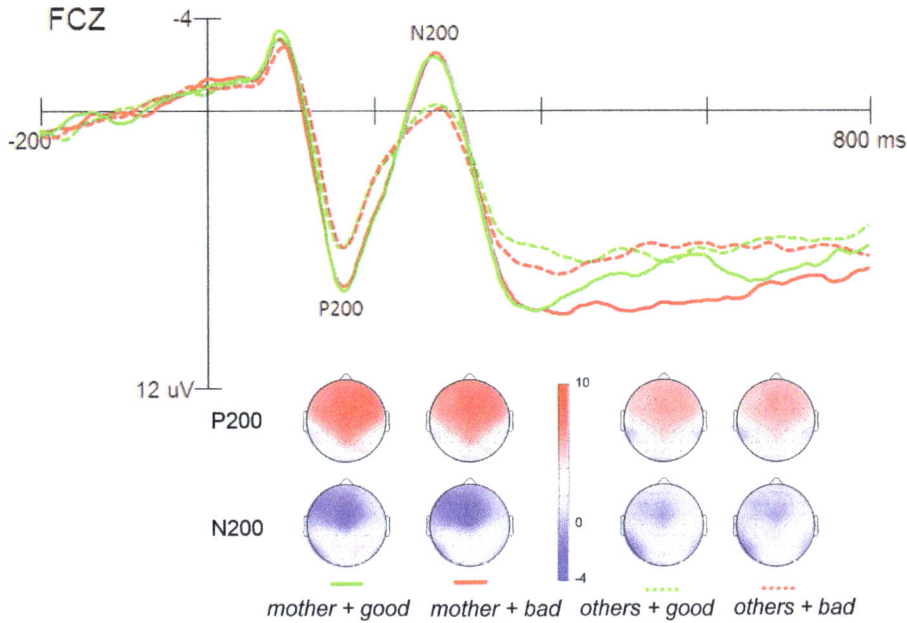

Figure 2. Grand averaged ERPs for target category words. The scalp topographies at peak latency for P200 and N200 of each condition are presented beneath.

N200. The peak amplitudes of the anterior N200 within 250–350 ms were entered into a four-way ANOVA. Main effect of target category, main effect of attribute, and the Category × Attribute interaction were not significant, all $Fs<1.8$, all $ps>.2$. However, a significant Category × Laterality interaction effect was found, $F_{(2,44)}=8.88$, $p=.001$, *partial* $\eta^2=.29$. Further analysis showed that the category effect was only significant over left area, $F_{(1,22)}=5.63$, $p=.027$, *partial* $\eta^2=.204$, with *mother* words eliciting larger N200 than *others* words in this area.

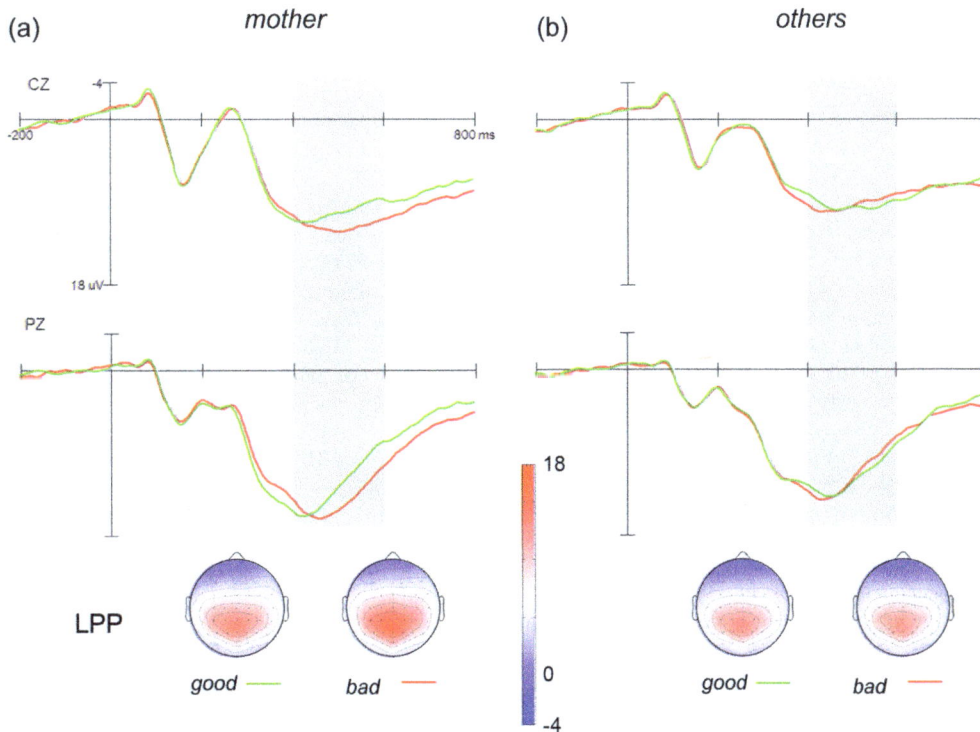

Figure 3. Grand averaged ERPs for target category words. The light gray shaded areas indicate the time window for the detection of the LPP component. The scalp topographies of each condition are presented beneath.

LPP. Mean amplitude of LPP was measured and submitted into a four-way ANOVA. The main effect of target category was significant, $F_{(1, 22)} = 19.41$, $p < .001$, $partial$ $\eta^2 = 0.47$, with $mother$ words elicited larger LPP than $others$ words ($mother$: $M = 10.24$ μV vs. $others$: $M = 8.47$ μV). The main effect of attribute was not significant, $F_{(1, 22)} = 1.40$, $p = .25$, $partial$ $\eta^2 = 0.06$. The category by attribute interaction was significant, $F_{(1, 22)} = 5.92$, $p = .024$, $partial$ $\eta^2 = 0.21$. Further analyses showed that $mother$ in the $mother + bad$ condition elicited a larger LPP ($M = 10.90$ μV) than in the $mother + good$ condition ($M = 9.59$ μV), $F_{(1, 22)} = 7.21$, $p = .014$, $partial$ $\eta^2 = 0.25$. By contrast, no significant difference was found in LPP mean amplitudes between the $others + bad$ ($M = 8.34$ μV) and $others + good$ conditions ($M = 8.61$ μV), $F_{(1, 22)} = 0.20$, $p = .66$, $partial$ $\eta^2 = 0.009$.

In addition to the $mother/others$ manipulation, since the majority of the sample were female and the "women are wonderful" effect is stronger in females than males [51], the gender ratio (female: male $= 14:9$) might have confounded the result. To rule it out, we averaged the data of female and male participants separately and then re-analyzed the original behavioral and ERPs result with gender (female vs. male) as a group factor. If the findings indeed reflected the maternal/others effect, then there should be no significant gender difference. Otherwise, if the findings were cofounded with the "women are wonderful" phenomenon, a gender effect should manifest on behavioral and/or neural response. The result showed that the gender effect was not significant after being entered into ANOVA tests. Moreover, adding this factor to analyses does not affect our major findings of either the behavioral or the ERPs results (including the P200, N200, and LPP components), which suggested that the gender factor did not affect the behavioral and neural response.

Discussion

The present study aimed to investigate attentional and evaluative processing of maternal stimuli. We examined whether there was an attentional preference to maternal information after controlling for familiarity, and we sought to reduce social desirability in the evaluations of maternal stimuli by using an implicit evaluative task and measuring electrophysiological responses. The behavioral data in the formal experiment, including accuracy and response time, supported the experimental control of stimulus familiarity. Target category effects were not significant for either measure, which would be difficult to explain if $mother$ words were more familiar than the $others$ words. Thus, the neural response to $mother$ words likely reflects the specificity of maternal stimulus processing instead of stimulus familiarity.

The behavioral results also suggested that participants indeed had a positive attitude towards maternal stimuli, which was consistent with previous findings [19–21]. That is, participants responded faster when $mother$ words were grouped with $good$ attributes than when they were grouped with bad attributes; whereas no significant difference was found between $others$ paired with $good$ or bad attributes.

The ERP results revealed two major findings. First, $mother$ words garnered more attention than non-specific $others$ words in both the early and late stages of processing. The P200/N200 and the LPP, respectively, were larger in amplitude for $mother$ than for $others$ words. Second, the positive attitude towards maternal stimuli emerged in the evaluative stage. The LPP amplitude was larger for the $mother + bad$ than $mother + good$ condition.

Previous research has consistently demonstrated that maternal stimuli, such as participants' mothers' faces, receive more attentional resources and deeper processing compared with $others$

stimuli, as shown by indexes such as looking time [17,18] and blood-oxygen-level-dependent (BOLD) signals [16]. Such preferences were usually attributed to familiarity. However, the present study extends this literature by showing that this kind of phenomenon occurs even after controlling for the level of familiarity. We believe that the selectively deep processing of maternal information was due to the critical role of mothers in human life and the relationships between the participants and their respective mothers.

The current study also revealed the temporal course for this attentional bias using ERPs. Compared with $others$, $mother$ elicited larger P200 and N200 components, suggesting that maternal information received considerable attention at an early stage of stimulus processing. Additionally, the augmented LPP amplitude for $mother$ compared with $others$ also reflected greater attentional resources allocation to $mother$ during later cognitive processing stages. Because the five items of maternal stimuli were specific and concrete, whereas the $others$ items are non-specific and abstract, it is possible that the attentional preference to maternal stimuli resulted from the concreteness of the words. However, we do not think so. Several empirical studies have shown that concrete words differ from abstract words at a late processing stage, with concrete words eliciting a larger N400 (between 300 and 550 ms) and a larger N700 (between 550 and 800 ms) than abstract words post stimulus onset, but not at the attentional stage (e.g., refs [52,53]). Therefore, the LPP difference to maternal stimuli indexes attention allocation to $mother$ and does not index the differences in word concreteness. Additionally, the attentional bias we observed is consistent with the results of previous studies where stimulus salience was operationalized as a function of the degree of self-relevance [31,54–58].

In the present study, the evaluative processing of mother was operationalized by the association between $mother$ words and evaluative attributes. Behavioral results from this study and other studies (e.g., refs [19–21]) suggest that people evaluate mother positively. In the $mother + bad$ condition, $mother$ words were assigned to negative attributes, which was incompatible with the intrinsic positive attitude towards the mother [19–21]. This evaluative incompatibility in the present study resulted in an augmented LPP. This finding was in line with earlier findings that the LPP reflects people's evaluations of social targets, such as people of different races or genders [40,41,59]. Additionally, the LPP latency was longer when incompatible evaluative information ($mother + bad$) is processed compared with the compatible evaluative information ($mother + good$), which is also in line with previous findings [41]. Our study shows that the evaluative processing of maternal stimuli occurs during a later stage of processing. For $others$ stimuli, however, the LPP amplitudes and latency were not significantly different between the $others + bad$ and $others + good$ conditions, which was consistent with earlier claims that people hold a neutral attitude towards non-specific others [42,43].

Given that the RTs in the $mother + bad$ condition were significantly longer than those in the $mother + good$ condition, two other potential factors might account for the ERP differences between these two conditions: overt motor response speed and task difficulty. We have two reasons for disagreeing with the former issue. First, participants carried out the same key-pressing responses to identical stimuli ($mother$ words) in both the $mother + bad$ and $mother + good$ conditions. Second, if the LPP amplitude difference was caused merely by the speed difference of the same motor response, there would be no significant difference in the amplitude of the ERP wave before a response between these two conditions. To directly test this hypothesis, we set the response point as the time zero and then measured and analyzed the amplitude of the ERP wave before the motor response over the centro-parietal area. The results revealed that the ERP wave in the *mother + bad* condition was larger than that in the *mother + good* condition, and no significant difference between the *others + bad* and *others + good* conditions. These results suggest that the differences in LPP amplitudes did not result from differences in overt motor response speed (please refer to Text S1 and Figure S1 for details).

Concerning the issue of task difficulty, the behavioral and neural findings between *mother + bad* and *mother + good* conditions might be due to differences in task difficulty. However, the source of this difficulty is worth noting. In the field of experimental psychology, task difficulty has been manipulated in several ways, including the stimulus characteristics [60,61], the physical effort required in the task [62], the understandability of the stimulus content [63], the length of time allotted to make a response [64,65], the number of cognitive operations needed to complete the task [66], the complexity of mental operations (e.g., [67]), and the strength of the inconsistency between different response tendencies [68,69]. In the current study, the differences in difficulty levels were not caused by the stimulus characteristics or the mental steps necessary for response implementation, but they varied as a function of the degree of mental inconsistency. That is, asking participants to respond to *mother* and *bad* words, the *mother + bad* condition creates a scenario in which automatic evaluation (i.e., associating maternal stimuli with positive descriptions) strongly conflicts with task-demand evaluation. This may have increased the task difficulty, thus leading to longer response times and larger LPP amplitudes compared to the *mother + good* condition, with no significant differences between *others + good* and *others + bad* conditions. Thus, even though our major findings might be interpreted in terms of task difficulty, we argue that these differences in difficulty levels between the *mother* conditions were the result of the internal positive attitude towards maternal stimuli.

Although the current study aimed to examine the maternal/other effect, it is possible that the "women are wonderful" effect [51], rather than the maternal/other effect, might explain our results. First, three of the five "*others*" items were masculine. Second, because the sample of the present study largely consisted of female participants and the "women are wonderful" effect is stronger in females than males [50], the gender ratio (female: male = 14:9) of the sample might have affected the result. However, we re-analyzed the data in order to rule out the potential effect of masculine words and the gender ratio of the sample. The first analysis showed that when we selectively made comparison between *mother* words and two gender-neutral *others* words, the results were essentially the same. Although the effect of category on the N200 amplitude was only significant over left hemisphere, we suggest this asymmetry may disappear in a larger sample. Alternatively, the attention to maternal information might depend more on left hemisphere, but we believe that this is unlikely because the contrast of N200 between *mother* words and all five *others* words did not show a left asymmetry. Regarding the low spatial resolution of ERP technique, future brain-imaging studies would be more appropriate for clarifying this issue. With respect to the gender ratio, a second analysis showed that the gender effect was not significant, i.e., it did not moderate the behavioral or the ERPs results. Thus, the results from these analyses both did not challenge our initial findings and interpretations.

The results suggest that both attentional and evaluative components are involved in processing maternal stimuli. The attentional distinction of *mother* from non-specific *others* occurs immediately after stimulus presentation, which is in line with the proposal that people spontaneously group their perceptions of others by relationship status [70]. The evaluative components contributed to the later processing of the maternal stimuli. The initial recognition and later evaluation of maternal stimuli probably jointly contribute to constructions of a complex representation of the mother, which in turn affects participants' cognition, emotion, motivation, and behaviors.

One limitation of the present study was that we only compared *mother* and *others* stimuli. We do not know whether such responses are specific to the mother or could be generalized to significant others, such as the father. The father's role as attachment figure has been emphasized recently (for a review, see [71]). It is likely that the processing of paternal stimuli involves cognitive and affective components similar to the processing of maternal stimuli. Future studies could extend our findings by adding another target, such as *father*, to the task design.

Another limitation was that we only tested adults. Thus, we could not test whether the current findings and conclusions can be generalized across different ages. Given that for most children, mothers are the primary attachment figures, whereas for adults the mother is generally ranked lower than romantic partners [9], it is possible that the processing of maternal stimuli is different between children and adults. However, this may not be the case, since there is some evidence that the neural activation evoked by maternal information is not modulated by age [72]. Thus, the response to the mother observed in the present study may also be generalizable to younger people. Future studies that examine the behavioral and neural response to maternal stimuli in children could help clarifying this issue.

In conclusion, our results indicate that maternal stimuli affect people's attentional and evaluative processing in a short time interval (less than one second). Such attentional preference and evaluative processing were not a result of stimulus familiarity or social desirability bias, but they were driven by the critical role of mother in human life. Moreover, we found that instead of using stimuli directly related to participants' own mother, such as the mother's face, just presenting symbolic stimuli that describe the mother elicits biased processing. This suggests that a more abstract, general, and typical mother concept—not just concrete and specific maternal information—can receive instant processing.

Author Contributions

Conceived and designed the experiments: LLW. Performed the experiments: LLW. Analyzed the data: LLW RLG. Wrote the paper: LLW RLG. Revised the paper: RLG JXZ HJC YLLL.

References

1. Murray L, Fiori-Cowley A, Hooper R, Cooper P (1996) The Impact of Postnatal Depression and Associated Adversity on Early Mother-Infant Interactions and Later Infant Outcome. Child Dev 67: 2512–2526.

2. Oweis A (2008) Maternal Depression and Infant Temperament Characteristics. MCN Am J Matern Child Nurs 33: 393–393.

3. Rautava S, Kalliomäki M, Isolauri E (2002) Probiotics During Pregnancy and Breast-feeding Might Confer Immunomodulatory Protection Against Atopic Disease in the Infant. J Allergy Clin Immunol 109: 119–121.

4. Yeung LTF, King SM, Roberts EA (2001) Mother-to-infant Transmission of Hepatitis C Virus. Hepatology 34: 223–229.

5. Hofer MA (1994) Early Relationships as Regulators of Infant Physiology and Behavior. Acta Paediatr 83: 9–18.

6. Bowlby J (1982) Attachment and loss. Vol. 1: Attachment (2nd Ed.). New York: Basic Books (new printing, 1999, with a foreword by Allan N. Schore; originally published in 1969).

7. Steeger CM, Gondoli DM (2013) Mother-Adolescent Conflict as a Mediator Between Adolescent Problem Behaviors and Maternal Psychological Control. Dev Psychol 49: 804–814.

8. Yap MB, Allen NB, O'Shea M, di Parsia P, Simmons JG, et al. (2011) Early Adolescents' Temperament, Emotion Regulation During Mother-child Interactions, and Depressive Symptomatology. Dev Psychopathol 23: 267–82.

9. Doherty NA, Feeney JA (2004) The Composition of Attachment Networks Throughout the Adult Years. Pers Relatsh 11: 469–488.

10. Antonucci TC, Akiyama H, Takahashi K (2004) Attachment and Close Relationships Across the Life Span. Attach Hum Dev 6: 353–370.

11. Mallers MH, Charles ST, Neupert SD, Almeida DM (2010) Perceptions of Childhood Relationships with Mother and Father: Daily Emotional and Stressor Experiences in Adulthood. Dev Psychol 46: 1651–61.

12. Field TM, Cohen D, Garcia R, Greenberg R (1984) Mother-stranger Face Discrimination by the Newborn. Infant Behav Dev 7: 19–25.

13. Bushneil IWR, Sai F, Mullin JT (1989) Neonatal Recognition of the Mother's Face. Br J Dev Psychol 7: 3–15.

14. Walton GE, Bower NJA, Bower TGR (1992) Recognition of Familiar Faces by Newborns. Infant Behav Dev 15: 265–269.

15. de Haan M, Nelson CA (1997) Recognition of the Mother's Face by Six-month-old Infants: a neurobehavioral study. Child Dev 68: 187–210.

16. Arsalidou M, Barbeau EJ, Bayless SJ, Taylor MJ (2010) Brain Responses Differ to Faces of Mothers and Fathers. Brain Cogn 74: 47–51.

17. Bushnell IWR (2001) Mother's Face Recognition in Newborn Infants: Learning and Memory. Infant Behav Dev 10: 67–74.

18. Pascalis O, de Schonen S, Morton J, Deruelle C, Fabre-Grenet M (1995) Mother's Face Recognition by Neonates: A Replication and an Extension. Infant Behav Dev 18: 79–85.

19. Dehart T, Pelham B, Fiedorowicz L, Carvallo M, Gabriel S (2011) Including Others in the Implicit Self: Implicit Evaluation of Significant Others. Self Identity 10: 127–135.

20. Zhou AB, Wu HF, Shi Z, Li Q, Liu PR, et al. (2010) The Contrastive Study of Mother-reference Effect in the Depth of Processing and Incidental Encoding Conditions. Psychological Exploration, 03: 39–44 (in Chinese).

21. Tottenham N, Shapiro M, Telzer EH, Humphreys KL (2012) Amygdala Response to Mother. Dev Sci 15: 307–319.

22. Luck SJ (2005) An Introduction to the Event-related Potential Technique. Cognitive neuroscience. Cambridge, Mass.: MIT Press. xii, 374 p.

23. Nosek BA, Banaji MR (2001) The Go/No-go Association Task. Soc Cogn 19: 625–666.

24. Banfield JF, van der Lugt AH, Munte TF (2006) Juicy Fruit and Creepy Crawlies: An Electrophysiological Study of the Implicit Go/NoGo Association Task. Neuroimage 31: 1841–1849.

25. van der Lugt AH, Banfield JF, Osinsky R, Münte TF (2012) Brain Potentials Show Rapid Activation of Implicit Attitudes Towards Young and Old People. Brain Res 1429: 98–105.

26. Hu X, Wu H, Fu G (2011) Temporal Course of Executive Control When Lying about Self- and Other-referential Information: An ERP Study. Brain Res 1369: 149–57.

27. Meixner JB, Rosenfeld JP (2010) Countermeasure Mechanisms in a P300-based Concealed Information Test. Psychophysiology 47: 57–65.

28. Chen AT, Weng XC, Yuan JJ, Lei X, Qiu J, et al. (2008) The Temporal Features of Self-referential Processing Evoked by Chinese Handwriting. J Cogn Neurosci 20: 816–827.

29. Keyes H, Brady N, Reilly RB, Foxe JJ (2010) My Face or Yours? Event-related Potential Correlates of Self-face Processing. Brain Cogn 72: 244–254.

30. Chen J, Yuan J, Feng T, Chen A, Gu B, et al. (2011) Temporal Features of the Degree Effect in Self-relevance: Neural Correlates. Biol Psychol 87: 290–295.

31. Chen J, Zhang Y, Zhong J, Hu L, Li H (2013) The Primacy of the Individual Versus the Collective Self: Evidence from an Event-related Potential Study. Neurosci Lett 535: 30–34.

32. Kok A (2001) On the Utility of P3 Amplitude as a Measure of Processing Capacity. Psychophysiology 38: 557–577.

33. Polich J (2007) Updating P300: An Integrative Theory of P3a and P3b. Clin Neurophysiol 118: 2128–48.

34. Herrmann CS, Knight RT (2001) Mechanisms of Human Attention: Event-related Potentials and Oscillations. Neurosci Biobehav Rev 25: 465–476.

35. Verleger R, Jaśkowski P, Wascher E (2005) Evidence for an Integrative Role of P3b in Linking Reaction to Perception. J Psychophysiol 19: 165–181.

36. Cacioppo JT, Crites SL, Berntson GG, G. H. Coles M (1993) If Attitudes Affect How Stimuli Are Processed, Should They Not Affect the Event-Related Brain Potential? Psychol Sci 4: 108–112.

37. Cacioppo JT, Crites SL, Gardner WL, Berntson GG (1994) Bioelectrical Echoes from Evaluative Categorizations: I. A Late Positive Brain Potential that Varies as a Function of Trait Negativity and Extremity. J Pers Soc Psychol 67: 115–125.

38. Ito TA, Cacioppo JT (2000) Electrophysiological Evidence of Implicit and Explicit Categorization Processes. J Exp Soc Psychol 36: 660–676.

39. Lust SA, Bartholow BD (2009) Self-reported and P3 Event-related Potential Evaluations of Condoms: Does What We Say Match How We Feel? Psychophysiology 46: 420–4.

40. Bartholow BD, Dickter CL, Sestir MA (2006) Stereotype Activation and Control of Race Bias: Cognitive Control of Inhibition and Its Impairment by Alcohol. J Pers Soc Psychol 90: 272–287.

41. Ito TA, Thompson E, Cacioppo JT (2004) Tracking the timecourse of social perception: the effects of racial cues on event-related brain potentials. Pers Soc Psychol Bull 30: 1267–1280.

42. Karpinski A (2004) Measuring Self-esteem Using the Implicit Association Test: The role of the other. Pers Soc Psychol Bull 30: 22–34.

43. Pinter B, Greenwald AG (2005) Clarifying the Role of the "Other" Category in the Self-esteem IAT. Exp Psychol 52: 74–9.

44. Anderson NH (1968) Likableness Ratings of 555 Personality-trait Words. J Pers Soc Psychol 9: 272–9.

45. Zhao C (2008) Wai Xian Zi Wo Zeng Qiang Yu Nei Yin Zi Wo Zeng Qiang De Shen Jing Ji Zhi Yan Jiu [Neural Research of Explicit Self-esteem and Implicit Self-esteem]. Unpublished mater's thesis, Capital Normal University, Beijing, China.

46. Semlitsch HV, Anderer P, Schuster P, Presslich O (1986) A Solution for Reliable and Valid Reduction of Ocular Artifacts, Applied to the P300 ERP. Psychophysiology 23: 695–703.

47. Eimer M (1997) An Event-related Potential (ERP) Study of Transient and Sustained Visual Attention to Color and Form. Biol Psychol 44: 143–60.

48. Wijers AA, Mulder G, Okita T, Mulder LJM, Scheffers MK (1989) Attention to Color: An Analysis of Selection, Controlled Search, and Motor Activation, Using Event-Related Potentials. Psychophysiology 26: 89–109.

49. Ito TA, Bartholow BD (2009) The Neural Correlates of Race. Trends Cogn Sci 13: 524–531.

50. Eagly AH, Mladinic A (1994) Are People Prejudiced Against Women? Some Answers From Research on Attitudes, Gender Stereotypes, and Judgments of Competence. Eur Rev Soc Psychol 5: 1–35.

51. Rudman LA, Goodwin SA (2004) Gender Differences in Automatic In-Group Bias: Why Do Women Like Women More Than Men Like Men? J Pers Soc Psychol 87: 494–509.

52. Barber HA, Otten LJ, Kousta ST, Vigliocco G (2013) Concreteness in Word Processing: ERP and Behavioral Effects in a Lexical Decision Task. Brain Lang 125: 47–53.

53. West WC, Holcomb PJ (2000) Imaginal, Semantic, and Surface-level Processing of Concrete and Abstract Words: An Electrophysiological Investigation. J Cogn Neurosci 12: 1024–1037.

54. Berlad I, Pratt H (1995) P300 in Response to the Subject's Own Name. Electroencephalogr Clin Neurophysiol 96: 472–4.

55. Ninomiya H, Onitsuka T, Chen C-H, Sato E, Tashiro N (1998) P300 in Response to the Subject's Own Face. Psychiatry Clin Neurosci 52: 519–522.

56. Gray HM, Ambady N, Lowenthal WT, Deldin P (2004) P300 as an Index of Attention to Self-relevant Stimuli. J Exp Soc Psychol 40: 216–224.

57. Miyakoshi M, Nomura M, Ohira H (2007) An ERP Study on Self-relevant Object Recognition. Brain Cogn 63: 182–9.

58. Tacikowski P, Nowicka A (2010) Allocation of Attention to Self-name and Self-face: An ERP Study. Biol Psychol 84: 318–324.

59. Osterhout L, Bersick M, McLaughlin J (1997) Brain Potentials Reflect Violations of Gender Stereotypes. Mem Cognit 25: 273–285.

60. Schevernels H, Krebs RM, Santens P, Woldorff MG, Boehler CN (2013) Task Preparation Processes Related to Reward Prediction Precede Those Related to Task-difficulty Expectation. Neuroimage, 84C: 639–647.

61. Kimura M, Takeda Y (2013) Task Difficulty Affects the Predictive Process Indexed by Visual Mismatch Negativity. Front Hum Neurosci 7: 267.

62. Fouriezos G, Bielajew C, Pagotto W (1990) Task-Difficulty Increases Thresholds of Rewarding Brain-Stimulation. Behav Brain Res 37: 1–7.

63. Lingnau A, Petris S (2013) Action Understanding Within and Outside the Motor System: The Role of Task Difficulty. Cereb Cortex 23: 1342–50.

64. Kaczkurkin AN (2013) The Effect of Manipulating Task Difficulty on Error-related Negativity in Individuals with Obsessive-compulsive Symptoms. Biol Psychol 93: 122–31.

65. Hughes ME, Johnston PJ, Fulham WR, Budd TW, Michie PT (2013) Stop-signal Task Difficulty and the Right Inferior Frontal Gyrus. Behav Brain Res 256: 205–13.

66. Kremlacek J, Kuba M, Kubova Z, Langrova J, Szanyi J, et al. (2013) Visual Mismatch Negativity in the Dorsal Stream is Independent of Concurrent Visual Task Difficulty. Front Hum Neurosci 7: 411.
67. Verner M, Herrmann MJ, Troche SJ, Roebers CM, Rammsayer TH (2013) Cortical Oxygen Consumption in Mental Arithmetic as a Function of Task Difficulty: A Near-infrared Spectroscopy Approach. Front Hum Neurosci 7: 217.
68. Green N, Bogacz R, Huebl J, Beyer AK, Kuhn AA, et al. (2013) Reduction of Influence of Task Difficulty on Perceptual Decision Making by STN Deep Brain Stimulation. Curr Biol 23: 1681–4.
69. Merola JL, Liederman J (1990) The Effect of Task Difficulty upon the Extent to Which Performance Benefits from Between-hemisphere Division of Inputs. Int J Neurosci 51: 35–44.
70. Sedikides C, Olsen N, Reis HT (1993) Relationships as Natural Categories. J Pers Soc Psychol 64: 71–82.
71. Bretherton I (2010) Fathers in Attachment Theory and Research: A Review. Early Child Dev Care 180: 9–23.
72. Tottenham N (2012) Human Amygdala Development in the Absence of Species-expected Caregiving. Dev Psychobiol 54: 598–611.

23

Enhanced Slow-Wave EEG Activity and Thermoregulatory Impairment following the Inhibition of the Lateral Hypothalamus in the Rat

Matteo Cerri*, Flavia Del Vecchio, Marco Mastrotto, Marco Luppi, Davide Martelli, Emanuele Perez, Domenico Tupone, Giovanni Zamboni, Roberto Amici

Department of Biomedical and NeuroMotor Sciences, Alma Mater Studiorum - University of Bologna, Bologna, Italy

Abstract

Neurons within the lateral hypothalamus (LH) are thought to be able to evoke behavioural responses that are coordinated with an adequate level of autonomic activity. Recently, the acute pharmacological inhibition of LH has been shown to depress wakefulness and promote NREM sleep, while suppressing REM sleep. These effects have been suggested to be the consequence of the inhibition of specific neuronal populations within the LH, i.e. the orexin and the MCH neurons, respectively. However, the interpretation of these results is limited by the lack of quantitative analysis of the electroencephalographic (EEG) activity that is critical for the assessment of NREM sleep quality and the presence of aborted NREM-to-REM sleep transitions. Furthermore, the lack of evaluation of the autonomic and thermoregulatory effects of the treatment does not exclude the possibility that the wake-sleep changes are merely the consequence of the autonomic, in particular thermoregulatory, changes that may follow the inhibition of LH neurons. In the present study, the EEG and autonomic/thermoregulatory effects of a prolonged LH inhibition provoked by the repeated local delivery of the GABA$_A$ agonist muscimol were studied in rats kept at thermoneutral (24°C) and at a low (10°C) ambient temperature (Ta), a condition which is known to depress sleep occurrence. Here we show that: 1) at both Tas, LH inhibition promoted a peculiar and sustained bout of NREM sleep characterized by an enhancement of slow-wave activity with no NREM-to-REM sleep transitions; 2) LH inhibition caused a marked transitory decrease in brain temperature at Ta 10°C, but not at Ta 24°C, suggesting that sleep changes induced by LH inhibition at thermoneutrality are not caused by a thermoregulatory impairment. These changes are far different from those observed after the short-term selective inhibition of either orexin or MCH neurons, suggesting that other LH neurons are involved in sleep-wake modulation.

Editor: Andrej A. Romanovsky, St. Joseph's Hospital and Medical Center, United States of America

Funding: This work has been supported by the grant PRIN 2008FY7K9S from the Ministero dell'Istruzione, dell'Università e della Ricerca (http://www.istruzione.it)- Italy (RA). The funders had no role in study design, data collection and analysis, decision to publish, or preparation of the manuscript.

Competing Interests: The authors have declared that no competing interests exist.

* Email: matteo.cerri@unibo.it

Introduction

The lateral hypothalamus (LH) is a complex network of several different kinds of neurons involved in many functions [1]. LH neurons are apparently able to evoke a behavioural response that is integrated and coordinated with an adequate level of autonomic activity. In fact, the pharmacological activation of LH neurons has been shown to promote active behaviour and locomotion [2], and to coherently induce an increase in sympathetic outflow [3]. Both effects can be the consequence of the activation of a subpopulation of LH neurons producing orexin [4].

Recently, it has been shown that the inhibition of LH neurons prevented rats from producing rapid eye movement (REM) sleep [5]. The cause of this complete absence of REM sleep was suggested to be the inhibition of the activity of a subpopulation of LH neurons which produces melanin-concentrating hormone (MCH) [5]. However, optogenetic inhibition of MCH neurons did not produce a significant reduction in REM sleep duration [6].

This supports the hypothesis that REM-on GABAergic (non-MCHergic/non-orexinergic) neurons, which have also been observed in the LH, play a role in the regulation of REM sleep appearance [7–9]. Additionally, the inhibition of neurons within the LH depressed waking and evoked an extended period of non-REM (NREM) sleep [5]. These observations partially fit with the reported effects of either optogenetic [8], or DREADD (designer receptors exclusively activated by designer drugs) silencing of orexin neurons [10], and the administration of a dual orexin receptor antagonist [11]. However, in these three cases of selective inhibition of orexinergic activity, wakefulness was not comparably suppressed to the level shown after muscimol injection within the LH [5], suggesting that the role played by LH neurons in arousal levels cannot be entirely ascribed to the orexin neurons. Furthermore, in the latter studies the increase in NREM sleep was not nearly as great as that shown after the inhibition of the entire LH neuronal population, and REM sleep was still present.

While the outcome of LH neurons inhibition (reducing wakefulness) fits well with the observed effect of LH neurons activation (promoting wakefulness), changes in autonomic functions induced by such inhibition have not yet been investigated.

Of particular interest is the role played by LH neurons in thermoregulation control. Since the activation of LH neurons produces an increase in thermogenesis [3], it can be hypothesized that LH neurons inhibition may result in a state of hypothermia. While a modest reduction in brain temperature (core temperature around 36°C), such as that described after peripheral injection of CCK [12], can favour both NREM sleep and REM sleep occurrence, during either spontaneous torpor [13–16] or centrally-induced deep hypothermia (Core temperature 22°C, 24°C) [17], [18], REM sleep appearance was inhibited. Therefore, the possibility that LH inhibition may induce a state of marked hypothermia could provide an alternative explanation for the inhibition of REM sleep appearance described by Clement et al., 2012.

In order to evaluate whether sleep changes induced by LH neurons inhibition are the mere consequence of a reduced thermogenesis and not of the inhibition of specific wake-sleep (WS) related neural substrates within the LH, the present study aims to investigate the effects induced on both the WS cycle and thermoregulation by the pharmacological inhibition of LH neurons. Moreover, since Clement and co-workers used a single administration of the GABA$_A$ agonist muscimol, leaving open the possibility that the relatively large vehicle volume and drug concentration might have caused an unwanted diffusion of the effects, we performed subsequent administrations of muscimol in small concentrations and volumes.

It is also critical to consider that neuronal inhibition can induce different effects according to the levels of neuronal activation preceding the inhibition. We therefore tested the effects of LH inhibition in different environmental conditions: at thermoneutrality, a condition that should not determine any specific activation of LH neurons, and during acute cold exposure, a condition that has been shown to increase the amount of wakefulness [19], and to induce a significant activation of LH neurons [20].

Here we show that the prolonged pharmacological inhibition of LH neurons almost abolished wakefulness and promoted a prolonged bout of NREM sleep characterized by an enhancement of slow-wave activity and by the absence of NREM-to-REM sleep transitions. A thermoregulatory impairment was observed when LH neurons were inhibited at an ambient temperature (Ta) of 10°C but not at Ta = 24°C.

Preliminary results of the experiments have been published in abstract form [21].

Materials and Methods

Ethical approval

The experiments were carried out with the approval of the Comitato Etico-Scientifico dell'Alma Mater Studiorum - University of Bologna (Ethical-Scientific Committee of the Alma Mater Studiorum - University of Bologna), in accordance with the European Union Directive (86/609/EEC) and under the supervision of the Central Veterinary Service of the Alma Mater Studiorum - University of Bologna and the National Health Authority. All efforts were made to minimize the number of animals used and their pain and distress.

Surgical Procedures

Male CD Sprague-Dawley rats (n = 12, Charles River Inc, Lecco, Italy) were deeply anaesthetized through the injection of diazepam (Valium; F. Hoffmann-La Roche ltd, Basel, Switzerland, 5 mg/kg, intramuscular) followed by ketamine-HCl (Ketavet; Parke-Davis, Detroit, MI, USA, 100 mg/kg, intraperitoneal), and placed in a stereotaxic apparatus (David Kopf Instruments, Tujunga, CA, USA) with the incisor bar set in order to keep the bregma and lambda on the same horizontal plane. Animals were surgically implanted with: i) electrodes for EEG and nuchal electromyographic (EMG) recording; ii) a catheter placed into the femoral artery for the telemetric recording of arterial pressure (AP) (PA-C40, DataSciences International, St.Paul, MN, USA); iii) a thermistor (B10KA303N, Thermometrics Corporation, Northridge, CA, USA) mounted inside a stainless-steel needle (21 gauge) stereotaxically implanted above the left anterior hypothalamus to record the deep brain temperature (T$_{brain}$); iv) two microinjection guide cannulas (C315G-SPC Plastics One Inc, Roanoke, VA, USA; internal cannula extension below guide: +3.5 mm), stereotaxically positioned in the left and the right LH. After surgery, animals received 20 ml/kg of saline subcutaneously and 0.25 ml of an antibiotic solution (penicillin G, 37500 IU; streptomycin-sulfate, 8750 IU) i.m. Animals recovered from surgery for at least one week, initially in their home cage and subsequently, for at least 3 days, in a Plexiglas cage with a stainless steel grid floor (wire diameter = 2 mm, inter-wire distance = 10 mm). The cage was positioned within a thermoregulated, sound-attenuated recording chamber where animals were kept throughout the experiment. The recording chamber was equipped with light and temperature controllers and acoustically insulated from the surroundings, so as to keep animals unaware of any activity outside the chamber. The recording chamber was located inside a Faraday-shielded room. Besides regular cage cleaning (at 9:00 am every day), operators entered the Faraday-shielded room only during the microinjection procedure. During recovery from surgery, animals were kept at an ambient temperature (Ta) of 24°C±0.5°C and under a 12:12 h light (L) - dark (D) cycle (light on at 09.00, 100 lux at cage level), and had free access to food and water. The recording chamber was also equipped with an infrared thermocamera (Thermovision A20, FLIR Systems, Boston, MA, USA) positioned under the stainless steel grid floor, to measure cutaneous temperature.

Experimental Protocols

After recovery from surgery (1 week to 10 days), animals were divided into two experimental groups. Animals in group A (n = 5) were recorded for 6 consecutive days in the following conditions: i) day 1, baseline, Ta = 24°C; ii) day 2, inhibitor injections (GABA$_A$ agonist muscimol, 1 mM, 100 nl, 1 bilateral injection/h starting at 11:00 h and ending at 16:00 h), Ta = 24°C; iii) day 3, recovery Ta = 24°C; iv) day 4, control, Ta = 24°C; v) day 5, saline vehicle injections (NaCl 0.9% w/v, 100 nl, 1 bilateral injection/h starting at 11:00 h and ending at 16:00 h), Ta = 24°C; vi) day 6, recovery, Ta = 24°C. Animals in group B (n = 7) were recorded for 6 consecutive days in the same conditions as those for group A with the exception that during both injection days (day 2 and day 5) animals were kept at Ta 10°C from 9:00 h to 17:00 h, the time period during which the injections were delivered.

Microinjection procedures

The microinjection system consisted of a Hamilton 5 µl gastight syringe (Hamilton Company, Bonaduz, Switzerland) positioned in an infusion pump (MA 01746, Harvard Apparatus, Holliston, MA, USA; infusion rate 0.3 µl/min) and connected to the internal cannula through one meter of microdialysis FEP tubing (ID

0.12 mm OD 0.65 mm, Microbiotech/se AB, Stockholm, Sweden).

The cannula and the tube were filled with either muscimol (Tocris Bioscience, Bristol, UK) dissolved in vehicle solution or vehicle solution only (commercially available sterile-pyrogen free saline for parenteral injection (0.9%), S.A.L.F. Bergamo, Italy), while the syringe and the initial part of the tube were filled with coloured mineral oil. The insertion of the internal cannula into the guide cannula was performed manually by an operator by opening the lid of the recording chamber, gently inserting the internal cannula in the guide cannula and locking the two together. Care was also taken to avoid removing the animal from the cage during the insertion of the cannula. Once the internal cannula was inserted, the lid of the recording chamber was closed. The pump and the syringe were located outside the recording chamber.

All microinjection procedures were performed as follows. At 10:55, the microinjecting cannula was inserted into the guide cannula. After closing the lid of the recording chamber, the first microinjection was performed. Ten minutes after the first injection, the lid of the recording chamber was opened again, the internal cannula extracted and inserted into the contralateral guide cannula. The lid was closed again, and the second microinjection was performed. After 10 more minutes, the recording chamber was opened and the cannula retrieved. This procedure was repeated for each of the 6 injections performed.

During each injection (average duration: 30 s±5 s), the volume injected (100 nl) was microscopically-assessed by the movement of the oil-liquid interface within the FEP tubing over a ruler. Compared to the single administration performed by Clement and co-workers [5] (muscimol, 1 μg/μl, 8.76 mM, in 300 nl), we thought that a sequence of injections (1 per hour) of a smaller volume (100 nl) and concentration (0.1 μg/μl, 1 mM) would reduce the possibilities of confounding effects induced by an unwanted diffusion to neuronal pools outside the LH.

Histology

At the end of the experiment, the injection site was marked with 80 nl of Fast Green 2% dye. Rats were anaesthetized with ketamine as described above and transcardially perfused (4% w/vol paraformaldehyde). The brain was extracted and postfixed overnight with 4% paraformaldehyde and then cryoprotected (30% w/vol sucrose). The brain was then sliced coronally on a cryostat (60 μm) and sections containing a dye spot were plotted on an atlas drawing [22] (Figure 1).

Signal Recording and Data Analysis

The EEG, EMG and T_{brain} signals were recorded by means of insulated copper wires connecting the headsocket to a swivel, amplified (Grass 7P511L, Astro-Med Inc, West Warwick (RI), USA), filtered (EEG: highpass 0.3 Hz, lowpass 30 Hz; EMG highpass 100 Hz, lowpass 1 KHz T_{brain} highpass 0.5 Hz), 12 bit digitalized (Micro MK 1401 II, CED, Cambridge, UK; acquisition rate: EEG: 1 KHz; EMG: 1 KHz; T_{brain}: 100 Hz) and acquired on a digital hard drive. AP signal was telemetrically recorded, amplified and digitally stored on a hard drive (acquisition rate: 500 Hz). Heart rate (HR) was derived from AP peak detection.

EEG power spectrum was calculated from a 4-sec-long 1-sec-sliding window. EEG total power and power bands (Delta (0.5–4.5 Hz), Theta (5.0–9.0 Hz), Sigma (11.0–15.0 Hz)) were normalized to the mean value (100%) of the day 1 (control) recording. A full EEG spectrum from 0.25 to 20 Hz for NREM sleep and wakefulness was also calculated and normalized according to the average state specific spectrum of day 1. Sleep stages were visually scored by an operator (one-second resolution), using a script

developed for Spike2 (sleepscore). Wakefulness, NREM sleep, and REM sleep were scored according to standard criteria based on EEG, EMG, and T_{brain} signals [19].

Digital images from the thermocamera were acquired at 1 frame/s and tail temperature (T_{tail}) was measured in the medial portion of the tail by analyzing the thermographic record (Thermocam Researcher, FLIR systems, Boston, MA, USA). Variations of T_{tail} were analyzed comparing the 10-min average value recorded one hour before the first injection with the 10-min average value recorded 1 hour after the first injection for all experimental groups. Paired t-test was used to compare the pre-injection levels of T_{tail} with the post-injection values. Unpaired t-test was used to compare T_{tail} variation induced by muscimol injection with the saline-induced variation.

Values are reported as mean ± SEM. A two-way ANOVA (SPSS 21.0) with repeated measures on both factors was used for the statistical analysis of the results of the injection day (i.e. day 2 or day 5) and, with a different time resolution, of the baseline day (i.e. day 1 or day 4) together with the recovery day (i.e. day 3 or day 6). The modified t-test (t^*) was used for both the pre-planned orthogonal and the pre-planned non-orthogonal contrasts [23], [24]. The α level of the non-orthogonal contrasts was adjusted using the sequential Bonferroni method [25].

For the analysis of the injection day, the Main Factors were defined as follows: i) the Factor "time" (which was considered for repeated measures) had 48 levels, corresponding to each 30-min interval of the whole 24-h period; ii) the Factor "Experimental Condition" (which was considered for repeated measures) had two levels (saline and muscimol). For each 30-min interval of the Factor "time", data were compared by means of the following orthogonal contrast: saline vs. muscimol.

For the analysis of the baseline day and recovery day, the Main Factors were defined as follows: i) the Factor "time" (which was considered for repeated measures) had 4 levels, corresponding to the L and D periods of both days; ii) the Factor "Experimental Condition" (which was considered for repeated measures) had two levels (saline and muscimol). For each level of the "time" Factor, orthogonal contrasts were used to compare saline and muscimol results. For each level of the "Experimental Condition" Factor, the following pre-planned non-orthogonal contrasts were tested: recovery day_L vs. baseline day_L; recovery day_D vs. baseline day_D. The statistical analysis of the cumulative amount of wakefulness, NREM sleep, and REM sleep during the injection day was carried out with a t-test. The statistical analysis for T_{tail} was carried out comparing the 10 minutes T_{tail} average 1 hour before the beginning of the microinjection procedure with the 10 minutes T_{tail} average 1 hour later with a paired t-test. For all comparisons, statistical significance was set at p<0.05.

Results

Effects on sleep

The 6-h inhibition of the LH neurons was characterized by a significant increase in the amount of NREM sleep at both Ta 24°C and Ta 10°C (Figure 2). At Ta 24°C, the amount of NREM sleep increased significantly during the injection period with a peak after the second injection (93.6±3.1%, $t^*_{(192)} = 4.43$, p<0.05 compared to saline) and remained significantly higher compared to saline for the entire period of injections.

At Ta 10°C, the injections of muscimol induced a significant increase in the amount of NREM sleep that peaked after the third injection (90.5±4.9%, $t^*_{(288)} = 5.52$, p<0.05 compared to saline). A significant negative peak in the amount of NREM sleep was observed between 20:00 h and 21:00 h and was associated with a

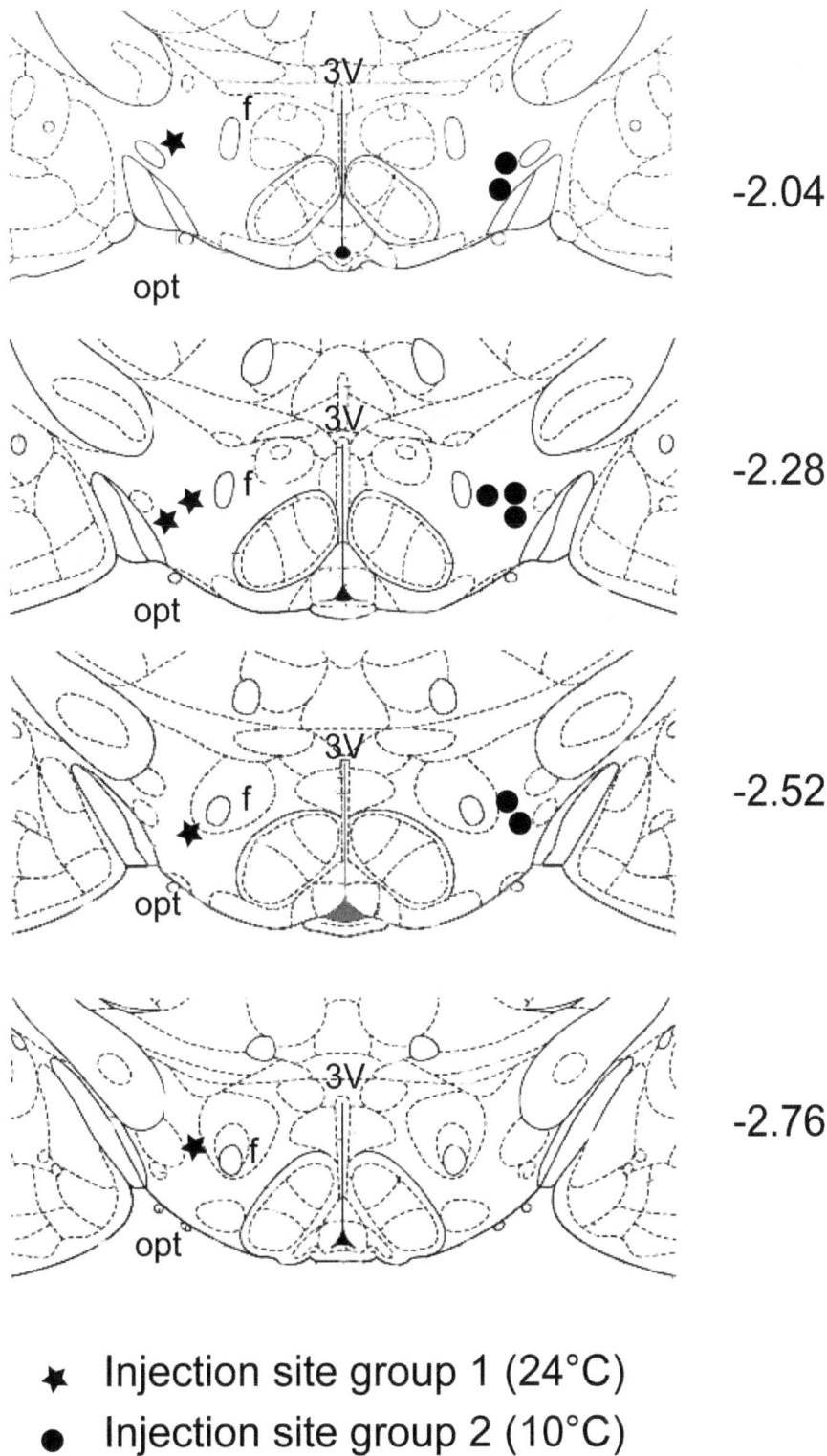

Figure 1. Injection Sites. The figure shows the location of the injection sites plotted on an atlas drawing [22]. Each injection was performed bilaterally but, for the sake of simplicity, is plotted monolaterally. Each slice refers to the antero-posterior distance in mm from Bregma, which is indicated on the right-hand side of each panel. The black stars, plotted on the left-hand side of each drawing, indicate the injection sites for group 1 animals (kept at an ambient temperature (Ta) of 24°C), while the black circles, plotted on the right-hand side of each drawing, indicate the injection sites for group 2 animals (exposed to Ta = 10°C during the injection period). 3V = third ventricle, f = fornex, opt = optic tract.

peak in the amount of wakefulness (70.6±9.1%, $t^*_{(288)}$ = 4.15, p< 0.05 compared to saline). On the recovery day after muscimol administration, no significant changes in the amount of NREM sleep were observed compared to the saline condition.

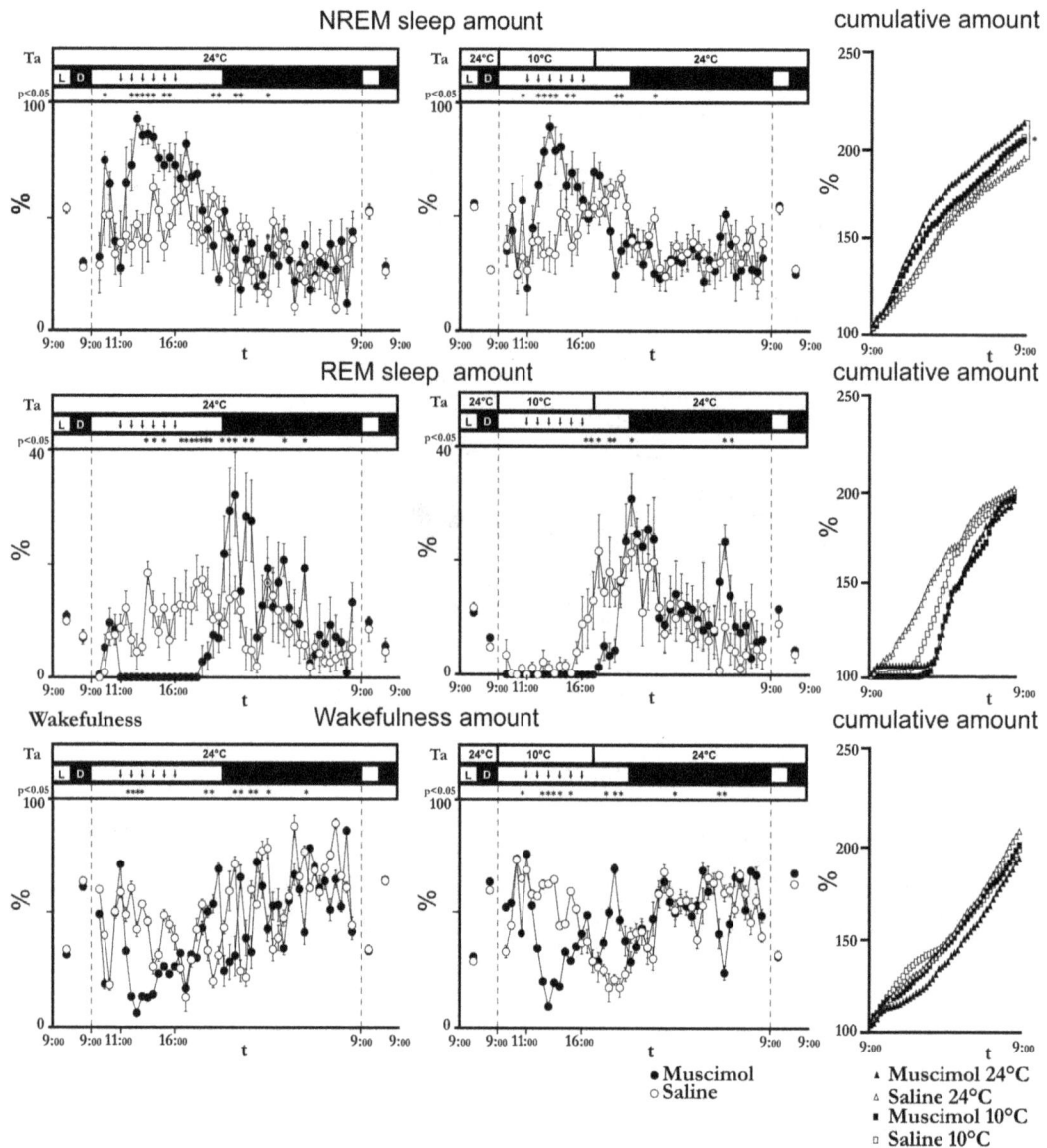

Figure 2. Sleep amount. The figure shows the time-course of the amount, expressed as the percentage of each epoch (12 h for Day 1, 3, 4, and 6; 30 min for day 2, and 5) of non-REM (NREM) sleep, REM sleep and wakefulness during the 6 experimental days (filled circles: days 1, 2 and 3; empty circles: days 4, 5 and 6) for group 1 animals (kept at an ambient temperature (Ta) of 24°C, left column) and group 2 animals (exposed to Ta = 10°C, from 9:00 to 17:00 of day 2, center column). The time resolution is 12 h for days 1, 3, 4, and 6 and 30 minutes for days 2 and 4. Vertical dashed lines divide consecutive experimental days. Each animal of each group was repeatedly injected with either the GABA$_A$ agonist muscimol (day 2, filled circles, 100 nl, 1 mM, 1 injection/h bilaterally) or saline (day 4, empty circles, 100 nl, 0, 9%, 1 injection/h bilaterally). Ta, light (L)/dark (D) cycle and statistical significance are plotted above each panel. Each down-pointing arrow marks an injection. Data are shown as mean ± SEM. * = p<0.05. In the right-hand column the cumulative amount (expressed as the percentage of the respective total amount during the day preceding the injection day) of NREM sleep, REM sleep and wakefulness during each injection day is shown. * = p<0.05.

During the 6-h period of LH neuron inhibition, the Delta power in NREM sleep was significantly higher both at 24°C and at 10°C, while Sigma power in NREM sleep was significantly lower compared to the saline condition (Figure 3). At Ta 24°C, Delta power increased rapidly after the first muscimol injection, reaching a peak after the third injection (138.3±12.0%, t*$_{(192)}$ = 2.59, p< 0.05 compared to saline), and returned to a normal level before the end of the injection period. On the other hand, Sigma power was drastically reduced after the first muscimol injection and remained very low for the entire period of injections (nadir: 40.3±5.8%, t*$_{(192)}$ = 5.48, p<0.05 compared to saline), slowly returning to normal at the end of the light period. At Ta 10°C, NREM sleep

Delta power rapidly increased after the first muscimol injection and remained significantly elevated for the entire injection period (peak 155.7±18.0%, t*$_{(240)}$ = 5.71, p<0.05 compared to saline). During the recovery day, Delta power showed a negative rebound; it was significantly lower compared to saline (Light period: 84.4±5.5%, t*$_{(20)}$ = 4.22, p<0.05 compared to saline; dark period: 83.9±7.3%, t*$_{(20)}$ = 3.32, p<0.05 compared to saline). Sigma power in NREM sleep was also drastically reduced, and remained significantly lower (nadir: 42.7±3.7%, t*$_{(288)}$ = 6.37, p<0.05 compared to saline) for a few hours after the last injection.

The EEG power spectrum in NREM sleep during the period of LH neuron inhibition showed a clear increase in the frequencies

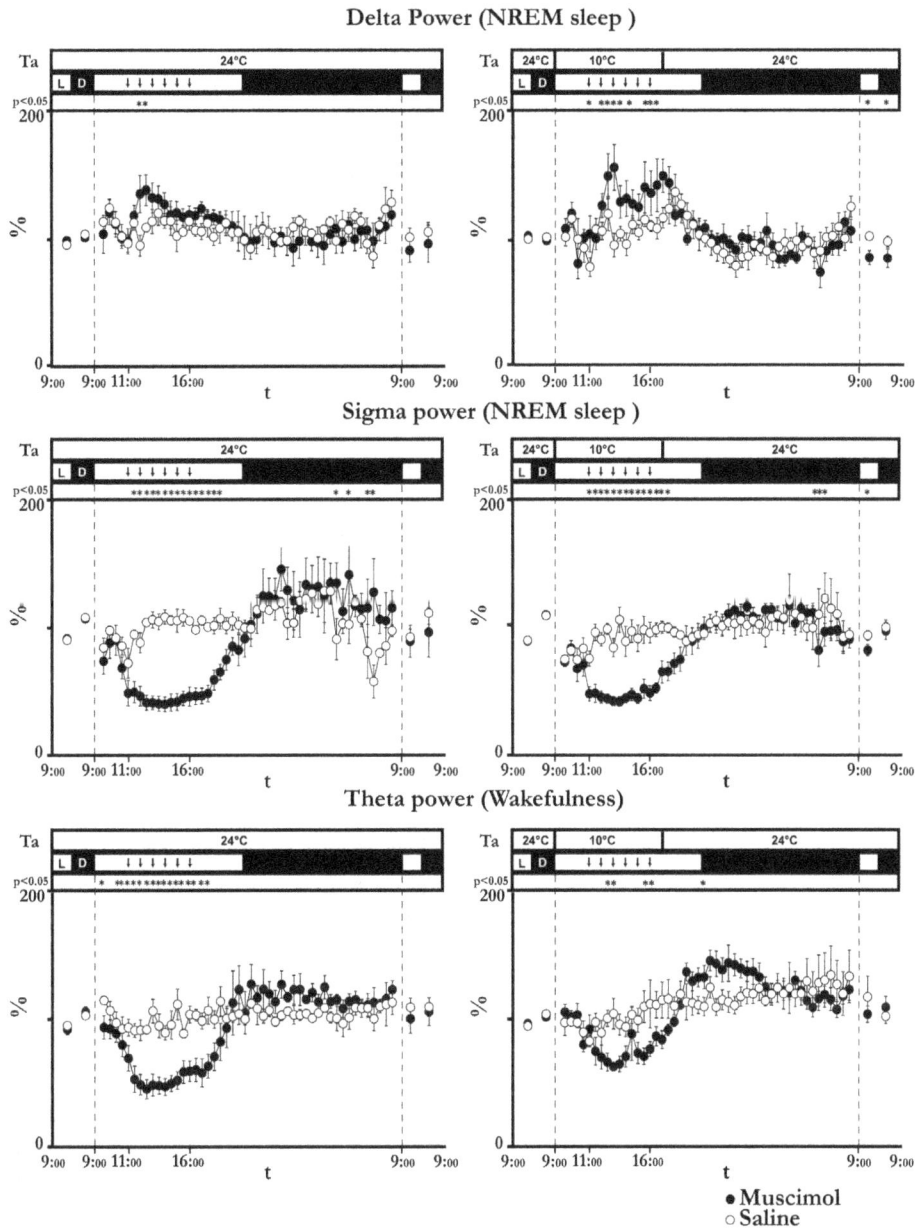

Figure 3. EEG power bands. The Figure shows the time-course of either Delta or Sigma power during non-REM (NREM) sleep and Theta power during wakefulness, during the 6 experimental days (filled circles: days 1, 2 and 3; empty circles: days 4, 5 and 6) for animals of group 1 (kept at an ambient temperature (Ta) of 24°C, left column) and for those of group 2 (exposed to Ta = 10°C from 9:00 to 17:00 of day 2, right column). Powers are normalized on the average EEG power of the day preceding the injection day and expressed as percentages. The time resolution is 12 h for days 1, 3, 4, and 6 and 30 minutes for days 2 and 4. Vertical dashed lines divide consecutive experimental days. Each animal of each group was repeatedly injected with either the GABA_A agonist muscimol (day 2, filled circles, 100 nl, 1 mM, 1 injection/h bilaterally) or saline (day 4, empty circles, 100 nl, 0, 9%, 1 injection/h bilaterally). Vertical dashed lines divide consecutive experimental days. Ta, light (L)/dark (D) cycle and statistical significance are plotted above each panel. Each downward arrow marks an injection. Data are shown as mean ± SEM. * = p<0.05.

below 2 Hz at Ta 24°C and below 3 Hz at Ta 10°C, and a drastic decrease in all the spectral components above 7 Hz was observed at both Tas (Figure 4).

REM sleep was totally suppressed during the prolonged inhibition of the LH neurons and for a few hours afterwards, at both Ta 24°C and Ta 10°C (Figure 2). Acute exposure to Ta 10°C with saline injections also resulted in an immediate drastic decrease in REM sleep amount, but at around 15:00 REM sleep appeared again. The amount of REM sleep lost during the injection period was fully recovered within the same day.

The changes in the amount of wakefulness induced by LH inhibition mirrored the effects on NREM sleep amount at both Ta 24°C and Ta 10°C (Figure 2). Theta power during wakefulness (Figure 3) was strongly decreased by the muscimol injections at both Ta 24°C (nadir: 47.4±6.8%, t*_{(192)} = 4.21, p<0.05 compared to saline) and Ta 10°C (nadir: 63.2±3.1%, t*_{(288)} = 2.13, p< 0.05 compared to saline), returning to normal levels a few hours after the last injections. Animals exposed to 10°C showed an increase in Theta power during the night following the LH

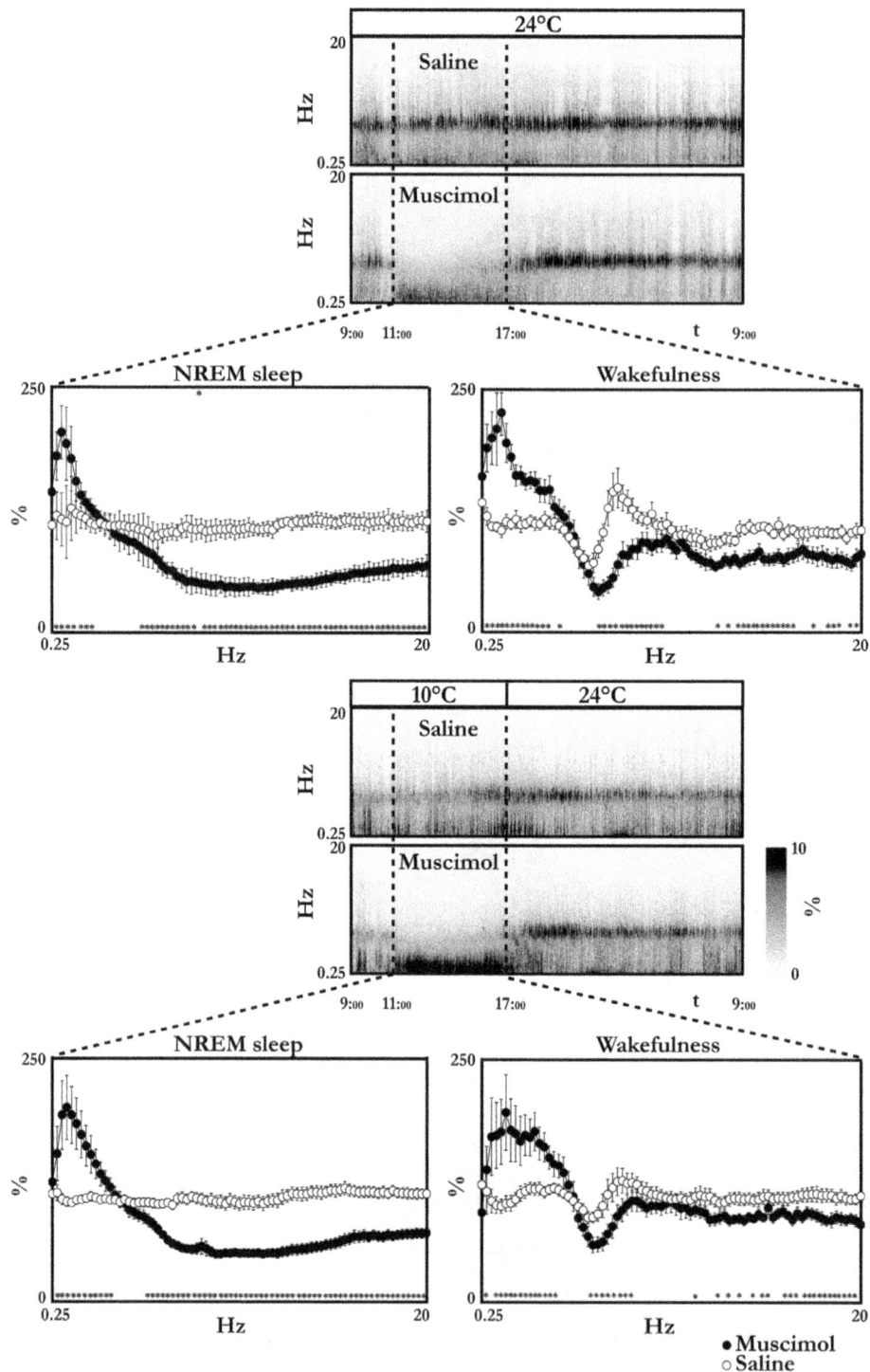

Figure 4. EEG spectra. The figure shows the time-course of the average EEG spectrum during the day of repeated injections of either the GABA_A agonist muscimol (100 nl, 1 mM, 1 injection/h bilaterally) or saline (100 nl, 0, 9%, 1 injection/h bilaterally) for group 1 animals (A and B) and for group 2 animals (E and F). EEG power is normalized on the average EEG power recorded during the day before the injection day and expressed as percentages. Ambient temperature is indicated above each panel. Vertical dashed lines indicate the injection period, from the first injection to 1 hour after the last injection. Panels C, D, G and H show the average EEG spectrum in non-REM sleep and in wakefulness during the injection period. Data are shown as mean ± SEM. * = p<0.05.

inhibition. No significant differences were observed during the recovery day.

The EEG power spectrum in wakefulness during the period of LH neuron inhibition showed a clear increase in the frequencies below 4 Hz at both Ta 24°C and Ta 10°C, and a drastic decrease in the frequency of the Theta band (Figure 4). Saline injections also produced a right-shift of the Theta region, which was around 1.5 Hz faster.

Effects on autonomic variables

At Ta 24°C, the repeated injection of saline produced a significant increase in T_{brain} compared to that observed during the injections of muscimol (peak: 37.8±0.3°C, $t^*_{(192)} = 5.20$, $p<0.05$) (Figure 5). At Ta 10°C, saline injection still produced an increase in T_{brain}, while muscimol injections evoked a decrease in T_{brain}, that reached a nadir of 35.5±0.2°C ($t^*_{(240)} = 8.42$, $p<0.05$ compared to saline) after 3 hours. T_{brain} returned rapidly towards physiological levels, but it remained significantly higher compared to the saline group for the rest of the day. No significant differences were observed in the recovery period. The decrease in T_{brain} was not caused by an increase in thermal dissipation, since the tail did not show any sign of vasodilation, but, rather, a modest but significant vasoconstriction (Figure 6), dropping from an average pre-injection value of 12.8±1.1°C to 11.8±1.1°C one hour after the first injection ($t_{(6)} = 2.59$, $p<0.05$). A significant reduction in T_{tail} was also observed at Ta 24°C, when T_{tail} dropped from an average pre-injection value of 31.1±0.3°C to 29.6±0.2°C one hour after the first injection ($t_{(4)} = 8.48$, $p<0.05$). The latter value was also significantly lower ($p<0.05$) compared to that observed one hour after the first saline injection (31.5±0.4°C; $t_{(5)} = 3.55$).

At Ta 24°C, HR was significantly higher following saline injections than following muscimol administration (Figure 5). The increase in HR induced by saline may be the result of the repeated microinjection procedure that, despite the care taken in trying to minimize the handling of the animal, may have disturbed the animal, resulting in a modest stress-induced hyperthermia. This effect was completely blocked by muscimol injection. At Ta 10°C, the acute cold exposure caused a rapid increase in HR that was only partially reversed by muscimol injections in a limited time window. No major effects on AP levels were observed following either muscimol or saline injections at both Tas.

Discussion

The results of the present study show that, as previously described [5], in the rat kept at normal laboratory temperature (Ta, 24°C) the prolonged inhibition of LH neurons produced a pronounced increase in NREM sleep and a total suppression of REM sleep. These effects were not likely to be the mere consequence of changes in body temperature, since no decrease in T_{brain} was observed following muscimol injection in animals kept at Ta 24°C, suggesting that LH neurons do not play a role in the basic maintenance of body temperature in a thermoneutral environment.

A novel finding is that NREM sleep enhancement was characterized by an increase in Delta power, due to a large enhancement of slow wave activity (SWA), with almost no activity in the faster frequencies of the EEG spectrum. We categorized this state as NREM sleep, although its peculiar spectral EEG characteristics may call for an *ad hoc* denomination. Moreover, the results show that these effects were also produced when the inhibition of LH neurons occurred during acute cold exposure, a condition which is known to interfere with sleep processes [19].

The lack of relevant bodily thermal changes following muscimol injection at Ta 24°C suggests that the effects observed on either NREM sleep or REM sleep were the consequence of the inhibition of LH neurons specifically involved in the regulation of wake-sleep processes. Although the orexin and the MCH neurons within the LH may represent the best candidates [26], [27], a role for non-orexin/non-MCH neurons cannot be disregarded [9].

In fact, the features of the NREM sleep occurring after the inhibition of the entire population of neurons within the LH by muscimol substantially differ from those described after the selective inhibition of subpopulations of neurons in the same area, especially the orexin and the MCH neurons. As far as the orexin neurons are concerned, while their fast acute optogenetic inhibition was shown to be sufficient to rapidly induce SWA [28], and systemic pharmacological antagonism of orexin was shown to produce an increase in NREM sleep in several mammals [29], the 1-h optogenetically-mediated inhibition of these neurons in mice was effective in providing an increase in NREM sleep amount only when delivered during the dark period, but not during the light period of the LD cycle (i.e. the period in which the effect was observed in the present study) [8].

Also, while a pharmacological blockade of orexin receptors was not shown to induce significant changes in the NREM sleep EEG power spectrum in humans [30], [31], in the present study the spectral EEG characteristics of both NREM sleep and wakefulness during the period of muscimol injection appeared to be different from their physiological counterpart. Although the EEG trace during LH inhibition did not show evident abnormalities, the EEG power spectrum during NREM sleep, in particular, presented a large increase below 2 Hz and a drastic reduction in the faster frequency regions. In addition, the EEG spectrum of wakefulness was characterized by an increase in the power of the low-frequency region that was concomitant with a mild reduction in the power of the fast-frequency region. These findings, together with the observation that the activity of orexin neurons undergoes a circadian modulation that should be at its lowest level during our injection period [32], suggest that the increase in NREM sleep and in SWA induced by muscimol injections may be the results of the inhibition of a wider neuronal population within the LH rather than just the orexin neurons.

The inhibition of LH neurons at Ta 10°C induced a relevant hypothermia, confirming the role of LH neurons in thermoregulation and apparently providing an explanation for the suppression of REM sleep. However, the fact that after muscimol delivery at Ta 24°C brain temperature remained at baseline levels suggests that an impairment in thermogenesis was unlikely to be the cause of the absence of REM sleep. Interestingly, the almost complete suppression of Sigma power during NREM sleep indicates the absence of any attempt to enter REM sleep, since it is known that the NREM to REM sleep transition is marked by a strong increase in Sigma power [33].

The suppression of REM sleep may therefore be considered to be the consequence of the inhibition of the activity of MCH neurons [27]. However, the optogenetic inhibition of these neurons did not affect REM sleep duration [6], suggesting that other neurons in the area besides the MCH positive are involved in the regulation of REM sleep appearance. It can be suggested that this third population of neurons may be the population of GABA-positive/MCH-and-orexina-negative REM-on neurons [9]. These neurons may induce REM sleep by an inhibitory projection to the ventrolateral part of the periaqueductal gray and to the dorsal deep mesencephalic nucleus GABAergic REM-off neurons [27].

The REM sleep suppression caused by LH neurons inhibition may resemble the REM sleep suppression induced by an inflammatory state [34]. In both conditions the suppression of REM sleep is concomitant with an increase in NREM sleep and in Delta power, but LH inhibition does not induce any increase in brain temperature, as usually seen after cytokine injection [34]. In consideration of the fact that the increase in brain temperature during inflammatory response has been shown to be separable from the concomitant thermoregulatory effects [35], it is possible to hypothesize that the neuronal population within the LH may be one of the areas mediating the effects of cytokines on sleep.

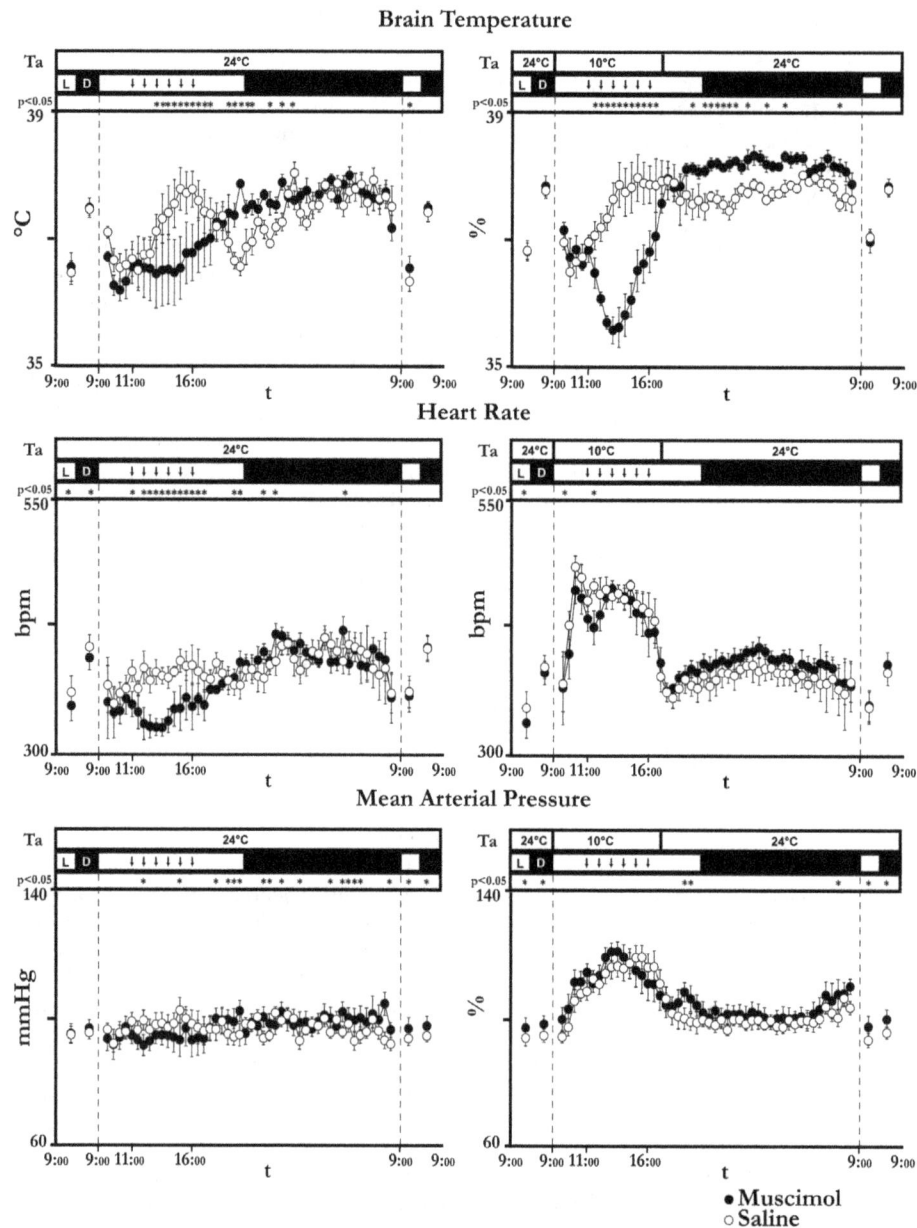

Figure 5. Autonomic parameters. The figure shows the time-course of brain temperature, heart rate and mean arterial pressure during the 6 experimental days (filled circles: days 1, 2 and 3; empty circles: days 4, 5 and 6) for animals of group 1 (kept at an ambient temperature (Ta) of 24°C, left column) and those of group 2 (exposed to Ta = 10°C from 9:00 to 17:00 of day 2, right column). The time resolution is 12 h for days 1, 3, 4, and 6 and 30 minutes for days 2 and 4. Vertical dashed lines divide consecutive experimental days. Each animal of each group was repeatedly injected with either the GABA$_A$ agonist muscimol (day 2, filled circles, 100 nl, 1 mM, 1 injection/h bilaterally) or saline (day 4, empty circles, 100 nl, 0, 9%, 1 injection/h bilaterally). Vertical dashed lines divide consecutive experimental days. Ta, light (L)/dark (D) cycle and statistical significance are plotted above each panel. Each downward arrow marks an injection. Data are visualized as mean ± SEM. * = p<0.05.

Our results also show that LH neurons have a limited role in regulating the activity of the autonomic nervous system.

LH inhibition failed to reverse the increase in HR and MAP caused by cold exposure and had limited effects on HR at Ta 24°C, suggesting that LH neurons are not involved in the thermoregulatory modulation of cardiovascular parameters.

Thermoregulation was more largely affected than cardiovascular regulation by LH neurons inhibition. At Ta 10°C, T_{brain} decreased significantly during the delivery of the first three injections, but this decrease was quickly reversed, despite the fact that the LH neurons were still actively inhibited, suggesting the

activation of a compensatory system. Since the decrease in T_{brain} was not caused by an increased thermal dissipation, it can only be explained by a reduced thermogenesis. It has been suggested that the orexin neurons within the LH are capable of amplifying an already active thermogenic drive, but have limited effects otherwise [4]. If this is the case, our data suggest that LH neurons, possibly the orexin neurons, are among the first responders that are activated to maintain a constant body temperature after cold exposure, potentiating the basic thermogenic drive, but they are not necessary for the maintenance of core temperature in a cold environment.

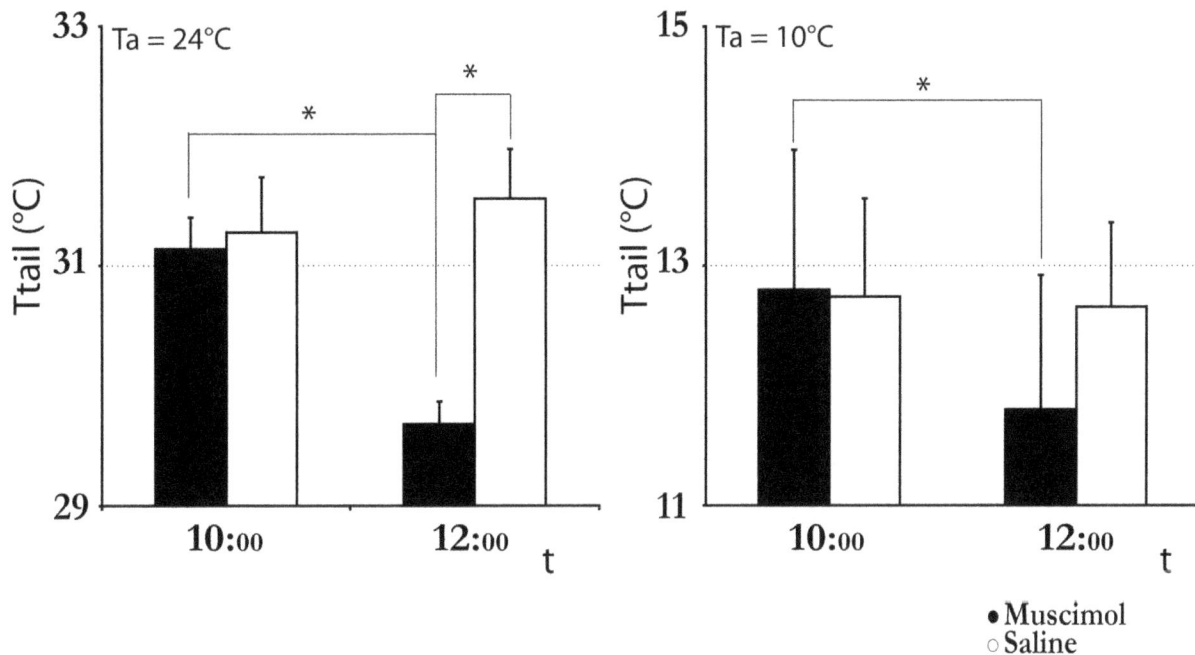

Figure 6. Tail temperature. The figure shows the average tail temperature measured from 9:50 to 10:00 (approximately 1 hour before the first injection) and from 11:50 and 12:00 (approximately 1 hour after the first injection of either muscimol (black bar) or saline (white bar)) at ambient temperature (Ta) = 24°C (on the left) or at Ta = 10°C (on the right). Data are shown as mean ± SEM. * = p<0.05.

At Ta 24°C, no decrease in T_{brain} was observed, suggesting that LH neurons may not play a role in the basic maintenance of body temperature in a thermoneutral environment. Unexpectedly, an increase in T_{brain} was observed during the injection of saline. This can be explained by the repeated injection procedure that, despite every effort on behalf of the experimenters, may have produced some distress in the animal. An alternative explanation may lie in the fact that orexin neurons have been shown to be activated by a decrease in pH [36]. Even if the volume of the saline injection was very small, the possibility that a transient reduction in extracellular pH may have resulted in an activation of orexin neurons cannot be ruled out, although it appears unlikely. It is worth noting that, whatever the cause of the saline-related increase in T_{brain}, the injection of muscimol suppressed it.

An increase in the vasoconstrictor tone in the tail blood vessels was induced by the muscimol injection both at Ta = 24°C and at Ta = 10 C°. The increased vasoconstriction may reveal the presence of a tonically-active inhibitory input originating in the LH and affecting other central areas involved in the regulation of cutaneous thermal conductance, such as the Preoptic Area [37] or the Raphe Pallidus [38]. Alternatively, it may be suggested that the reduction in the thermogenic drive induced by the inhibition of LH neurons immediately triggered a compensatory response that was sufficient to avoid hypothermia at Ta = 24°C but not at Ta = 10°C.

In conclusion, the results of our study show that: i) the acute inhibition of neurons within the LH induced a large increase in NREM sleep with enhanced SWA, and suppressed both REM sleep and the EEG activity characterizing the NREM to REM sleep transition; ii) these effects cannot be merely ascribed to the inhibition of either orexin or MCH neurons within the LH, suggesting a role for non-orexin/non-MCH neurons; iii) neurons located within the LH are involved in a first line of cold defense, but are not apparently essential for the maintenance of body temperature.

Acknowledgments

The authors wish to thank Ms. Melissa Stott for reviewing the English.

Author Contributions

Conceived and designed the experiments: MC GZ RA. Performed the experiments: MC FD MM DM. Analyzed the data: MC FD ML. Contributed to the writing of the manuscript: MC EP DT GZ RA.

References

1. Berthoud HR, Munzberg H (2013) The lateral hypothalamus as integrator of metabolic and environmental needs: from electrical self-stimulation to opto-genetics. Physiol Behav 104: 29–39.

2. Li FW, Deurveilher S, Semba K (2011) Behavioural and neuronal activation after microinjections of AMPA and NMDA into the perifornical lateral hypothalamus in rats. Behav Brain Res 224: 376–386.

3. Cerri M, Morrison SF (2005) Activation of lateral hypothalamic neurons stimulates brown adipose tissue thermogenesis. Neuroscience 135: 627–638.

4. Tupone D, Madden CJ, Cano G, Morrison SF (2011) An orexinergic projection from perifornical hypothalamus to raphe pallidus increases rat brown adipose tissue thermogenesis. J Neurosci 31: 15944–15955.

5. Clement O, Sapin E, Libourel PA, Arthaud S, Brischoux F, et al. (2012) The lateral hypothalamic area controls paradoxical (REM) sleep by means of descending projections to brainstem GABAergic neurons. J Neurosci 32: 16763–16774.

6. Jego S, Glasgow SD, Herrera CG, Ekstrand M, Reed SJ, et al. (2013) Optogenetic identification of a rapid eye movement sleep modulatory circuit in the hypothalamus. Nat Neurosci 16: 1637–1643.

7. Hassani OK, Henny P, Lee MG, Jones BE (2010) GABAergic neurons intermingled with orexin and MCH neurons in the lateral hypothalamus discharge maximally during sleep. Eur J Neurosci 32: 448–457.

8. Tsunematsu T, Tabuchi S, Tanaka KF, Boyden ES, Tominaga M, et al. (2013) Long-lasting silencing of orexin/hypocretin neurons using archaerhodopsin induces slow-wave sleep in mice. Behav Brain Res 255: 64–74.

9. Sapin E, Berod A, Leger L, Herman PA, Luppi PH, et al. (2013) A very large number of GABAergic neurons are activated in the tuberal hypothalamus during paradoxical (REM) sleep hypersomnia. PLoS One 5: e11766.

10. Sasaki K, Suzuki M, Mieda M, Tsujino N, Roth B, et al. (2011) Pharmacogenetic modulation of orexin neurons alters sleep/wakefulness states in mice. PLoS One 6: e20360.

11. Betschart C, Hintermann S, Behnke D, Cotesta S, Fendt M, et al. (2013) Identification of a novel series of orexin receptor antagonists with a distinct effect on sleep architecture for the treatment of insomnia. J Med Chem 56: 7590–7607.

12. Kapas L, Obal F, Jr, Alfoldi P, Rubicsek G, Penke B, et al. (1988) Effects of nocturnal intraperitoneal administration of cholecystokinin in rats: simultaneous increase in sleep, increase in EEG slow-wave activity, reduction of motor activity, suppression of eating, and decrease in brain temperature. Brain Res 438: 155–164.

13. Walker JM, Garber A, Berger RJ, Heller HC (1979) Sleep and estivation (shallow torpor): continuous processes of energy conservation. Science 204: 1098–1100.

14. Harris DV, Walker JM, Berger RJ (1984) A Continuum of Slow-Wave Sleep and Shallow Torpor in the Pocket Mouse Perognathus longimembris. Physiological Zoology 57: 428–443.

15. Krilowicz BL, Glotzbach SF, Heller HC (1988) Neuronal activity during sleep and complete bouts of hibernation. Am J Physiol 255: R1008–1019.

16. Deboer T, Tobler I (1994) Sleep EEG after daily torpor in the Djungarian hamster: similarity to the effect of sleep deprivation. Neurosci Lett 166: 35–38.

17. Cerri M, Mastrotto M, Tupone D, Martelli D, Luppi M, et al. (2013) The inhibition of neurons in the central nervous pathways for thermoregulatory cold defense induces a suspended animation state in the rat. J Neurosci 33: 2984–2993.

18. Tupone D, Madden CJ, Morrison SF (2013) Central activation of the A1 adenosine receptor (A1AR) induces a hypothermic, torpor-like state in the rat. J Neurosci 33: 14512–14525.

19. Cerri M, Ocampo-Garces A, Amici R, Baracchi F, Capitani P, et al. (2005) Cold exposure and sleep in the rat: effects on sleep architecture and the electroencephalogram. Sleep 28: 694–705.

20. Takahashi Y, Zhang W, Sameshima K, Kuroki C, Matsumoto A, et al. (2013) Orexin neurons are indispensable for prostaglandin E2-induced fever and defence against environmental cooling in mice. J Physiol 591: 5623–5643.

21. Del Vecchio F, Al-Jahmany A, Amici R, Cerri M, Luppi M, et al. (2012) Effects on sleep of the inhibition of the lateral hypothalamus in the rat. J Sleep Res S358: 571.

22. Paxinos G, Watson C (2007) The rat brain in stereotaxic coordinates. San Diego: Elsevier.

23. Wallenstein S, Zucker CL, Fleiss JL (1980) Some statistical methods useful in circulation research. Circ Res 47: 1–9.

24. Winer BJ, Brown DR, Michels KM (1991) Statistical principles in experimental design. Boston: McGraw-Hill.

25. Holm S (1979) A simple sequentially rejective multiple test procedure. Scand J Stat 6: 65–70.

26. de Lecea L, Huerta R (2014) Hypocretin (orexin) regulation of sleep-to-wake transitions. Front Pharmacol 5: 16.

27. Luppi PH, Peyron C, Fort P (2013) Role of MCH neurons in paradoxical (REM) sleep control. Sleep 36: 1775–1776.

28. Tsunematsu T, Kilduff TS, Boyden ES, Takahashi S, Tominaga M, et al. (2011) Acute optogenetic silencing of orexin/hypocretin neurons induces slow-wave sleep in mice. J Neurosci 31: 10529–10539.

29. Brisbare-Roch C, Dingemanse J, Koberstein R, Hoever P, Aissaoui H, et al. (2007) Promotion of sleep by targeting the orexin system in rats, dogs and humans. Nat Med 13: 150–155.

30. Bettica P, Squassante L, Groeger JA, Gennery B, Winsky-Sommerer R, et al. (2012) Differential effects of a dual orexin receptor antagonist (SB-649868) and zolpidem on sleep initiation and consolidation, SWS, REM sleep, and EEG power spectra in a model of situational insomnia. Neuropsychopharmacology 37: 1224–1233.

31. Fox SV, Gotter AL, Tye SJ, Garson SL, Savitz AT, et al. (2013) Quantitative Electroencephalography Within Sleep/Wake States Differentiates GABAA Modulators Eszopiclone and Zolpidem From Dual Orexin Receptor Antagonists in Rats. Neuropsychopharmacology 38: 2401–2408.

32. Estabrooke IV, McCarthy MT, Ko E, Chou TC, Chemelli RM, et al. (2001) Fos expression in orexin neurons varies with behavioral state. J Neurosci 21: 1656–1662.

33. Capitani P, Cerri M, Amici R, Baracchi F, Jones CA, et al. (2005) Changes in EEG activity and hypothalamic temperature as indices for non-REM sleep to REM sleep transitions. Neurosci Lett 383: 182–187.

34. Krueger JM, Johannsen L (1989) Bacterial products, cytokines and sleep. J Rheumatol Suppl 19: 52–57.

35. Krueger JM, Takahashi S (1997) Thermoregulation and sleep. Closely linked but separable. Ann N Y Acad Sci 813: 281–286.

36. Williams RH, Jensen LT, Verkhratsky A, Fugger L, Burdakov D (2007) Control of hypothalamic orexin neurons by acid and CO2. Proc Natl Acad Sci U S A 104: 10685–10690.

37. Tanaka M, McKinley MJ, McAllen RM (2013) Role of an excitatory preoptic-raphe pathway in febrile vasoconstriction of the rat's tail. Am J Physiol Regul Integr Comp Physiol 305: R1479–1489.

38. Cerri M, Zamboni G, Tupone D, Dentico D, Luppi M, et al. (2010) Cutaneous vasodilation elicited by disinhibition of the caudal portion of the rostral ventromedial medulla of the free-behaving rat. Neuroscience 165: 984–995.

24

Thoughts of Death Modulate Psychophysical and Cortical Responses to Threatening Stimuli

Elia Valentini[1,2]*, Katharina Koch[1,2], Salvatore Maria Aglioti[1,2]

1 Sapienza Università di Roma, Dipartimento di Psicologia, Roma, Italy, 2 Fondazione Santa Lucia, Istituto di Ricovero e Cura a Carattere Scientifico, Roma, Italy

Abstract

Existential social psychology studies show that awareness of one's eventual death profoundly influences human cognition and behaviour by inducing defensive reactions against end-of-life related anxiety. Much less is known about the impact of reminders of mortality on brain activity. Therefore we explored whether reminders of mortality influence subjective ratings of intensity and threat of auditory and painful thermal stimuli and the associated electroencephalographic activity. Moreover, we explored whether personality and demographics modulate psychophysical and neural changes related to mortality salience (MS). Following MS induction, a specific increase in ratings of intensity and threat was found for both nociceptive and auditory stimuli. While MS did not have any specific effect on nociceptive and auditory evoked potentials, larger amplitude of theta oscillatory activity related to thermal nociceptive activity was found after thoughts of death were induced. MS thus exerted a top-down modulation on theta electroencephalographic oscillatory amplitude, specifically for brain activity triggered by painful thermal stimuli. This effect was higher in participants reporting higher threat perception, suggesting that inducing a death-related mind-set may have an influence on body-defence related somatosensory representations.

Editor: Benjamin Thompson, University of Waterloo, Canada

Funding: E. Valentini is supported by the Avvio alla Ricerca Sapienza grant scheme. S. M. Aglioti was funded by the European Union Information and Communication Technologies Grant (VERE project, FP7-ICT-2009-5, Prot. Num. 257695) and the Italian Ministry of Health (grant RC11.G and RF-2010-2312912). The funders had no role in study design, data collection and analysis, decision to publish, or preparation of the manuscript.

Competing Interests: The authors have declared that no competing interests exist.

* Email: elia.valentini@uniroma1.it

Introduction

"[...] Death, the most dreaded of evils, is therefore of no concern to us; for while we exist death is not present, and when death is present we no longer exist. Epicurus (Letter to Menoeceus, 43–44).

Awareness of unavoidable death has a powerful impact on cognition and human behaviour [1]. The terror management theory (TMT) has shown that pondering on one's own mortality promotes stereotypical thinking as well as a defensive attitude towards one's own values and beliefs [2]. An important asset of the TMT is the hypothesis that cultural and personality factors may act as mediators of the anxiogenic effects caused by the awareness of death. In particular, the hypothesis that increased self-esteem makes an individual less prone to anxiety or thoughts about death has received much experimental support (e.g. [3–6]). Other authors have shown how priming thoughts about one's death induces negative emotions (e.g. anxiety), provokes avoidance of self-focused states [7], and leads individuals high in neuroticism to avoid physical sensations, including pleasurable ones [8].

Although there is general agreement that thoughts of death significantly affect cognition and human behaviour, only a few studies have investigated how thoughts of death influence cortical representation of sensory information. Noteworthy here are studies that investigated the effect of death-content accessibility on bold signal or event-related potentials (ERPs) amplitudes [9–11] and on its interaction with neural processes linked to social-affective categorization of facial expressions [12], as well as with observation of others' pain [13]. More specifically, using fMRI, Quirin et al. [10] reported that accessibility to thoughts of death induced higher activation of structures usually associated with emotion regulation, such as the amygdala and the anterior cingulate cortex (ACC). More recently, Klackl et al. [11] reported larger late positive potential amplitudes associated with death-related words, a finding that may be interpreted as indexing preferential mortality salience effects on emotion regulation. Nevertheless, these results are in contrast with evidence of decreased ACC and insular activity for death-related words in the context of a linguistic Stroop task [9]. Surprisingly, although a relationship between mortality salience effects and implicit anxiogenic mechanisms has been acknowledged in previous studies, there is currently no evidence linking the effects of mortality salience to representation of threatening sensory information within the central nervous system.

Here, we sought to determine whether thoughts of death can influence perceptual ratings and cortical representations associated to threatening sensory stimuli. Combining a paired stimulation design with electroencephalography (EEG), we explored the effects of mortality salience on ERPs and oscillatory theta activity elicited by pairs (S1–S2) of laser thermal painful stimuli, before and after the induction of a cognitive mind-set (i.e., a mental disposition). Pairs of auditory stimuli, matched in subjective intensity with the painful radiant thermal stimuli, were used to explore the effects on perception and neural representation of non-painful stimuli. Paired stimulation was conceived as a minimalist approach to induce a repetition suppression effect (e.g. [14]). Indeed, most of studies investigating short-term habituation of EEG responses evoked by radiant heat stimulation reported a dramatic reduction of response magnitude to repeated identical stimuli already at the level of the second stimulus, with no further decrement in response to the following stimuli (e.g. [15,16]). The second stimulus of each pair was therefore designed as a test stimulus and conceived as a minimal measure of basic sensitization/habituation processes.

We hypothesized that mortality salience interferes with phasic cortical responses to repeated threatening sensory stimuli by exerting a top-down allocation of attentional resources regardless of sensory stimulation salience that leads to stimulus detection and attentional orientation processes [17], and thus impairing the reduction of response amplitude observed to repeated stimulation at short fixed inter-stimulus interval (e.g. [18,19]).

Overall, the present design enabled us to isolate the effects of mortality salience from i) the sole salience or novelty of the sensory stimulation, ii) the variability of the neural responses prior to the mind-set induction, and thus iii) disclose cognitive/emotional top-down modulations of cortical representation of threat contingent upon accessibility to death thoughts.

Methods

Ethics statement

Participants gave written informed consent and were debriefed at the end of the experiment. All experimental procedures were approved by the Fondazione Santa Lucia local ethics committee and were in accordance with the standards of the Declaration of Helsinki.

Participants

Twenty right-handed healthy participants (12 females) aged between 21 and 33 (mean $\pm$ SD, 24.5$\pm$4.4) participated in the study. All had normal or corrected-to-normal vision and were naïve as to the purpose of the experiment. None of the participants had a history of neurological or psychiatric illnesses or conditions that could potentially interfere with pain sensitivity (e.g. drug intake or skin diseases).

Personality measures

Preliminary screening and selection of volunteers was conducted using self-report measures of personality traits that could potentially interfere with the effect of the applied mind-set induction on perception and cortical arousal. The Beck Depression Inventory (BDI) [20] and the State-Trait Anxiety Inventory (STAI) [21] were administered to obtain an index of individual psychopathological symptoms of depression and anxiety, respectively. Participants who scored higher than 17 on the BDI and higher or lower than two standard deviations (SD) on the STAI were not allowed to enter the study [22]. These cut-off scores determined the preliminary exclusion of two participants.

Nociceptive and auditory stimulation

The nociceptive heat stimuli were pulses generated by an infrared neodymium yttrium aluminium perovskite (Nd:YAP) laser with a wavelength of 1.34 μm (Electronical Engineering, Florence, Italy). Duration of the laser pulses was 5 ms. These pulses selectively and directly activate the Aδ and C-fiber nociceptive terminals located in the superficial layers of the skin [23]_EN-REF_4. The laser beam was transmitted via an optic fiber and its diameter was set at approximately 7 mm ($\approx$38 mm^2) by focusing lenses. Laser pulses were delivered on a square area (5$\times$5 cm) defined on the left hand dorsum prior to the beginning of the experimental session. He-Ne laser indicated the area to be stimulated. To prevent increases in baseline skin temperature and fatigue or sensitization of the nociceptors, the position of the laser beam was changed after each pulse. An infrared thermometer (precision $\pm$0.3°C) was used to measure the temperature of the stimulated skin area before and during the experiment (group-average intensity of 34.2$\pm$0.7°C). Temperature fluctuations never exceeded 0.8 SD°C within participants.

During a familiarization and calibration procedure on the quality of the sensation associated with radiant heat stimuli, participants were instructed to define the intensity of the sensation using both a numerical rating scale (NRS) and a visual-analogue scale (VAS). For both of these methods, intensity was defined as how strong the sensation was. Participants were instructed to verbally rate intensity of painful stimuli according to the NRS from not intense or barely intense (0–10) to low intense (21–40), moderately intense (41–60), highly intense (61–80) and extremely intense (81–100). Participants were allowed to give decimal ratings over the entire numerical scale. The energy of the stimulus was adjusted using a staircase procedure. The procedure required one increase (increasing) series and one decrease (decreasing) series in steps of 0.5 Joules (J), followed by an increase (increasing) series in steps of 0.25 J until the target intensity of the nociceptive-related sensation was reported (i.e. pricking/burning sensation; [24]). Lastly, energies within 0.5 J below and above the energy eliciting the pricking/burning sensation were delivered to test the reliability of the intensity ratings. Eventually, all the calibrated stimuli were defined as painful by the participants and perceived as threatening. As our objective was to establish a perceptual similarity between laser heat- and auditory-related percepts, once the target intensity was found and the corresponding laser energy calibrated (group-average intensity of 4.5$\pm$0.4 J), participants were required to self-adjust the intensity of the auditory stimulation to match the intensity of the nociceptive stimulus using the same criteria as the NRS for the nociceptive stimuli (see [19,25] for a detailed description). This procedure was applied to create a threatening experience similar to the one induced by somatosensory nociceptive stimuli, by asking the participants to focus on the most simple aspect of somatosensory nociceptive sensation: its magnitude. By matching the two types of sensory stimuli according to their magnitude we obtained a match of the salience of sensory stimulation and reduced the complexity of a matching procedure based on cognitive/affective aspects of the stimuli (e.g. unpleasantness), while obtaining a comparable level of threat for auditory stimuli during the experiment. Auditory stimuli were short tones of 800 Hz frequency (50 ms; 5 ms as the rising and falling time of the tone) emitted by a loudspeaker placed in front of the participants' left hand ($\approx$50 cm from the participant and $\approx$50 cm from the midline). Once auditory intensity was calibrated (group-average intensity of 81.8$\pm$3.6 dB; measured at the subject's left ear), participants underwent a brief learning procedure during which the NRS anchors were transferred onto the experimental VAS. If a significant discrepancy was noticed between NRS ratings during calibration and VAS judgments during learning, the calibration procedure was repeated.

During this procedure the participants received paired stimuli (at a fixed interval of 1 s) to accurately match the two modalities according to the requirements of the experimental design.

EEG recording

EEG recordings were obtained from sixty tin electrodes (Electro-cap International - ECI) placed according to the positions of the 10–20 International System. Three surface electrodes were positioned for the vertical, horizontal electro-oculography (EOG) recording below the right eye and at the right and left ocular canthi and one electrode at the left mastoid for electromyography recording (EMG). The reference was on the nose and the ground at AFz. Electrode impedance was kept below 5 kΩ. The EEG signal was amplified and digitized at 1000 Hz.

Design and experimental procedure

Participants underwent two separate experimental sessions (on two different days, same time of day). In both sessions, participants were submitted to four recording blocks (Fig. 1, top panel). The first two blocks had no cognitive manipulation (condition *pre*) and served as a baseline condition to compare with the modulatory effects of the following cognitive manipulation (condition *post*). After the first two blocks, participants were randomly assigned to one of two mind-set conditions (cf. [26,27]). The order in which the mind-sets were administered in the two experimental sessions was counterbalanced across participants (Fig. 1, top panel, centre). Following the typical TMT paradigm, participants were asked to write down their thoughts in a short questionnaire consisting of two open questions that focused either on the possibility of their own death ('Mortality Salience'-*MS*) or the contingency of having failed an important exam ('Exam Salience'-*ES*). The *ES* mind-set induction was meant to trigger a negative valence state similar to that induced by the *MS* condition; thus, it controlled for the specific effects of mortality salience on human behaviour [27,28]. Importantly, *ES* was selected as the control condition after a preliminary pilot survey in which several different mind-sets used in the experimental TMT literature were compared along different dimensions in a sample of 100 respondents. *ES* was judged as the condition most similar to *MS* (thus, not significantly different from it) across several parameters, e.g. arousal, valence, threat, puzzlement (see Material S1). Participants had 5 min to answer the questions, after which they were exposed to a distraction period. This was based on the notion that to observe the implicit effects associated with mortality salience the individual should be distracted from the salience of this mental content [29]. The distraction period lasted 15 min during which participants completed the Positive and Negative Affect Schedule (PANAS, [30]) and the State Anxiety Inventory (STAI-Y, [31]), and were asked to play with a brain-shaped Rubik's cube before undergoing the EEG again (20 minutes in total). Administration of the questionnaires was repeated immediately after the last two blocks to check for carry-over effects caused by the mind-set induction on participants' self-reported state mood and anxiety.

Participants were comfortably seated in a temperature-controlled room (25 C°) with their hands resting on a table, ≈40 cm from the body midline. A wooden frame blocked the sight of their left arm and the laser device. Participants were asked to relax and fixate the center of the computer screen placed in front of them. The background of the computer screen was black throughout the experiment. Each block lasted between 7 and 12 min and there was a 5 min pause between blocks 1 and 2 and blocks 3 and 4 (Fig. 1, top panel). In each block, 20 pairs of stimuli (S1–S2, a pair), 10 per each sensory modality, were delivered in a pseudo-random fashion (no more than three consecutive pairs belonging to the same modality) or near the left hand dorsum at a constant inter-stimulus interval (ISI) of 1 s. Thus, each participant was subjected to 80 trials (40 pairs and 80 single stimuli per modality) in each experimental session. Between each laser pulse of a nociceptive pair, the laser beam was manually displaced by at least 1 cm along a proximal-distal line on the hand dorsum [15]. The direction of this displacement was balanced in each block (10 pairs in the proximal direction and 10 pairs in the distal direction). A proximal-distal spatial displacement was used to minimize the role of variations in thickness and innervations of the irradiated skin [32] in affecting the strength of the nociceptive input.

Each pair formed a single experimental trial (Fig. 1, bottom panel) in which S1 was considered the conditioning stimulus and S2, the test stimulus. The timing of each trial was as follows; a white fixation cross on the computer screen (3 s) was followed by a yellow fixation cross that alerted the participants to relax all their muscles and avoid eye movements before the impending stimulation (6–12 s). Nociceptive and auditory stimuli composing the pair were delivered at 1 s inter-stimulus intervals and jittered during this time window. After the delivery of each pair of stimuli a yellow fixation cross appeared on the screen (3 s) to signal participants to wait to report their sensations. Participants were asked to rate both intensity and threat for each stimulus in the pair (i.e., provide two ratings for S1 and two for S2) using the right hand to move a mouse and position a pointer on a 101 point electronic visual-analogue scale (VAS) on the screen, within 15 s from its appearance. At the bottom of this scale, zero was represented by the label "not intense at all" for the intensity assessment and "not threatening at all" for the threat assessment. At the top of this scale, 100 was represented by the label "extremely intense" or "extremely threatening". Intensity and threat ratings were asked in a pseudo-random order (repeated no more than three times within each block). Threat was defined during the brief learning procedure and was meant to distinguish the sensory-discriminative dimension associated with the magnitude of the sensation from a cognitive-affective dimension related to interpretation of its homeostatic meaning. Threat ratings were measuring participants' interpretations of the stimuli as indicating imminent danger, warning of an incoming unpleasant state. According to the trial timeline, the inter-trial interval thus ranged between 24 and 30 s. During *pre* and *post* blocks, the group's average skin temperature was 34.2±0.7°C and 34.3±0.9°C, respectively.

Data analysis

State mood and anxiety. Scores obtained on the PANAS and STAI scales were analyzed using the Wilcoxon matched pairs test to compare scores obtained immediately after *MS* and *ES* inductions as well as at the end of the experiment. The level of significance was set at $P<0.05$.

Psychophysics. The calibration procedure was aimed at improving participants' ability to detail their sensations and concurrently counteract the ordinal nature of the VAS scale by increasing within and between subjects reliability [33]. This approach allowed for the normal distribution of intensity ratings in all conditions across the two different sensory modalities. Indeed, participants could be clustered in three different ranges of perceived intensity: a lower bound, corresponding to a sensation of low intensity (21–40; mean and SD = 34.7±4.1; n=4), a middle range corresponding to moderate intensity (41–60; 51.7±6.4; n=10) and an upper bound corresponding to high intensity (61–80; 71.1±7.5; n=6).

The factor Time (two levels: *pre* and *post*) was split in order to feed an analysis of covariance (ANCOVA) with a continuous

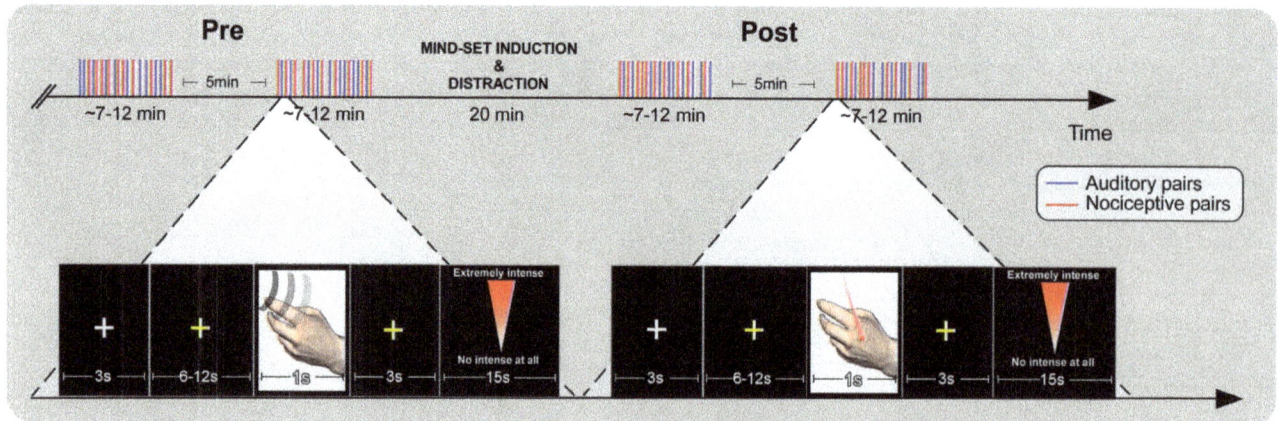

Figure 1. Experimental design. EEG activity and subjective ratings of intensity and threat of sensory stimulation were collected in two separate experimental sessions during which participants underwent a 'Mortality Salience' (MS) or an 'Exam Salience' (ES) mind-set induction (top panel, central). The order of MS and ES was counter-balanced across participants. ERPs elicited by either nociceptive somatosensory stimuli delivered to the hand dorsum (top panel, red) or by auditory stimuli delivered in the same area (top panel, blue) were recorded in four blocks. The first two blocks were free from cognitive manipulation (condition 'Pre', top left) whereas the following two blocks (condition 'Post', top right) were preceded by the mind-set induction (5 min) and a distraction period (20 min) during which participants completed the Positive and Negative Affect Schedule and the State Anxiety Inventory. In each block, 20 pairs of stimuli (S1–S2, a pair), 10 per each sensory modality, were delivered in a pseudorandom order. The stimuli composing a pair were separated by 1 s inter-stimulus interval. Each pair established a single trial which started with a fixation cross on the screen (3 sec), followed by a yellow fixation cross (6–13 sec) in which the pair was jittered (bottom panel). Three seconds after receiving each pair of stimuli, participants were required to rate (on a 101-point electronic visual-analogue scale) the intensity and threat of each stimulus in the pair (thus providing two ratings for S1 and two for S2 within a 15 sec time window). This procedure allowed determining whether any modulation was exerted by the mind-set induction on the cortical responses and perception associated with nociceptive and auditory stimuli.

predictor *pre* and a categorical predictor Mind-set (two levels: *MS* and *ES*) of the response pattern observed in the *post* mind-set induction measures (i.e., the dependent variables). ANCOVA was carried out separately on ratings obtained in each sensory modality (auditory and nociceptive). Analysis of covariance is the most powerful statistical approach for experiments in which subjects are assigned randomly to treatment groups, regardless of whether there is a bias due to the initial measurement, because it allows reducing within group error variance (i.e. it strongly reduces between-subject variability from the treatment comparison) [34–37]. Finally, we computed *post-pre* change scores for both *MS* and *ES* conditions; they were compared using t-tests for paired dependent samples. The level of significance was set at $P<0.05$. Partial eta squared ($p\eta^2$) as measures of effect size of significant main effects and interactions are reported.

EEG preprocessing. EEG data were preprocessed with Vision Analyzer software (Brain Products, v. 1.05). They were first downsampled to 250 Hz, transformed to the average reference [38], DC detrended and band-pass filtered from 0.5 to 30 Hz. Data were then segmented into epochs using a time window ranging from 1 s before the first stimulus (S1) to 1 s after the second stimulus (S2) of each pair (total epoch duration: 3 s). Epoched data were further processed using EEGLAB (v. 12.x; [39]) and Letswave 5 (http://nocions.webnode.com/). EOG and EMG artifacts were subtracted using independent component analysis (ICA; [40]).

EEG Analysis in the time domain. Epochs belonging to the same experimental condition (*ES pre, ES post, MS pre, MS post*) were averaged and time-locked to the onset of the first stimulus of each pair. This procedure yielded eight average waveforms, one for each experimental condition and sensory modality (nociceptive and auditory respectively). For each individual average waveform, the relative peak amplitude of the late nociceptive and auditory evoked potentials (NEPs and AEPs respectively) elicited by S2 was

extracted (mean of 10 ms around the peak). For NEPs N1, the mean of the activity in the range of the observed topography was extracted (130–180 ms). The NEP N1 wave was measured at the temporal and central electrodes contralateral to the stimulated side (T8 and C4), referenced to Fz (see [41,42]). It was defined as the negative deflection preceding the N2 wave, which appears as a positive deflection in this montage. The N2 and P2 waves were measured at the vertex (Cz) referenced to the common average. The N2 wave was defined as the most negative deflection after stimulus onset. The P2 wave was defined as the most positive deflection after stimulus onset. For AEPs, N1 and P2 waves were measured at the vertex (Cz) referenced to the common average. The N1 wave was defined as the most negative deflection after stimulus onset. The P2 wave was defined as the most positive deflection after stimulus onset.

ANCOVA was carried out separately on the extracted S2 NEP and AEP amplitudes. Then, whole-waveform t-tests (i.e. the entire EEG signal in a given epoch) were performed to assess point-by-point amplitude differences within each mind-set (*pre* vs. *post*) and the differences between the two mind-sets during *pre* and *post* induction (*MS* vs. *ES*) on the S2 evoked activity. The threshold for statistical significance was set at $P<0.05$. Furthermore, differences in amplitude intervals were considered as significant only when they lasted at least 10 ms, a temporal cluster used to account for multiple comparisons. The maximal *t* value (signed) in each relevant time interval is reported. These analyses allowed testing the relevant differences within (*pre-post* increase vs. decrease in amplitude) and between (increase vs. decrease in amplitude within *MS* or *ES* conditions). The finding of a difference in ERPs amplitude between *pre* and *post*, regardless of the mind-set induction, points to an unspecific mind-set effect on repetition suppression. Conversely, the finding of a difference during *post*-induction trials only when there was no difference during *pre*-induction trials suggests a specific effect of mind-set on repetition suppression.

EEG Analysis in the time-frequency domain. Time-frequency representations (TFRs) were computed using a Morlet wavelet in which the initial spread of the Gaussian envelope was set at 0.15 and the central frequency of the wavelet at 3 Hz. The transform expressed the oscillation amplitude as a function of time and frequency, regardless of its phase [43]. Averaging these estimates across trials discloses both phase-locked and non-phase-locked modulations of signal amplitude. Across-trial averaging of these time–frequency representations produced a spectrogram of the average EEG oscillation amplitude as a function of time and frequency. For each estimated frequency, results were displayed as an event-related percentage (ER%) increase or decrease in oscillation amplitude relative to a pre-stimulus reference interval (-0.6 to -0.2 s before the onset of S1), according to the following formula: $ER_{t,f} \% = [A_{t,f} - R_f]/R_f$, where $A_{t,f}$ is the signal amplitude at a given time t and at a given frequency f, and R_f is the signal amplitude averaged within the reference interval [44]. Recent studies confirmed that the theta and gamma frequency bands (e.g. [45,46]) reflect aspecific and specific information related to pain perception. Here we focused on the theta frequency range (3–8 Hz). Thus, one time-frequency region of interest (ROIs) was defined in the spectrograms obtained at Cz, where the main spectral events maximally express their magnitude. The time-frequency limits of the time-frequency ROI (3–8 Hz and 100–500 ms) were defined according to previous studies (e.g. [47,48]). Within the time-frequency ROI, ER% amplitudes were extracted by computing the mean of the 10% pixels displaying the highest activity in the given time-frequency range. This "top 10%" summary measure reflects the higher ER% values within each window of interest to reduce the noise introduced by including near-to-zero values. This approach, which was successfully used to analyze both EEG [15] and fMRI data [49,50], proved suitable to disclose condition-specific effects [19,51–53]. For point-by-point t-tests, the same data analysis approach implemented in the time domain was used in the time-frequency domain; the only exception was the temporal cluster chosen for significance: amplitude intervals were considered as significant only when they lasted more than 20 ms.

Additional analyses. Gender, age, measures of mood and anxiety as well as ratings of intensity and threat were used as categorical or continuous covariates in separate ANCOVAs in which, together with *pre* mind-set activity, their contribution to the significant differences observed between *MS* and *ES* summary measures was tested.

In addition, observed differences were further assessed by testing the moderating effect of an amplitude response profile (ARP) in each individual. This was at variance with the use of the sole regressor pre for S2 activity, as the ARP was calculated as the difference of S1–S2 activity in *pre* blocks. Specifically, participants were split into low and high amplitude suppressors (*lows*, *highs*) according to the median value of the mean activity recorded in the *pre* mind-set induction blocks. *Lows* and *highs*, classified according to a median split procedure, were considered as two levels of a categorical predictor (Suppressors), which entered ANCOVA with the continuous regressor *pre*, the categorical predictor Mind-set (two levels: *MS* and *ES*) and S2 peak amplitudes as the dependent variable. All the additional analyses were computed only on the neural activities affected by Mindset according to the main ANCOVA analyses.

Results

State mood and anxiety

Pre and *post* state mood and anxiety score distributions were not significantly different between *MS* and *ES* conditions immediately after mind-set induction (PANAS positive: $Z = 0.59$, $P = 0.55$; PANAS negative: $Z = 1.54$, $P = 0.12$; State anxiety: $Z = 1.54$, $P = 0.12$) or at the end of the experimental session (PANAS positive: $Z = 0.67$, $P = 0.50$; PANAS negative: $Z = 0.12$, $P = 0.91$; State anxiety: $Z = 0.35$, $P = 0.72$).

Thus, there was no difference in aware feelings of mood or anxiety between the two different mind-sets, which suggests a similar activation of proximal defenses [54].

Nociceptive intensity and threat

All the stimuli were perceived as painful by participants. The ANCOVA on intensity and threat ratings at S2 revealed that the covariate *pre* was significant for the analysis of intensity and threat ($F(1, 37) = 410.33$, $P < 0.001$; $p\eta^2 = 0.92$ and $F(1, 37) = 638.78$, $P < 0.01$; $p\eta^2 = 0.94$, respectively). When adjusting for the effect of the ratings obtained in the *pre* blocks, a significant main effect of Mind-set was observed in intensity and threat ratings in the *post* blocks ($F(1, 37) = 9.92$, $P < 0.01$; $p\eta^2 = 0.21$ and $F(1, 37) = 11.88$, $P < 0.01$; $p\eta^2 = 0.24$, respectively). This effect was accounted for by higher ratings of intensity and threat in *MS* trials than in *ES* trials, as confirmed by the paired t-tests performed on *post - pre* change scores ($t(19) = 3.93$, $P < 0.01$, and $t(19) = 4.37$, $P < 0.001$ respectively) (Fig. 2, left panel). Importantly, when controlling for the effect of the three ranges of perceived intensity (21–40; 41–60; 61–80), the ANCOVA showed neither a main effect ($F(2, 33) = 1.07$, $P = 0.38$) nor its interaction with the factor Mind-set ($F(2, 33) = 0.34$, $P = 0.71$), thus suggesting that neither the range of intensity alone nor its combination with the experimental conditions explained the observed effects.

Auditory intensity and threat

All auditory stimuli were detected by participants during the experiment. The ANCOVA on intensity and threat ratings at S2 revealed that the covariate *pre* was significant for the analysis of intensity and threat ($F(1, 37) = 224.22$, $P < 0.001$; $p\eta^2 = 0.86$ and $F(1, 37) = 676.22$, $P < 0.001$; $p\eta^2 = 0.95$, respectively). When adjusting for the effect of the ratings obtained in the *pre* blocks, no significant main effect of Mind-set was observed in intensity ratings ($F(1, 37) = 0.93$, $P = 0.34$), but a significant effect was observed in judgments of threat ($F(1, 37) = 6.21$, $P = 0.02$; $p\eta^2 = 0.14$). This effect was accounted for by higher ratings of threat in *MS* trials than *ES* trials, as confirmed by the paired t-tests performed on *post-pre* change scores, in which differences associated with the judgment of threat reached significance ($t(19) = 4.37$, $P < 0.001$); the higher relative increase of intensity following *MS* was not significant ($t(19) = 1.47$, $P = 0.15$) (Fig. 2, right panel).

Nociceptive evoked potentials

Grand average waveforms and global field power (GFP) of nociceptive evoked potentials (NEPs) are displayed in Fig. 3. Nociceptive stimuli delivered before (Fig. 3; left panel) and after (Fig. 3; right panel) mind-set induction elicited maximal N2 and P2 waves at the scalp vertex (electrode Cz) and N1 activity corresponding to a lower amplitude topography contralateral to the stimulated body limb.

At Cz, the t-tests performed on S2-ERPs revealed no difference between *MS* and *ES* mind-sets on *pre* and *post* respectively ($t_{19} = -1.40$; $P = 0.45$; $t_{19} = -2.37$; $P = 0.25$). However, the

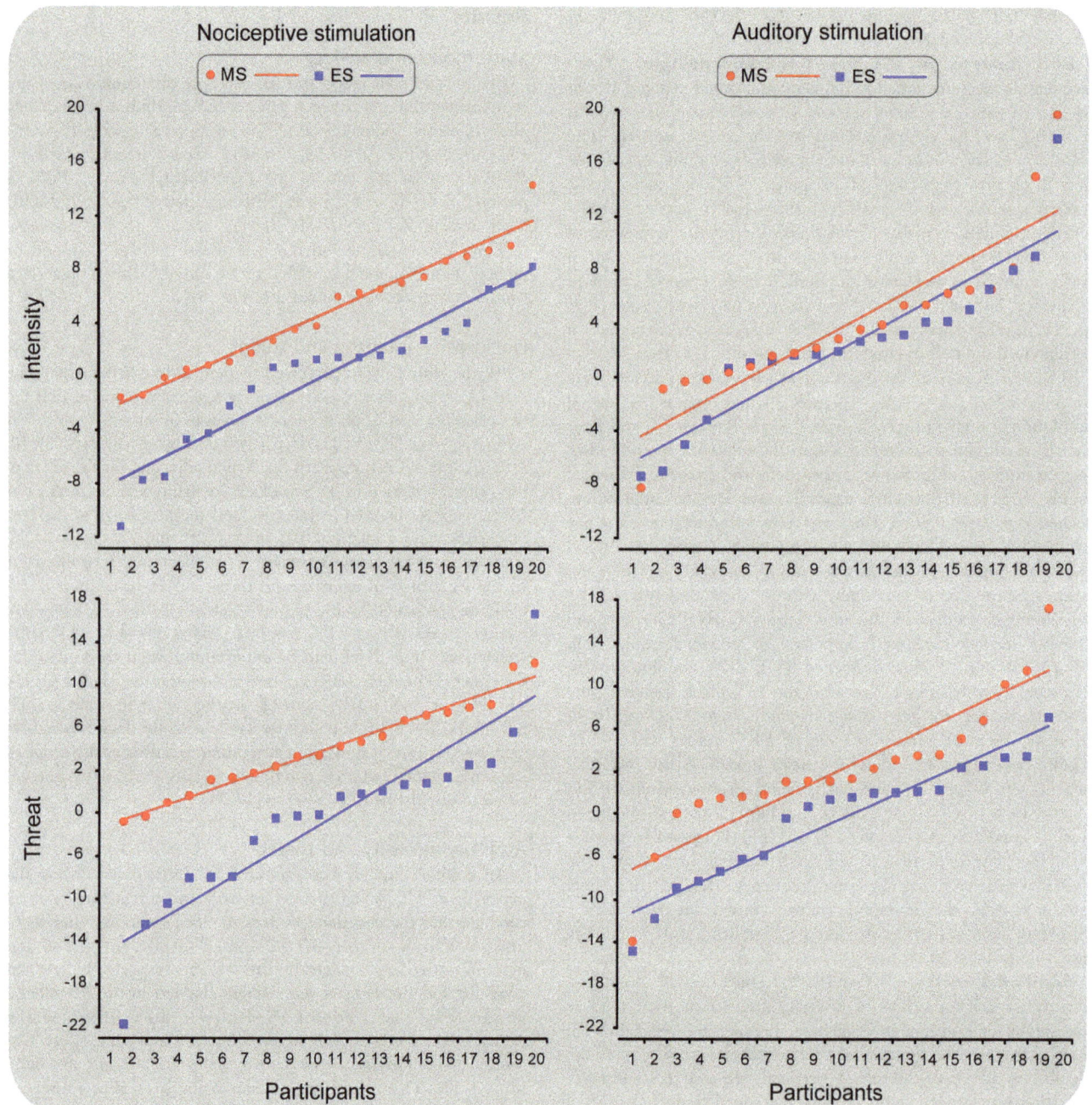

Figure 2. Scatterplots of mindset-induced changes (Post-Pre) in rating intensity and threat of S2 for both nociceptive and auditory stimuli. The x axis shows each participants' ratings as a function of increased range of intensity and threat. The corresponding average ratings of intensity and threat are displayed on the y axis. Negative and positive values indicate lower and higher ratings following mind-set induction. Individual data were fitted by a linear function. An increase of both intensity and threat was observed during the MS condition, especially in the nociceptive modality (left panel).

within mind-set t-test revealed a significant difference between *pre* and *post* mind-set induction activity during both *MS* ($t_{19} = 3.35$; $P = 0.005$) and *ES* ($t_{19} = 3.77$; $P = 0.009$) sessions, which was accounted for by lower amplitudes in the N2 wave range after both *MS* and *ES* induction with respect to the *pre* mind-set induction. Importantly though, the ANCOVA on N2 and P2 peak amplitudes confirmed that once *pre* was regressed from *post* no effect of mind-set could be detected (N2: $F(1, 37) = 0.20$, $P = 0.66$; P2: $F(1, 37) = 0.62$, $P = 0.15$, respectively). In both cases, there was an effect of the covariate *pre* ($F(1, 37) = 46.99$, $P<0.001$;

$p\eta^2 = 0.56$, and $F(1, 37) = 26.76$, $P<0.001$; $p\eta^2 = 0.42$), suggesting that the N2 wave amplitude reduction observed in *post* was likely due to a general effect of habituation.

At C4, the t-tests performed on S2-ERPs revealed no difference between *MS* and *ES* mind-sets in the *pre* and *post* conditions respectively ($t_{19} = 2.20$; $P = 0.28$; $t_{19} = -2.06$; $P = 0.40$). Similarly, at T8 the t-tests performed on S2-ERPs revealed no difference between *MS* and *ES* mind-sets in the *pre* and *post* condition respectively ($t_{19} = -1.85$; $P = 0.40$; $t_{19} = -0.64$; $P = 0.33$). Furthermore, the within mind-set t-test also revealed no significant

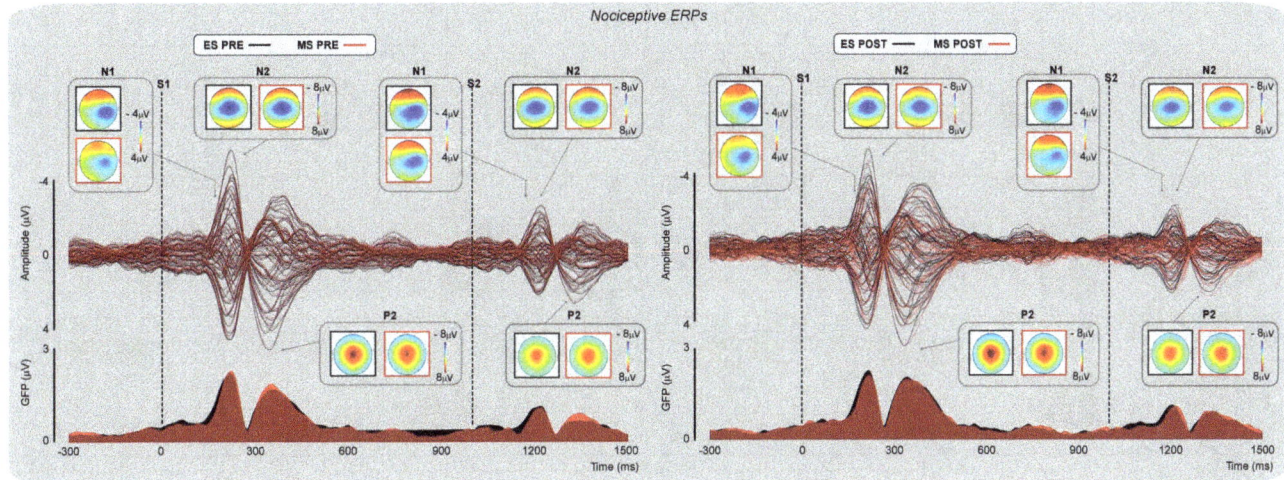

Figure 3. Nociceptive evoked potentials (NEPs). Group-level average scalp topographies of NEPs (upper and lower panel) and global field power (GFP; lower panel) elicited by stimulation of the left hand dorsum before and after mind-set induction (left and right panel respectively). Butterfly plots show ERPs from 60 channels superimposed in 20 participants. NEPs were elicited by pairs of nociceptive stimuli delivered at a fixed 1 s ISI. Representative scalp topographies of each NEP during ES (black) and MS (red) conditions are shown in the insets. Note the amplitude reduction between S1- and S2-related activity.

difference between *pre* and *post* at C4 (*ES*: $t_{19} = 1.40$; $P = 0.36$; *MS*: $t_{19} = -0.32$; $P = 0.46$) or T8 (*ES*: $t_{19} = -0.004$; $P = 0.60$; *MS*: $t_{19} = -1.19$; $P = 0.50$). ANCOVA confirmed no effect in the early N1 peak amplitudes, at either C4 ($F(1, 37) = 0.26$, $P = 0.61$) or T8 $F(1, 37) = 0.09$, $P = 0.52$. The covariate *pre* was significant at both C4 ($F(1, 37) = 44.65$, $P < 0.001$; $p\eta^2 = 0.55$) and T8 ($F(1, 37) = 64.90$, $P < 0.001$; $p\eta^2 = 0.64$).

Analysis of the N2 amplitude differences as a function of the amplitude response profile (ARP) revealed that there was no significant interaction between ARP and type of Mind-set ($F(1, 35) = 2.31$, $P = 0.14$); however, there was a significant main effect of the ARP ($F(1, 35) = 8.08$, $P < 0.01$), which was explained by lower amplitudes in *highs* than *lows*. This finding likely explains why differences in N2 amplitudes were found only during within mind-set t-tests and not between mind-sets t-tests and ANCOVA. This result also suggests the differences found in the N2 amplitudes were not specific to the influence of *MS* or *ES* mind-sets but partly driven by between-subject differences in inherent neural habituation/dishabituation profiles.

Auditory evoked potentials

Grand average waveforms and global field power (GFP) of auditory evoked potentials (AEPs) are displayed in Fig. 4. Auditory stimuli delivered before (Fig. 4; left panel) and after (Fig. 4; right panel) mind-set induction elicited N1 and P2 waves that were maximal at the scalp vertex (electrode Cz). At Cz, the t-tests performed on S2-ERPs revealed no difference between *MS* and *ES* mind-sets in *pre* and *post* respectively ($t_{19} = -2.46$; $P = 0.23$; $t_{19} = -3.02$; $P = 0.17$). In addition, no significant difference between *pre* and *post* was revealed by the within mind-set t-test during the *MS* ($t_{19} = 3.21$; $P = 0.11$) or *ES* ($t_{19} = 3.92$; $P = 0.10$) sessions. However, similar to the results obtained with the nociceptive ERPs, the ANCOVA on N1 and P2 peak amplitudes confirmed no significant effect of Mind-set ($F(1, 37) = 2.13$, $P = 0.15$ and $F(1, 37) = 2.17$, $P = 0.15$, respectively). In both cases, there was an effect of the covariate *pre* ($F(1, 37) = 86.50$, $P < 0.001$; $p\eta^2 = 0.70$, and $F(1, 37) = 68.02$, $P < 0.001$; $p\eta^2 = 0.80$).

Analysis of the N1 amplitude differences as a function of ARP revealed no significant interaction between behaving as *lows* or

highs and type of Mind-set induction ($F(1, 35) = 1.00$, $P = 0.32$) and no significant main effect of the ARP ($F(1, 35) = 0.71$, $P = 0.40$). This control analysis showed that the lack of influence of Mind-set induction on the auditory N1 was not related to individual variability in response amplitude.

Nociceptive oscillatory activity

Grand average spectrograms of nociceptive-related brain activity (as measured at Cz referenced to the common average) both before (Fig. 5, panel A, top) and after (Fig. 5, panel A, bottom) mind-set induction. At Cz, the t-tests performed on the S2-ER% revealed no difference in *pre* mind-set activity ($t_{19} = 0.63$; $P = 0.53$; Fig. 5, top right graph) but highlighted a significant difference in the *post* mind-set activity at the level of the theta band ROI ($t_{19} = 2.55$; $P = 0.02$), which was accounted for by a higher ER% magnitude after *MS* than *ES* induction (233 ± 9 vs. 208 ± 6) (Fig. 5, panel B, bottom). This difference peaked at 262 ms (range: 239–290 ms) and at 5 Hz (3.3–6.8 Hz). The within mind-set t-test revealed no significant difference between *pre* and *post* during the *MS* condition ($t_{19} = -0.96$; $P = 0.35$; Fig. 5, panel A, right), but there was a trend to a significant reduction of S2 ER% magnitude (237 ± 10 vs. 208 ± 6) following *ES* induction ($t_{19} = -2.11$; $P = 0.05$; Fig. 6, panel A, left). The ANCOVA on ER% S2 magnitude revealed a significant effect of mind-set ($F(1, 37) = 4.70$, $P = 0.03$; $p\eta^2 = 0.11$). Moreover, regressing out the *pre* mind-set activity had no significant effect on the model, i.e., it did not help address the *post* mind-set differences ($F(1, 37) = 0.33$, $P = 0.57$). In other words, the ANCOVA confirmed the difference evidenced by the t-tests, which was entirely explained by higher ER% magnitude in the theta band following the *MS* than the *ES* mind-set (ER% least squares means, *MS* vs. *ES*, 234 ± 8 vs. 207 ± 8; Fig. 5, panel B, bottom).

Analysis of ER% magnitude differences as a function of ARP revealed no significant interaction between behaving as *lows* or *highs* and type of Mind-set ($F(1, 37) = 0.37$, $P = 0.55$) nor a significant main effect of the ARP ($F(1, 37) = 0.60$, $P = 0.44$). At the same time, the introduction of this factor in the ANCOVA model did not affect the significance of the factor Mind-set ($F(1, 37) = 4.72$, $P = 0.03$; $p\eta^2 = 0.12$). This finding suggests that the

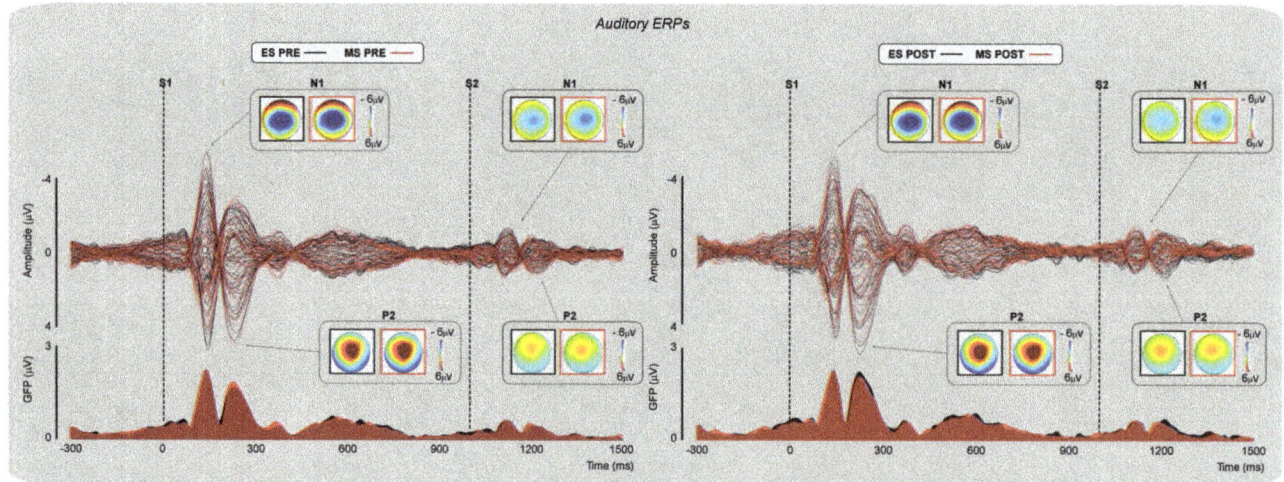

Figure 4. Auditory evoked potentials (AEPs). Group-level averages, scalp topographies, and global field power (GFP) of AEPs elicited by stimulation of the left hand dorsum before and after mindset induction (upper and lower panel respectively). Butterfly plots show ERPs from 60 channels superimposed in 20 participants. ERPs were elicited by pairs of nociceptive stimuli delivered at a fixed 1 s ISI. Representative scalp topographies of each AEP component during ES (black) and MS (red) conditions are shown in the insets. Note the significant amplitude reduction between S1- and S2-related activity.

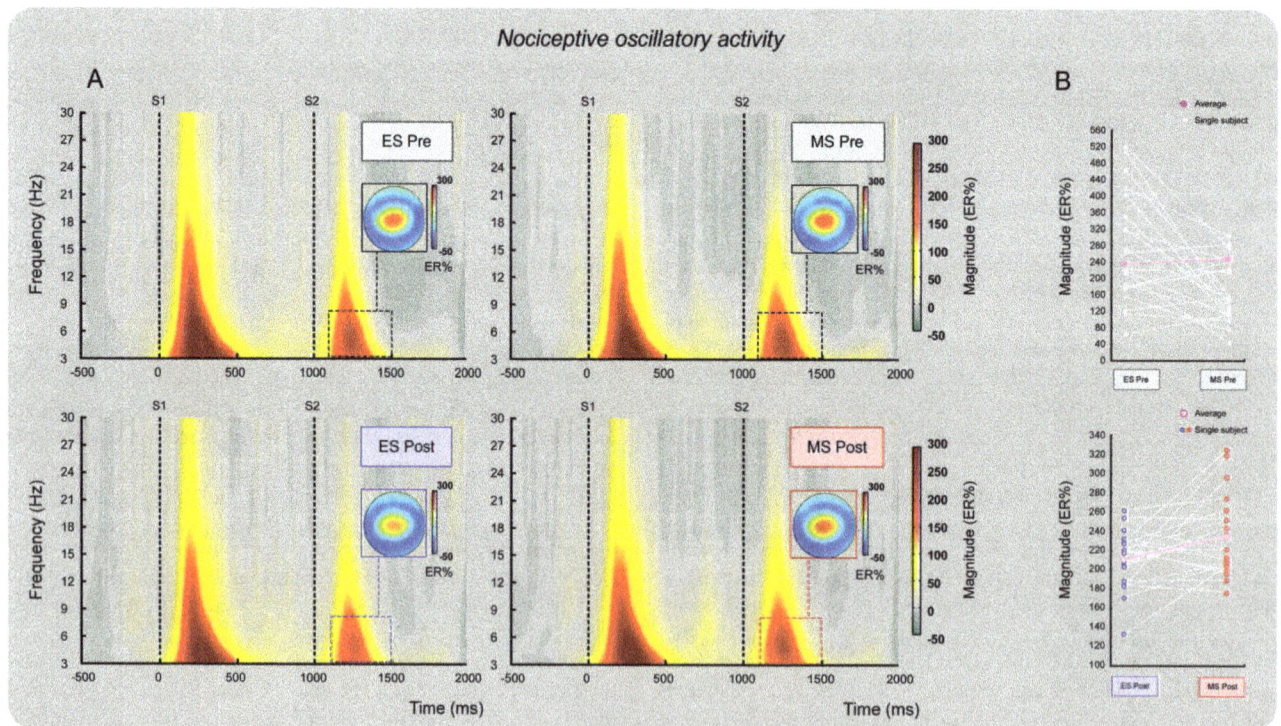

Figure 5. Effect of the two mind-sets induction on the nociceptive S2-ER% oscillatory activity at Cz. Grand average time-frequency representation of nociceptive-related oscillatory activity (as measured at Cz) both before (panel A, top) and after (panel A, bottom) mind-set induction. The a priori identified theta time-frequency ROI was used to extract the "top 10%" of the signal amplitude increase (ER%) relative to the pre-stimulus interval (−0.6 to −0.2 sec before onset of S1). Note the decrease of signal magnitude at S2 following ES mind-set induction (panel A, bottom left). No similar decrease occurred after MS mind-set induction (panel A, bottom right). Panel B: the y axes show single subject and group means of oscillatory amplitude (ER%) before (top) and after (bottom) mind-set induction. Higher ER% magnitude after MS than ES mind-set induction (233±9 vs. 208±6 ER%) (bottom) was detected both by t-test and ANCOVA. ANCOVA revealed that this difference was entirely explained by the modulatory effect of MS on S2 even when regressing out Pre activity. The difference peaked at 262 ms (range: 239–290 ms) and 5 Hz (3.3–6.8 Hz).

genuine modulation of oscillatory ER% magnitude was due to the induction of a cognitive mind-set and that the specific effect of mortality salience was reliable regardless of the inherent neural habituation/dishabituation profile of each individual.

Auditory oscillatory activity

Grand average spectrograms of auditory-related brain activity (as measured at Cz referenced to the common average) both before (Fig. 6; panel A, top) and after (Fig. 6; panel A, bottom) mind-set induction. At Cz, the t-tests performed on S2-ER% revealed no difference in either *pre* mind-set ($t_{19} = 1.55$; $P = 0.14$) or *post* mind-set activity ($t_{19} = 0.46$; $P = 0.65$) at the level of the theta band ROI (Fig. 6; panel A, top and bottom, respectively). The within mind-set t-test also revealed no significant difference in either the *ES* ($t_{19} = -0.10$; $P = 0.92$) or *MS* condition ($t_{19} = 0.73$; $P = 0.47$) (Fig. 6, panel A, left and right, respectively). The ANCOVA on ER% S2 magnitude confirmed the lack of effect of Mind-set ($F(1, 37) = 0.38$, $P = 0.54$) and no significant contribution of the covariate *pre* to the model variability ($F(1, 37) = 1.05$, $P = 0.31$).

Analysis of ER% magnitude differences as a function of the ARP revealed no significant interaction between behaving as *lows* or *highs* and type of Mind-set induction ($F(1, 35) = 0.72$, $P = 0.40$) or a significant main effect of the ARP ($F(1, 35) = 1.55$, $P = 0.22$). This control analysis showed that the lack of influence of mind-set induction on the auditory theta ER% was not related to individual variability in response profile.

Covariance of oscillatory activity with subjective ratings and demographics

ANCOVA revealed that, following the induction of mortality salience, the ER% magnitude increased concomitantly with the increase in ratings of threat. That is, the higher the rating of threat attributed to the S2 nociceptive stimulus, the higher the theta ER% magnitude (Fig. 7, left). Moreover, the ER% magnitude increase co-varied with the participants' age, that is, the older the participant, the greater the increase in magnitude regardless of the type of mind-set applied (Fig. 7, right). In addition there was no co-variation of the nociceptive related ER% magnitude with state mood and anxiety measures (lowest $F = 1.55$; lowest $P = 0.22$).

Discussion

Here, we provide evidence that reminders of one's own mortality have a preferential effect on perceptual judgments (Fig. 2) as well as on cortical spectral activity (Fig. 5) associated with the processing of somatosensory nociceptive input. Furthermore, the effect observed on cortical activity covaried significantly with participants' ratings of threat and their age (Fig. 7). More specifically, we found that the effect of Mind-set on intensity ratings was significant for nociceptive stimuli (Fig. 2, top left) but not for auditory stimuli (Fig. 2, top right). Conversely, the increase in threat ratings following reminders of mortality affected individual's judgments of both nociceptive and auditory stimuli (Fig. 2, bottom left and right). The analyses of ERPs revealed a reduction of the negativity following mind-set induction. However, such decrement became insignificant when the S2 amplitudes

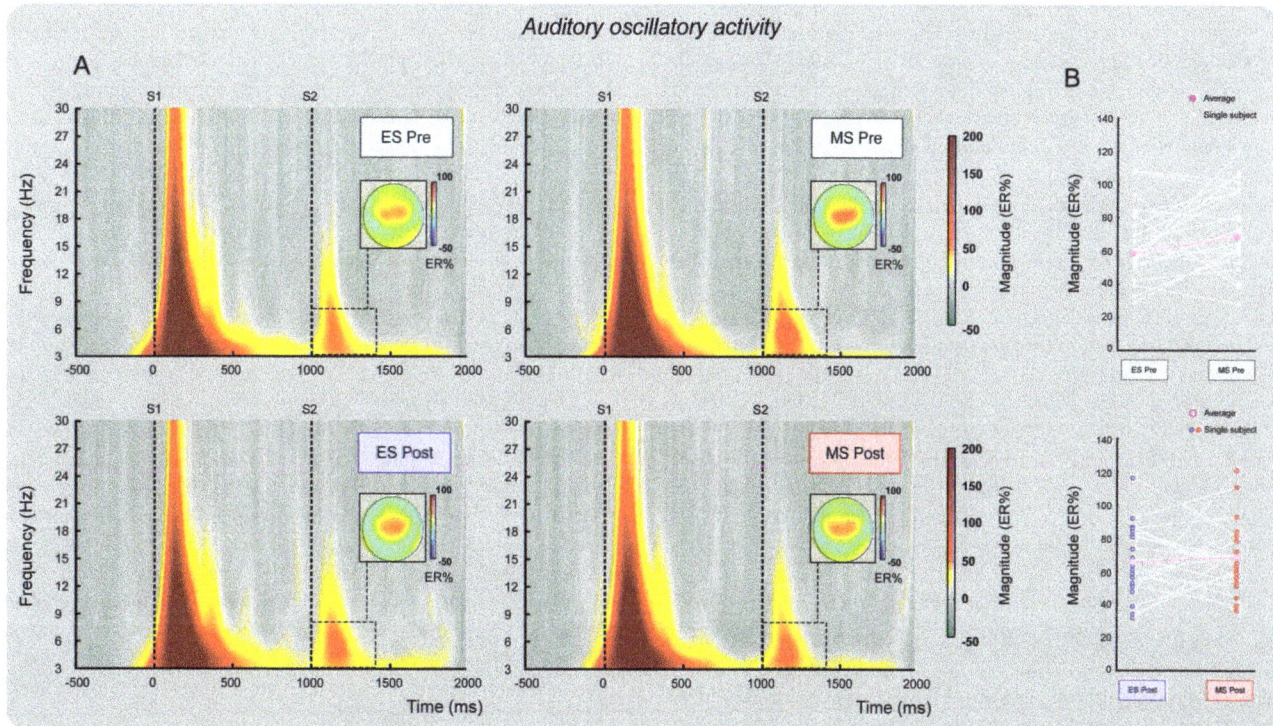

Figure 6. There was no effect of mind-set induction on the auditory S2-ER% oscillatory activity at Cz. Grand average time-frequency representation of nociceptive-related oscillatory activity (as measured at Cz) both before (panel A, top) and after (panel A, bottom) mind-set induction. The a priori identified theta time-frequency ROI was used to extract the "top 10%" of signal amplitude increase (ER%) relative to the pre-stimulus interval (-0.6 to -0.2 sec before the onset of S1). Note the decrease of signal magnitude at S2 following mind-set inductions (panel A, bottom left and right). Panel B: the y axes show single subject and group means of oscillatory amplitude (ER%) before (top) and after (bottom) mind-set inductions.

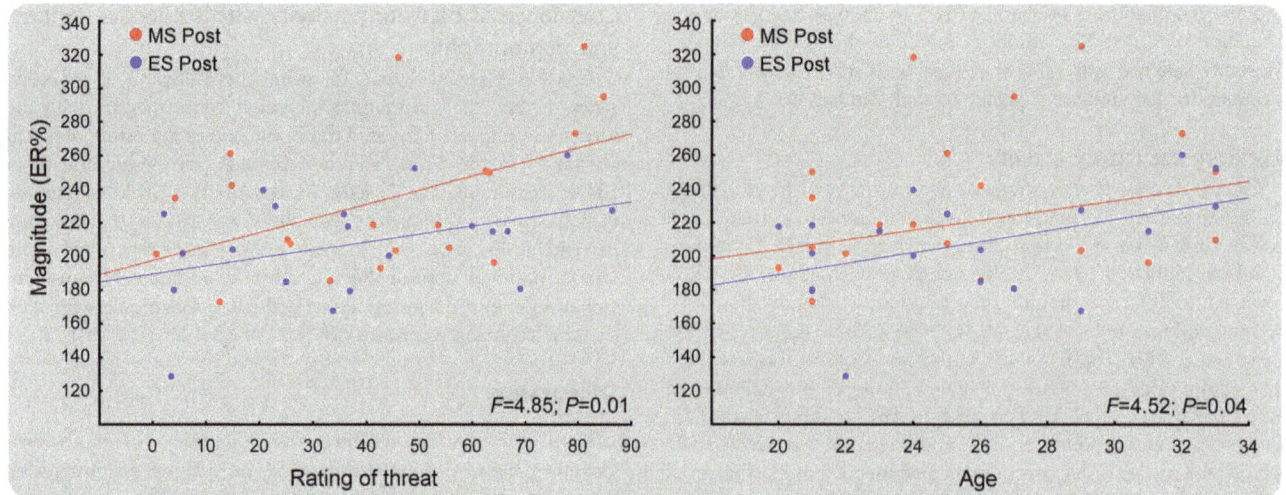

Figure 7. Covariation of nociceptive ER% with subjective ratings (left) and demographics (right). In each scatterplot both MS (red) and ES (blue) conditions are represented with their respective fits. The scatterplot at the left shows that the higher the rating of threat attributed to nociceptive S2, the higher the magnitude of theta activity. More importantly, the different slopes indicate that the increase in the ER% was higher after MS than ES mind-set induction. Similarly, the scatterplot on the right shows that the higher the participant's age the higher the magnitude of theta activity. Note in this case the nearly parallel relationship between the two slopes, which indicates that the effect of age modulated the two mindsets equally.

recorded before the mind-set induction were regressed out. Furthermore, the effect of Mind-set observed on the nociceptive evoked N2 became insignificant when the variability associated with individual differences in response amplitude was regressed out, thus suggesting that the amplitude reduction was due to habituation and inter-individual variations in response amplitude.

Importantly, the analyses of oscillatory ER% magnitude provided a statistical difference between the two mind-sets. We found higher nociceptive-related theta activity elicited by S2 following reminders of death than following reminders of a failed exam (Fig. 5, panels A and B); no such effect was found in the auditory theta activity (Fig. 6, panels A and B). Note that regressing out the S2 ER% observed before the mind-set induction did not explain the post-induction difference, which was thus entirely explained by higher ER% magnitude in the theta band following mortality salience but not exam salience (Fig. 5, panel B, bottom). Interestingly, this top-down impairment of the expected magnitude suppression at S2 covaried with the participants' perception of threat, that is, the higher the rating of threat attributed to the nociceptive stimulus, the higher the theta ER% magnitude (Fig. 7, left). Moreover, the ER% magnitude increase covaried with the participants' age, that is, the older the participant, the greater the increase in magnitude regardless of the type of mind-set applied (Fig. 7, right).

The interaction between mortality salience and brain representation of threatening somatosensory input

Here we explored the selective effect of inducing a mortality salience mind-set on the perception of nociceptive stimuli and on the magnitude of evoked potentials and oscillatory EEG activity associated with them. We focused on evoked vertex potentials (N1, N2, and P2 NEPs; N1 and P2 AEPs) and oscillatory responses in the theta band (3–8 Hz). The paired stimulation design served to test whether a significant top-down modulation (indexed by S2-related responses) associated with the contextual relevance of accessibility to death thoughts could revert the amplitude

suppression phenomenon associated with the reduced salience of the repeated sensory input.

The effects reported here can be distinguished as mind-set specific (i.e., the modulation of nociceptive theta ER%) vs. mind-set unspecific (i.e., the modulation of NEP N2 and AEP N1). The phase-locked N1, N2, and P2 nociceptive-evoked potentials (especially the vertex N2-P2 waves) include low frequencies in the delta/theta band (1–8 Hz) [15,47], and particularly in the delta range [47]. Nevertheless, recent studies reported that theta (e.g., [46]) and even alpha spectral activity [45,55] may contribute to the above components. Thus, there are at least three reasons why the TF representation in the theta band may not entirely account for variations in the magnitude of LEPs. First, different parameters of TF signal decomposition may bring about subtle different results in terms of involved frequencies. Second, and independent of the first reason, the latency and magnitude of the TF decomposition cannot be related only to the contribution of each one of these responses in isolation nor captures solely the phase-locked information (although most of the information represented in the theta band is phase-locked). Third, all sensory evoked responses are contributed by activities in the range of delta and alpha frequencies and not only by the theta frequency band [56]. As we detailed above, the theta oscillatory activity reported in the present study can be considered as a general representation of the late vertex activity evoked in the time domain which only partially represents each specific time-locked nociceptive evoked potential. It has been speculated that activity in the theta range may serve as a biomarker of pain processing [55,57] and more generally as an index of abnormal neural processing in psychiatric and neurological diseases [58].

It is possible that, as theta activity can be particularly sensitive to the intra- and inter-individual short-term variations of salient sensory information perceived as threatening, and ultimately ensuing in the experience of pain (e.g., [46]), it could be sensitive to the unaware involuntary top-down cognitive/emotional modulation exerted by reminders of mortality. However, according to the TMT theory, such modulation would not be mediated by self-reported negative mood or anxiety. Yet, as correctly argued by Tritt et al. in a recent insightful review [59], this notion cannot rely on a statistical null effect (namely, the absence of differences in ratings of mood between mind-sets). In addition, the idea that defense mechanisms triggered by mortality salience are based on a specific death–related "potential for anxiety" mechanism rather than on a more general anxiety mechanism did not receive enough evidence yet. Therefore, a more biologically plausible explanation should be advocated that is grounded on brain mechanisms evolutionarily developed to resolve uncertainty in the environment (and so avoid unexpected events) [60], basically mediated by a general anxiety system [59].

Despite such theoretical debate, our current results provide evidence in favor of the TMT by showing that the effect of mortality salience on nociceptive theta ER% was not associated with positive and negative affect or anxiety because the self-reported measures did not explain the variance associated with the mind-set effect and did not covary with the observed effects (cf. Results section). Nevertheless, the fact that following mortality salience the ER% magnitude increased concomitantly with the increase in ratings of threat (Fig. 7, left) suggests that the motivational state associated to the reminders of mortality increased arousal and vigilance in the participants. Tritt et al. [59] proposed that biological underpinnings of mortality salience might not be unique but rather a particular expression of a more general set of biological responses to uncertainty. In this respect, the findings obtained in our preliminary survey (see Material S1) support the notion that self-reported measures of general anxiety and emotions may be strongly influenced by mind-sets different from reminders of mortality (e.g. the possibility of becoming paralyzed or being abandoned). These authors suggest that a brain-based anxiety system exists, which is responsible for the biological processes subtending mortality salience and, more generally, threat defense phenomena. This would also explain the specific sensitivity of brain responses to somatosensory threatening stimuli to the top-down modulation exerted by mortality salience. The fact that no mediation of self-reported anxiety on the neural measures was found in the present study, by no means implies that future studies will be unable to identify automatic, implicit and unconscious anxiety mediation of mortality salience effects on the neural correlates of bodily threat.

Methodological and theoretical considerations

Several aspects of the methods applied here are worth discussion to foster future research in this area. We implemented a calibration procedure in which the intensity of auditory stimulation was adjusted to match the intensity of the laser stimulation. The self-adjusting calibration approach is reported in detail in previous publications [19,25]. In short, participants were asked to abstain from a separate assessment of auditory sensation and, instead, attempt to equalize their perception of the auditory stimulus in relation to the nociceptive one. However, it must be noted that, despite the attempt to match the perceptual magnitude between the two modalities, the auditory stimulation could not be fully comparable with somatosensory heat stimulation (for it did likely not activate mechano-nociceptors in the ear). In spite of the fact that auditory stimuli were salient and perceived as threatening, they did not induce pain. Thus, whether the effects observed in this study would be replicated using a nociceptive and/or painful stimulus in a sensory modality other than somatosensory remains an open question. However, it should be noted that it may not be possible to induce pain by selectively activating nociceptors in non-somatosensory modalities (i.e. auditory, visual, and olfactory). Despite this criticality, the finding that participants

attributed some degree of threat to auditory stimuli, and that this was modulated by reminders of mortality, reflects the success of the perceptual calibration procedure (Fig. 2), thus substantiating the methodological sensitivity of the control sensory stimulation used. Nevertheless, our results cannot provide conclusive modality specific effects, and different sensory stimuli acquiring homeostatic significance/behavioural relevance for the body could exert similar effects at the level of brain responses. In addition, the effect size of the significant difference in the theta oscillatory activity was small ($p\eta^2 = 0.11$), thus suggesting that this finding should be considered as a preliminary observation in need of replication.

The specificity and sensitivity of the effects of mortality salience on theta activity concomitant to somatosensory threatening stimuli is supported by the effects associated with the induction of a failed exam mind-set, a control condition which was suggested to be most comparable to mortality salience across several cognitive/affective dimensions (see Material S1). The biological underpinnings of mortality salience may be not mapped on a specific neural system but rather on a set of areas representing the neural reactivity to uncertainty [59]. It should be emphasized that death was not rated as the worst option in several of the measured circumstances. Indeed, self-reported ratings of negativity, alarm, threat, and significance were higher for other mind-sets (e.g. becoming paralyzed or being abandoned) than for reminders of mortality.

Another important aspect of the methodology adopted in the present study was the use of a within subject design, which contrasts with classical social psychology studies [27,28]. To the best of our knowledge only two neuroscientific studies [10,11] applied a within- rather than a between-subjects experimental design. Between-subjects designs do not take into account individual differences in responsiveness to the mind-set induction, hence the participation of an individual in repeated tests in each experimental condition increases the statistical power and precision of the study, as well as it reduces the amount of participants required in a study.

Although the age range of the sample recruited in the present study was limited, an interaction between the cognitive mind-set inductions and the age of the participants (namely, the older the participant the larger the effects of the mind-sets) is consistent with the differential effect of mortality salience across different ages [27,61]. Yet, future studies with a more representative age group will determine whether the age-related differences reported here are actually a result of developmental changes over the life span and whether the effect may be specific to a cognitive mind-set specifically associated to reminders of mortality or whether it would be an unspecific effect, as observed in the current study.

To conclude, our findings support the hypothesis that reminders of mortality have a modulatory effect on the perception of threatening somatosensory stimuli and their associated neural responses. Importantly, this effect becomes stronger the more the stimuli are judged as threatening, suggesting an influence of death-related thoughts on somatosensory representation.

Acknowledgments

The authors thank Dr. Enea Francesco Pavone for technical support.

Author Contributions

Conceived and designed the experiments: EV KK SMA. Performed the experiments: EV KK. Analyzed the data: EV. Contributed reagents/materials/analysis tools: EV KK SMA. Wrote the paper: EV KK SMA.

References

1. Kastenbaum R, Costa PT Jr (1977) Psychological perspectives on death. Annu Rev Psychol 28: 225–249.
2. Rosenblatt A, Greenberg J, Solomon S, Pyszczynski T, Lyon D (1989) Evidence for terror management theory: I. The effects of mortality salience on reactions to those who violate or uphold cultural values. J Pers Soc Psychol 57: 681–690.
3. Greenberg J, Simon L, Pyszczynski T, Solomon S, Chatel D (1992) Terror management and tolerance: does mortality salience always intensify negative reactions to others who threaten one's worldview? J Pers Soc Psychol 63: 212–220.
4. Greenberg J, Solomon S, Pyszczynski T, Rosenblatt A, Burling J, et al. (1992) Why do people need self-esteem? Converging evidence that self-esteem serves an anxiety-buffering function. J Pers Soc Psychol 63: 913–922.
5. Harmon-Jones E, Simon L, Greenberg J, Pyszczynski T, Solomon S, et al. (1997) Terror management theory and self-esteem: evidence that increased self-esteem reduces mortality salience effects. J Pers Soc Psychol 72: 24–36.
6. Pyszczynski T, Greenberg J, Solomon S, Arndt J, Schimel J (2004) Why do people need self-esteem? A theoretical and empirical review. Psychol Bull 130: 435–468.
7. Arndt J, Greenberg J, Simon L, Pyszczynski T, Solomon S (1998) Terror management and self-awareness: Evidence that mortality salience provokes avoidance of the self-focused state. Pers Soc Psychol Bull 24: 1216–1227.
8. Goldenberg JL, Hart J, Pyszczynski T, Warnica GM, Landau M, et al. (2006) Ambivalence toward the body: death, neuroticism, and the flight from physical sensation. Pers Soc Psychol Bull 32: 1264–1277.
9. Han S, Qin J, Ma Y (2010) Neurocognitive processes of linguistic cues related to death. Neuropsychologia 48: 3436–3442.
10. Quirin M, Loktyushin A, Arndt J, Kustermann E, Lo YY, et al. (2012) Existential neuroscience: a functional magnetic resonance imaging investigation of neural responses to reminders of one's mortality. Soc Cogn Affect Neurosci 7: 193–198.
11. Klackl J, Jonas E, Kronbichler M (2013) Existential neuroscience: neurophysiological correlates of proximal defenses against death-related thoughts. Soc Cogn Affect Neurosci 8: 333–340.
12. Henry EA, Bartholow BD, Arndt J (2010) Death on the brain: effects of mortality salience on the neural correlates of ingroup and outgroup categorization. Soc Cogn Affect Neurosci 5: 77–87.
13. Luo S, Shi Z, Yang X, Wang X, Han S (2013) Reminders of mortality decrease midcingulate activity in response to others' suffering. Soc Cogn Affect Neurosci.
14. Todorovic A, de Lange FP (2012) Repetition suppression and expectation suppression are dissociable in time in early auditory evoked fields. J Neurosci 32: 13389–13395.
15. Iannetti GD, Hughes NP, Lee MC, Mouraux A (2008) Determinants of laser-evoked EEG responses: pain perception or stimulus saliency? J Neurophysiol 100: 815–828.
16. Ronga I, Valentini E, Mouraux A, Iannetti GD (2013) Novelty is not enough: laser-evoked potentials are determined by stimulus saliency, not absolute novelty. J Neurophysiol 109: 692–701.
17. Legrain V, Mancini F, Sambo CF, Torta DM, Ronga I, et al. (2012) Cognitive aspects of nociception and pain: bridging neurophysiology with cognitive psychology. Neurophysiol Clin 42: 325–336.
18. Fruhstorfer H, Soveri P, Jarvilehto T (1970) Short-term habituation of the auditory evoked response in man. Electroencephalogr Clin Neurophysiol 28: 153–161.
19. Valentini E, Torta DM, Mouraux A, Iannetti GD (2011) Dishabituation of laser-evoked EEG responses: dissecting the effect of certain and uncertain changes in stimulus modality. J Cogn Neurosci 23: 2822–2837.
20. Beck AT, Steer RA, Brown GK (1996) Manual for the Beck Depression Inventory II (BDI-II). San Antonio, TX: Psychology Corporation.
21. Spielberger CD, Gorssuch RL, Lushene PR, Vagg PR, Jacobs GA (1983) Manual for the State-Trait Anxiety Inventory.
22. Gontkovsky ST, Vickery CD, Beatty WW (2004) Construct validity of the 7/24 spatial recall test. Appl Neuropsychol 11: 75–84.
23. Cruccu G, Pennisi E, Truini A, Iannetti GD, Romaniello A, et al. (2003) Unmyelinated trigeminal pathways as assessed by laser stimuli in humans. Brain 126: 2246–2256.
24. Plaghki L, Mouraux A (2005) EEG and laser stimulation as tools for pain research. Curr Opin Investig Drugs 6: 58–64.
25. Valentini E, Liang M, Aglioti SM, Iannetti GD (2012) Seeing touch and pain in a stranger modulates the cortical responses elicited by somatosensory but not auditory stimulation. Hum Brain Mapp 33: 2873–2884.
26. Arndt J, Greenberg J, Solomon S, Pyszczynski T, Simon L (1997) Suppression, accessibility of death-related thoughts, and cultural worldview defense: exploring the psychodynamics of terror management. J Pers Soc Psychol 73: 5–18.
27. Burke BL, Martens A, Faucher EH (2010) Two decades of terror management theory: a meta-analysis of mortality salience research. Pers Soc Psychol Rev 14: 155–195.
28. Hayes J, Schimel J, Arndt J, Faucher EH (2010) A theoretical and empirical review of the death-thought accessibility concept in terror management research. Psychol Bull 136: 699–739.
29. Pyszczynski T, Greenberg J, Solomon S (1999) A dual-process model of defense against conscious and unconscious death-related thoughts: an extension of terror management theory. Psychol Rev 106: 835–845.
30. Watson D, Clark LA, Tellegen A (1988) Development and validation of brief measures of positive and negative affect: the PANAS scales. Journal of personality and social psychology. 54: 1063–1070.
31. Spielberger CD, Gorsuch RL, Lushene R, Vagg PR & Jacobs GA (1983) Manual for the State-Trait Anxiety Inventory, Palo Alto, CA.
32. Schlereth T, Magerl W, Treede R (2001) Spatial discrimination thresholds for pain and touch in human hairy skin. Pain 92: 187–194.
33. Carlsson AM (1983) Assessment of chronic pain. I. Aspects of the reliability and validity of the visual analogue scale. Pain 16: 87–101.
34. Dimitrov DM, Rumrill PD Jr (2003) Pretest-posttest designs and measurement of change. Work 20: 159–165.
35. Rausch JR, Maxwell SE, Kelley K (2003) Analytic methods for questions pertaining to a randomized pretest, posttest, follow-up design. J Clin Child Adolesc Psychol 32: 467–486.
36. Porter AC, Raudenbush SW (1987) Analysis of covariance: Its model and use in psychological research. Journal of Counseling Psychology 34: 383–392.
37. Senn S (2006) Change from baseline and analysis of covariance revisited. Stat Med 25: 4334–4344.
38. Lehmann D, Skrandies W (1980) Reference-free identification of components of checkerboard-evoked multichannel potential fields. Electroencephalogr Clin Neurophysiol 48: 609–621.
39. Delorme A, Makeig S (2004) EEGLAB: an open source toolbox for analysis of single-trial EEG dynamics including independent component analysis. Journal of Neuroscience Methods 134: 9–21.
40. Jung TP, Makeig S, Humphries C, Lee TW, McKeown MJ, et al. (2000) Removing electroencephalographic artifacts by blind source separation. Psychophysiology 37: 163–178.
41. Tarkka IM, Treede RD (1993) Equivalent electrical source analysis of pain-related somatosensory evoked potentials elicited by a CO_2 laser. J Clin Neurophysiol 10: 513–519.
42. Hu L, Mouraux A, Hu Y, Iannetti GD (2010) A novel approach for enhancing the signal-to-noise ratio and detecting automatically event-related potentials (ERPs) in single trials. Neuroimage 50: 99–111.
43. Mouraux A, Iannetti GD (2008) Across-trial averaging of event-related EEG responses and beyond. Magnetic Resonance Imaging 26: 1041–1054.
44. Pfurtscheller G, Lopes da Silva FH (1999) Event-related EEG/MEG synchronization and desynchronization: basic principles. Clinical Neurophysiology 110: 1842–1857.
45. Zhang ZG, Hu L, Hung YS, Mouraux A, Iannetti GD (2012) Gamma-band oscillations in the primary somatosensory cortex–a direct and obligatory correlate of subjective pain intensity. J Neurosci 32: 7429–7438.
46. Schulz E, Tiemann L, Schuster T, Gross J, Ploner M (2011) Neurophysiological coding of traits and states in the perception of pain. Cereb Cortex 21: 2408–2414.
47. Mouraux A, Guerit JM, Plaghki L (2003) Non-phase locked electroencephalogram (EEG) responses to CO2 laser skin stimulations may reflect central interactions between A partial partial differential- and C-fibre afferent volleys. Clinical Neurophysiology 114: 710–722.
48. Ploner M, Gross J, Timmermann L, Pollok B, Schnitzler A (2006) Pain suppresses spontaneous brain rhythms. Cerebral Cortex 16: 537–540.
49. Iannetti GD, Niazy RK, Wise RG, Jezzard P, Brooks JC, et al. (2005) Simultaneous recording of laser-evoked brain potentials and continuous, high-field functional magnetic resonance imaging in humans. Neuroimage 28: 708–719.
50. Mitsis GD, Iannetti GD, Smart TS, Tracey I, Wise RG (2008) Regions of interest analysis in pharmacological fMRI: how do the definition criteria influence the inferred result? Neuroimage 40: 121–132.
51. Torta DM, Liang M, Valentini E, Mouraux A, Iannetti GD (2012) Dishabituation of laser-evoked EEG responses: dissecting the effect of certain and uncertain changes in stimulus spatial location. Exp Brain Res 218: 361–372.
52. Valentini E, Betti V, Hu L, Aglioti SM (2013) Hypnotic modulation of pain perception and of brain activity triggered by nociceptive laser stimuli. Cortex 49: 446–462.
53. Hu L, Peng W, Valentini E, Zhang Z, Hu Y (2013) Functional features of nociceptive-induced suppression of alpha band electroencephalographic oscillations. J Pain 14: 89–99.

54. Greenberg J, Pyszczynski T, Solomon S, Simon L, Breus M (1994) Role of consciousness and accessibility of death-related thoughts in mortality salience effects. J Pers Soc Psychol 67: 627–637.

55. Schulz E, Zherdin A, Tiemann L, Plant C, Ploner M (2012) Decoding an individual's sensitivity to pain from the multivariate analysis of EEG data. Cereb Cortex 22: 1118–1123.

56. Luck SJ (2005) An introduction to the event-related potential technique. Cambridge, MA: MIT Press.

57. Walton KD, Dubois M, Llinas RR (2010) Abnormal thalamocortical activity in patients with Complex Regional Pain Syndrome (CRPS) type I. Pain 150: 41–51.

58. Schulman JJ, Cancro R, Lowe S, Lu F, Walton KD, et al. (2011) Imaging of thalamocortical dysrhythmia in neuropsychiatry. Front Hum Neurosci 5: 69.

59. Tritt SM, Inzlicht M, Harmon-Jones E (2012) Toward a Biological Understanding of Mortality Salience (And Other Threat Compensation Processes). Social Cognition 30: 715–733.

60. Hirsh JB, Inzlicht M (2008) The devil you know: neuroticism predicts neural response to uncertainty. Psychol Sci 19: 962–967.

61. Maxfield M, Pyszczynski T, Kluck B, Cox CR, Greenberg J, et al. (2007) Age-related differences in responses to thoughts of one's own death: mortality salience and judgments of moral transgressions. Psychol Aging 22: 341–353.

25

Representation of Cognitive Reappraisal Goals in Frontal Gamma Oscillations

Jae-Hwan Kang[1], Ji Woon Jeong[2], Hyun Taek Kim[2], Sang Hee Kim[1]*, Sung-Phil Kim[3]*

1 Department of Brain and Cognitive Engineering, Korea University, Seoul, Republic of Korea, **2** Department of Psychology, Korea University, Seoul, Republic of Korea, **3** Department of Human and Systems Engineering, Ulsan National Institute of Science and Technology, Ulsan, Republic of Korea

Abstract

Recently, numerous efforts have been made to understand the neural mechanisms underlying cognitive regulation of emotion, such as cognitive reappraisal. Many studies have reported that cognitive control of emotion induces increases in neural activity of the control system, including the prefrontal cortex and the dorsal anterior cingulate cortex, and increases or decreases (depending upon the regulation goal) in neural activity of the appraisal system, including the amygdala and the insula. It has been hypothesized that information about regulation goals needs to be processed through interactions between the control and appraisal systems in order to support cognitive reappraisal. However, how this information is represented in the dynamics of cortical activity remains largely unknown. To address this, we investigated temporal changes in gamma band activity (35–55 Hz) in human electroencephalograms during a cognitive reappraisal task that was comprised of three reappraisal goals: to decease, maintain, or increase emotional responses modulated by affect-laden pictures. We examined how the characteristics of gamma oscillations, such as spectral power and large-scale phase synchronization, represented cognitive reappraisal goals. We found that left frontal gamma power decreased, was sustained, or increased when the participants suppressed, maintained, or amplified their emotions, respectively. This change in left frontal gamma power appeared during an interval of 1926 to 2453 ms after stimulus onset. We also found that the number of phase-synchronized pairs of gamma oscillations over the entire brain increased when participants regulated their emotions compared to when they maintained their emotions. These results suggest that left frontal gamma power may reflect cortical representation of emotional states modulated by cognitive reappraisal goals and gamma phase synchronization across whole brain regions may reflect emotional regulatory efforts to achieve these goals. Our study may provide the basis for an electroencephalogram-based neurofeedback system for the cognitive regulation of emotion.

Editor: Antonella Gasbarri, University of L'Aquila, Italy

Funding: This research was supported by both the Mid-career Researcher Program (NRF-2012R1A2A2A04047239) and the Brain Research Program (NRF-2006-2005112) through the National Research Foundation of Korea funded by the Ministry of Science, ICT & Future Planning. The funders had no role in study design, data collection and analysis, decision to publish, or preparation of the manuscript.

Competing Interests: The authors have declared that no competing interests exist.

* Email: spkim@unist.ac.kr (SPK); sangheekim.ku@gmail.com (SHK)

Introduction

An individual's ability to regulate emotional responses to external stimuli or internal mental representations relates not only to that individual's mental health but also to many social problems [1–3]. Accordingly, cognitive regulation of emotion, which refers to cognitive processes involved in influencing the onset, offset, intensity, or quality of emotional responses [4], has emerged as an important topic in many disciplines (i.e., psychology, psychiatry, and social neuroscience). Emotion regulation processes can be categorized based on whether they occur before or after an emotion is generated: antecedent-focused emotion regulation is applied earlier to alter the trajectory of emotion responses before they arise, whereas response-focused emotion regulation is applied later to modulate the emotional response after the emotion is generated [5]. Our study focuses on cognitive reappraisal, one type of antecedent-focused emotion regulation strategy. Cognitive reappraisal is considered an effective emotion regulation strategy and has received relatively more scientific attention than others have because it generally requires

fewer cognitive demands and induces no memory impairment [6,7].

Over the past decades, many neuropsychological studies have investigated how emotion regulation strategies modulate neural responses to emotional events. To this end, they directly measured brain activity during emotion regulation using various methods, such as electroencephalogram (EEG), magnetoencephalogram (MEG), and functional magnetic resonance imaging (fMRI). Studies using EEG have shown a close relationship between the arousal level modulated by an emotional stimulus and the amplitude of the late positive potential (LPP), which arises approximately 300 to 400 ms after stimulus onset, and persists throughout the duration of stimulus presentation [8,9]. Other studies have demonstrated the LPP as an indicator of emotional perception [8,10,11], and suggested that it is modulated by a network of cortical and subcortical regions related to visual and emotional information processing [12]. Emotion regulation decreased LPP amplitude when individuals downregulated their emotional response to negative stimuli [13,14].

Ochsner and colleagues proposed a functional architecture underlying cognitive regulation of emotion that consists of both a voluntary top-down cognitive control system implemented in the prefrontal cortex (PFC) and the dorsal anterior cingulate cortex (dACC), and an automatic bottom-up emotional appraisal system implemented in subcortical structures, including the amygdala and the insula [15]. Many fMRI studies have indicated that interactions between the control system and the appraisal system play a key role in cognitive control of emotion [16–20]. These studies showed that regulation of emotions using cognitive control strategies to downregulate emotional responses increased blood oxygenation level-dependent (BOLD) activity in the PFC and dACC, and decreased BOLD activity in the amygdala and the insula. This inverse relationship between frontal cortical and subcortical areas was predominantly observed in cognitive reappraisal tasks [15,21,22], and was directly related to the performance of emotion regulation [23].

In addition to this inverse relationship of the BOLD activity in the amygdala and the insula, PFC activity—particularly in the medial prefrontal cortex (mPFC)—has been implicated in the integration of emotional state information [24]. Additionally, Quirk and Beer suggested that the role of the mPFC in emotion regulation was to maintain regulation goals and transfer them to other cortical areas [25]. Urry and colleagues reported that mPFC BOLD activity increased, was sustained, or decreased according to the reappraisal goal of increasing, maintaining, or decreasing emotional responses, respectively [26]. A similar finding was reported by Ochsner and colleagues who showed differences in mPFC BOLD activity between the increase and decrease conditions [15].

These findings suggest that cognitive reappraisal goals may be represented and maintained in PFC during emotion regulation. It is likely that dynamic interactions between the control system and the appraisal system underlie the representation of reappraisal goals in PFC [27]. However, the dynamics of cortical activity representing goal information during cognitive reappraisal remain unclear, largely because of the limited temporal resolution of fMRI. Because the time scale of the dynamic interactions between the appraisal system and the control system is much smaller than the dynamics of the BOLD signal, faster methods, such as EEG or MEG, may be required to investigate the temporal dynamics of PFC activity. However, few EEG/MEG studies have shown neural correlates of cognitive reappraisal goals. Therefore, this study aims to locate the representation of reappraisal goals in the temporal patterns of EEG oscillations during a cognitive reappraisal task. We posit that such representation of cognitive reappraisal goals in EEG activity would provide a basis for developing an online neurofeedback paradigm for the enhancement of emotion regulation ability.

In particular, we focused on gamma oscillations in EEG in relation to cognitive reappraisal goals. Although little is known about the direct relationship between gamma oscillations and cognitive reappraisal, there have been substantial findings to lead us to investigate gamma oscillations. First, gamma oscillations in EEG are known to be highly correlated with BOLD activity [28,29]. Therefore, it is likely that reappraisal goals represented in BOLD activity in PFC would be reflected in gamma oscillations. Second, the induced gamma activity has been used as an important tool to understand the neural mechanism underlying emotional processing [30]. A number of studies showed that emotional stimuli induced higher gamma power compared to neutral stimuli [31–34]. Martini and colleague has revealed that unpleasant stimuli increased gamma power in the frontal regions as well as large-scale gamma phase synchronization across frontal and temporal regions [35]. Popov and colleague have revealed the increased gamma power and local cross-frequency coupling of

alpha and gamma oscillations in the mPFC during cognitive reappraisal to decrease emotions in response to unpleasant stimuli [36]. Third, gamma oscillations are known to be associated with cognitive processes that can be recruited during the manipulation of emotion regulation, such as attention, memory [37,38] and emotion intelligence [39,40]. For instance, Müller and colleagues reported that gamma power increased during selective attention to emotional stimuli compared to neutral ones [33]. Recent studies have suggested that gamma oscillations are implicated in emotional intelligence that assesses how well a person understands self-emotion or mindfulness that refers to non-judgmental awareness of internal and external emotions [39–43].

Given that these findings suggest a close relationship between gamma oscillations and emotional and cognitive processes, we investigated two characteristics of gamma oscillations—spectral power and large-scale phase synchronization—during cognitive regulation of emotion. Specifically, we tested the following hypotheses to address how gamma oscillations would be modulated during cognitive reappraisal. First, we hypothesized that frontal gamma power would vary with different reappraisal goals. While it was uncertain whether increasing/decreasing emotions would increase/decrease gamma power, frontal gamma power might be affected by reappraisal goal information in PFC activity and/or emotional and cognitive processing outcomes directed by these goals. Second, we hypothesized that large-scale gamma phase synchronization over the whole brain would increase during cognitive reappraisal. As large-scale phase synchronization in scalp EEG reflects the engagement of brain-wide neural networks to support cognitive control [35,44,45], we expected that gamma phase synchronization would reflect cognitive regulatory efforts, and thus increase during cognitive reappraisal to increase or decrease emotional responses.

Materials and Methods

Participants

Twenty healthy young adults (9 men, 11 women; mean age = 22.4 ± 2.41 years) participated in the study. All participants were right-handed and had normal or corrected-to-normal vision without any self-reported neurological or neuropsychological disorders. The Institutional Review Board (IRB) of Korea University approved this study, and all participants provided written informed consent after the study procedure had been explained to them.

Experimental procedure

Emotion regulation tasks and stimuli. We devised a cognitive reappraisal task with three different reappraisal goals: to decrease, maintain, or increase emotional responses [46]. In each epoch, participants were provided with a visual cue about a reappraisal goal before they responded to a stimulus. These visual cues were displayed on a screen and consisted of an up arrow, down arrow, and dash to indicate the increase, decrease, and maintain conditions respectively. In the increase condition, the participants were asked to amplify the intensity of their emotional response to a presented stimulus. In the maintain condition, the participants were asked to respond naturally to a stimulus by being aware of their feeling and maintaining it. In the decrease condition, the participants were asked to reduce the intensity of their emotional response. The cognitive reappraisal strategy the participants used was the self-focused strategy [15], in which the participants changed their level of self-relevance to a stimulus; in other words, they attempted to feel more or less involved in the event depicted in the presented stimulus.

Each participant was presented with 132 emotional pictures selected from an in-house affective picture set. The picture set consisted of an equal number of positive and negative pictures. The pictures were selected based on normative ratings in valence (1 to 7; unpleasant to pleasant) and arousal (1 to 7; calm to exciting), where the ratings were obtained from a separate group of 50 healthy participants who did not participate in this emotion regulation study. For our study, we selected a set of emotional stimuli based on these normative ratings in arousal and valence such that pictures with high arousal level and both positive and negative valence were selected. The average (± standard deviation [SD]) normative ratings in valence of the selected stimuli were 2.59±1.05 for negative and 5.29±1.19 for positive pictures. The normative ratings in valence were significantly different between selected positive and negative pictures ($p<0.01$). The average normative ratings in arousal of the selected stimuli were 4.60±1.42 for negative and 4.60±1.39 for positive pictures, respectively. The normative ratings in arousal of the selected stimuli were significantly higher than for neutral pictures (average: 3.65±1.35) contained in the in-house affective picture set ($p<0.01$). The participants never saw the same picture twice during the experiment.

Task procedure. The task consisted of four blocks with a 5-min inter-block break. A total of 132 epochs containing all six conditions (3 reappraisal conditions×2 valence conditions) were randomly assigned to each block. A single epoch was composed of five consecutive periods (see Fig. 1). First, an epoch began with a blank screen presented for 1000 ms. Second, a visual cue appeared on the screen for 2000 ms to indicate a reappraisal goal. During this period, the participants acknowledged the meaning of the presented reappraisal goal and prepared to regulate their emotional response. Third, a 200-ms blank screen appeared again before stimulus onset. Fourth, an emotional picture was displayed on the screen for 4000 ms. During this period, the participants regulated their emotional response to the presented picture in accordance with the previously presented regulatory instruction cue. Picture presentation was pseudo-random, and no more than three pictures of the same valence condition were shown during consecutive epochs. Fifth, after the picture disappeared, assessment of the presented picture occurred. The participants were presented with a five-scale rating screen for 1500 ms to assess the valence level (1 = unpleasant to 5 = pleasant), followed by another rating screen for 1500 ms to assess the arousal level (1 = very low to 5 = very high). The participants rated the picture's five-scale valence and arousal levels by pressing one of five buttons on the computer keyboard.

EEG recording. Scalp EEG was recorded using 13 wet electrodes and the Grass Model 12A5 amplifier (Grass-Telefactor; An Astro-Med, Inc., West Warwick, Rhode Island, USA). The electrode locations (F3/z/4, C3/z/4, P3/z/4, O1/2, and T5/6) were determined according to the International 10–20 system. The EEG signal recorded from each electrode was sampled at 512 Hz, referenced to the right earlobe (A2), grounded using an electrode placed on the forehead (AFz), and re-referenced to the average activity of both earlobe electrodes. The vertical electro-oculogram (vEOG) was recorded 1 cm below the right eye. Over the recording session, the impedance of each electrode was maintained below 5 KΩ. The EEG signal was digitized and then filtered using both a band-pass filter (0.1 to 100 Hz) to eliminate high-frequency noise and a notch filter at 60 Hz to attenuate power-line noise. To avoid the influence of edge effects arising from signal filtering and wavelet transform, the filtered EEG signal was first segmented into epochs of 6000 ms, starting 1000 ms before stimulus onset to 5000 ms after stimulus onset, passed through a series of signal processing steps with this extra data length, and then truncated back to the exact epoch length of 200 ms before to 4000 ms after stimulus onset. For the elimination of epochs contaminated by artifacts, such as eye movements, we performed independent component analysis (ICA) followed by visually inspecting EEG signals simultaneously with the vEOG. This noise reduction process removed an average of 40.4±25.7 contaminated epochs per participant, resulting in an average of 157.6±25.7 total epochs per participant.

Gamma band activity analysis. Since this study investigated how gamma band activity (GBA) was modulated during cognitive reappraisal tasks, we analyzed two primary aspects of GBA: spectral power and large-scale gamma phase synchronization. First, time-varying spectral power was estimated in the time-frequency domain by convoluting the EEG signal with the complex Morlet wavelet (see Equation 1) [47].

$$w(t, f_0) = A \cdot e^{-(-t^2/2\sigma_t^2)} \cdot e^{2i\pi f_0 t} \quad with \quad A = \sqrt{\frac{1}{\sigma_t\sqrt{\pi}}} \quad (1)$$

The transform using the complex Morlet wavelet characterized higher frequency components with a fine temporal resolution and lower frequency components with a more precise frequency resolution [47]. For example, with the constant ratio of seven, the complex Morlet wavelet transform yielded the following resolutions in the time-frequency (TF) plane: SDs = 5 Hz, 31.8 ms with a 35-Hz wavelet; SDs = 7.86 Hz, 20.3 ms with a 55-Hz wavelet.

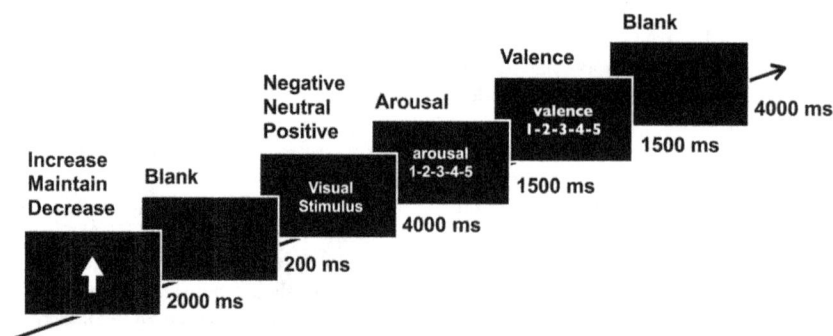

Figure 1. Timeline of the cognitive reappraisal task. Three regulatory instructions—increase, maintain, and decrease—were indicated by the up-arrow, dash, and down-arrow, respectively. After a 200 ms blank period, a 4000 ms visual emotional stimulus appeared for the cognitive reappraisal task. For the arousal and valence rating of the stimulus, two 5-point scale screens followed for 3000 ms each.

This property provided an advantage to analyzing relatively high-frequency GBA with finer time resolutions. For each epoch, time-varying power in a given frequency band was calculated using the absolute value of the convolution of the EEG signal with the wavelet. Power values were log-transformed and normalized by subtracting the mean power value in the baseline period and then dividing by the standard deviation of the power value in the baseline period. The baseline period was the 200-ms period during the blank screen before stimulus onset. The gamma power analyzed in this study was the average of the power values in the gamma band ranging from 35 to 55 Hz.

Second, phase synchronization between a pair of EEG signals recorded from two different electrodes was estimated using the phase-locking value (PLV) [48,49]. Electroencephalogram signals were filtered using a zero phase-lag finite impulse response (FIR) band-pass filter with a 2-Hz bandwidth, a central frequency (f_0) ranging from 35 to 55 Hz, and a 1-Hz frequency step [48,50]. The filtered signals were then transformed using the complex Morlet wavelet (with parameters identical to above) to obtain estimates of instantaneous phases. An instantaneous PLV for time instant (t) and for the frequency (f) between a pair of EEG signals at channels n and m was calculated as (see Equation 2),

$$PLV_{nm}(t,f_0) = \frac{1}{K}\sum_{k=1}^{K} \left| e^{j(\varphi_n(t,f_0,k) - \varphi_m(t,f_0,k))} \right| \quad (2)$$

where K is the number of trials and n, m, t, f, and k are instantaneous phases for the kth epoch. The instantaneous PLV ranged from zero (i.e., no phase coupling) to one (i.e., perfect phase coupling). To obtain a normal distribution, the calculated PLV was Fisher's z-transformed [51].

Statistical analyses. To identify what caused significant differences in frontal gamma power and when it occurred, we performed a three-way repeated-measures analysis of variance (RMANOVA) with the factors of reappraisal goals (i.e., decrease, maintain, increase), valence types (i.e., negative, positive), and frontal laterality (i.e., left, midline, right) on the gamma power data. This analysis was repeatedly applied to each 20-ms time window that moved from stimulus onset to stimulus offset (i.e., 4000 ms after onset). We also conducted post-hoc analyses using one-paired t-tests to assess the differences within the 20 ms within each factor. All analyses were conducted using Bonferroni adjustments of the p-value. We also investigated significant differences in the PLVs across reappraisal goals in two steps. In the first step, we performed a randomization test with 200 surrogate data sets to assess whether the instantaneous PLVs for each EEG pair exhibited a significant difference [48,50]. If the original instantaneous PLV was significantly higher than the distribution of the surrogate instantaneous PLVs ($p<0.01$), we determined that the instantaneous PLV indicated significant phase synchronization. Otherwise, we did not include that instantaneous PLV in the next step. Following the randomization test, we averaged the significant instantaneous PLVs across the frequencies (21 frequencies over 35 to 55 Hz) for each time instant. In the second step, we tested the difference in PLVs between two different reappraisal goals (i.e., increase vs. maintain and maintain vs. decrease) for a given EEG channel pair. To investigate overall PLV patterns over time and to avoid possible misinterpretations by analyzing the PLV in an overly short time interval, we divided an epoch into 11 segments, including one baseline segment with a 200-ms duration and 10 post-stimulus segments each with a 400-ms duration. We then calculated the average time of the frequency-averaged instantaneous PLVs in each segment. Using

these time-frequency-averaged PLVs from all the epochs, we repeatedly performed one-tail paired t-tests to determine differences between two reappraisal goals in each segment.

Results

Topographic map of gamma power associated with the three reappraisal goals

For an overall view of time-varying gamma activity, we built time-varying topographic maps of gamma power per cognitive reappraisal goal, as shown in Figure 2. We observed the maximum gamma power over the parietal-occipital regions irrespective of regulatory goals, which is consistent with our previous study [52]. Gamma power over the whole brain appeared to be higher and more sustained in the increase condition than in the other conditions. Additionally, gamma power in the frontal regions in the decrease condition was reduced compared to the other conditions.

Spectral power and statistical analyses

Three-way RMANOVA (3 reappraisal goals × 2 valence levels × 3 frontal laterality positions) were conducted in the 20-ms time windows without overlap during the presentation of stimuli to identify whether and when significant differences for the within-factors occurred. The analysis revealed that stimuli began to induce significant main effects of reappraisal goals and frontal laterality after the 2000 ms after stimulus onset, while there was no significant main effect of valence levels and no interactions within all combinations across factors for all frontal channels and time windows ($p<0.01$). Figure 3 depicts the temporal patterns of the frontal gamma power for the different reappraisal goals. The analysis of temporal patterns showed that frontal gamma power began to diverge according to the cognitive reappraisal goals at approximately 2000 ms after stimulus onset. Additionally, it is noteworthy that compared to the baseline level (marked by the horizontal lines at the zero level in Fig. 3), gamma power at the left frontal region (F3) increased, decreased, or did not change. We assigned two separate time segments, including the windows with significant main effects, to a mid-period (1926 to 2453 ms) and a late-period (3293 to 3625 ms), and performed a post-hoc analysis with Bonferroni adjustment in these segments.

In the post-hoc analysis, we compared gamma power in the mid-period and late-period across reappraisal goals at each frontal channel (see Fig. 4). In the mid-period, the left frontal activity (F3) showed more differences across conditions compared to the mid (Fz) and right (F4) frontal activities. At the F3 channel, gamma power exhibited a monotonic pattern (i.e., decrease<maintain<increase) with a significant difference between the decrease and maintain conditions (paired t-test: $t(19) = 2.53$; $p<0.05$) and a marginally significant difference between the maintain and increase conditions, $t(19) = 2.19$, $p = 0.065$. At the Fz channel, gamma power in the increase condition was significantly higher than in the maintain condition, $t(19) = 3.37$, $p<0.001$, and decrease condition, $t(19) = 2.92$, $p<0.05$, but there was no difference between the maintain and decrease conditions, $t(19) = 1.00$, $p = 0.166$. At the F4 channel, no significant difference was observed between any pairing of reappraisal conditions ($p>0.05$). In the late-period, gamma power in the increase condition was higher than that in the decrease condition at all three channels but this difference reached significance only at Fz: F3, $t(19) = 2.26$, $p = 0.063$; Fz, $t(19) = 2.85$, $p = 0.015$, and F4, $t(19) = 2.21$, $p<0.060$. In addition, gamma power in the increase condition was significantly higher than in the maintain condition at Fz, $t(19) = 3.91$, $p<0.01$, and F4, $t(19) = 3.09$, $p<0.01$. In summary,

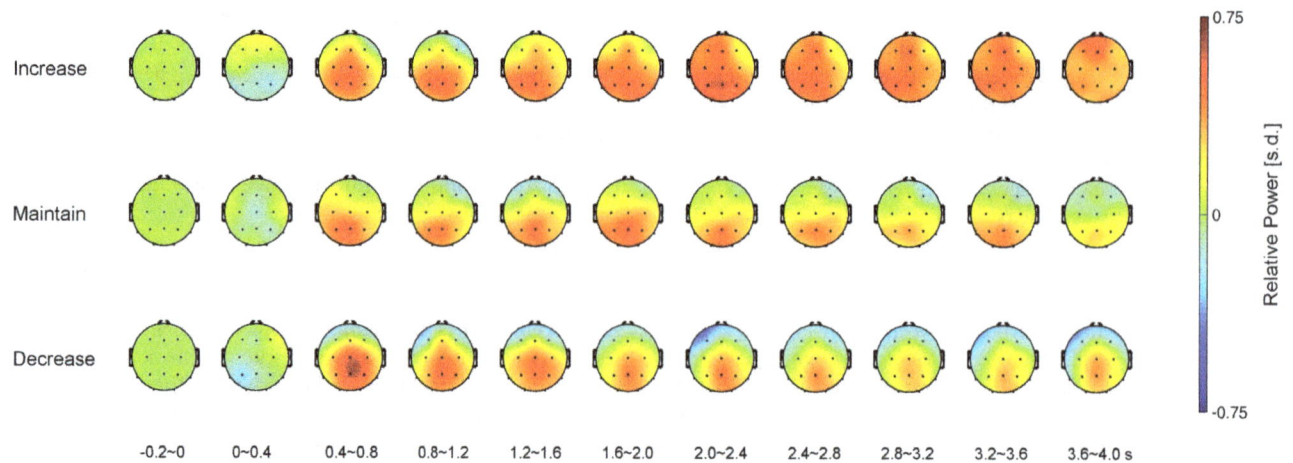

Figure 2. Time-varying topographic maps of gamma power in three different cognitive reappraisal conditions. Gamma power in each of the 13 EEG channels (see small black dots) was subtracted from the mean of the baseline power and divided into the standard deviation of the baseline power, resulting in the relative power. Bottom labels represent the time windows based on visual stimulus onset (increase, top; maintain, mid; decrease, bottom).

only the mid-period gamma power in the left frontal region (F3) showed a monotonically increasing pattern consistent with the reappraisal goals (i.e., decrease<maintain<increase).

The RMANOVA revealed that neither the main effect of valence type nor the interaction between reappraisal goals reached level of significance. We performed further statistical analyses to clarify whether negative and positive stimuli modulated similar or different patterns of gamma power during the mid-period and late-period using one-paired t-tests. For negative stimuli, the gamma power for both the increase and maintain conditions was larger than for the decrease condition at the F3 channel during the mid-period; this difference was marginally significant for the maintain condition and significant for the increase condition (decrease vs. maintain, $t(19) = 2.15$, $p = 0.066$; decrease vs. increase $t(19) = 2.52$, $p<0.05$). At the Fz channel, the gamma power for the increase condition was significantly higher than for the decrease, $t(19) = 2.69$, $p<0.01$, and maintain conditions, $t(19) = 2.17$, $p< 0.05$, during the mid-period. During the late-period, more pronounced gamma power for the increase condition compared to the other conditions was obtained at the Fz channel with a significant difference (ps<0.01), and at the F4 channel with a marginally significant difference (ps<0.065), while the statistical differences across reappraisal goals disappeared at the F3 channel (ps>0.1). The positive stimuli elicited smaller differences in gamma power across the reappraisal goals than the negative stimuli, although both induced a similar pattern of gamma activity. Again, gamma power for the increase condition was higher than that for the other conditions at the F3 channel during the mid-period (increase vs. maintain $t(19) = 2.17$, $p = 0.063$; increase vs. decrease $t(19) = 2.69$, $p<0.05$). There were no significant differences across reappraisal goals during the late-period (ps>0.07). In sum, the negative stimuli generated more enhanced differences in gamma power across reappraisal goals than the positive stimuli.

Gamma phase synchrony

We also tested how gamma phase synchronization across the brain varied across reappraisal goals. From the statistical analysis of PLV differences across different reappraisal goals in each time segment (paired t-tests, $p<0.01$; see Methods and Materials), we constructed a series of topographic maps for the phase-synchronized EEG channel pairs that exhibited significant differences in

PLVs between a pair of reappraisal conditions (see Fig. 5). We observed that relatively more EEG pairs showed higher PLVs in the decrease condition than in the maintain condition, predominantly from 1200 to 2400 ms after stimulus onset. Across all time segments after stimulus onset, 28 pairs showed higher PLVs in the decrease condition, whereas only two pairs showed higher PLVs in the maintain condition. We also found relatively more EEG pairs showing higher PLVs in the increase condition than in the maintain condition, predominantly from 800 to 1200 ms, and 2000 to 3200 ms. Across all time segments, 37 pairs showed higher PLVs with the increase condition, whereas no pair showed higher PLVs with the maintain condition. Between the increase and decrease conditions, few EEG pairs showed significant differences in PLVs.

Discussion

In this study, we investigated how gamma oscillations in human EEG varied with cognitive reappraisal goals to decrease, maintain, or increase emotional responses to external visual stimuli. We analyzed two aspects of gamma oscillations: spectral power and large-scale phase synchronization. We found that frontal gamma power was modulated by reappraisal goals whereby it increased, sustained, or decreased with the regulatory goals of increasing, maintaining, or decreasing emotional responses, respectively. This linear modulation of frontal gamma power with reappraisal goals appeared in the left frontal region during the period of 1926 to 2453 ms after viewing an emotional picture. Regarding large-scale phase synchronization, there were more phase-synchronized pairs of gamma oscillations over the whole brain for the decrease and increase goal conditions compared to the maintain goal condition.

We also observed maximum gamma power over the parietal region regardless of cognitive reappraisal goals. Parietal neural activity related to emotional processing has been largely studied using the LPP. Previous studies have reported that variations in LPP amplitudes were modulated by emotional stimuli [8,10,11] and emotion regulation tasks [9,13,14,53]. Overall, the LPP amplitude was enhanced by emotional stimuli relative to neutral stimuli, and downregulated by cognitive reappraisal. These phenomena were found predominantly in centro-parietal regions and were associated with the degree of attention and the

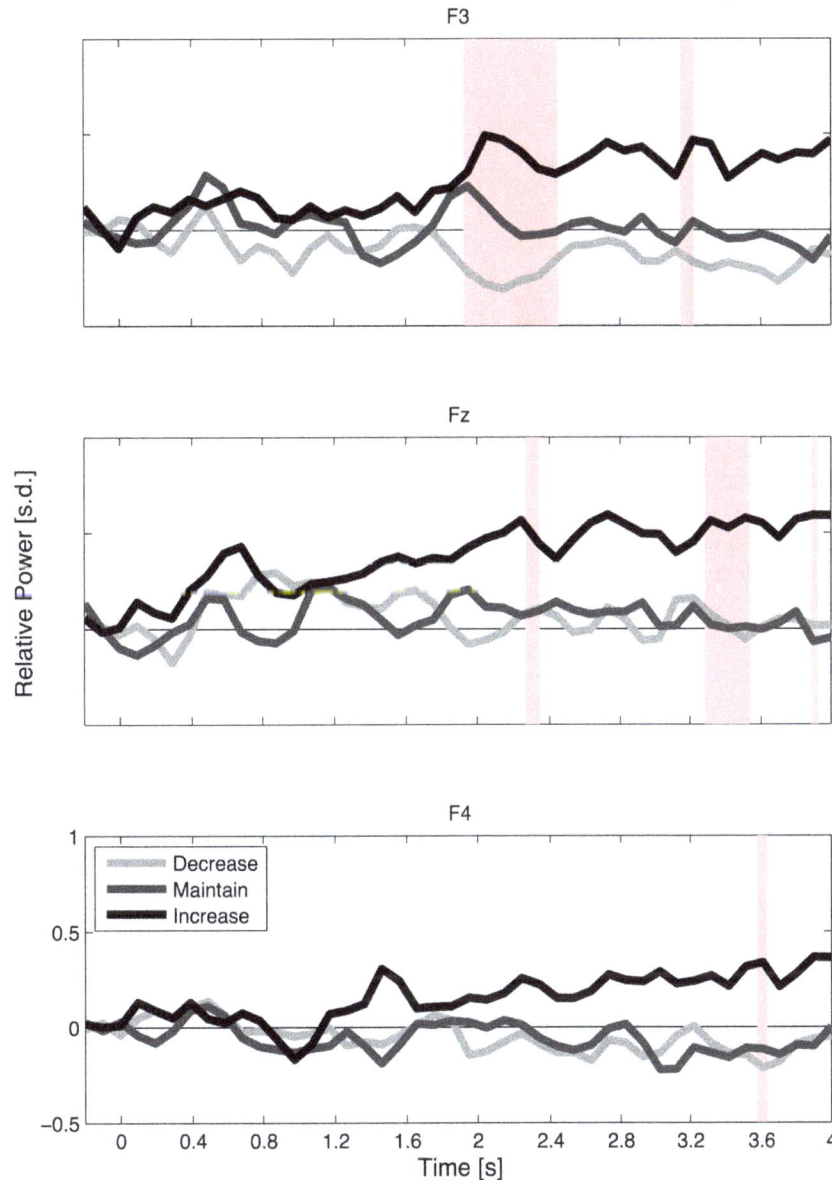

Figure 3. Temporal changes in frontal gamma power. Time-varying gamma activity at the left (F3, top), mid (Fz, mid), and right (F4, bottom) frontal regions during the cognitive reappraisal tasks. Lines indicate the decrease (light gray), maintain (dark gray), and increase (black) conditions. The light red areas in each panel indicate the significant difference durations ($p < 0.01$).

reappraisal of emotional stimuli [13,23,54]. However, there is a lack of evidence for the association of neural mechanisms underlying LPP modulation with the control system of emotion regulation implemented in the frontal cortex. In line with this perspective, Hajcak and colleagues recently addressed the importance of the frontal cortex for emotion regulation, and the necessity of investigating the relationship between gamma oscillations and individual differences in emotional response and regulation [13].

In contrast to the parietal LPP, a close relationship between the frontal cortex and emotion regulation processes has been revealed based on the results from many fMRI studies [15,26,55–57]. Ochsner and colleagues showed that both up and downregulation of negative emotion activated the PFC and the ACC [15]. Additionally, they revealed that upregulation of negative emotion activated the left-hemisphere, whereas downregulation of negative

emotion activated both hemispheres. Using both positive and negative stimuli, Kim and Hamann reported that PFC activity was increased by the regulatory condition and that positive upregulation involved left PFC regions, whereas negative downregulation involved right PFC regions [57]. Furthermore, Urry and colleagues showed that the activity in Brodmann area (BA) 10, a region of the mPFC, was linearly correlated with regulatory goals (i.e., decrease<maintain<increase) [26]. These results suggest that mPFC activity might be associated with regulatory goals for cognitive emotion regulation.

In general, the mPFC has been implicated in a wide range of cognitive tasks, such as mentalizing, problem solving, explicit processing of internal information, emotion regulation, and emotional task execution [24,25,58–60]. According to the gateway hypothesis proposed by Burgess and colleagues, the mPFC is engaged in the goal-directed coordination of stimulus-independent

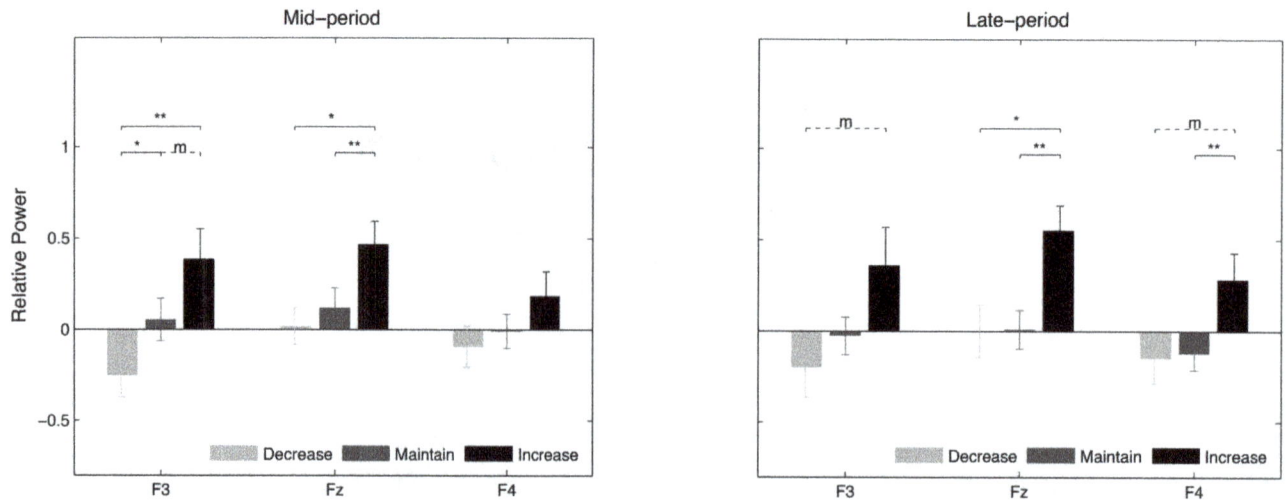

Figure 4. Statistical results in the mid and late interval. Comparison of frontal gamma power across three cognitive reappraisal goals (decrease, light black; maintain, dark gray; increase, black) in the mid (left) and late (right) interval. The error bars indicate standard error of the mean (SEM).

thought (SIT) and stimulus-oriented thought (SOT) when predetermined actions fail to achieve a goal [58]. They also suggested that the function of the mPFC is "metacognition" (i.e., referring to one's own thoughts in a consciously controlled and goal-directed mode) and evaluation, monitoring, or manipulation of internally generated information [58]. The mPFC has also been implicated in cognitive emotion regulation. Olsson and Ochsner reported that the mPFC was involved in the integration of information about internal body states and in the categorization of emotional states [24]. Quirk and Beer suggested that the role of the mPFC in emotion regulation is maintaining the goal of downregulating emotion and transferring this information to the orbitofrontal cortex (OFC), which then effects the suppression of amygdala activity [25]. These previous studies suggest that the mPFC

integrates emotional state information and manipulate a regulatory goal during cognitive reappraisal.

The timing of frontal gamma power modulation during cognitive reappraisal suggests that this modulation reflects a closed-loop system including feedback from the appraisal system. We observed frontal gamma power modulation approximately 2000 ms after stimulus onset. If frontal gamma power solely represented the top-down control process, it should have appeared much earlier than 2000 ms (i.e., top-down emotion regulation effectively reduced the LPP that typically appears 300 to 800 ms) [13]. Therefore, it is likely that our observation of frontal gamma power modulation reflects the maintenance of reappraisal goals by the PFC that is supported by closed-loop information transfer between the control and appraisal systems.

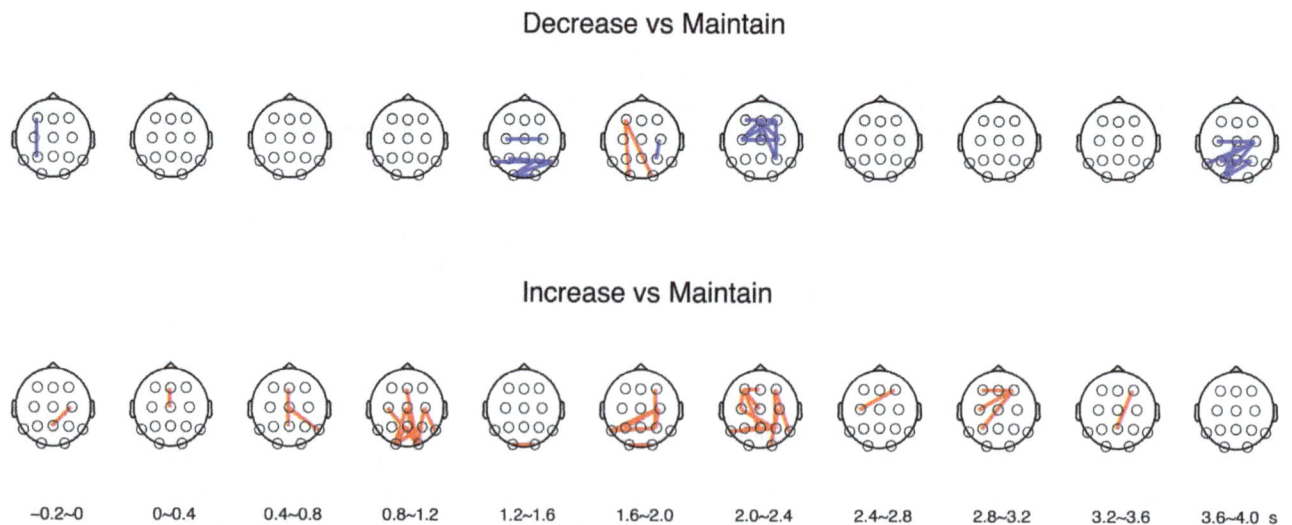

Decrease vs Maintain

Increase vs Maintain

−0.2~0   0~0.4   0.4~0.8   0.8~1.2   1.2~1.6   1.6~2.0   2.0~2.4   2.4~2.8   2.8~3.2   3.2~3.6   3.6~4.0 s

Figure 5. Differences of degree in PLV pairs between cognitive reappraisal conditions. The top panel shows the comparison between the decrease and maintain conditions (red: maintain>decrease; blue: maintain<decrease). The bottom panel depicts the comparison of the degree of PLV in all possible pairs between the increase and maintain conditions (red: increase>maintain; blue: increase<maintain). Significance level is $p < 0.01$. Bottom labels represent the time windows based on visual stimulus onset.

It is also noteworthy that frontal gamma power modulation appeared only during the middle interval, from 1926 to 2453 ms after stimulus onset. Notably, both the significant difference of frontal gamma power across reappraisal goals and the increase of gamma phase synchronization for regulatory efforts occurred simultaneously in this period. After this period, such a difference of frontal gamma power became insignificant and gamma phase synchronization began to decrease (see Fig. 5). This observation suggests that frontal gamma power might reflect cortical representation of emotional states modulated by cognitive reappraisal processes involving regulatory efforts indicated by increases in gamma phase synchronization.

Our results showed the left frontal lateralization of gamma power during cognitive appraisal. Several neuroimaging studies has suggested that left frontal regions was more involved in emotional processing than right frontal regions by showing that differences in BOLD activity modulated by pleasant and unpleasant stimuli were bigger in the left DLPFC than in the right DLPFC [61,62]. Considering the positive correlations between gamma oscillations and BOLD activity [28,29], our results may suggest that left frontal gamma oscillations reflect the cortical representation of emotional states in the left DLPFC modulated by the reappraisal goals.

Overall, we also found strong gamma phase synchronization across EEG channels during cognitive reappraisal that may be an indicator of increased functional connectivity during reappraisal trials. In general, large-scale phase synchronization between brain oscillations represents communication between distant neural assemblies [63]. Furthermore, increased gamma phase synchronization has been observed in many cognitive tasks, including visual perception [47,49,50], learning [64], emotional processing [35], and emotion regulation [36]. These studies indicate that conscious cognitive efforts, such as cognitive reappraisal, elicit increases in large-scale gamma phase synchronization in the brain. Our findings are also in line with previous fMRI studies showing an increased functional coupling between cortical and subcortical regions during conscious reappraisal of emotions [21,27,65].

Furthermore, we observed that gamma phase synchronization appeared earlier in the increase condition than in the decrease condition (see Fig. 5). We surmise that this temporal difference might be related to the level of regulatory difficulty. Previous studies reported that decreasing emotion was more difficult than increasing emotion [15,57], owing to the difficulty of reversing emotional reactivity. Therefore, it is likely that faster gamma phase synchronization in the increase condition compared to the decrease condition was due to the relatively easy and fast execution of emotion regulation.

Despite these robust effects of frontal gamma activity associated with cognitive reappraisal, there are still several limitations to our study that should be addressed by future work. First, since we mainly focused on the temporal variations of brain oscillations modulated by different stimulus types and reappraisal goals, the number of EEG channels was insufficient to represent variations of local gamma power and global gamma phase synchronization. In fact, this limitation kept us from applying EEG source localization methods to investigate gamma oscillation sources in the frontal cortex and other regions. Additionally, it would be interesting to examine functional connectivity between localized sources that are related to emotional regulatory processes. Second, we excluded neutral stimuli in this study to ensure the presence of emotional responses in all cognitive reappraisal conditions. The use of neutral stimuli might be confusing in our study, as it would have been difficult for participants to manipulate their emotional responses to neutral stimuli without evoked emotions. Thus, neutral stimuli might result in unexpected cognitive processes irrelevant to emotion regulation when participants attempt to reappraise their responses. However, the exclusion of neutral stimuli in our study raises the issue of confirmation of emotional responses modulated by the pictures, because the participants' responses between emotional and neutral stimuli might have provided support for the validity of emotional responses elicited by the different picture set. To partially resolve this issue, we selected a set of pictures from the in-house picture database with high-arousal normative ratings. This database was standardized in terms of ratings in arousal and valence, and we carefully collected pictures such that their arousal ratings were clearly higher than for the neutral pictures ($p<0.01$). In addition, a recent study by Ahn and colleagues on emotional memory effects, using the same stimuli as in our study, showed that these emotional pictures were recalled better than neutral pictures one week after presentation, supporting the notion that this picture set elicited emotional responses in participants [16]. However, to completely confirm the induction of emotional experiences by our stimulus set, it would be necessary to use neutral stimuli together with emotional ones in future studies.

In addition, previous studies have reported stimulus-preceding negativity (SPN), an ERP component, which was generally elicited before the onset of stimulus during the emotion regulation [14,66]. According to these studies, the SPN amplitude during the preparation period was modulated by emotion regulation conditions. Therefore, it would be interesting to investigate in future studies how neural oscillations (particularly gamma oscillations) are modulated by cognitive reappraisal during this preparation period.

Identifying neural correlates of emotion regulation processes may aid in the development of new methods for the treatment of emotion-related psychiatric disorders. For example, a cognitive training program that provides neurofeedback may assist patients in regulating their emotional responses in real-time. In fact, recent studies have demonstrated the feasibility of providing online feedback for emotion regulation by presenting the amygdala activity from BOLD signals in real time [67–69]. However, current fMRI-based methods possess critical weaknesses, including a significant time delay from neural activity to presentation, and environmental restrictions during the magnetic resonance (MR) scanning (e.g., the subject must lie inside the scanner). In contrast, an EEG-based method can provide greater mobility and a finer time resolution that is critical for online feedback. Recent advances in the development of dry and mobile EEG sensors would add practicality to the use of EEG in neurofeedback applications. However, little effort has been made to utilize EEG signals for neurofeedback of emotion regulation, predominantly because of the lack of evidence for EEG correlates of regulation goals. However, our results indicating the representation of regulatory goals in frontal gamma activity of EEG may provide a new opportunity to develop effective neurofeedback training systems for emotion regulation.

Author Contributions

Conceived and designed the experiments: HTK SPK. Performed the experiments: JWJ SHK. Analyzed the data: JHK. Wrote the paper: JHK.

References

1. Bonanno GA, Papa A, Lalande K, Westphal M, Coifman K (2004) The importance of being flexible: the ability to both enhance and suppress emotional expression predicts long-term adjustment. Psychological Science 15: 482–487. doi:10.1111/j.0956-7976.2004.00705.x.

2. Davidson RJ (2000) Dysfunction in the Neural Circuitry of Emotion Regulation– A Possible Prelude to Violence. Science 289: 591–594. doi:10.1126/science.289.5479.591.

3. Phillips ML, Ladouceur CD, Drevets WC (2008) A neural model of voluntary and automatic emotion regulation: implications for understanding the pathophysiology and neurodevelopment of bipolar disorder. Mol Psychiatry 13: 833–857. doi:10.1038/mp.2008.65.

4. Gross JJ (1998) Antecedent- and response-focused emotion regulation: divergent consequences for experience, expression, and physiology. Journal of Personality and Social Psychology 74: 224–237.

5. Gross JJ (1998) The emerging field of emotion regulation: An integrative review. Review of general psychology 2: 271.

6. Gross JJ (2002) Emotion regulation: affective, cognitive, and social consequences. Psychophysiology 39: 281–291.

7. Hayes JP, Morey RA, Petty CM, Seth S, Smoski MJ, et al. (2010) Staying cool when things get hot: emotion regulation modulates neural mechanisms of memory encoding. Front Hum Neurosci 4: 230. doi:10.3389/fnhum.2010.00230.

8. Cuthbert BN, Schupp HT, Bradley MM, Birbaumer N, Lang PJ (2000) Brain potentials in affective picture processing: covariation with autonomic arousal and affective report. Biological Psychology 52: 95–111.

9. Hajcak G, Nieuwenhuis S (2006) Reappraisal modulates the electrocortical response to unpleasant pictures. Cognitive, Affective, & Behavioral Neuroscience 6: 291–297.

10. Keil A, Bradley MM, Hauk O, Rockstroh B, Elbert T, et al. (2002) Large-scale neural correlates of affective picture processing. Psychophysiology 39: 641–649.

11. Schupp HT, Cuthbert BN, Bradley MM, Cacioppo JT, Ito T, et al. (2000) Affective picture processing: the late positive potential is modulated by motivational relevance. Psychophysiology 37: 257–261.

12. Liu Y, Huang H, McGinnis-Deweese M, Keil A, Ding M (2012) Neural Substrate of the Late Positive Potential in Emotional Processing. Journal of Neuroscience 32: 14563–14572. doi:10.1523/JNEUROSCI.3109-12.2012.

13. Hajcak G, MacNamara A, Olvet DM (2010) Event-Related Potentials, Emotion, and Emotion Regulation: An Integrative Review. Developmental Neuropsychology 35: 129–155. doi:10.1080/87565640903526504.

14. Moser JS, Krompinger JW, Dietz J, Simons RF (2009) Electrophysiological correlates of decreasing and increasing emotional responses to unpleasant pictures. Psychophysiology 46: 17–27. doi:10.1111/j.1469-8986.2008.00721.x.

15. Ochsner KN, Ray RD, Cooper JC, Robertson ER, Chopra S, et al. (2004) For better or for worse: neural systems supporting the cognitive down- and up-regulation of negative emotion. NeuroImage 23: 483–499. doi:10.1016/j.neuroimage.2004.06.030.

16. Davidson RJ (2002) Anxiety and affective style: role of prefrontal cortex and amygdala. Biol Psychiatry 51: 68–80.

17. Goldin PR, McRae K, Ramel W, Gross JJ (2008) The Neural Bases of Emotion Regulation: Reappraisal and Suppression of Negative Emotion. Biol Psychiatry 63: 577–586. doi:10.1016/j.biopsych.2007.05.031.

18. Kim H, Somerville LH, Johnstone T, Alexander AL, Whalen PJ (2003) Inverse amygdala and medial prefrontal cortex responses to surprised faces. NeuroReport 14: 2317–2322. doi:10.1097/01.wnr.0000101520.44335.20.

19. Ochsner KN, Bunge SA, Gross JJ, Gabrieli JDE (2002) Rethinking feelings: an FMRI study of the cognitive regulation of emotion. J Cogn Neurosci 14: 1215–1229. doi:10.1162/089892902760807212.

20. Phan KL, Fitzgerald DA, Nathan PJ, Moore GJ, Uhde TW, et al. (2005) Neural substrates for voluntary suppression of negative affect: A functional magnetic resonance imaging study. Biol Psychiatry 57: 210–219. doi:10.1016/j.biopsych.2004.10.030.

21. Banks SJ, Eddy KT, Angstadt M, Nathan PJ, Phan KL (2007) Amygdala-frontal connectivity during emotion regulation. Social Cognitive and Affective Neuroscience 2: 303–312. doi:10.1093/scan/nsm029.

22. Urry HL, van Reekum CM, Johnstone T, Davidson RJ (2009) Individual differences in some (but not all) medial prefrontal regions reflect cognitive demand while regulating unpleasant emotion. NeuroImage 47: 852–863. doi:10.1016/j.neuroimage.2009.05.069.

23. Hajcak G, Moser JS, Simons RF (2006) Attending to affect: Appraisal strategies modulate the electrocortical response to arousing pictures. Emotion 6: 517–522. doi:10.1037/1528-3542.6.3.517.

24. Olsson A, Ochsner KN (2008) The role of social cognition in emotion. Trends in Cognitive Sciences 12: 65–71. doi:10.1016/j.tics.2007.11.010.

25. Quirk GJ, Beer JS (2006) Prefrontal involvement in the regulation of emotion: convergence of rat and human studies. Current Opinion in Neurobiology 16: 723–727. doi:10.1016/j.conb.2006.07.004.

26. Urry HL, van Reekum CM, Johnstone T, Kalin NH, Thurow ME, et al. (2006) Amygdala and ventromedial prefrontal cortex are inversely coupled during regulation of negative affect and predict the diurnal pattern of cortisol secretion among older adults. Journal of Neuroscience 26: 4415–4425. doi:10.1523/JNEUROSCI.3215-05.2006.

27. Stein JL, Wiedholz LM, Bassett DS, Weinberger DR, Zink CF, et al. (2007) A validated network of effective amygdala connectivity. NeuroImage 36: 736–745. doi:10.1016/j.neuroimage.2007.03.022.

28. Foucher JR, Otzenberger H, Gounot D (2003) The BOLD response and the gamma oscillations respond differently than evoked potentials: an interleaved EEG-fMRI study. BMC Neuroscience 4: 22. doi:10.1186/1471-2202-4-22.

29. Magri C, Schridde U, Murayama Y, Panzeri S, Logothetis NK (2012) The Amplitude and Timing of the BOLD Signal Reflects the Relationship between Local Field Potential Power at Different Frequencies. Journal of Neuroscience 32: 1395–1407. doi:10.1523/JNEUROSCI.3985-11.2012.

30. Onton J, Makeig S (2009) High-frequency Broadband Modulations of Electroencephalographic Spectra. Front Hum Neurosci 3: 61. doi:10.3389/neuro.09.061.2009.

31. Keil A, Gruber T, Müller MM (2001) Functional correlates of macroscopic high-frequency brain activity in the human visual system. Neuroscience and Biobehavioral Reviews 25: 527–534.

32. Müller MM, Keil A, Gruber T, Elbert T (1999) Processing of affective pictures modulates right-hemispheric gamma band EEG activity. Clin Neurophysiol 110: 1913–1920.

33. Müller MM, Gruber T, Keil A (2000) Modulation of induced gamma band activity in the human EEG by attention and visual information processing. Int J Psychophysiol 38: 283–299.

34. Balconi M, Lucchiari C (2008) Consciousness and arousal effects on emotional face processing as revealed by brain oscillations. A gamma band analysis. Int J Psychophysiol 67: 41–46. doi:10.1016/j.ijpsycho.2007.10.002.

35. Martini N, Menicucci D, Sebastiani L, Bedini R, Pingitore A, et al. (2012) The dynamics of EEG gamma responses to unpleasant visual stimuli: From local activity to functional connectivity. NeuroImage 60: 922–932. doi:10.1016/j.neuroimage.2012.01.060.

36. Popov T, Steffen A, Weisz N, Miller GA, Rockstroh B (2012) Cross-frequency dynamics of neuromagnetic oscillatory activity: Two mechanisms of emotion regulation. Psychophysiology 49: 1545–1557. doi:10.1111/j.1469-8986.2012.01484.x.

37. Kaiser J, Lutzenberger W (2003) Induced Gamma-Band Activity and Human Brain Function. neuroscientist 9: 475–484. doi:10.1177/1073858403259137.

38. Joormann J, Yoon KL, Siemer M (2010) Cognition and emotion regulation. Emotion regulation and psychopathology: A transdiagnostic approach to etiology and treatment: 174–203.

39. Tolegenova AA, Kustubayeva AM, Matthews G (2014) Personality and Individual Differences. Pers Individ Dif 65: 75–80. doi:10.1016/j.paid.2014.01.028.

40. Jaušovec N, Jaušovec K (2010) Emotional intelligence and gender: A neurophysiological perspective: 109–126.

41. Berkovich-Ohana A, Glicksohn J, Goldstein A (2012) Mindfulness-induced changes in gamma band activity - implications for the default mode network, self-reference and attention. Clin Neurophysiol 123: 700–710. doi:10.1016/j.clinph.2011.07.048.

42. Chambers R, Gullone E, Allen NB (2009) Mindful emotion regulation: An integrative review. Clinical Psychology Review 29: 560–572. doi:10.1016/j.cpr.2009.06.005.

43. Chiesa A, Serretti A, Jakobsen JC (2013) Mindfulness: Top–down or bottom–up emotion regulation strategy? Clinical Psychology Review 33: 82–96. doi:10.1016/j.cpr.2012.10.006.

44. Bhattacharya J, Petsche H, Feldmann U, Rescher B (2001) EEG gamma-band phase synchronization between posterior and frontal cortex during mental rotation in humans. Neuroscience Letters 311: 29–32.

45. Gandal MJ, Edgar JC, Klook K, Siegel SJ (2012) Gamma synchrony: Towards a translational biomarker for the treatment-resistant symptoms of schizophrenia. Neuropharmacology 62: 1504–1518. doi:10.1016/j.neuropharm.2011.02.007.

46. Ahn HM, Kim SA, Hwang IJ, Jeong JW, Kim H-T, et al. (2013) The effect of cognitive reappraisal on long-term emotional experience and emotional memory. J Neuropsychol: n/a–n/a. Available: http://www.scopus.com/inward/record.url?eid=2-s2.0-84889991377&partnerID=40&md5=e6f7a283dd661f70291e218446fb1210.

47. Tallon-Baudry C, Bertrand O, Delpuech C, Pernier J (1996) Stimulus specificity of phase-locked and non-phase-locked 40 Hz visual responses in human. J Neurosci 16: 4240–4249.

48. Lachaux JP, Rodriguez E, Martinerie J, Varela FJ (1999) Measuring phase synchrony in brain signals. Hum Brain Mapp 8: 194–208.

49. Rodriguez E, George N, Lachaux JP, Martinerie J, Renault B, et al. (1999) Perception's shadow: long-distance synchronization of human brain activity. Nature 397: 430–433. doi:10.1038/17120.

50. Trujillo LT, Peterson MA, Kaszniak AW, Allen JJB (2005) EEG phase synchrony differences across visual perception conditions may depend on recording and analysis methods. Clinical Neurophysiology 116: 172–189. doi:10.1016/j.clinph.2004.07.025.

51. Penny WD, Duzel E, Miller KJ, Ojemann JG (2008) Testing for nested oscillation. Journal of Neuroscience Methods 174: 50–61. doi:10.1016/j.jneumeth.2008.06.035.

52. Kang J-H, Ahn HM, Jeong JW, Hwang I, Kim H-T, et al. (2012) The modulation of parietal gamma oscillations in the human electroencephalogram

with cognitive reappraisal. NeuroReport 23: 995–999. doi:10.1097/WNR.0b013e32835a6475.

53. Moser JS, Most SB, Simons RF (2010) Increasing negative emotions by reappraisal enhances subsequent cognitive control: A combined behavioral and electrophysiological study. Cognitive, Affective, & Behavioral Neuroscience 10: 195–207. doi:10.3758/CABN.10.2.195.

54. Krompinger JW, Moser JS, Simons RF (2008) Modulations of the electrophysiological response to pleasant stimuli by cognitive reappraisal. Emotion 8: 132–137. doi:10.1037/1528-3542.8.1.132.

55. Ghashghaei HT, Hilgetag CC, Barbas H (2007) Sequence of information processing for emotions based on the anatomic dialogue between prefrontal cortex and amygdala. NeuroImage 34: 905–923. doi:10.1016/j.neuroimage.2006.09.046.

56. Ghashghaei HT, Barbas H (2002) Pathways for emotion: interactions of prefrontal and anterior temporal pathways in the amygdala of the rhesus monkey. Neuroscience 115: 1261–1279.

57. Kim SH, Hamann S (2007) Neural correlates of positive and negative emotion regulation. J Cogn Neurosci 19: 776–798. doi:10.1162/jocn.2007.19.5.776.

58. Burgess PW, Simons JS, Dumontheil I, Gilbert SJ, Duncan J, et al. (2005) Measuring the mind: Speed, control, and age.

59. Gilbert SJ, Spengler S, Simons JS, Steele JD, Lawrie SM, et al. (2006) Functional specialization within rostral prefrontal cortex (area 10): a meta-analysis. J Cogn Neurosci 18: 932–948. doi:10.1162/jocn.2006.18.6.932.

60. Ramnani N, Owen AM (2004) Anterior prefrontal cortex: insights into function from anatomy and neuroimaging. Nat Rev Neurosci 5: 184–194. doi:10.1038/nrn1343.

61. Herrington JD, Mohanty A, Koven NS, Fisher JE, Stewart JL, et al. (2005) Emotion-Modulated Performance and Activity in Left Dorsolateral Prefrontal Cortex. Emotion 5: 200–207. doi:10.1037/1528-3542.5.2.200.

62. Miller GA, Crocker LD, Spielberg JM, Infantolino ZP, Heller W (2013) Issues in localization of brain function: the case of lateralized frontal cortex in cognition, emotion, and psychopathology. Frontiers in integrative neuroscience 7. doi:10.3389/fnint.2013.00002/abstract.

63. Fell J, Axmacher N (2011) The role of phase synchronization in memory processes. Nat Rev Neurosci 12: 105–118. doi:10.1038/nrn2979.

64. Gruber T, Keil A, Müller MM (2001) Modulation of induced gamma band responses and phase synchrony in a paired associate learning task in the human EEG. Neuroscience Letters 316: 29–32.

65. Wager TD, Davidson ML, Hughes BL, Lindquist MA, Ochsner KN (2008) Prefrontal-Subcortical Pathways Mediating Successful Emotion Regulation. Neuron 59: 1037–1050. doi:10.1016/j.neuron.2008.09.006.

66. Thiruchselvam R, Blechert J, Sheppes G, Rydstrom A, Gross JJ (2011) Biological Psychology. Biological Psychology 87: 84–92. doi:10.1016/j.biopsycho.2011.02.009.

67. Hamilton JP, Glover GH, Hsu J-J, Johnson RF, Gotlib IH (2010) Modulation of subgenual anterior cingulate cortex activity with real-time neurofeedback. Hum Brain Mapp 32: 22–31. doi:10.1002/hbm.20997.

68. Johnston SJ, Boehm SG, Healy D, Goebel R, Linden DEJ (2010) Neurofeedback: A promising tool for the self-regulation of emotion networks. NeuroImage 49: 1066–1072. doi:10.1016/j.neuroimage.2009.07.056.

69. Zotev V, Krueger F, Phillips R, Alvarez RP, Simmons WK, et al. (2011) Self-Regulation of Amygdala Activation Using Real-Time fMRI Neurofeedback. PLoS ONE 6: e24522. doi:10.1371/journal.pone.0024522.t003.

26

Towards an Optimization of Stimulus Parameters for Brain-Computer Interfaces Based on Steady State Visual Evoked Potentials

Anna Duszyk[1][*][◑], Maria Bierzyńska[3][◑], Zofia Radzikowska[1], Piotr Milanowski[2], Rafał Kuś[2], Piotr Suffczyński[2], Magdalena Michalska[2], Maciej Łabęcki[2], Piotr Zwoliński[4], Piotr Durka[2]

1 University of Social Sciences and Humanities, Warsaw, Poland, 2 University of Warsaw, Faculty of Physics, Warsaw, Poland, 3 Nencki Institute of Experimental Biology PAS, Warsaw, Poland, 4 Warsaw Memorial Child Hospital, Department of Neurosurgery, Warsaw, Poland

Abstract

Efforts to construct an effective brain-computer interface (BCI) system based on Steady State Visual Evoked Potentials (SSVEP) commonly focus on sophisticated mathematical methods for data analysis. The role of different stimulus features in evoking strong SSVEP is less often considered and the knowledge on the optimal stimulus properties is still fragmentary. The goal of this study was to provide insight into the influence of stimulus characteristics on the magnitude of SSVEP response. Five stimuli parameters were tested: size, distance, colour, shape, and presence of a fixation point in the middle of each flickering field. The stimuli were presented on four squares on LCD screen, with each square highlighted by LEDs flickering with different frequencies. Brighter colours and larger dimensions of flickering fields resulted in a significantly stronger SSVEP response. The distance between stimulation fields and the presence or absence of the fixation point had no significant effect on the response. Contrary to a popular belief, these results suggest that absence of the fixation point does not reduce the magnitude of SSVEP response. However, some parameters of the stimuli such as colour and the size of the flickering field play an important role in evoking SSVEP response, which indicates that stimuli rendering is an important factor in building effective SSVEP based BCI systems.

Editor: Gennady Cymbalyuk, Georgia State University, United States of America

Funding: This research was financed from Polish funds for science and the project "Optimisation of stimuli for SSVEP-based Brain Computer Interfaces based on psychophysiology of phenomenon" realized within the Ventures Programme of Foundation for Polish Science, operated within the Innovative Economy Operational Programme (IE OP) 2007–2013 within European Regional Development Fund. The funders had no role in study design, data collection and analysis, decision to publish, or preparation of the manuscript.

Competing Interests: The authors have declared that no competing interests exist.

* Email: aduszyk@st.swps.edu.pl

◑ These authors contributed equally to this work.

Introduction

Individuals with neuromuscular disorders such as multiple sclerosis, amyotrophic lateral sclerosis, and locked-in syndrome have no voluntary control of their muscles and are often unable to communicate. Brain Computer Interface (BCI) systems give them an opportunity to have contact with the external world and accomplish simple, everyday activities. BCI systems are most frequently based on recordings of the brain's electrical activity from the scalp (electroencephalogram, EEG) because of the relatively low price and portability. In this study we investigated a BCI system based on the Steady State Visual Evoked Potentials (SSVEP) phenomenon.

SSVEPs can be detected mainly in EEG signals recorded from above the visual areas of the scalp as a response to stimulation with light flickering with fixed frequency [1]. During such stimulation, increases in EEG power at the frequency of stimulation can be observed. SSVEPs are detected at stimulus frequency, its harmonics and subharmonics [2]. The SSVEP spectrum shows characteristic peaks which are relatively stable over time [3], [2]. Stimuli eliciting SSVEP can be characterized by different properties which affect the strength of the response, like colour and shape.

Perception of visual stimuli depends on characteristics of the human nervous system. In order to explain presented results we need first to describe briefly the operating principles of the visual system, because its features influence the processing of particular stimuli. SSVEP generation is as an outcome of stimulation repeated with certain frequency, so motion perception seems to be the prime to generate this type of response.

The human visual system consists of three parallel information processing pathways: Parvocellular (PC), Magnocellular (MC), and Koniocellular (KC) [4]. Each of them is responsible for processing specific physical parameters of the stimulus and is characterized by different temporal and spatial resolutions (see: [4], [5]). The magnocellular pathway originates from L and M cones in the retina. It is sensitive to differences in achromatic contrast and motion [6], and carries information about depth [4]. The receptive fields of the MC pathway are relatively large [7] and exhibit a transient response to changes in retinal stimulation, which begins and ends quickly [8]. The PC pathway mainly carries information about colour (red and green) and shape [9].

Receptive fields of this pathway are typically half the size of magnocellular fields [4] and exhibit a more sustained response to changes in retinal stimulation [8]. The KC pathway carries information about blue and yellow colour and reacts to spectral stimuli [10]. Visual pathways play a crucial role in the formation of SSVEPs at the cortical level. We expected that stimuli processed by the MC pathway (e.g. brighter and larger), which is responsible for perception of motion, would evoke the biggest SSVEP amplitude.

Colour seems to be the most evident feature to be examined, because the visual pathways process different colours in different ways. Experiments performed by Regan in 1966 (see also [1]) showed that blue, red, and yellow stimuli presented at certain frequencies evoke SSVEPs with different magnitudes. Red stimuli gave the strongest response in 11 Hz, while blue stimuli were less sensitive to frequencies and gave the strongest response in 13 Hz. SSVEP elicited by yellow stimuli was least dependent on frequency and gave the lowest response. An impact of frequency and different colour interaction was shown by Gerloff [11]. A checkerboard with different combinations of hues and flickering with frequencies ranging from 6 to 17 Hz was used to evoke SSVEPs. However, results of this study do not allow for inference on the relation of stimulation colour to amplitude of SSVEP and are characterized by large intra- and inter-subject variability.

A review of 59 papers written by Zhu in 2010 [12] indicates that green, black, gray, red, and white are currently the most commonly used stimuli colours in SSVEP-based BCIs. However, it is not known which of these colours is best for SSVEP-based BCIs, as none of these experiments directly investigated the influence of colour on strength of the SSVEP response.

Knowledge about the influence of stimulus size on SSVEP response seems to be crucial in the design of graphic user interfaces, because the size of a single flickering field determines the number of simultaneously presented stimuli. Another important parameter of stimuli used in SSVEP-BCI's is the distance between flickering fields. Knowledge about the influence of these parameters on brain response is crucial for an optimal design of BCI systems.

As for the shapes and patterns of the stimuli, Zhu [12] concluded that checkerboards, squares, and rectangles are the most common in BCI-related studies. However, author concludes that no general conclusion can be drawn about their influence on the strength of SSVEP response. In an experiment from 2007 [13], plain stimuli gave stronger SSVEP response than checkerboards and striped stimuli. Due to different shapes of receptive fields in successive stages of information processing in the visual system, one can hypothesize that square stimuli will evoke better response than circular ones [14]. Spatial attention is another factor that can influence the SSVEP response. Amplitude of the response can change as a function of the user's concentration on the stimulus [15], [16], [17]. It is generally assumed that presence of a fixation point minimizes undesired eye movements and helps users to concentrate on the chosen stimulus [18]. Environmental conditions should also be considered; for example it was shown that a darkened room has positive influence on the strength of the SSVEP response [19].

On the other hand, it seems that a stimulus evoking strong SSVEP response in particular single trial is not identical to the most optimal stimulus in BCI systems. A selection of stimulus parameters to BCI systems ought to take into account both the physiological and psychological processes. It is known that high intensity stimulus evokes the strongest response of sensory systems. However, the stronger stimulus is perceive, the faster a user gets tired and the weaker focus of attention becomes. It seems that a

compromise to both point of view: to maximize a strength of cerebral response and minimalize a fatigue and displeasure. Based on physiological research we hypothesized that the big and fair stimuli evoke magnitude of SSVEP, but we were interested in whether in case of long and tiring stimulation less aggressive stimuli give better results.

Overall, the existing state of the art does not clarify which choices of stimuli features are the best for SSVEP-based BCIs. Nevertheless, many studies conclude that experimental design and paradigm are crucial in developing efficient BCI systems [5], [20].

In this study we investigate the parameters of stimuli, which positively affect the magnitude of SSVEP response measured by EEG. The experimental paradigm was designed to simulate a real BCI system as close as possible. Block of trials lasted ~45 minutes, which is a period of time sufficient to write a short massage by potential BCI-user. The goal was to measure the strength of the SSVEP response related to parameters of the stimuli as well as to the psychological factors such as focus of attention, motivation and tiredness. In two experiments we systematically measure the SSVEP response to stimuli with varying parameters, including colour, size, shape, inter-stimulus distance, and presence or absence of a fixation point.

Materials and Methods

Results presented in this paper come from two consecutive experiments. Experiment I was a test of five stimulus parameters that could potentially influence the magnitude of SSVEP response over a relatively wide range of their values. Based upon its results, three parameters with narrowed ranges were chosen for the second experiment conducted on a larger group of subjects.

1. Participants

In Experiment I, five young adults ($M_{age} = 25.8$; SD $= 1.79$) of both sexes were examined. 20 subjects participated in Experiment II ($M_{age} = 27.2$; SD $= 3.3$). All subjects were screened for photogenic epilepsy, neurological and psychiatric disorders, and use of medications known to adversely affect EEG recording. No financial compensation was given. All participants were informed about the experiment procedure and signed a written consent.

2. Experimental setup

Both experiments were carried out in a darkened room with windows curtained. Two desk lamps were the only light sources. Subjects were sitting on a chair one meter from the center of the display. Experiments were divided into sessions. Lengths of the breaks between sessions were controlled by the participant. Each session lasted 45 minutes and each trial included 4 seconds of stimulation and a 6 second rest period. Each of the presented stimuli was repeated 30 times.

Four stimuli were presented simultaneously and subjects were asked to concentrate on the one indicated by an auditory cue. The schematic sequence of events is presented in Fig. 1. Experiment I consisted of 4 s long stimulation periods interleaved by 6 s long resting periods. The screen was black during the rest period. In order to create experimental conditions corresponding to the SSVEP paradigm used in BCI systems, all four fields were simultaneously active (each flickering at a different frequency) during the stimulation intervals. Four frequencies of stimulation (14, 17, 25, and 30 Hz) were chosen on the basis of the results obtained by Kuś [21]. Investigated parameters (colour, size, etc.) were software controlled and randomly presented on an LCD screen, while the flickering was generated by the underlaid LEDs. Stimuli were presented on a hybrid device [22] constructed at the

Faculty of Physics, University of Warsaw in order to optimize stability of stimuli rendering. The device consists of an array of LEDs underlaid below an LCD screen (195 mm high and 350 mm wide), where the LEDs highlight precisely determined area of the screen. Each of the four squares displayed on the LCD screen is highlighted by a group of LEDs, flickering with frequencies controlled by the software. Using such a device eliminates problems with monitor refresh rate and at the same time enables full control of stimulus appearance.

3. Experiment I

The first experiment was designed to investigate the influence of five parameters — shape, colour, distance between stimuli, size, and presence or absence of the fixation point — on the magnitude of SSVEP response. Four sizes (angular size in degrees) were investigated: $\sim0.57°$, $\sim1.49°$, $\sim2.6°$, and ~3.72. Stimuli were organized in three different inter-stimulus distance settings: next to each other (no distance $=0°$), centered on each stimulus area (medium distance $= \sim2.3°$), and on the opposite points of the presentation area (long distance $= \sim4.93°$). The five examined colours were chosen from the RGB model: blue, red, green, white, and yellow. The luminance of white and yellow stimuli was 30 lx, green - 20 lx, red - 12 lx, blue – 4 lx, and black background - 2 lx. Two stimuli shapes were used: square and circle (both had equal surface areas). The absence and presence of a fixation point located in the middle of each flickering field was also examined. A detailed description of the investigated stimuli is listed in Table 1. This experiment consisted of six sessions of 45 minutes each.

4. Experiment II

Based upon the results of Experiment I, we chose three parameters for further investigation in Experiment II and conducted it on a larger population using more restricted ranges of variability. We did not further investigate the shape and inter-stimulus distance, because these parameters showed no significant influence on the response in Experiment I. We restricted the variability of remaining parameters to the following ranges: colours yellow, white, and red, sizes $\sim2.6°$ and $\sim3.72°$. Additionally presence/absence of fixation point was tested due

to participants' suggestion that it had helped them to concentrate This parameter was a substitute of signs which are located in the flickering field in real BCI systems. Detailed parameters of selected stimuli are given in Table 2. Presented stimuli were circular as this shape evoked slightly stronger SSVEP-response; however, this difference was not statistically significant.

5. Data acquisition

The EEG data acquisition was performed using the EasyCap EEG positioning system and a 32-channel Porti 7 amplifier made by TMSI. It was connected to the computer via a USB interface using optical fiber. The scalp area was prepared before placing the electrodes and conductive gel was used in order to reduce skin impedance.

The data was recorded with a 1024 Hz sampling rate. Skin impedance was maintained below 5k Ohms. 20 electrodes were used. 19 electrodes were placed in a 10–20 system and there was one additional electrode FCz. Averaged signal from mastoids (M1 and M2 electrodes) was used as a reference. The ground electrode was placed on the chest near the breastbone area. Dedicated software was used for data acquisition and stimuli presentation. This software is available on terms of the GPL license from http://git.braintech.pl and http://braintech.pl/svarog.

6. Ethics statement

The project was approved by the Research Ethics Committee at University of Social Sciences and Humanities in Warsaw, Poland. All participants declared the absence of neurological and mental illnesses, and were screened against the photosensitive epilepsy with the standard clinical EEG test. Informed, written consent was obtained from all of the participants.

7. Data analysis

7.1. Signal pre-processing. Seven channels from occipital and parietal areas were chosen for analysis: O1, O2, Pz, P3, P4, P7, and P8, all down-sampled to 128Hz. Placement of these electrodes corresponds to primary (O1 and O2) and secondary visual areas, thus the signal collected from these areas should be the most significant in terms of SSVEP response energy (Pastor,

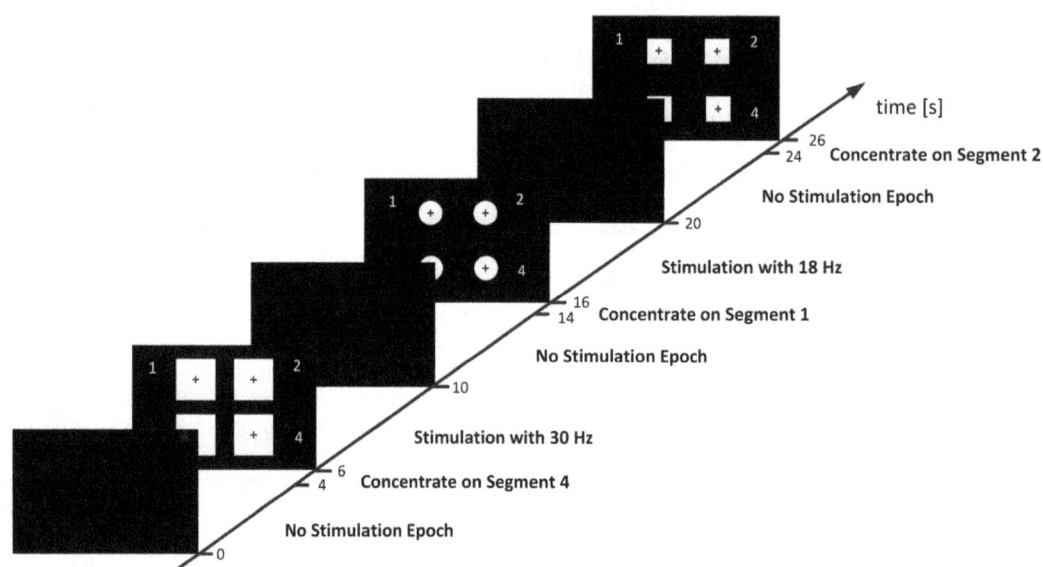

Figure 1. Time course of the experimental paradigm.

Table 1. Parameters of the stimulus used in Experiment I.

Tested parameter	Dimension	Inter-stimulus distance	Fixation point	Stimulus colour	Shape
Size	~0.57°, ~1.49°, ~2.60°, ~3.72°	~4.76°, ~3.50°, ~2.30°, ~1.26°	yes	white	square
Inter-stimulus distance	~2.60°	0° , ~2.30°, ~5.27°	yes	white	square
Colour	~2.60°	~2.30°	yes	white, red, green, yellow, blue	square
Absence of fixation point	~2.60°	~2.30°	no	white	square
Shape	~2.60°	~2.30°	yes	white	circle, square

2003). Downsampling was conducted using a Chebyshev type I filter of order 8. Next, from specified channels, two classes of segments were extracted: 4s long epochs of signal recorded during the visual stimulation with frequency f denoted as x_f^+ and 4s long epochs measured before the onset of stimulation with frequency f, marked as x_f^-.

7.2. Frequency domain filtering. We expected that the most prominent changes in EEG signal during the visual stimulation would be observed at the stimulation frequency. Therefore, all segments in both classes were band-pass filtered by means of a 3rd order elliptic filter with pass-band centered at the given frequency stimulation f. The width of the pass- band was 2 Hz. The level of the filter peak-to-peak ripple in the pass-band was 0.04 dB, whereas the minimum stop-band attenuation was 40 dB. The filtered time series are denoted as y_f^+ and y_f^-.

7.3. Spatial filtering. It is important to combine information carried in analyzed channels to estimate the SSVEP response. Analyzing each channel separately can be misleading, as the SSVEP changes significantly not only from subject to subject but also as far as topology is concerned. This means that to observe the SSVEP, one should take into account several electrodes at once. To estimate the montage of EEG, which amplifies the magnitude of the SSVEP response, we used the Common Spatial Patterns (CSP) method. CSP estimates a spatial filter, that is, a linear combination of channels, which is optimal for discrimination between two different experimental conditions (for a full method description see [23], [24], [25]) in terms of variance. Here the signals y_f^+ and y_f^- were used to set the CSP filter for each stimulation frequency f separately. Applying the CSP filter to original signals from both classes y_f^+ and y_f^- results in two one-dimensional signals z_f^+ and z_f^- which differ mostly in terms of variance. The signal z_f^+ has a large variance when there was a response (at a given frequency) and z_f^- has a small variance when no response was present.

7.4. Measures of SSVEP response. The estimation of magnitude of SSVEP was performed in two steps:

Assessment of the power spectrum $P^\alpha(f), \alpha \in \{-,+\}$ of the signals z_f^+ and z_f^- was conducted using the Welch method with Hanning window of 1 s length with a 3/4 second overlap. It is known that the spectral power of EEG decreases as the frequency increases. This property implies that response to high-frequency SSVEP has lower absolute power than response to low-frequency stimulation. Therefore, SSVEP strength can be better measured as a relative increase of power at the stimulation frequency or its harmonic, in respect to its baseline value (spontaneous EEG activity). The quantity, which measures the relative increase or decrease of EEG power in Event Related Spectral Perturbation [26], is defined as follows:

$$\text{ERSP}_f = \frac{\overline{P_f^+} - \overline{P_f^-}}{\overline{P_f^-}}$$

where $\overline{P^\alpha}(f)$ is the $P^\alpha(f)$ averaged over experiment realizations with given stimulation frequency f. ERSPs reflect stimulus-induced changes in spectral power within a particular frequency band.

7.5. Statistical inference. The statistical significance of difference for estimated ERSPs in each tested group was calculated using the Friedman test [27]. For every subject, each tested group consisted of ERSPs determined for one frequency. If the test indicated a statistically significant difference, a post-hoc Wilcoxon signed-rank [28] test was performed to check which condition differed from others. During these calculations, a single hypothesis was tested multiple times, therefore we applied the Bonferroni correction to account for multiple comparisons, dividing the significance level by the number of comparisons done in each group [29].

Results

This section presents the results of statistical analysis of differences in the magnitude of SSVEP response elicited by different stimuli. As described in the "Data Analysis" section, the magnitude of the response was quantified as the relative change of

Table 2. Parameters of the stimulus used in Experiment II.

Tested parameter	Dimension	Inter-stimulus distance	Fixation point	Stimulus colour	Shape
Size	~2.60°, ~3.72°	~2.30°, ~1.26°	yes	white	circle
Colour	~2.60°	~2.30°	yes	white, red, yellow	circle
Absence of fixation point	~2.60°	~2.30°	no	white	circle

spectral power in the corresponding frequency band and calculated after applying the optimal common spatial filter (see Section "Data Analysis"). Both of these analysis methods are commonly used in SSVEP-based BCI systems, so the presented results can be directly compared and applied to BCI systems.

There were 30 repetitions of recorded SSVEP response for each subject and each combination of stimuli parameters and frequency. This allowed for a separate assessment of the statistical significance of changes for each subject. Investigation of inter-subject variability was beyond the scope of this study, so we decided to concentrate on the mean effects. All of the results presented in this section were obtained by pooling together measurements for each combination of stimuli parameters and frequencies obtained from all of the subjects.

1. Effect of colour on magnitude of SSVEP response

The impact of colours presented in Experiment I on mean SSVEP was examined using the Friedman test, indicating significant differences across all frequencies ($\chi^2(4) = 29.96$; $p < 0.001$). Mean ERSP for all participants (Fig. 2) showed that the weakest response is evoked by blue stimuli.

Decrease of SSVEP for stimulation with blue squares was significant in comparison with all other colours. Differences between other colours were not significant in tests conducted on mean results for all subjects. The results of statistical analysis are shown in Table 3.

In Experiment II, differences between yellow, white, and red stimuli were tested (Fig. 3). The Friedman test did not reveal statistically significant results: $\chi^2(2) = 4.44$; in.

2. Effect of stimulus size on magnitude of SSVEP response

In Experiment I, stimulus size examination showed a strong linear effect on SSVEPs (Fig. 4). This was confirmed using the Friedman test performed on mean values for each subject ($\chi^2(3) = 43.81$; $p < 0.001$). The relative power increased with the size of the stimulus. Post hoc comparisons revealed significant differences between SSVEP

magnitudes when side length of 41 pixels was compared to the three other sizes (detailed results of post hoc tests are given in Table 4).

In Experiment II, Friedman tests performed for all frequencies confirmed a significant effect of size ($\chi^2(1) = 5.16$; $p < 0.05$). Larger stimuli induced higher SSVEP response (mean ERSP = 8.53) for all frequencies as compared to the response evoked by smaller stimuli (mean ERSP = 5.76) (Fig. 5).

3. Effect of fixation point absence on magnitude of SSVEP response

The mean value of SSVEPs decreased to 9.7 when a fixation point was used during stimuli presentation, compared to 11.4 for stimuli presented without a fixation point (Fig. 6). However, Friedman tests performed on all frequencies indicated that this difference was not significant ($\chi^2(1) = 0.27$; in.). Nevertheless, presence of fixation point was taken into consideration in further analysis, because participants reported that it had helped them to concentrate on given field; also, presence of the fixation point corresponds to signs (i.e. letters) appearing in real BCI systems.

In Experiment II, larger SSVEP response was visible for stimuli without a fixation point (mean ERSP = 6.43) than with one (5.76) (Fig. 7). However, comparisons performed across all frequencies revealed no effect of this parameter.

4. Effect of stimuli shape on the magnitude of SSVEP response

Shape did not significantly affect SSVEP magnitude: $\chi^2(1) = 0.39$; in. Although the effect of shape was not significant, circles evoked higher SSVEP amplitude than squares (Fig. 8). Accordingly, we used this shape in the second experiment.

5. Effect of distance between stimuli on magnitude of SSVEP response

The influence of distance between stimuli on SSVEP magnitude was examined among all frequencies using Friedman tests, indicating no significant differences: $\chi^2(2) = 1.52$; in. (Fig. 9)

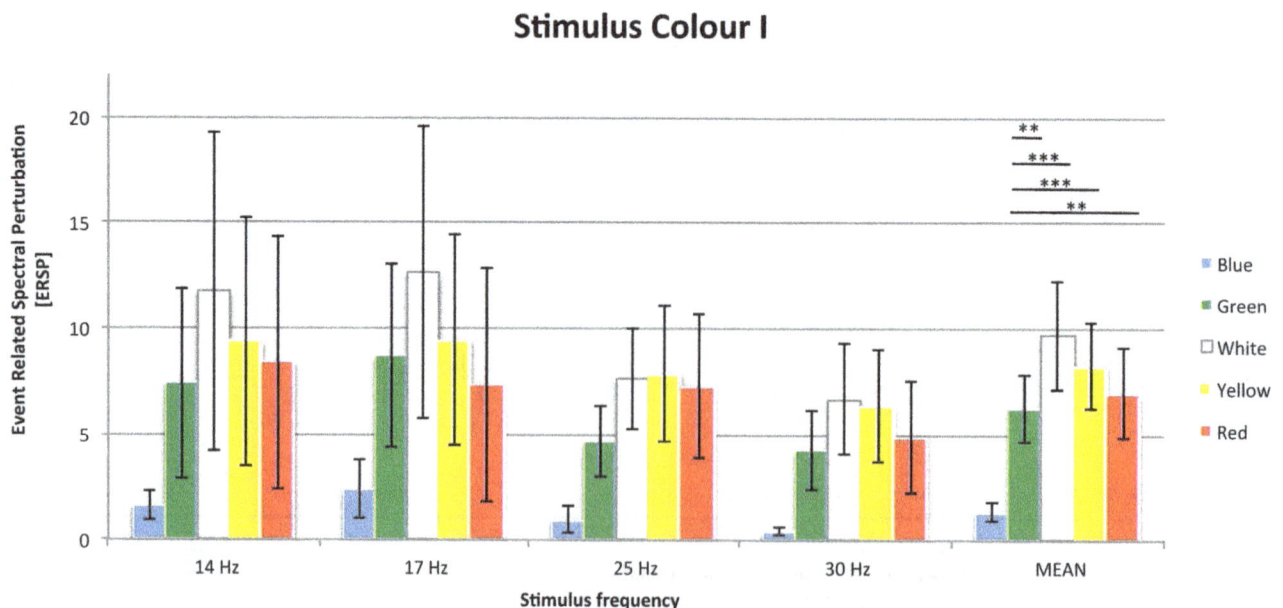

Figure 2. Relative power increase for SSVEP response to different colours of stimuli. Mean computed for all the subjects. Error bars indicate standard error of the mean (SEM). Horizontal lines above the bars indicate statistically significant differences on the level of p<0.001 (***), p<0.01 (**), and p<0.05 (*).

Table 3. The results of post-hoc Wilcoxon signed-rank for comparison of SSVEP magnitude pairs evoked by different coloured stimuli in experiment I.

	yellow	blue	red	green	white
yellow	-	$\chi2(1) = 19,24; p<0,001$	in.	in.	in.
blue	$\chi2(1) = 19,24; p<0,001$	-	$\chi2(1) = 11,88; p<0,01$	$\chi2(1) = 13,36; p<0,01$	$\chi2(1) = 19,25; p<0,001$
red	in.	$\chi2(1) = 11,88; p<0,01$	-	in.	in.
green	in.	$\chi2(1) = 13,36; p<0,01$	in.	-	in.
white	in.	$\chi2(1) = 19,25; p<0,001$	in.	in.	-

Discussion

To the best of our knowledge, this experiment was the first complex study on the optimization of stimuli features used in SSVEP based BCI systems. In contrast to numerous studies regarding data analysis and technical aspects of BCI system operation, there are few articles on the relevance of stimulation parameters. On the basis of neurophysiological knowledge it can be expected that proper choice of the features of the flickering field could strengthen neural response and ease response detection. This in turn could improve efficiency of SSVEP-based BCIs. On the other hand, the balance between the strong neural response and usability (not tiring, comfortable conditions of long stimulation) seems to be necessary. The existing state of art does not unequivocally answer which choices of stimuli features are best for SSVEP based BCIs. Nevertheless, some authors claim that experimental design and paradigm are crucial for developing efficient BCI systems [5], [20]. In the current study we decided to investigate parameters of the stimuli affecting SSVEP response. Five parameters were investigated for SSVEP based BCIs: colour, size, shape, fixation point presence, and inter-stimulus distance, of which three showed an influence on the strength of SSVEP response. Finding the best stimulus parameters for BCI systems was the main goal of this study. We put a great effort into designing an experimental procedure as similar as possible to BCI. In particular, to include possible interferences between frequencies

appearing simultaneously in real BCI systems, we applied four simultaneously flickering fields with different frequencies.

Due to their basic functions (e.g. temporal and spatial resolution), it is suspected that the three visual pathways play a crucial role in SSVEP formation. However, their role is still not well identified [2]. Researchers presume that the strength of SSVEP depends on the cortical location and stimuli appearance [30], [5]. Presented results indicate that every set of parameters evokes SSVEP response, but the largest amplitude was elicited after stimulation characterized by qualities that are processed by the MC pathway (e.g., large plain stimulus with bright colour). One of the tested parameters, which significantly improved the SSVEP response, was the colour of flickering square. Five different colours were used: white, green, red, blue, and yellow, with a black background. We put great effort into the applicability of chosen stimuli in BCI technology. For that reason the selection of stimuli hues and their luminance was based on the RGB model. Stimulation with white and yellow light evoked the largest amplitude. Different colours caused differences in luminance and contrast of the stimulation - white and yellow were the brightest. The obtained results could be explained by the contrast response function [31], which shows the impact of contrast value on V1 neuron firing rates. According to Albrecht [31] the magnitude of neuron activity exponentially increases as the contrast intensifies. In the case of a high contrast, the response saturates. Assuming that the results were an effect of brightness on the strength of

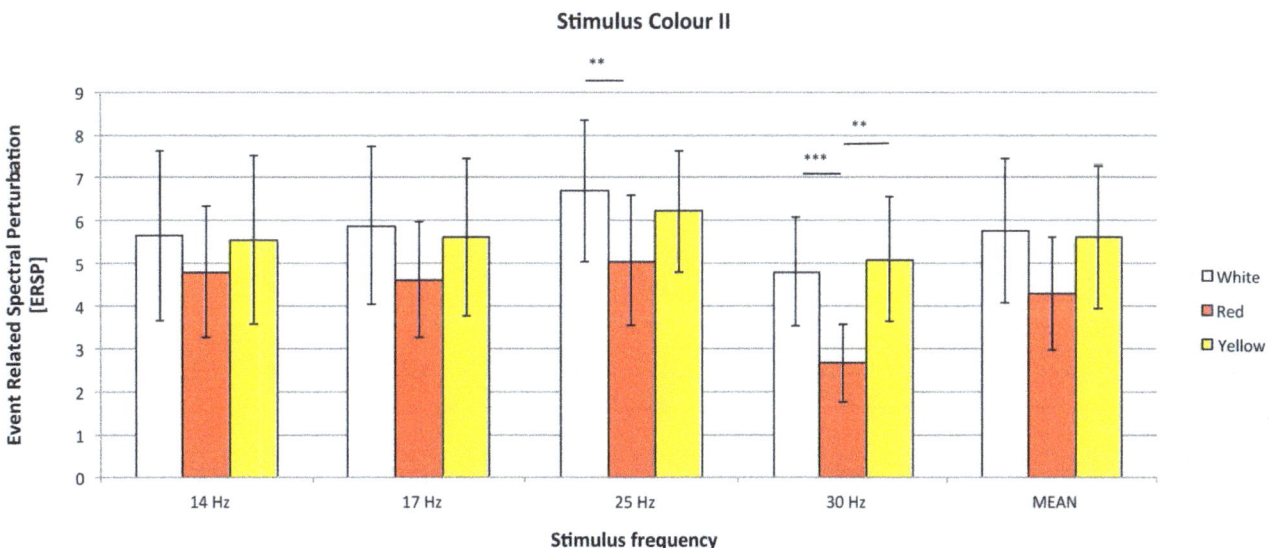

Stimulus Colour II

Figure 3. SSVEP responses to stimuli of different colours; organization of the plot as in Figure 2.

Stimulus Size I

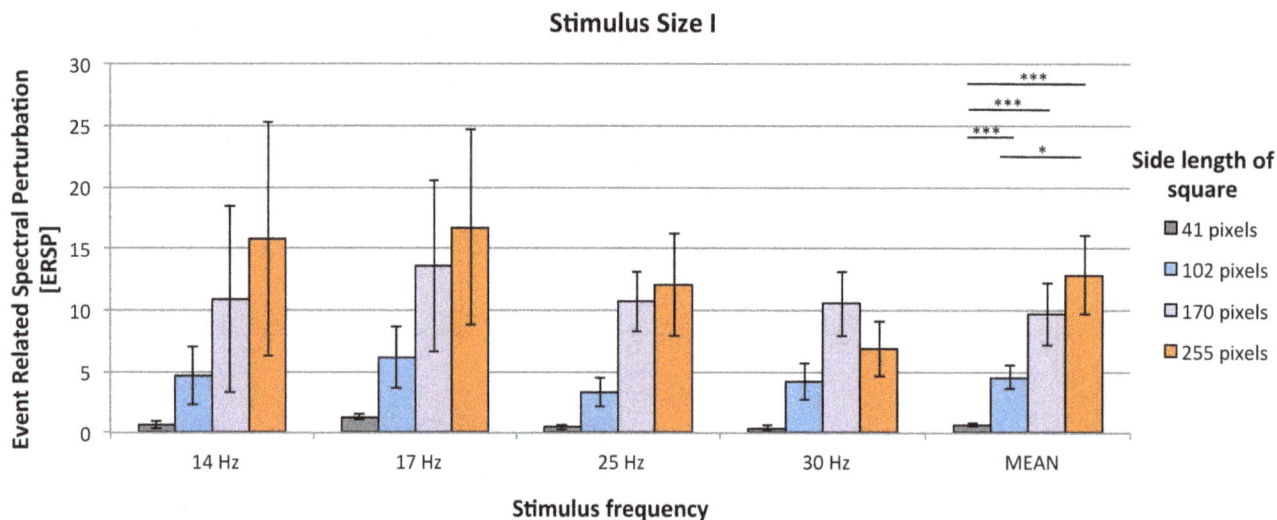

Figure 4. SSVEP responses to stimuli of different sizes; organization of the plot as in Figure 2.

SSVEP response, increase of amplitude might be explained by the properties of the MC pathway. One of its characteristics is high sensitivity to luminance changes of perceived objects or better perception of brighter stimulus as compared to the PC pathway [32]. Considering colour as a variable differentiating stimulus, it may be difficult to point to one hypothesis. The MC pathway is not sensitive to changes of hues [32], [9]. The PC pathway is responsible for detection and processing of information about perceived light wavelength, but its temporal resolution is approximately five cycles per second [33], [4]. It can be suspected that dark colours (blue, green) evoke lower SSVEP response in comparison to bright colours (white, yellow) because of the contrast between stimuli and the background (black) [6], [34]. The contrast was not fixed, so bright stimuli were easier to differentiate from the background.

The next parameter tested in this study was the size of the stimulus. The largest square was most effective for SSVEP - based BCI, as it evoked the highest response amplitude. These results are in line with a visual evoked potentials experiment [35] in which the influence of stimulus parameter on the visual gamma-band response was analyzed. The results showed that large stimuli evoked larger response amplitude. The authors explain this phenomenon by the assumption that larger stimuli activate larger cortical areas in the retinotopic visual cortices than smaller stimuli do [35]. Similar results were obtained by Ng [36]. In his study the size of examined stimuli ranged from 0.67 to 8.9 degrees (visual angle). The amplitude of SSVEP response grew in direct proportion with the size of the stimulus. We suspected that big

and fair stimuli could make subject tired with time and the SSVEP could be reduced. Nevertheless, in case of big stimulus and white/ yellow field neural response was stronger in compare to SSVEP evoked by more pleasant ones.

Inter-stimulus distance and shape in this study revealed no significant effect on SSVEP magnitude. We suspected that presence of the other flickering fields in the visual field could hinder focus on cued square and affect SSVEP response. The magnitude of this response is strongly modulated by attention [17]. In our experiment, all tested distances were within human visual field, so in every condition all four squares were perceived. The results showed that interfering flickering stimuli do not have any impact on tested potentials. A significant impact of distance was showed by Ng [36]. The most accurate stimuli were placed at a distance of more than 5 degrees apart. This study differs methodologically from our experiment. We directly measured increase in magnitude in SSVEP response, while Ng used a classifier.

The presence of a fixation point lowered the strength of SSVEP response, but the mean differences were insignificant. That was contrary to our research hypothesis, and the effect was significant only in the case of two frequencies (17 and 25 Hz). These results can be explained on the psychophysiological level by properties of the visual pathways. When a fixation point is present, a person focuses on the center of the stimulus. The center of the visual field is dominated by the PC pathway, which has low temporal resolution [37]. Therefore, focusing attention on the center may

Table 4. The results of post-hoc Wilcoxon signed-rank for comparison of SSVEP magnitude evoked by different sized stimuli in experiment II.

	~0.57°	~1.49°	~2.60°4	~3.72°
~0.57°	-	$\chi2(1) = 18,34$; p<0,001	$\chi2(1) = 26,19$; p<0,001 in.	in. $\chi2(1) = 26,19$; p<0,001;
~1.49°	$\chi2(1) = 18,34$; p<0,001	-	in.	$\chi2(1) = 8,55$; p<0,05
~2.60°	$\chi2(1) = 26,19$; p<0,001 in.	in.	-	in.
~3.72°	$\chi2(1) = 26,19$; p<0,001; in.	$\chi2(1) = 8,55$; p<0,05	in.	-

Stimulus Size II

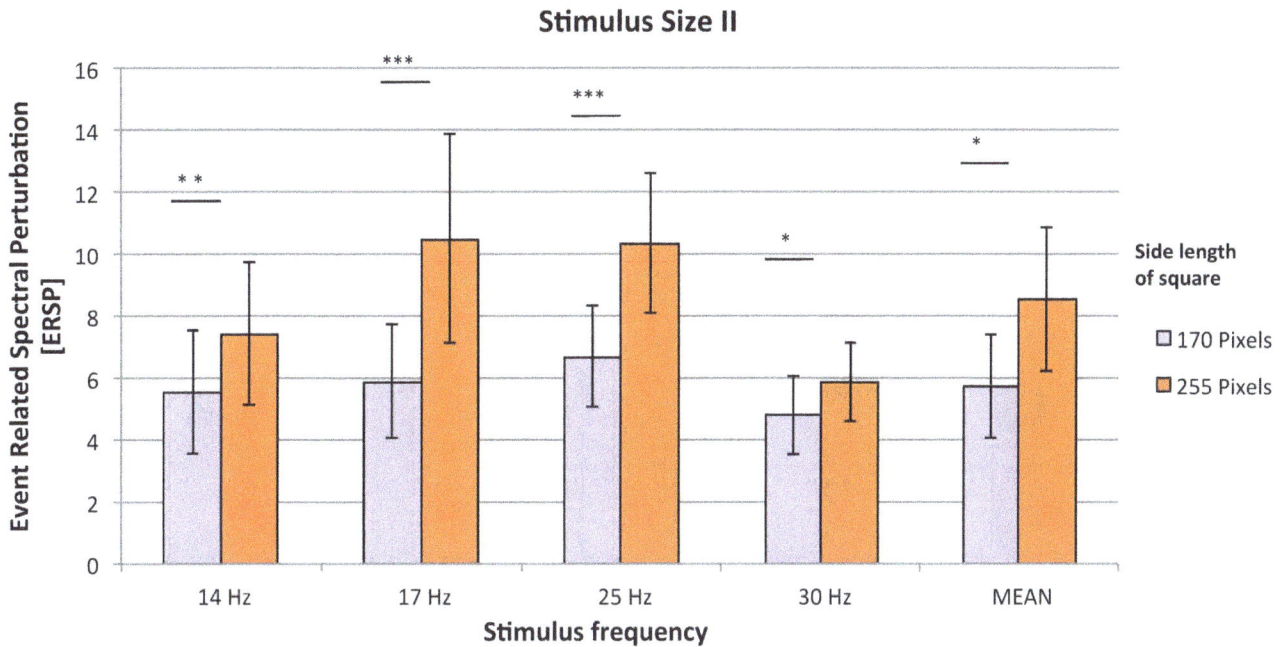

Figure 5. SSVEP responses to stimuli of different sizes; organization of the plot as in Figure 2.

lower subject's sensitivity to flickering. This phenomenon can explain the inconsistencies with psychological theories.

Conclusions

This experiment, to the best of our knowledge, was the first detailed study examining specific parameters of stimuli and their relation to SSVEP magnitude. We showed the significant impact of some features of flickering field on the amplitude of the response. Based on our results, it seems that the best stimuli for

BCI systems should be as bright and large as possible. The significant advantage of such parameters is an increase of SSVEP response, but they have disadvantages as well. If large fields are used, it can limit the amount of command buttons available in the menu panel of BCI systems. Also, very bright hues can be tiring to use for long periods of time.

A robust optimization should also take into account the possible interactions between the different parameters of the stimuli; in this work varied each parameter separately, which relates to the assumption of the lack of interactions. However, testing this

Fixation Point I

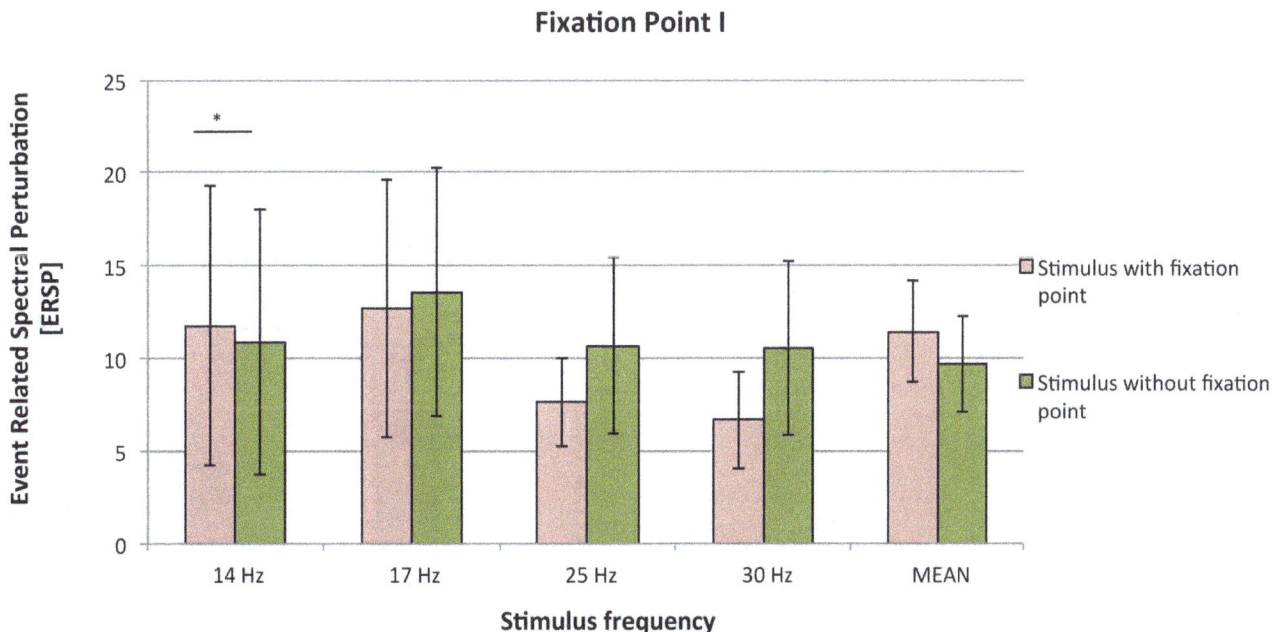

Figure 6. SSVEP responses to stimuli with and without fixation point; organization of the plot as in Figure 2.

Fixation Point II

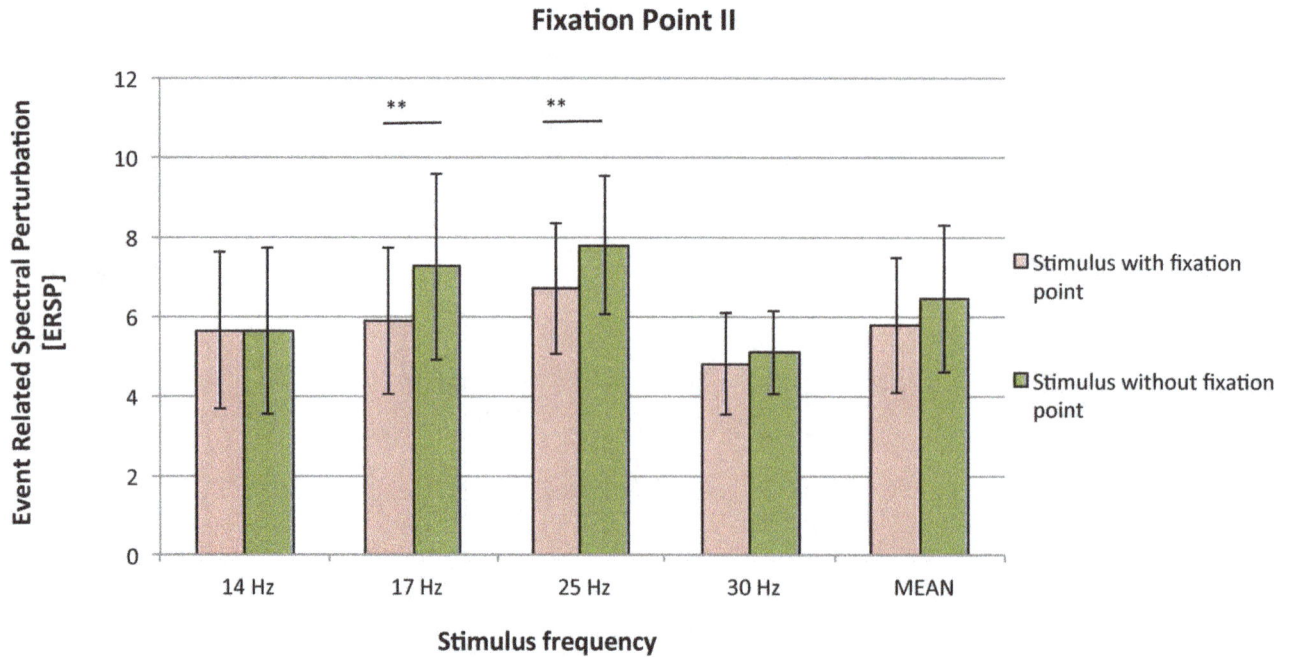

Figure 7. SSVEP responses to stimuli with and without fixation point; organization of the plot as in Figure 2.

hypothesis directly would require a large amount of repetitions of the experiment with different combinations of parameters. On the other hand, the main assumption which drove the experimental design, as mentioned in the Introduction, was proximity to the real-world application of BCI, including a significant duration of each stimulation to simulate possible adaptation and fatigue. In such setup a complete search of the solution space would require up to dozens days of signal collection for each participant, which exceeded the possibilities and aims of this research.

Optimal selection of the parameters of SSVEP stimuli appears to be one of the major factors influencing the efficiency of SSVEP-based BCI systems. The results presented in this paper provide a solid foundation upon which studies on the usability of particular designs of SSVEP based BCIs can be planned. In particular, further research should take into consideration the contrast between stimulus and background, as well as response specificity and maybe also possible interactions between different stimuli features.

Stimulus Shape

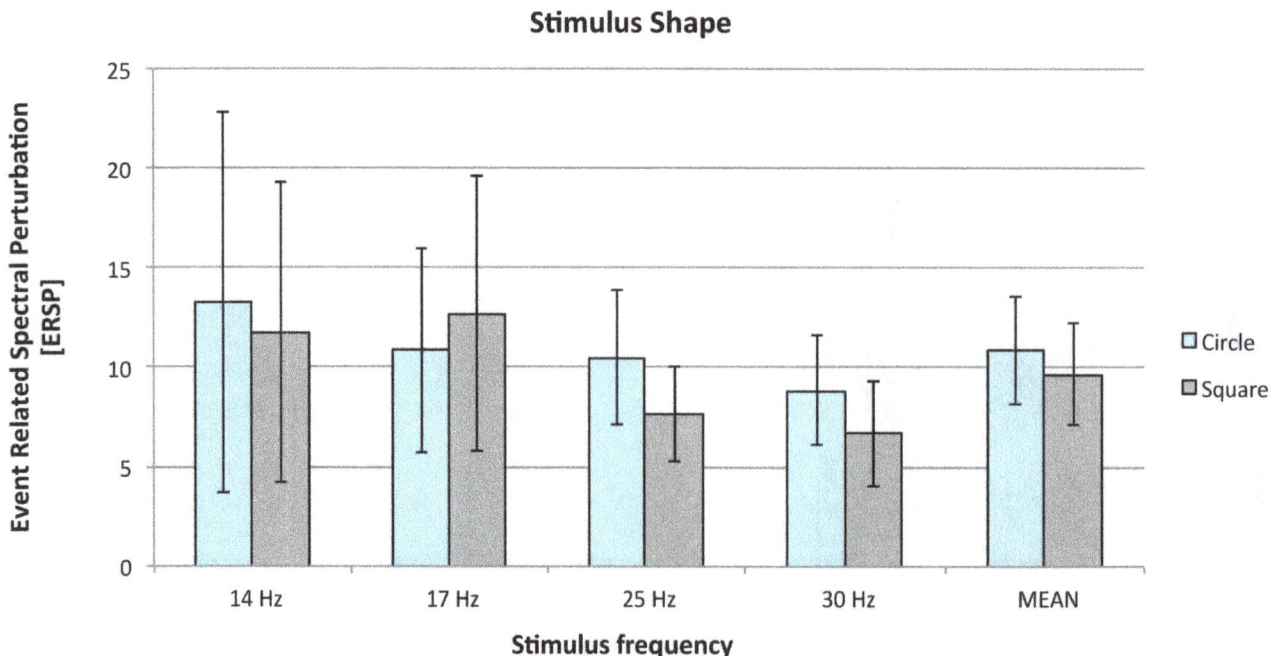

Figure 8. SSVEP responses to circle and square stimuli; organization of the plot as in Figure 2.

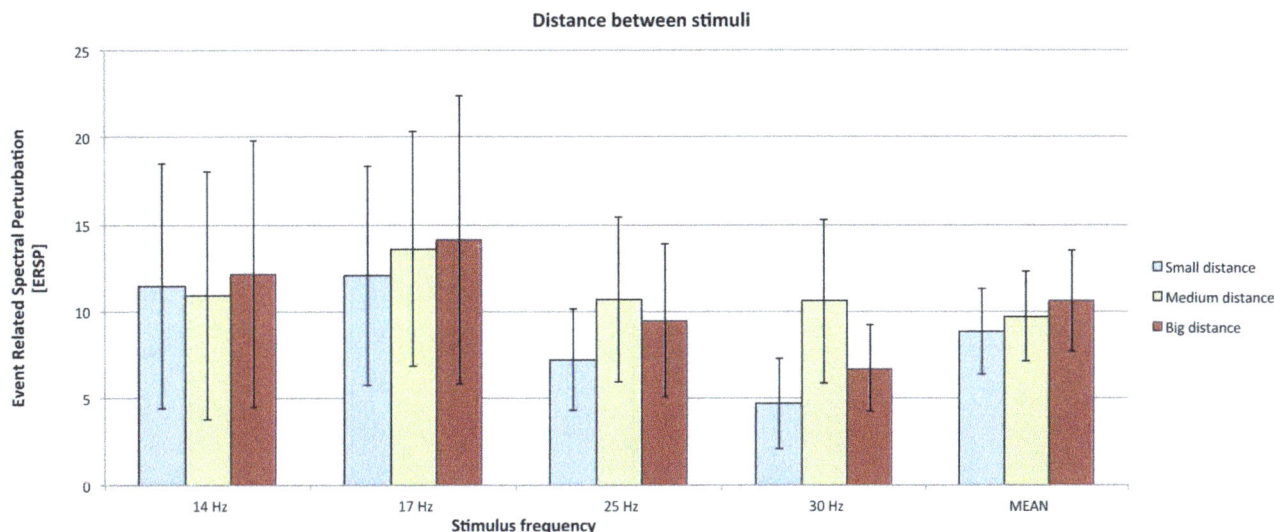

Figure 9. SSVEP responses to circle and square stimuli; organization of the plot as in Figure 2.

Author Contributions

Conceived and designed the experiments: AD MB ZR PS PD. Performed the experiments: AD MB ZR ML. Analyzed the data: PM RK. Contributed reagents/materials/analysis tools: PM RK. Wrote the paper: AD MB ZR RK PM PS PD. Designed the software: MM. Selected and screened the participants against photosensitive epilepsy: PZ.

References

1. Regan D (1975) Recent advances in electrical recording from the human brain. Nature 6 (253): 401–407.
2. Vialatte F, Maurice M, Dauwels J, Cichocki A (2008) Steady State Visual Evoked Potentials in the Delta Range (0.5-5 Hz). In proc. 15th International Conference on Advances in Neuroinformation Processing.
3. Regan D (1977) A high frequency mechanism which underlies visual evoked potentials. Electroencephalogr Clin Neurophysiol 25 (3): 231–237.
4. Kaplan E (2003) The M, P and K Pathwayof the Primate Visual System. In: Chalupa, LN editor. The Visual Neuroscience.Cambridge: MIT Press. pp. 481–483.
5. Vialatte F, Maurice M, Dauwels J, Cichocki A (2010) Steady- state visually evoked potentials: Focus on essential paradigms and future perspectives. Prog Neurobiol 90: 418–438.
6. Kaplan E, Shapley RM (1986) The primate retina contains two types of ganglion cells, with high and low contrast sensitivity. Proc.Natl. Acad. Sci. USA 83: 2755–2757.
7. Croner LJ, Kaplan E (1995) Receptive Fields of P and M ganglion cells across the primate retina. Vis Res, 35: 7–24.
8. Purpura K, Tranchina D, Kaplan E, Shapley RM (1990) Light adaptation in the primate retina: analysis of changes in gain and dynamics of monkey retinal ganglion cells. Vis Neurosci 4: 75–93.
9. MacLeod DI, Boynton A (1979) Chromaticity diagram showing cone excitation by stimuli of equal luminance. J Opt Soc Am 69: 1183–1186.
10. Cheong SK, Tailby C, Solomon SG, Martin PR (2013) Cortical like receptive fields in the lateral geniculate nucleus of marmoset monkeys. J Neurosci 33 (16): 6864–76.
11. Gerloff M, Schilling M (2012) Subject response variability in terms of colour and frequency of capacitive SSVEP measurements. IEEE Trans Biomed Eng 57: 95–98.
12. Zhu D, Bieger J, Molina GG, Aart RM (2010) A Survey of Stimulation Methods Used in SSVEP-Based BCIs. Computational Intelligence and Neuroscience 1: 702357.
13. Allison B, Wolpaw E, Wolpaw J (2007) Brain-computer interface systems: progress and prospects. Expert Rev Med Devices 4 (4): 463–474.
14. Regan D (2000) Human Perception of Objects: Early Visual Processing of Spatial Form Defined by Luminance, Color, Texture, Motion, and Binocular Disparity. Sunderland: Sinauer Associates, Inc. 577 p.
15. Allison B, McFarland D, Schalk G, Zheng S, Moore M, et al. (2008) Towards an independent brain–computer interface using steady state visual evoked potentials. Clin. Neurophysiol 119: 399–408.
16. Hoffmann U, Fimbel EJ, Keller T (2009) Brain-computer interface based on high frequency steady-state visual evoked potentials: A feasibility study. In Proc. 4th International IEEE/EMBS Conference on Neural Engineering NER 09, pp. 466–469.

17. Kelly S, Lalor E, Finucane C, McDarby G, Reilly R (2005) Visual spatial attention control in an independent brain-computer interface. IEEE Trans Biomed Eng 52 (9): 1588–1596.
18. Summers RJ, Meese TS (2009) The influence of fixation points on contrast detection and discrimination of patches of grating: masking and facilitation. VR 49: 1894–1900.
19. Wang N, Qian T, Zhuo Q, Gao X (2010) Discrimination between idle and work states in BCI based on SSVEP. In proc. 2nd International Advanced Computer Control Conference 4: 355–358.
20. Wolpaw JR, Birbaumerc N, McFarlanda DJ, Pfurtschellere G, Vaughana TM (2002) Brain– computer interfaces for communication and control. Clin Neurophysiol 113: 767–791.
21. Kuś R, Duszyk A, Milanowski P, Łabęcki M, Bierzyńska M, Radzikowska Z, Michalska M, Zygierewicz J, Suffczyński P, Durka PJ (2013) On the Quantification of SSVEP Frequency Responses in Human EEG in Realistic BCI Conditions. PLoS ONE 8 (10).
22. Durka P, Kus R, Zygierewicz J, Michalska M, Milanowski P, et al. (2012) User-centered design of brain-computer interfaces: OpenBCI. pl and BCI Appliance. Bulletin of the Polish Academy of Sciences, Technical Sciences 60 (3): 427–431.
23. Fukunaga K (1990) Introduction to Statistical Pattern Recognition, 2nd edn. San Diego: Academic Press. 396 p.
24. Ramoser H, Müller-Gerking J, Pfurtscheller G (2000) Optimal spatial filtering of single trial EEG during imagined hand movement. IEEE Trans Neural Syst Rehabil Eng 8 (4): 441–446.
25. Blankertz B, Tomioka R, Lemm S, Kawanabe M, Müller KR (2008) Optimizing spatial filters robust EEG single-trial analysis. IEEE Trans. Signal Process 25 (1): 41–56.
26. Makeig S (1993) Auditory Event-Related Dynamics of the EEG Spectrum and Effects of Exposure to Tones. Electroencephalography and Clinical Neurophysiology 86: 283–293.
27. Friedman M (1937) The use of ranks to avoid the assumption of normality. Unplicit in the analysis of variance. JASA 32: 675–701.
28. Wilcoxon M (1945) Individual Comparisons by Ranking Methods. Biometrics Bull 1(6): 80–83.
29. Hevre A (2007) Bonferoni and Sidak corrections for multiple comparisons. In: Salkind N J editor, California: Thousand Oaks. pp. 103–107.
30. Pastor M, Artieda J, Arbizu J, Valencia M, Masdeu J (2003) Human cerebral activation during steady-state visual-evoked responses. Journal of Neuroscience 23(37): 621–627.
31. Albrecht DG, Hamilton DB (1982) Striate cortex of monkey and cat: contrast response function. J Neurophysiol 48: 217–237.
32. Lee BB, Pokorny J, Smith VC, Martin PR, Valberg A (1990) Luminance and chromatic modulation sensitivity of macaque ganglion cells and human observers. J Opt Soc Am A 7: 2223–2236.
33. Holcomb A (2009) Seeing slow and seeing fast: two limits on perception. Trends Cogn Sci 13(5): 216–221.

34. Lotto RB, Purves D (2000) An empirical explanation of color contrast. PNAS 97(23): 12834–12839.

35. Busch N, Debener S, Kranczioch C, Engelb AK, Herrmann CS (2004) Size matters: effects of stimulus size, duration and eccentricity on the visual gamma-band response. Clin. Neurophysiol 115(8): 1810–1820.

36. Ng K, Bradley A, Cunnington R (2012) Stimulus specificity of a steady-state visual-evoked potential-based brain-computer interface. Journal of Neural engineering 9(3): doi 036008.

37. Kalloniatis M, Luu Ch (2007) Temporal Resolution. In: Kolb H, Fernandez E, Nelson R editors. Webvision: The Organisation of the Retina and Visual System. Salt Lake City: University of Utah Health Sciences Center. Available: http://www.ncbi.nlm.nih.gov/books/NBK11530/. Accessed 2014 Sep 20.

Permissions

Contributors

Wim J. R. Rietdijk
Department of Applied Economics, Erasmus School of Economics, Erasmus University Rotterdam, Rotterdam, The Netherlands

Ingmar H. A. Franken
Institute of Psychology, Erasmus University Rotterdam, Rotterdam, The Netherlands

A. Roy Thurik
Department of Applied Economics, Erasmus School of Economics, Erasmus University Rotterdam, Rotterdam, The Netherlands
Panteia, Zoetermeer, The Netherlands
GSCM-Montpellier Business School, Montpellier, France

Paul C. Baier
Department of Neurology, University of Kiel, Kiel, Germany
Department of Clinical Neurophysiology, University of Göttingen, Göttingen, Germany

Magdalena M. Brzózka, Sven P. Wichert and Michael C. Wehr
Department of Psychiatry, Ludwig-Maximilian-University, Munich, Germany

Ali Shahmoradi, Lisa Reinecke and Christina Kroos
Research Group Gene Expression, Max Planck Institute of Experimental Medicine, Göttingen, Germany

Henrik Oster
Circadian Rhythms Group, Max Planck Institute of Biophysical Chemistry, Göttingen, Germany
Medical Department I, University of Lübeck, Lübeck, Germany

Reshma Taneja
Department of Physiology, National University of Singapore, Singapore, Singapore

Johannes Hirrlinger
Research Group Gene Expression, Max Planck Institute of Experimental Medicine, Göttingen, Germany
Carl-Ludwig Institute of Physiology, University of Leipzig, Leipzig, Germany

Moritz J. Rossner
Department of Psychiatry, Ludwig-Maximilian-University, Munich, Germany
Research Group Gene Expression, Max Planck Institute of Experimental Medicine, Göttingen, Germany

Luiz R. G. Britto
Departamento de Fisiologia e Biofı́sica, Instituto de Ciênmcias Biomédicas, Universidade de São Paulo, São Paulo, São Paulo, Brazil

Erika R. Kinjo, Guilherme S. V. Higa and Alexandre H. Kihara
Departamento de Fisiologia e Biofı́sica, Instituto de Ciênmcias Biomédicas, Universidade de São Paulo, São Paulo, São Paulo, Brazil
Núcleo de Cognição e Sistemas Complexos, Centro de Matemática, Computac,ão e Cognição, Universidade Federal do ABC, São Bernardo do Campo, São Paulo, Brazil

Edgard Morya
Instituto Internacional de Neurociência de Natal Edmond e Lily Safra, Natal, Rio Grande do Norte, Brazil

Angela C. Valle
Laboratório de Neurociências - LIM 01, Departamento de Patologia, Faculdade de Medicina, Universidade de São Paulo, São Paulo, São Paulo, Brazil

Chenhong Li
College of Biomedical Engineering, South-Central University for Nationalities, Wuhan, People's Republic of China

Junfeng Gao
College of Biomedical Engineering, South-Central University for Nationalities, Wuhan, People's Republic of China
School of Life Science and Technology, University of Electronic Science and Technology of China, Chengdu, People's Republic of China

Hongjun Tian
Nanjing Fullshare Superconducting Technology Co., Ltd., Nanjing, People's Republic of China

Yong Yang
School of Information Technology, Jiangxi University of Finance and Economics, Nanchang, People's Republic of China

Xiaolin Yu
Department of Information Engineering, Officers College of CAPF, People's Republic of China

Nini Rao
School of Life Science and Technology, University of Electronic Science and Technology of China, Chengdu, People's Republic of China

Fengqiong Yu, Rong Ye, Lei Zhang and Chunyan Zhu
Laboratory of Cognitive Neuropsychology, Department of Medical Psychology, Anhui Medical University, Hefei, China

Shiyue Sun
School of Humanities and Social Sciences, Beijing Forestry University, Beijing, China
Luis Carretié
Faculty of Psychology, Universidad Autónoma de Madrid, Madrid, Spain

Yi Dong
Anhui Mental Health Center, Hefei, China

Yuejia Luo
Institute of Social and affective Neuroscience, Shenzhen University, Shenzhen, China

Kai Wang
Laboratory of Cognitive Neuropsychology, Department of Medical Psychology, Anhui Medical University, Hefei, China
Department of Neurology, the First Affiliated Hospital of Anhui Medical University, Hefei, China

Fabrizia Caminiti, Simona De Salvo, Maria Cristina De Cola, Margherita Russo, Placido Bramanti and Rosella Ciurleo
IRCCS Centro Neurolesi "Bonino-Pulejo", Messina, Italy,

Silvia Marino
IRCCS Centro Neurolesi "Bonino-Pulejo", Messina, Italy,
Department of Biomedical Sciences and Morphological and Functional Imaging, University of Messina, Messina, Italy

Lauren Harms, Juanita Todd, Timothy W. Budd, Deborah M. Hodgson and Patricia T. Michie
School of Psychology, University of Newcastle, Callaghan, NSW, Australia
Priority Centre for Translational Neuroscience and Mental Health Research, University of Newcastle, Newcastle, NSW, Australia
Schizophrenia Research Institute, Darlinghurst, NSW, Australia
Hunter Medical Research Institute, Newcastle, NSW, Australia

W. Ross Fulham and Ulrich Schall
Priority Centre for Translational Neuroscience and Mental Health Research, University of Newcastle, Newcastle, NSW, Australia
Schizophrenia Research Institute, Darlinghurst, NSW, Australia
Hunter Medical Research Institute, Newcastle, NSW, Australia
School of Medicine and Public Health, University of Newcastle, Callaghan, NSW, Australia

Michael Hunter
School of Psychology, University of Newcastle, Callaghan, NSW, Australia
Priority Centre for Translational Neuroscience and Mental Health Research, University of Newcastle, Newcastle, NSW, Australia
Hunter Medical Research Institute, Newcastle, NSW, Australia

Crystal Meehan
School of Psychology, University of Newcastle, Callaghan, NSW, Australia
Priority Centre for Translational Neuroscience and Mental Health Research, University of Newcastle, Newcastle, NSW, Australia
Schizophrenia Research Institute, Darlinghurst, NSW, Australia

Markku Penttonen
Department of Psychology, University of Jyvaskyla, Jyvaskyla, Finland

Katerina Zavitsanou
School of Psychiatry, Faculty of Medicine, University of New South Wales, Sydney, NSW, Australia
Neuroscience Research Australia, Randwick, NSW, Australia

Chandramohan Wakade, Raymond Chong and Eric Bradley
Department of Physical Therapy, Georgia Regents University, Augusta, Georgia, United States of America

Bobby Thomas
Department of Pharmacology and Toxicology and Neurology, Georgia Regents University, Augusta, Georgia, United States of America

John Morgan
Department of Neurology, Georgia Regents University, Augusta, Georgia, United States of America

Yatin Mahajan, Chris Davis and Jeesun Kim
The MARCS Institute, University of Western Sydney, Penrith, New South Wales, Australia

Matthias A. Reinhard, Wolfram Regen, Chiara Baglioni, Christoph Nissen, Bernd Feige, Dieter Riemann and Kai Spiegelhalder
Department of Psychiatry and Psychotherapy, University Medical Center Freiburg, Freiburg, Germany

Jürgen Hennig
Department of Diagnostic Radiology, University Medical Center Freiburg, Freiburg, Germany

Evonne Low, Nathan J. Stevenson, Vicki Livingstone, C. Anthony Ryan, Conor O. Bogue and Geraldine B. Boylan
Neonatal Brain Research Group, Irish Centre for Fetal and Neonatal Translational Research, Department of Paediatrics and Child Health, University College Cork, Cork, Ireland

Sean R. Mathieson and Janet M. Rennie
Elizabeth Garrett Anderson Institute for Women's Health, University College London Hospital, London, United Kingdom

Xingwei An
Department of Biomedical Engineering, Tianjin University, Tianjin, China
Neurotechnology Group, Berlin Institute of Technology, Berlin, Germany

Dong Ming
Department of Biomedical Engineering, Tianjin University, Tianjin, China

Benjamin Blankertz
Neurotechnology Group, Berlin Institute of Technology, Berlin, Germany

Johannes Höhne
Neurotechnology Group, Berlin Institute of Technology, Berlin, Germany
Machine Learning Group, Berlin Institute of Technology, Berlin, Germany

Mathias Weymar and Alfons O. Hamm
Department of Biological and Clinical Psychology, University of Greifswald, Greifswald, Germany

Jaroslaw M. Michalowski
Faculty of Psychology, University of Warsaw, Warszawa, Poland

Qiuling Luo and Lulu Qu
School of Psychology, Center for the Study of Applied Psychology, South China Normal University, Guangzhou, China

Yang Wang
School of Psychology, Center for the Study of Applied Psychology, South China Normal University, Guangzhou, China
Department of Psychology, The Chinese University of Hong Kong, Hong Kong, S.A.R., China

Chen Qu
Department of Psychology, The Chinese University of Hong Kong, Hong Kong, S.A.R., China

Xuebing Li
Key Laboratory of Mental Health, Institute of Psychology, Chinese Academy of Sciences, Beijing, China

Fahmida A. Chowdhury and Mark P. Richardson
Institute of Psychiatry, Psychology and Neuroscience, King's College London, London, United Kingdom
Centre for Epilepsy, King's College Hospital, London, United Kingdom

Wessel Woldman and John R. Terry
College of Engineering, Mathematics and Physical Sciences, University of Exeter, Exeter, United Kingdom

Thomas H. B. FitzGerald
Institute of Psychiatry, Psychology and Neuroscience, King's College London, London, United Kingdom
Wellcome Trust Centre for Neuroimaging, UCL, London, United Kingdom

Robert D. C. Elwes and Lina Nashef
Centre for Epilepsy, King's College Hospital, London, United Kingdom

Katherine K. M. Stavropoulos and Leslie J. Carver
Psychology Department, University of California San Diego, La Jolla, California, United States of America

Seul-Ki Yeom, Siamac Fazli and Seong-Whan Lee
Department of Brain and Cognitive Engineering, Korea University, Seoul, Republic of Korea,

Klaus-Robert Müller
Machine Learning Group, Berlin Institute of Technology, Berlin, Germany

Odysseas Papazachariadis and Stefano Ferraina
Department Physiology and Pharmacology, Sapienza University Rome, Rome, Italy,

Vittorio Dante
Istituto Superiore di Sanitá (ISS), Rome, Italy,

Paul F. M. J. Verschure
Laboratory for Synthetic, Perceptive, Emotive and Cognitive Systems, Center of Autonomous Systems and Neurorobotics, ICREA-Universitat Pompeu Fabra, Barcelona, Spain,

Paolo Del Giudice
Istituto Superiore di Sanitá (ISS), Rome, Italy,
INFN, Rome, Italy

Caitlin Chicoine and Levi Hargrove
Rehabilitation Institute of Chicago, Center for Bionic Medicine, Chicago, IL, United States of America

Todd Parrish
Northwestern University, Feinberg School of Medicine, Chicago, IL, United States of America

Sean Deeny and Arun Jayaraman
Rehabilitation Institute of Chicago, Center for Bionic Medicine, Chicago, IL, United States of America

Northwestern University, Feinberg School of Medicine, Chicago, IL, United States of America

Tatiana Selchenkova, Alexandra Corneyllie, Fabien Perrin and Barbara Tillmann
Lyon Neuroscience Research Center, Auditory Cognition and Psychoacoustics Team, Centre National de la Recherche Scientifique, Unité Mixte de Recherche 5292, Institut National de la Santéet de la Recherche Médicale, Unité 1028, University Lyon 1, Lyon, France

Clément François
Cognition and Brain Plasticity Group, Bellvitge Biomedical Research Institute, L'Hospitalet de Llobregat (Barcelona), Barcelona, Spain
Department of Basic Psychology, University of Barcelona, Barcelona, Spain
Attention, Perception and Acquisition of Language Lab, Hospital Sant Joan de Déu, Barcelona, Spain

Daniele Schön
Aix-Marseille Université, Institut de Neurosciences des Systémes, Marseille, France
Institut National de la Santéet de la Recherche Me´ dicale, Unité 1106, Marseille, France

Álvaro Costa, Enrique Hortal, Eduardo Iáñ ez and José M. Azorín
Brain-Machine Interface Systems Lab, Miguel Herna´ndez University, Elche, Spain

Jianxin Zhang
Key Laboratory of Mental Health, Institute of Psychology, Chinese Academy of Sciences, Beijing, China

Lili Wu, Ruolei Gu, Huajian Cai and Yu L. L. Luo,
Key Laboratory of Behavioral Science, Institute of Psychology, Chinese Academy of Sciences, Beijing, China

Matteo Cerri, Flavia Del Vecchio, Marco Mastrotto, Marco Luppi, Davide Martelli, Emanuele Perez, Domenico Tupone, Giovanni Zamboni and Roberto Amici
Department of Biomedical and NeuroMotor Sciences, Alma Mater Studiorum - University of Bologna, Bologna, Italy

Elia Valentini, Katharina Koch and Salvatore Maria Aglioti
Sapienza Universita` di Roma, Dipartimento di Psicologia, Roma, Italy
Fondazione Santa Lucia, Istituto di Ricovero e Cura a Carattere Scientifico, Roma, Italy

Jae-Hwan Kang and Sang Hee Kim
Department of Brain and Cognitive Engineering, Korea University, Seoul, Republic of Korea

Ji Woon Jeong and Hyun Taek Kim
Department of Psychology, Korea University, Seoul, Republic of Korea

Sung-Phil Kim
Department of Human and Systems Engineering, Ulsan National Institute of Science and Technology, Ulsan, Republic of Korea

Anna Duszyk and Zofia Radzikowska
University of Social Sciences and Humanities, Warsaw, Poland

Piotr Milanowski, Rafał Kuś, Piotr Suffczyński, Magdalena Michalska, Maciej Łabö cki and Piotr Durka
University of Warsaw, Faculty of Physics, Warsaw, Poland
Maria Bierzyńska
Nencki Institute of Experimental Biology PAS, Warsaw, Poland,

Piotr Zwoliński
Warsaw Memorial Child Hospital, Department of Neurosurgery, Warsaw, Poland

Index

www.ingramcontent.com/pod-product-compliance
Lightning Source LLC
Chambersburg PA
CBHW061331190326
41458CB00011B/3961